Family Practice Obstetrics
Second Edition

Family Practice Obstetrics
Second Edition

Edited by

Stephen D. Ratcliffe, M.D., M.S.P.H.
Professor and Family Practice Program Director
Department of Family and Preventive Medicine
University of Utah School of Medicine
Salt Lake City, Utah

Elizabeth G. Baxley, M.D.
Professor
Department of Family and Preventive Medicine
University of South Carolina School of Medicine
Columbia, South Carolina

Janis E. Byrd, M.D.
Clinical Associate Professor
Department of Family Medicine
University of Wisconsin Medical School
Madison, Wisconsin

Ellen L. Sakornbut, M.D.
Professor
Department of Family Medicine
University of Tennessee, Memphis, College of Medicine
Memphis, Tennessee

HANLEY & BELFUS, INC. / Philadelphia

BS

Publisher: HANLEY & BELFUS, INC.
Medical Publishers
210 South 13th Street
Philadelphia, PA 19107
(215) 546-7293; 800-962-1892
FAX (215) 790-9330
Web site: http://www.hanleyandbelfus.com

Note to the reader: Although the information in this book has been carefully reviewed for correctness of dosage and indications, neither the authors nor the editors nor the publisher can accept any legal responsibility for any errors or omissions that may be made. Neither the publisher nor the editors make any warranty, expressed or implied, with respect to the material contained herein. Before prescribing any drug, the reader must review the manufacturer's current product information (package inserts) for accepted indications, absolute dosage recommendations, and other information pertinent to the safe and effective use of the product described.

Library of Congress Cataloging-in-Publication Data

Family Practice Obstetrics / edited by Stephen D. Ratcliffe . . . [et. al.]—2nd ed.
    p. ; cm.
  Includes bibliographical references and index.
  ISBN 1-56053-359-5 (alk. paper)
    1. Obstetrics—Handbooks, manuals, etc. 2. Family medicine—Handbooks, manuals, etc.
I. Ratcliffe, Stephen D., 1952– II. Handbook of pregnancy and perinatal care in family
practice.
    [DNLM: 1. Obstetrics—Handbooks. 2. Family Practice—Handbooks. WQ 39 F198 2000]
  RG531.F36 2000
618.2—dc21

                                             00-039604

FAMILY PRACTICE OBSTETRICS, 2nd edition   ISBN 1-56053-359-5

Last digit is the print number: 9 8 7 6 5 4 3 2 1

10/29/03

Contents

Contributors

Louise Acheson, M.D., M.S.
Associate Professor of Family Medicine, Assistant Professor of Reproductive Biology, Case Western Reserve University and University Hospitals of Cleveland, Cleveland, Ohio

Patricia Adam, M.D., M.S.P.H.
Assistant Professor, Department of Family Practice and Community Health, University of Minnesota, Minneapolis, Minnesota

Elizabeth G. Baxley, M.D.
Professor, Department of Family and Preventive Medicine, University of South Carolina School of Medicine, Columbia, South Carolina

V. Leigh Beasley, M.D.
Department of Family and Preventive Medicine, University of South Carolina School of Medicine, Columbia, South Carolina

Jennifer Bell, M.D.
Clinical Instructor, Department of Family and Preventive Medicine, University of Utah School of Medicine, Salt Lake City, Utah

Janis E. Byrd, M.D.
Clinical Associate Professor, Department of Family Medicine, University of Wisconsin Medical School, Madison, Wisconsin

Matthew K. Cline, M.D.
Associate Professor of Family Medicine, Anderson Family Practice Residency, Medical University of South Carolina, Anderson, South Carolina

James R. Damos, M.D.
Clinical Professor, Department of Family Medicine, University of Wisconsin–Baraboo Family Practice Rural Training Program, Baraboo, Wisconsin

Mark Deutchman, M.D.
Professor, Department of Family Medicine, University of Colorado Health Sciences Center, Denver, Colorado

Patricia Fontaine, M.D.
Associate Professor, Department of Family Practice and Community Health, University of Minnesota, Minneapolis, Minnesota

Ina May Gaskin, C.P.M., M.A.
Midwife, The Farm, Summertown, Tennessee

Dwenda Gjerdingen, M.D.
Professor, Department of Family Practice, University of Minnesota, St. Paul, Minnesota

Robert Gobbo, M.D.
Department of Family Practice, Sutter Merced Medical Center, Merced, California

Debra Hobbins, M.S.N., A.P.R.N.
Nurse Practitioner, Department of Primary Care, Veterans Administration Health Care System, Salt Lake City, Utah

John C. Houchins, M.D.
Assistant Professor, Department of Family and Preventive Medicine, University of Utah School of Medicine, Salt Lake City, Utah

Elizabeth Joy, M.D.
Associate Professor, Department of Family and Preventive Medicine, University of Utah School of Medicine, Salt Lake City, Utah

Ita M. Killeen, M.D.
Clinical Associate Professor, Department of Family and Preventive Medicine, University of Utah; Student Health Service, Montana State University, Bozeman, Montana

Roger Kimber, M.D.
Associate Director, Family and Community Medicine Residency Program, Penn State University/Good Samaritan Hospital, Lebanon, Pennsylvania

Walter L. Larimore, M.D.
Clinical Professor, Department of Community and Family Medicine, University of South Florida College of Medicine, Tampa, Florida

James Sloan Manning, M.D.
Associate Professor, Department of Family Medicine, University of Tennessee, Memphis, College of Medicine, Memphis, Tennessee

Donald Marquardt, M.D., Ph.D.
Private Practice of Family Medicine, Cedar Rapids, Iowa

Neil J. Murphy, M.D., FACOG, FAAFP
Women's Health Service, South Central Foundation, Alaska Native Medicine Center, Anchorage, Alaska

Carol Osborn, M.D.
Assistant Professor, Department of Family and Preventive Medicine, University of Utah School of Medicine, Salt Lake City, Utah

Patricia A. Payne, CNM, MPH
Research Associate, Cecil G. Sheps Center for Health Services Research, Adjunct Faculty, Department of Family Medicine, University of North Carolina at Chapel Hill School of Medicine, Chapel Hill, North Carolina

Kent Petrie, M.D.
Assistant Clinical Professor, Department of Family Medicine, University of Colorado Health Sciences Center, Denver, Colorado

Stephen D. Ratcliffe, M.D., M.S.P.H.
Professor and Family Practice Program Director, Department of Family and Preventive Medicine, University of Utah School of Medicine, Salt Lake City, Utah

Ellen L. Sakornbut, M.D.
Professor, Department of Family Medicine, University of Tennessee, Memphis, College of Medicine, Memphis, Tennessee

Osman Sanyer, M.D.
Assistant Professor, Department of Family and Preventive Medicine, University of Utah School of Medicine, Salt Lake City, Utah

William G. Sayres, Jr., M.D.
Clinical Instructor, Department of Family Medicine, University of Washington School of Medicine, Seattle, Washington

Ted Schultz, M.D.
Clinical Instructor, Department of Family and Preventive Medicine, University of Utah School of Medicine, Salt Lake City, Utah

Joseph B. Stanford, M.D., M.S.P.H.
Assistant Professor, Department of Family and Preventive Medicine, University of Utah School of Medicine, Salt Lake City, Utah

David Turok, M.D.
Clinical Instructor, Department of Family and Preventive Medicine, University of Utah School of Medicine, Salt Lake City, Utah

Preface to the First Edition

The experience of birth is not fundamentally a medical event for families, and it should not be so for the physicians who attend these families. The inclusion of a new child in the life of a family has a profound effect on the actions, needs, and perspectives of family members, and the inclusion of birth care in the professional life of the family physician has far-reaching implications for the breadth and scope of that physician's practice and the perspective achieved in the care of families. As family physicians, we contribute something in return to our patients and their families from our longitudinal and comprehensive experience.

Family physicians render care to pregnant patients in a variety of settings, including managed care, and rural and inner city sites. Although a major focus of recent family medicine literature has been placed on low-intervention birthing appropriate to the care of the "low-risk" patient, the definition of what is "low risk" may vary according to one's perspective. Indeed, in some settings, family physicians are more likely to be providing care to high-risk and indigent populations than are their obstetric colleagues. The reasons that many of these patients would be considered high-risk are often issues of lifestyle, health habits, and poor access to health care. Thus, it is appropriate that physicians trained with an emphasis on prevention and continuity of care should become critical providers of care in these settings.

Regardless of the risk status, a comprehensive approach to birth care, including assessment and management of psychosocial and biomedical risk factors, has merit for all women and families. This approach needs to be patient-centered, prevention-oriented, and educational. This approach to care is at the heart of what we do as family physicians. In addition, since we see a wide range of patients with differing needs and levels of function, we are accustomed to making decisions about the use of simple or conservative measures versus more intensive management, consultation or referral, and invasive procedures. This is of special interest in the care of pregnant women, since most are healthy and not in need of extensive intervention. In fact, we must recognize that some interventions, which have in many settings become standard therapy, may not improve and may worsen patient outcomes. These are critical issues in the care of patients who are in large part healthy.

This text was written to assist family physicians and other maternity care practitioners in providing comprehensive information from a primary care perspective. Although a number of obstetric texts are available, our experience as family physician educators was that they were not ideally suited for family physicians. Traditional obstetric texts encompass a great deal of information about complicated obstetrics, but often have little information about the common medical and psychosocial problems that affect our patients in their pregnancies. The evolution of birth care as it is practiced by family physicians mandates skills that encompass all aspects surrounding birth, including the preconception and postpartum period. An approach that emphasizes a physician-centered, technical approach to the normal experience of birth is poorly adapted to training family physicians. Nonetheless, since family physicians continue to provide birth care in settings where there are no obstetric consultants available, this text would be incomplete if it did not significantly address complications and emergencies. In addition, the approach to many topics provides information about preconception care and the medical care of pregnant women useful to the family physician who does not provide birth care as well.

We have attempted to provide an evidence-based approach to areas of controversy and empiric practice. Randomized controlled trials (RCTs) are referenced whenever possible and are identified as such. Citations have been provided for both original studies and review articles depending on the type of information presented. We have utilized sources such as The Cochrane Pregnancy and Childbirth Database because of the critical approach in analyzing RCTs, both published and unpublished. In some instances, evidence is limited to descriptive information or case control studies owing to the infrequent nature of the problem or the difficulty in performing RCTs.

As the specialty of Family Medicine has matured, it has become clear that the work of a family physician takes place in a characteristic process. All components of this process are not unique to our discipline, but the total content is best conceived, taught, and modeled from its own practitioners. The work presented here was written by family physicians for the use of family physicians and for our nurse midwifery and obstetric colleagues. More importantly, it was written for the benefit of our patients, who have allowed us the wondrous privilege of caring for them at their births. It was our experience with patients that convinced us that we should be present at births, and it is our continued experience that causes us to examine the content and quality of their care.

Preface to the Second Edition

The basic tenets of the first edition provide the foundation of the second edition. This book is intended for family physicians and other practitioners who strive to provide maternity services in a *patient-* and *family-centered* manner. We have continued to emphasize the use of the *best evidence* to guide our practices. We aim to present a balanced approach to disease prevention and health promotion with an ability to anticipate and respond to obstetric urgencies and emergencies.

What is new in the second edition? In terms of content, we have added new sections that address alternative medicine and prenatal care (Chapter 2, section F), exercise in pregnancy (Chapter 3, section G), persistent occiput posterior (Chapter 16, section G), evaluation and management of infection in the newborn (Chapter 18, section E), and return to work issues (Chapter 20, section G). We have added an entire new chapter on commonly encountered mental health problems in pregnancy. The original content has been updated and expanded in its depth, although we have maintained a succinct format to allow quick access to key clinical information.

Our intention was to present the highest level of medical evidence in the form of randomized controlled trials to support recommendations throughout this text. We have once again extensively drawn upon the Cochrane Library for much of the evidence. The reader is directed to Appendix D where an in-depth explanation of clinical effectiveness as measured by "number needed to treat" is presented. This concept is emphasized throughout the book.

Finally, we have doubled the number of authors who have contributed to the second edition, including three nurse midwives. We hope that our collective effort will contribute to the safety and well-being of our patients and will increase the satisfaction and enjoyment of providing maternity care.

Stephen D. Ratcliffe, M.D., M.S.P.H.
Elizabeth G. Baxley, M.D.
Janis E. Byrd, M.D.
Ellen L. Sakornbut, M.D.

Acknowledgments

We first acknowledge the substantial work and scholarship that our contributing authors have made to create this book. We thank them and their families. Marc Hoenig, Judi Weston, Lois Silk, Val Smith, and Kristen Christensen deserve our thanks for their substantial contributions to this book that included collecting and cross-referencing thousands of references and the creation of figures and tables. Kristen also played a central role in expertly assembling each chapter. We acknowledge the significant support of the Department of Family and Preventive Medicine of the University of Utah in providing the technical expertise of the persons named above. We thank our publisher, Hanley & Belfus, and its talented editor Natasha Andjelkovic for their support and patience.

We wish to dedicate this book to two people. Dr. Jim Halford was one of the pioneers of family medicine who served for many years as the Program Director of the Family Practice Residency in Anderson, South Carolina. He taught several of the writers of this text the meaning of *family-centered maternity care* long before this phrase became in vogue. Dr. F. Marian Bishop is one of the founders of Family Medicine. Her dedication to the establishment and growth of our discipline has been extraordinary. It is a privilege to dedicate this text to these rarest of individuals.

Finally, we must single out each member of our immediate families and thank them for the many sacrifices they made in order for us to complete this work. Thank you for your unwavering support and love.

Stephen D. Ratcliffe, M.D., M.S.P.H.
Elizabeth G. Baxley, M.D.
Janis E. Byrd, M.D.
Ellen L. Sakornbut, M.D.

CHAPTER 1

Obstetric Risk Assessment

SECTION A.
PRECONCEPTION RISK ASSESSMENT

Joseph B. Stanford, M.D., M.S.P.H.
Debra Hobbins, M.S.N., A.P.R.N., N.P.

Preconception care is preventive care delivered before pregnancy. The purpose of preconception care is to identify and modify medical, social, and behavioral risks, with the goals to improve maternal and infant outcomes of pregnancy and to optimize the long-term health of the woman and the child.[30] Preconception care encompasses risk assessment through history taking, physical examination, and laboratory testing. It aims for risk reduction through education, medical management, and appropriate referral.[16,37]

I. Goals of Preconception Care
The specific goals of preconception care are to:
• Stress the advantages of and encourage planned pregnancies.
• Identify thoroughly and systematically risk factors that could affect a woman's reproductive outcomes and long-term health and the long-term health of her offspring.
• Provide individualized patient education.
• Initiate appropriate preventive and therapeutic interventions.[1,8,37]

II. Rationale for Preconception Care
The primary rationale for preconception care is twofold. First, planned or wanted pregnancies are associated with better pregnancy outcomes.[12] Second, many interventions to reduce pregnancy risk must be applied early in fetal development or before conception for maximum effectiveness.[24,26,50] The critical phases of early cell differentiation and organogenesis take place during the first few weeks after conception, before many women know they are pregnant. Abnormal development may result from infectious, nutritional, chemical, thermal, environmental, pharmacologic, and physiologic insults to the embryo early in pregnancy.

Preconception care also recognizes linkages between a woman's overall health, family planning needs, her childbearing health, and her child's health across the life span, rather than treating each pregnancy as an isolated event.[52] For example, stopping smoking before or during pregnancy can have a lifetime of positive effects for mother and child. Recognizing partner and family influences also is integral to preconception care. Preconception care is a concept fully concordant with the philosophical orientation of family physicians.

III. Evidence to Support Preconception Care as a Comprehensive Strategy
Preconception care as a comprehensive strategy is a relatively new concept. Much research remains to be done on its benefits and risks, which components may or may not be effective, and how to deliver it optimally. Some elements of preconception care,

such as giving oral folic acid supplements to all women[13] and maintaining a euglycemic state in diabetic women in early pregnancy,[6] have been studied and found to improve perinatal outcomes. The effectiveness of preconception care as an integrated strategy has not been shown by randomized controlled trials, however, and the Cochrane Library concludes that currently there are insufficient or inadequate quality data on which to base a recommendation for practice to offer integrated preconception care to all women.[22] There are some potential risks from preconception care, including the potential to reinforce a woman's unrealistic expectations for a perfect outcome of pregnancy or to impose the provider's values on a woman's reproductive choices.[16]

Despite this lack of systematic evidence, preconception care promises a high potential for improvement in maternal and infant outcomes. This promise is based on strong evidence for some of its components, an extensive body of data on better outcomes for planned or wanted pregnancies,[12] and the potential to help women make informed decisions about their health and their reproduction.[24] Professional and public health consensus endorses preconception care.[1,12,48,49] The U.S. Public Health Service Expert Panel on the Content of Prenatal Care suggests that the most important part of prenatal care is the preconception visit. The panel states that all women who can get pregnant are candidates for preconception care.[49] The March of Dimes Committee on Perinatal Health states that a preconception visit should be a standard part of an annual medical visit for all women of childbearing age.[35] The *Healthy People 2010 Objectives: Draft for Public Comment* has a specific goal to increase the proportion of providers of primary care to women of reproductive age who provide preconception counseling routinely.[38]

IV. Models of Care
There are at least three models for delivering preconception care.
- Comprehensive visit: The comprehensive visit or series of visits occurs with a health care provider with preconception care being the major focus of the encounter.
- Opportunistic preconception visit: Preconception care occurs during a visit to a health care provider for other reasons, whether for preventive care, family planning, or management of acute or chronic illness.
- Community-based initiatives: Components of preconception care may be delivered as community-based initiatives.

V. The Comprehensive Preconception Care Visit
The formal preconception visit is similar in intensity and content to the initial prenatal visit. This visit consists of a systematic identification of risks through a comprehensive health assessment that includes age; nutrition assessment; gynecologic, obstetric, medical, surgical, dental, family, and psychosocial histories; physical examination; and laboratory tests. Based on risks identified, clinicians provide individualized education, and appropriate preventive and therapeutic interventions are initiated. These components are listed in Tables 1, 2, and 3 and are described subsequently.

A. Preconception History
1. Age

At greater than 35 years of age, women are at increased risk of subfertility because of decreased ovarian and cervical function.[54] They also have an increased risk of chromosomal abnormalities, such as trisomies 21, 18, and 13, thought to result from an increased incidence of nondisjunction during oocyte formation.[43] At age 35, the risk of a live birth with a significant chromosomal abnormality is about 1 in 200; this risk rises to 1 in 20 at age 45. At greater than 35 years of age, women also may have an increased risk of gestational diabetes, hypertension, and placental abnormalities.[50] Teen mothers, especially younger than age 16,

TABLE 1. Preconception Health Assessment: History

Age
  Maternal age < 15 or > 35 years
  Paternal age > 35 years
Nutrition history
  Body mass index (weight/height)
  Diet, supplements
  Exercise
  Anorexia, bulimia, pica
Gynecologic history
  Menarche and menstrual cycles
  Family planning methods
  Uterine or cervical malformations
  Gynecologic surgery or procedures
  DES exposure (as fetus)
  Subfertility
Obstetric history
  Gestational diabetes
  Preeclampsia
  Prior fetal loss
  Birth-related complications
  Cesarean section
  Preterm birth
  Birth of child < 5.5 or > 9 lb
  Child with birth defect
  Neonatal complications or death
Medical history
  Infectious diseases
    Exposure/immunity
      Immunization status (especially
        tetanus, rubella, hepatitis B)
      Rubella (proven immunity?)
      Varicella
      Human parvovirus B19 (Fifth disease)
      Cytomegalovirus
      Toxoplasmosis (cat?)
      Tuberculosis
    Sexually transmitted infections
      Trichomonas
      Human papillomavirus
      Papanicolaou smear history
      Pelvic inflammatory disease
      Chlamydia
      Gonorrhea
      Syphilis
      Herpes simplex virus
      Hepatitis B
      HIV
  Environmental
    Radiation exposure
    Hyperthermia > 38.9° C (102° F)
    Home—oven cleaners, paint, bleach,
      wood finishing items
    Work—pesticides, cytotoxins, heavy metals,
      gases, solvents, radiation, vibrating machines
  Medications
    Prescription teratogens*
      Lithium
      Isotretinoin (Accutane) and retinoids
      Anticonvulsant medications
      Warfarin (Coumadin)
      Androgenic steroids
      Medroxyprogesterone (Provera)
      Angiotensin-converting enzyme inhibitors

Medical history *(cont.)*
  Medications *(cont.)*
    Over-the-counter teratogens*
      Vitamin A, > 10,000 IU/d
      Aspirin
      Ibuprofen
      Some herbs
  Chronic disease
    Congenital disease
    Diabetes
    Seizure disorder
    Asthma
    Recurrent urinary tract infection
    Renal disease
    Anemia
    Thyroid disease
    Autoimmune disease
    Chronic hypertension
    Thromboembolic disease
    Heart disease
    Pulmonary hypertension
    Marfan's syndrome
    Cancer
    Other chronic disease
  Surgical history
  Dental health
Family history (woman and partner)
  Diabetes
  Birth defects
  Mental retardation
  Fragile X syndrome
  Hemophilia
  Consanguinity
  Other heritable conditions
Consider genetic carrier testing:
  Sickle-cell anemia: African, African-American,
    Middle Eastern, Indo-Pakistani, Mediterranean
  Tay-Sachs: Ashkenazi Jew, French-Canadian, Cajun
  Cystic fibrosis: White
  α-thalassemia: African, Southeast Asian, Filipino
  β-thalassemia: African, Mediterranean, Southeast
    Asian, Indo-Pakistani, Asian, African-American
Psychosocial history
  Desire for pregnancy
  Housing
  Home environment
  Family/social support
  Violence
  Cultural beliefs and issues
  Alcohol, tobacco
  Recreational, intravenous drugs
  Caffeine (> 300 mg/d)
  Life stresses
Financial concerns: income, insurance coverage,
  copays and deductibles, government assistance
Employment: nature of, hours, prolonged standing,
  physical stress
Leave policies: illness, pregnancy, childbirth, post-
  partum, infant care
Partner
  Relationship, support
  Tobacco, alcohol, drug use

* Partial listing.
DES = diethylstilbestrol; HIV = human immunodeficiency virus.

TABLE 2. Preconception Health Assessment: Physical Examination and Laboratory Tests

Physical Examination	Laboratory Tests	Laboratory Tests
In all patients:	In all patients:	As indicated:
Height	Blood type, Rh factor	Tuberculosis (PPD)
Weight	Antibody titer	Genetic testing
Blood pressure	(direct Coombs)	Hemoglobin electrophoresis
Pulse	Hemoglobin/hematocrit	Drug screen
Brief dental examination	Rubella titer	Toxoplasma titer
Thyroid examination	Syphilis serology	Cytomegalovirus titer
Cardiac examination	Urinalysis	Varicella-zoster titer
Respiratory examination	Papanicolaou smear	Herpes simplex
Breast examination	Chlamydia	Toxicology screen (illicit drugs)
Pelvic examination	Gonorrhea	Lead level
Pelvimetry	Hepatitis B surface antigen	Drug screen
As indicated:	HIV antibody (offered,	Thyroid function studies
Ophthalmoscopic examination	with individualized	Hemoglobin A_{1C}
Neurologic examination	counseling and	Others as indicated
Lower extremities	woman's consent)	

HIV = human immunodeficiency virus; PPD = purified protein derivative.

have an increased risk of low-birth-weight infants, prematurity, and infant mortality, although much of this risk may be due to associated socioeconomic disadvantages rather than age per se.[31]

Advanced paternal age (> 35 years) is associated with new autosomal dominant or single gene mutations, such as neurofibromatosis, achondroplastic dwarfism, and Apert's syndrome.[16,43] The absolute incidence of autosomal dominant disease as a consequence of new mutations among infants whose fathers are 40 years old is 0.3%.[39] There also is an increased risk of common birth defects with advanced paternal age that may be related to new and previously unrecognized dominant mutations.[28]

2. Nutritional status

Extremely overweight or underweight women may have difficulty conceiving.[54] Obesity at conception is linked to increased risk of neural tube defects, independent of folic acid intake,[53] and to increased risk of gestational diabetes. Women underweight at conception are at increased risk of preterm birth and low-birth-weight infants.[1]

All women who are capable of becoming pregnant should consume 0.4 mg/d of folic acid during the first 6 weeks of gestation to reduce the risk of neural tube defects and orofacial clefts in offspring.[13] There is no reduction in neural tube defects in infants born to women who initiated folic acid supplementation after 6 weeks' gestation.[45] Women who have previously given birth to an infant affected by a neural tube defect should be offered preventive treatment of 4.0 mg/d of folic acid at least 1 month before they plan to conceive and continuing through the first 3 months of pregnancy.[14] Folic acid, the synthetic version of folate, is twice as absorbable as folate. Folic acid now is added to all enriched cereal grain products[15]; dietary sources of folate include dried beans and peas, spinach, asparagus, broccoli, wheat germ, and citrus fruits and juices.

It is prudent to assess a woman's diet and, if necessary, refer her for dietary counseling. Iron supplements of 30 to 60 mg/d of elemental iron are appropriate for anemic women.[25] Zinc deficiency is associated with congenital malformations. Zinc is found in animal protein or supplements, but currently there is insufficient evidence to recommend routine supplementation.[34] A calcium intake of 1200 to 1500 mg/d, obtained in four to five glasses of milk, during early adulthood can prepare for the needs of fetal bone and teeth mineralization, can minimize a

TABLE 3. Preconception Counseling and Interventions

Individualized Education	Immunizations	
Partner influence on pregnancy outcome	MMR, varicella, oral polio—contraindicated in pregnancy; delay conception for 3 months after immunization	
Abuse can occur or escalate during pregnancy; resources to help		
Age-associated risks of pregnancy	Tetanus-diphtheria okay in pregnancy; booster devery 10 yr	
Healthy diet		
Zinc, 15 mg/d, animal protein	Hepatitis B if indicated	
Avoid vitamin A supplements > 8000 U/d; avoid liver; β-carotene and all vegetables are okay		
	Possible Referrals	**Possible Prescriptions**
Regular exercise 15–30 min daily, interspersed with rest, water	Nutrition counselor (especially weight or eating disorders)	Folic acid, 0.4–1 mg daily (4.0 mg daily if history of neural tube defects)
Appropriate weight for height	Natural family planning counselor to monitor mucus discharge to identify fertile period	Prenatal vitamins as indicated
Plans for childbearing		
Keep menstrual calendar		
Family planning methods		If iron deficiency anemia, iron, 30–60 mg daily (elemental)
Discontinuing contraception	Counselor for relationship issues	
Identifying fertile period—monitoring mucus discharge or OTC urine hormonal testing	Addiction treatment	Calcium supplements to attain total 1200 mg daily
Subfertility after 12 months of random intercourse or 6 months of fertility-focused intercourse	Genetic counseling and carrier testing	Consider changing or weaning off prescription medications
Risk factors for sexually transmitted infections	Medical specialist for comanagement and control of chronic disease	
Smoking risks and cessation		Contraceptive method
Alcohol and illicit drugs risks and cessation	Infertility specialist	Treatment of infection
Limit OTC medications	Perinatologist to quantify risk of identified conditions	
Limit caffeine to 300 mg/d or less		
Avoid hot tub/saunas, treat fever		
Environmental exposures and risks		
Hyperthermia risks		
Control of chronic illness		
Information on genetic conditions		
Lifestyle and employment risks		
Health insurance, benefits, copays		
Family leave policies		
Importance of dental hygiene		
Physical examination and laboratory findings		

OTC = over-the-counter; MMR = measles, mumps, rubella.

woman's risk of osteoporosis, and may reduce the risk of pregnancy-induced hypertension in women at high risk for the condition or with low calcium intake.[9] Routine use of prenatal vitamins is not recommended, but many providers prescribe prenatal vitamins preconceptionally because of the difficulty of determining a patient's nutritional status.[55]

3. Exercise

Exercise is to be encouraged as part of wellness care, but caution should be taken not to increase rapidly activity that was not engaged in before pregnancy. Exercise should be engaged in on a regular basis, with periods of strenuous activity ideally limited to 15 to 20 minutes and with adequate hydration. Non–weight-bearing exercises, such as swimming, cycling, and brisk walking, are safe from the preconception period throughout the entire pregnancy. There no longer is a recommended pregnancy heart rate or maximum core temperature.[2]

4. Gynecologic history

An abnormal menstrual history may indicate subfertility requiring further evaluation and indicates that the date of the last menstrual period is less reliable in determining gestational age of pregnancy.[54] Abnormalities of the cervix or uterus may inhibit conception or maintenance of pregnancy.

A contraceptive history is valuable for providing anticipatory guidance in planning pregnancy and on the return to fertility after discontinuing contraception. After discontinuing oral contraceptives, the probability of conception is reduced for the first few cycles in approximately 20% of women. Some women have reduced conception rates for at least six cycles.[17] After discontinuing medroxyprogesterone (Depo-Provera), the average time to conception is 9 to 10 months, but in heavier women, the delay of return to fertility may be 18 months.[17]

5. Obstetric history

Factors that contribute to earlier poor pregnancy outcomes often increase risk for future pregnancies and may imply the need for more intensive monitoring during pregnancy.[3,16] A history of preterm labor is a strong risk factor for recurrence of preterm labor. Clinicians should attempt to identify underlying treatable conditions that may have contributed to the previous episode of preterm labor.[24] Three or more spontaneous abortions are sufficient to recommend karyotyping for the woman and her partner as well as an evaluation for thrombophilia (see Chapter 7, section E). Women with a previous cesarean section should be counseled about vaginal birth after cesarean section.

6. Medical history

a. Infectious disease: Exposure or immunity to infectious diseases, including sexually transmitted infections, needs to be investigated. Sexual risk behavior for acquiring sexually transmitted infections should be identified and discussed.[16,48]

b. Environmental exposures: Radiographs in the first trimester delivering less than 5 rad to the fetus have not been found to be teratogenic. Ovarian dose has been used as an approximation of fetal exposure. A chest radiograph delivers 8 mrad to the ovary, a cholecystogram delivers 300 mrad, an upper gastrointestinal series delivers 558 mrad, an intravenous pyelogram delivers 407 mrad, and a barium enema delivers 805 mrad.[28] It is prudent to minimize x-ray exposure throughout pregnancy.

Preconception toxic exposures may result in infertility, spontaneous abortions, or congenital malformations in offspring (see Chapter 4, section A). In some cases, these toxic, mutagenic, teratogenic, and carcinogenic effects may not become apparent until childhood or adulthood in the form of behavioral disorders and neoplasms.[10] Temperatures greater than 38.9°C during the first 4 to 14 weeks of pregnancy have been associated with growth deficiencies, central nervous system defects, and a variety of orofacial malformations. Exposure to a hot tub, sauna, or fever during early pregnancy is associated with neural tube closure defects, with hot tubs having the highest adjusted relative risk, 2.8 (95% confidence interval, range 1.2 to 6.5). Electric blankets are not associated with increased risk.[28]

c. Medications: All prescription and over-the-counter drugs, including herbal preparations, should be reviewed for possible adverse effects in pregnancy. Women should be informed about medications with teratogenic potential (see Table 1 for partial list) to enable them to plan carefully for pregnancy. The woman may be able to modify, substitute, or eliminate these drugs preconceptionally.[28]

Excessive amounts of water-soluble vitamins have not been linked to adverse pregnancy outcomes. Women should be counseled to avoid vitamin A supplementation greater than 8000 units/d before and in the 7 weeks after conception because of the association with and increased incidence of craniofacial, central nervous system, thymic, urogenital, and congenital heart defects. These cautions do not apply to β-carotene. It is prudent to limit the intake of foods high in vitamin A, such as liver.[41]

d. Chronic disease: Pregnancy poses a high risk of mortality for mother, fetus, or both for some women with certain chronic diseases. Maternal mortality rates for cardiac disease are as follows: primary pulmonary hypertension, 50%; Eisenmenger's syndrome, 30% to 70%; Marfan's syndrome, 25% to 50%; peripartum cardiomyopathy, 15% to 60%; mitral stenosis with atrial fibrillation, 14% to 17%; aortic valve disease, 10% to 20%; tetralogy of Fallot, 12%; and coarctation of the aorta, 5%.[44] The perinatal mortality rate for moderate and severe renal disease is 10%, with a 57% and 100% risk of preterm birth.[19] During preconception counseling, the provider should discuss with the woman and her partner in detail, in lay terms, the nature of her disease and spell out the risks associated with pregnancy. This discussion may require telephone consultation with a maternal-fetal medicine specialist to quantify the risk. Referral for treatment, amelioration, or cure is imperative.

In preexisting diabetes (not gestational diabetes), teratogenesis is related to first-trimester hyperglycemia.[40] Women with diabetes need education about the importance of developing and continuing good general health practices and optimal glycemic control before conception and throughout pregnancy.[21] Other chronic illnesses also should be under control before conception.[8]

7. Surgical history

A history of previous surgeries and any complications is of interest for the potential impact should surgical intervention become necessary during pregnancy or birth.

8. Dental health

Evidence links periodontal disease to preterm labor. It is prudent to encourage optimal dental hygiene and repair as indicated before pregnancy.[18]

9. Family history

Clinicians should ask all couples about personal or family histories of birth defects, mental retardation, consanguinity, and genetic diseases.[3] It has been estimated that all individuals carry five to seven lethal recessive genes.[51] Some genetic conditions cluster by race, and screening can be offered for carrier status (see Table 1).[16] Preconception education about genetic conditions provides the couple with information to understand the opportunities for antenatal diagnosis, its limitations, and the risks involved so that the couple can consider their reproductive options and make knowledge-based decisions about the reproductive risks they are willing to take.[16]

10. Psychosocial history

A brief discussion of the woman's desire for pregnancy and factors associated with that desire is appropriate. Housing, home environment, family and social support, and safety need to be addressed. Cultural and extended family issues surrounding childbearing merit exploration and may alert the family physician to potential marital problems, parenting issues, grandparental beliefs, and influences that may affect the woman's psychosocial status (see Chapter 4).[30]

a. Domestic violence: All women should be screened for domestic violence. It is estimated that 17% to 37% of pregnant women experience domestic violence, making this condition more common than gestational diabetes, hypertension, and birth defects together (see Chapter 4, section F).[5,36] Victims may have placental separation; perinatal hemorrhage; rupture of the uterus, liver, or spleen; and preterm birth. This topic can be incorporated into a routine history with questions such as "In the last year has anyone punched, kicked, or physically hurt you?" or "Have you ever been in a relationship with someone who hurt you?"[5,36] Women should be aware that domestic violence often escalates during pregnancy and that there are resources to help.

  b. Alcohol: It is crucial to review the use of alcohol. Fetal alcohol syndrome is more prevalent than Down syndrome and spina bifida and is the leading cause of mental retardation.[48] Because alcohol is a known teratogen and no amount has been proven safe, many providers counsel for complete abstinence.[1] Alcohol use also is associated with stillbirth, low-birth-weight infants, and spontaneous abortion.

  c. Smoking: Smoking is a leading preventable cause of low birth weight and increases risks of spontaneous abortion, preterm labor, and the incidence of upper respiratory infections and deaths from sudden infant death syndrome in infants.[1] Smoking cessation programs in pregnancy are effective in improving at least some of these outcomes.[33]

  d. Recreational and intravenous drug use: Recreational and intravenous drug use carries an overall increased risk of nutritional deficiencies. Marijuana may contribute to low birth weight, preterm birth, and congenital malformations,[16] although the evidence for this association is not strong.[7] Cocaine or crack use has been associated with placental abruption, preterm birth, intrauterine growth restriction, low birth weight, decreased head circumference, congenital malformations, central nervous system dysfunction in newborns, and an increased incidence of sudden infant death syndrome. Heroin can cause altered fetal growth and intrauterine growth restriction, and increased risk of behavioral and school-related problems; the fetus exposed to heroin or, more frequently, methadone, has a 50% to 95% chance of experiencing the neonatal withdrawal syndrome, or neonatal abstinence syndrome.[7] Intravenous drug abuse is associated with serious sequelae, such as subacute bacterial endocarditis, hepatitis B, and human immunodeficiency virus infection.[7]

      Women who have a recent history of substance abuse require increased surveillance during pregnancy. Some providers advocate random or routine toxicology screening, discussed with the woman in advance. Providers should be aware of the legal requirements in their jurisdiction related to suspected or confirmed drug use by pregnant women.

  e. Caffeine: To date, a link between caffeine and birth defects has not been shown definitively. High levels of caffeine use have been linked to spontaneous abortion, however, and concerns linger about possible long-term neurobehavioral effects on offspring. It is wise to advise women to limit caffeine intake during pregnancy.[23] Some authors recommend a limit of 300 mg/d—the amount of caffeine in 2 cups of coffee, 7 cups of tea, 15 cups of cocoa, or 3 32-oz cola drinks.[37]

  f. Employment and financial concerns: Employment and financial concerns should be discussed preconceptionally. Long work hours, work-related stress, strenuous physical work, and prolonged standing may contribute to preterm birth.[16,29] Ascertaining the nature of employment provides clues about exposure to environmental toxins and work hazards.

Pregnancy and childbirth frequently are the first major medical expenses a woman and her partner incur and may be underestimated. It is appropriate to encourage the woman and her partner to investigate insurance coverage, copays, and deductibles as well as employer family leave policies that are applicable during pregnancy, childbirth, and the postpartum period and for infant care.[1,16]

11. Partner involvement

Partner involvement in preconception care contributes to the emotional well-being of the couple and is important for family, genetic, and psychosocial histories. It provides an opportunity to educate the partner as well as the woman about the potential influences of their lifestyle and health status on future pregnancy and to enlist partner support for lifestyle modifications recommended for the woman.[48] In addition, smoking and alcohol use by the father are implicated independently in low birth weight and subfertility.[16] Partner promiscuity or intravenous drug abuse puts the woman and fetus at risk for all sexually transmitted infections.

It may be beneficial to conduct portions of the preconception visit with the partner present. It is crucial, however, that the woman be interviewed without her partner present for questions related to reproductive history, sexually transmitted infection, and domestic violence or abuse. Confidentiality of the woman's history must be maintained in this regard.

B. Preconception Physical Examination and Laboratory Testing

1. Physical examination

The physical examination items listed in Table 2 are targeted to detect conditions that are most likely to affect pregnancy and birth. If chronic diseases such as those listed in Table 1 are identified by history or examination, further evaluation beyond what is listed in Table 2 may be necessary. For example, a woman with a significant heart murmur before pregnancy may require diagnostic echocardiography.

2. Laboratory testing

The tests listed in Table 2 for all patients are essentially the same tests that have been done traditionally at the first prenatal visit. In some cases, doing these tests before conception may indicate conditions that should be treated before conception. If the testing is done within a few months of conception, it may not be necessary to repeat the tests at the first prenatal visit. Urine culture during pregnancy has been shown to be effective to detect asymptomatic bacteriuria, but it is not known if urine culture before conception has any benefit. Evidence does not support screening for asymptomatic bacterial vaginosis during a preconception visit.[11] Additional laboratory tests, some of which specifically are listed in Table 2, may be considered based on risk factors identified in the history and physical examination.

C. Preconception Counseling and Interventions

1. Individualized education

All risks identified through the history, physical examination, and laboratory testing should be discussed with the woman so that she has an understanding of their potential impact. Potential interventions likewise should be identified and recommended. Some interventions may be initiated best before conception (e.g., taking folic acid, controlling chronic disease such as diabetes), and others may take the form of increased surveillance in pregnancy (e.g., preterm labor or gestational diabetes). Routine counseling to reduce risk in pregnancy should be offered to all women; this has been discussed previously relative to the associated areas and is summarized in Table 3.

2. Immunizations

A woman should be up to date on immunizations before becoming pregnant. Live virus vaccines (measles, mumps, rubella [MMR]; varicella; and oral polio) should not be given during pregnancy, and pregnancy should be avoided for 3 months after receiving them.[32]

3. Referral

In some cases, referral may be advisable for further specialized counseling; this could include referrals to manage identified risks, to assist in quantifying risks, or to assist in achieving pregnancy.

4. Prescriptions

Folic acid, available over the counter, should be prescribed specifically to all women who may become pregnant. Other prescriptions should be individualized to the woman's medical needs.

5. Proception

Many women who want to conceive prefer methods that are more accurate than random intercourse or guessing based on calendar calculations of when to have intercourse.[46] Basal body temperature is an ineffective means to identify the time of fertility prospectively.[42] Techniques of natural family planning or fertility awareness can be used to time coitus effectively to the approximately 6 days per menstrual cycle that women normally are fertile.[20] Such techniques are best learned from a trained instructor.[47] Some clinicians or women use urinary luteinizing hormone test kits, which are available over the counter, but these kits provide a restricted window of 1 to 2 days of identified fertility, and there is a significant chance of missing the most fertile days altogether.[20] An over-the-counter system has become available in the United States that identifies fertile days based on urinary luteinizing hormone, urinary estrogen, and calculations from previous cycle lengths (The ClearPlan Easy Fertility Monitor, Unipath, Princeton, NJ).

D. Resources for Preconception Care

Many organizations provide guidelines for preconception care, patient questionnaires that can be used to streamline the process of obtaining a preconception history, and educational materials for preconception patient education, including the American Academy of Family Physicians, the American College of Obstetricians and Gynecologists, and the American College of Nurse Midwives. In many locations, a *pregnancy risk* telephone consultation service is available to obtain the latest information on risks from preconception or gestational exposures to drugs or environmental toxins.

VI. Incorporating Preconception Care into Primary Care

From the point of view of an individual patient, the comprehensive preconception care visit (or series of visits) may be an optimal way to receive the benefits of preconception care. Few women currently present specifically for such visits before becoming pregnant, however. For the benefits of preconception care to reach the widest number of women possible, preconception care needs to be delivered in other ways.

A. Opportunistic Preconception Care

One recommended approach to make preconception care widely available to women is to provide opportunistic preconception care at visits to health care providers for other reasons.[1,4] Obvious opportunities for adding preconception care are visits for pregnancy testing, family planning, and gynecologic preventive care. For some women, visits for management of chronic disease, such as diabetes, seizures, or psychiatric conditions, may be more important for some components of preconception care. For example, only one third of diabetic women seek preconception care, so it is important that some form of preconception counseling takes place at each routine visit.[27] Any visit with a woman of childbearing potential should be viewed as an opportunity to address at least some component of preconception care.

It is not possible or desirable to provide all components of preconception care during a visit that has been scheduled for another purpose. The primary care provider must prioritize the components of preconception care and decide which ones have sufficient priority to include within the time available, given the other needs to be addressed at the visit. This prioritization should be individualized to the woman's needs. Components of preconception care that are likely to be key for most women include family planning; tobacco, alcohol, or illicit drug use; adequate intake of folate; and relationship with her partner.

A challenge arises in addressing preconception care with women that currently do not desire pregnancy. Issues of family planning are paramount for these women if they are sexually active. It is also important for them to recognize the ways that they can improve their own health whether or not they become pregnant in the future. Even when pregnancy occurs unexpectedly, optimal health and nutrition (such as adequate intake of folic acid) improve outcomes.

B. Community-Based Preconception Care

An additional approach to reaching women with preconception care is community-based intervention. This intervention may include educational initiatives (e.g., public awareness campaigns about smoking in pregnancy) or public health interventions (e.g., fortifying cereal products with folic acid). This approach may prove more effective than clinic-based care for some components of preconception care.

C. Preconception Care Is Primary Preventive Care

To be delivered optimally, preconception services must be prioritized and integrated within the existing structure of clinical visits for all reasons and, ideally, integrated within all care of the woman and her family members across the life span. A comprehensive approach also includes community-based initiatives. Preconception care is an integral part of primary preventive care for the woman and her family. Many of the components of preconception care are well known to family physicians and already are an established part of preventive care that currently is provided. The concept of preconception care offers a compelling structure and rationale for these preventive services, emphasizing that in most cases better outcomes are achieved by paying attention to these components before pregnancy. Further research is needed to understand the importance of the various components of preconception care and how best to integrate these components into primary care and public health. Meanwhile, it is the task of the family physician to prioritize and integrate the components of preconception care individually for each woman.

References

1. ACOG: Preconceptional Care. Washington, DC, American College of Obstetricians and Gynecologists, 1995.
2. ACOG Technical Bulletin: Exercise During Pregnancy and the Postpartum Period. Washington, DC, American College of Obstetricians and Gynecologists, 1994.
3. ACOG Technical Bulletin: Preconceptional Care. No. 205, 1995.
4. Adams M, Bruce C, Shulman H, et al: PRAMS working group: Pregnancy planning and preconception counseling. Obstet Gynecol 82:955–959, 1993.
5. AMA: Violence against women: Relevance for medical practitioners. JAMA 267:3184–3189, 1992.
6. American Diabetes Association: Preconception care of women with diabetes. Diabetes Care 20:S40–S43, 1997.
7. Andres R: Social and illicit drug use in pregnancy. In Resnik RCR (ed): Maternal Fetal Medicine. Philadelphia, WB Saunders, 1999, pp 145–164.
8. Apgar B: Pregnancy. In Johnson BE, Johnson CA, Murray JL, Apgar BA (eds): Women's Health Care Handbook. Philadelphia, Hanley & Belfus, 1996, pp 136–153.

9. Atallah A, Hofmeyr G, Duley L: Calcium supplementation during pregnancy for preventing hypertensive disorders and related problems. Cochrane Review The Cochrane Library, Issue 1, Oxford, Update Software, 2000.
10. Berkowitz G: Occupational exposures and reproduction. In Current Obstetric Medicine. St. Louis, Mosby-Year Book, 1993, pp 51–81.
11. Brocklehurst P, Hannah M, McDonald H: Interventions for treating bacterial vaginosis in pregnancy. Cochrane Review The Cochrane Library, Issue 1, Oxford, Update Software, 2000.
12. Brown S: The Best Intentions: Unintended Pregnancy and the Well Being of Children and Families. Washington, DC, National Academy Press, 1995.
13. Centers for Disease Control and Prevention: Recommendations for the use of folic acid to reduce the number of cases of spina bifida and other neural tube defects. MMWR 41:1–7, 1992.
14. Centers for Disease Control and Prevention: Knowledge and Use of Folic Acid by Women of Childbearing Age. Atlanta, GA, Centers for Disease Control and Prevention, 1997.
15. Centers for Disease Control and Prevention: Preventing Neural Tube Defects: A Prevention Model and Resource Guide. Atlanta, GA, Centers for Disease Control and Prevention, 1998.
16. Cefalo R, Bowes W, Moos M: Preconception care: A means of prevention. Ballieres Clin Obstet Gynaecol 3:403–416, 1995.
17. Chez R: Control of human reproduction: Contraception, sterilization and pregnancy termination. In Scott Jr DP, Hammond CB, Spellacy WN, Gordon JD (eds): Danforth's Handbook of Obstetrics and Gynecology. Philadelphia, Lippincott-Raven, 1996, pp 321–331.
18. Dasanayake AP: Poor periodontal health of the pregnant woman as a risk factor for low birth weight. Ann Periodontol 3:206–212, 1998.
19. Davison J: Renal disorders. In Creasy RK, Resnik R (eds): Maternal-Fetal Medicine. Philadelphia, WB Saunders, 1999, pp 873–894.
20. Dunson D, Baird D, Wilcox A, et al: Day-specific probabilities of clinical pregnancy based on two studies with imperfect measures of ovulation. Hum Reprod 14:1835–1839, 1999.
21. Elixhauser A, Weschler JM, Kizmmiller JL, et al: Cost benefit analysis of preconception care for women with established diabetes mellitus. Diabetes Care 16:1146–1157, 1993.
22. Enkin M, Keirse MJNC, Renfrew M: A Guide to Effective Care in Pregnancy and Childbirth, 2nd ed. Oxford, Oxford University Press, 1995.
23. Eskenazi B: Caffeine—filtering the facts. N Engl J Med 341:1688, 1999.
24. Fontaine P, Sayres W: Obstetric risk assessment. In Ratcliffe SD, Byrd JB, Sakornbut EL (eds): Handbook of Pregnancy and Perinatal Care in Family Practice: Science and Practice. Philadelphia, Hanley & Belfus, 1996, pp 1–14.
25. Freightner J: Routine iron supplementation during pregnancy. Publications Canada, The Canadian Task Force on the Periodic Health Examination. 1994, pp 64–71.
26. Gjerdingen DK, Fontaine P: Preconception health care: A critical task for family physicians. J Am Board Fam Pract 4:237–250, 1991.
27. Janz N, Herman WH, Becker MP, et al: Diabetes and pregnancy. Diabetes Care 18:157–165, 1995.
28. Jones K: Effects of therapeutic, diagnostic and environmental agents. In Creasy, RK, Resnik R (eds): Maternal-Fetal Medicine. Philadelphia, WB Saunders, 1999, pp 132–144.
29. Klebanoff M, Shiono P, Carey J: The effect of physical activity during pregnancy on preterm delivery and birthweight. Am J Obstet Gynecol 163:1450, 1990.
30. Leavitt C: Preconception health promotion. Prim Care 20:537–549, 1993.
31. Lee KS, Ferguson RM, Corpuz M, et al: Maternal age and incidence of low birth weight at term: A population study. Am J Obstet Gynecol 158:84–89, 1988.
32. Lee S, Ewert DP, Frederick PD: Resurgence of congenital rubella syndrome in the 1990s: Report on missed opportunities and failed prevention policies among women of childbearing age. JAMA 267:2616–2620, 1992.
33. Lumley J, Oliver S, Waters E: Interventions for promoting smoking cessation during pregnancy. Cochrane Review The Cochrane Library, Issue 1, Oxford, Update Software, 2000.
34. Mahomed K: Zinc supplementation in pregnancy. Cochrane Review The Cochrane Library, Issue 1, Oxford, Update Software, 2000.
35. March of Dimes Birth Defects Foundation: Toward Improving the Outcome of Pregnancy: The 90s and Beyond. White Plains, NY, March of Dimes, 1993.
36. McFarlane J, Parker B, Soeken K: Assessing for abuse during pregnancy. JAMA 267:3176–3178, 1992.
37. Moos M: March of Dimes Nursing Modules: Preconceptional Health Promotion. White Plains, NY, Education & Health Promotion Deptartment, 1994.
38. Public Health Service: Healthy People 2010 Objectives: Draft for Public Comment. Washington, DC, Office of Disease Prevention and Health Promotion, U.S. Deptartment of Health and Human Services, 1998.
39. Risch N, Reich EW, Wishnick MM: Spontaneous mutation and parental age in humans. Am J Hum Genet 41:218–248, 1987.

40. Rodgers B: Efficacy of preconception care of diabetic women in a community setting. J Reprod Med 41:422–426, 1996.
41. Rothman K, Moore LL, Singer MR, et al: Teratogenicity of high vitamin A intake. N Engl J Med 333:1369–1373, 1995.
42. Royston P: Identifying the fertile phase of the menstrual cycle. Stat Med 10:221–240, 1991.
43. Scioscia A: Prenatal genetic diagnosis. In Creasy RK, Resnik R (eds): Maternal-Fetal Medicine. Philadelphia, WB Saunders, 1999, pp 40–62.
44. Shabetai R: Cardiac diseases. In Creasy RK, Resnik R (eds): Maternal-Fetal Medicine. Philadelphia, WB Saunders, 1999, pp 793–819.
45. Shaw G, Lammer EJ, Wasserman CR, et al: Risks of orofacial clefts in children born to women using multivitamins containing folic acid periconceptionally. Lancet 346:393–396, 1995.
46. Stanford JB, Lemaire JC, Thurman PB: Women's interest in natural family planning. J Fam Pract 46:65–71, 1998.
47. Stanford JB, Thurman PB, Lemaire JC: Physicians' knowledge and practices regarding natural family planning. Obstet Gynecol 94:672–678, 1999.
48. Swan L: Preconceptual obstetric risk assessment and health promotion. Am Fam Phys 51:1875–1885, 1995.
49. Task Force on Prenatal Care: Caring for Our Future: The Content of Prenatal Care. Washington, DC, Public Health Service, U.S. Department of Health and Human Services, U.S. Government Printing Office, 1989.
50. Taysi K: Preconceptional counselling. Obstet Gynecol Clin North Am 15:167–178, 1988.
51. Vogel F: Human Genetics. New York, Springer, 1995.
52. Walker L: Toward an integrative science of women's health. Obstet Gynecol Neonat Nurs 25:379–382, 1996.
53. Werler M, Louik C, Shapiro S: Pre-pregnant weight in relation to risk of neural tube defects. JAMA 275:1089–1092, 1996.
54. Weschler T: Taking Charge of Your Fertility: The Definitive Guide to Natural Birth Control and Pregnancy Achievement. New York, HarperCollins, 1995.
55. Yu S, Keppel KG, Singh GK: Preconceptional and prenatal multivitamin-mineral supplement use in the 1988 National Maternal and Infant Health Study. Am J Public Health 86:240–242, 1996.

SECTION B.
ANTENATAL RISK ASSESSMENT

Janis E. Byrd, M.D.

The assessment of risk in pregnancy has become a standard part of modern maternity care, and providers are expected to identify risk factors in a timely manner and provide appropriate interventions and referral.[6] In designing a system for assessing risk, the clinician first should study the epidemiology of the problems and validate prevention and intervention strategies by prospective studies.[4] In obstetric risk assessment as in many other areas of health care, few randomized controlled trials to evaluate individual components of risk assessment have been carried out. Instead, risk assessment began based on observations and assumptions about what clinicians thought would improve outcomes for mothers and later for infants. Risk assessment, at least in part, was an attempt to decide who should receive *specialist* care and deliver in the new hospitals that were being built after World War I. In Chapter 3, available data on specific problems are given. This section focuses on goals, methods, and problems in antenatal risk assessment.

I. Goals
The purpose of initial evaluation of risk factors for pregnancy complications is to plan for special risk care, consultation, or referral and to provide for treatment of disease conditions. Continuous assessment throughout the pregnancy is necessary for early detection of symptomatic and asymptomatic complications.

II. Tools
The standard tools for risk assessment are the history (medical, obstetric, social, family, and psychological), physical examination, and laboratory or medical imaging tests.

TABLE 4. Prenatal High Risk Scoring Form*

Reproductive History		Associated Conditions		Present Pregnancy	
Age	< 16 = 0 ☐	Previous	= 1 ☐	Bleeding	
	16–35 = 0 ☐	gynecologic		< 20 wk	= 1 ☐
	> 35 = 2 ☐	surgery		> 20 wk	= 3 ☐
		Chronic renal	= 2 ☐	Anemia < 10 g/dL	= 1 ☐
Parity	1–4 = 0 ☐	disease		Prolonged	= 1 ☐
	5+ = 2 ☐	Gestational diabetes	= 1 ☐	pregnancy	
Past obstetric history		Diabetes mellitus	= 3 ☐	(42 wk)	
Habitual abortion/	= 1 ☐	Cardiac disease	= 3 ☐	Hypertension	= 2 ☐
infertility		Other medical		Premature	= 2 ☐
PPH/manual	= 1 ☐	disorders (chronic		rupture of	
removal		bronchitis, lupus),		membranes	
Infant > 9 lb	= 1 ☐	score according	= 1–3 ☐	Polyhydramnios	= 2 ☐
(4082 g)		to severity		Small for dates	= 3 ☐
Infant < 5 lb 8 oz	= 1 ☐			Multiple pregnancy,	
(2500 g)				breech, mal-	= 3 ☐
PIH/hypertension	= 1 ☐			presentation	
Previous cesarean	= 2 ☐			RH isoimmuni-	= 3 ☐
Stillbirth or	= 3 ☐			zation	
neonatal death					
Prolonged labor or	= 1 ☐				
difficult delivery					
Category score_____		Category score_____		Category score_____	
Total risk score		1st visit_____		Total at 36 weeks =	

(Record scores box on prenatal sheet)
Note.   Low risk   =   0–2
        High risk   =   3–6
        Extreme risk   =   > 7

* Score each question as indicated. Total each category score at first visit. Repeat at 30 weeks.
PPH = postpartum hemorrhage; PIH = pregnancy-induced hypertension.
Adapted from Lefevre M, Williamson HA, Hector M: Obstetric risk assessment in rural practice. J Fam Pract 28:691–695, 1989.

Special risk-scoring systems or forms may be used to organize these data and prompt the provider. To be effective, any system must be linked to action. Only risks for conditions that respond to intervention and for which resources are available should be included. Identified risks should be placed on a problem list along with a plan for intervention and follow-up. Systems also need to be simple to use and reliable when used by multiple providers. The system should show correlation between increasing risk score and worsening perinatal outcome.

III. Problems With Risk-Scoring Systems
A. Application to Low-Risk Pregnancies
Sensitivity, specificity, and positive predictive value (PPV) are used most often to evaluate antenatal risk-scoring systems. The first problem arises because all adverse outcomes in obstetrics are uncommon. When the prevalence of a problem is low, the PPV is low and the specificity is high. This situation can be altered by raising or lowering the threshold arbitrarily, separating high- from low-risk, and thus changing the proportion of women who receive routine versus intensive antenatal care.[7] Wilson and Schifrin[8] suggested the extreme position that no pregnancy is low risk and recommended a single standard of maternal and fetal evaluation for all pregnancies. Their assumption was that this approach would lower the perinatality rate further. Others have found that this maximum strategy approach may be detrimental and produce poorer outcomes in low-risk women (see Chapter 13, section A).[1,5]

TABLE 5. Prenatal Risk Factors

Cardiovascular and renal		Anatomic abnormalities	
Moderate-to-severe toxemia	10	Uterine malformation	10
Chronic hypertension	10	Incomplete cervix	10
Moderate-to-severe renal disease	10	Abnormal fetal position	10
Severe heart disease, class II-IV	10	Polyhydramnios	10
History of eclampsia	5	Small pelvis	5
History of pyelonephritis	5	**Miscellaneous**	
Class I heart disease	5	Abnormal cervical cytology	10
Mild toxemia	5	Multiple pregnancy	10
Acute pyelonephritis	5	Sickle cell disease	10
History of cystitis	1	Age > 35 or < 15 years	5
Acute cystitis	1	Viral disease	5
History of toxemia	1	Rh sensitivity only	5
Metabolic		Positive serology	5
Diabetes	10	Severe anemia (< 9 g hemoglobin)	5
Previous endocrine ablation	10	Excessive use of drugs	5
Thyroid diabetes	5	History of TB or PPD > 10mm	5
Prediabetes	5	Weight 100 or 200 lb	5
Family history of diabetes	1	Pulmonary disease	5
Previous history		Flu syndrome (severe)	5
Previous fetal exchange	10	Vaginal spotting	5
transfusion of Rh		Mild anemia (9–10.9 g hemoglobin)	1
Previous stillbirth	10	Smoking > 1 pack per day	1
Postterm (42 weeks)	10	Alcohol (moderate)	1
Previous premature infant	10	Emotional problem	1
Previous neonatal death	10		
Previous cesarean section	5		
Habitual abortion	5		
Infant >10 lb	5		
Multiparity > 5	5		
Epilepsy	5		
Fetal anomalies	1		

TB = tuberculosis; PPD = purified protein derivative.
Courtesy of Calvin J. Hobel, M.D., et al, from the Division of Perinatal Medicine, Department of Obstetrics and Pediatrics, Harbor General and the University of California Los Angeles School of Medicine.

B. Application to Different Populations

The second problem is related closely to the first in that not all populations are identical. Many risk-scoring systems were developed in tertiary centers in populations different from the one in which they are being used. A few have been reevaluated in rural or low-risk settings. Lefevre et al.[3] evaluated the Coopland (Manitoba) system (Table 4) in a rural population and found a PPV of 45% with a sensitivity of 11% and a specificity of 98%. Kelly et al.[2] compared the Goodwin and Hobel systems (Tables 5 and 6) and found PPVs of 29% to 37% in low-risk patients.

C. Real Versus Theoretic Risks

The third problem is the separation of real from theoretic risks. In high-risk populations, most pregnant women have good outcomes, whereas in low-risk populations, 20% or more have adverse outcomes. Because about 75% of the population generally is classified as low risk by most systems, about half the perinatal morbidity and mortality comes from the low-risk group.[8] This situation occurs because many risks develop intrapartum independently of prior antenatal risks, and some risks are not identifiable at this time.

D. Variable Outcome Measures

Outcome measures vary in number and specificity. Most measures include perinatal mortality, morbidity (respiratory distress syndrome, intraventricular hemorrhage),

TABLE 6. Antepartum Fetal Risk Score

Baseline Data			Obstetric History	
Age > 35 years	1		Abortion	
Age > 40 years	2		Stillbirth	
Para 0	1		Neonatal death	
Para 6+	2		Surviving premature infant	
Interval < 2 years	1		Antepartum hemorrhage	
Obesity (> 200 lb [> 90 kg])	1		Toxemia	
Diabetes B, C, D	2		Difficult midforceps deliver	
Diabetes F	3		Cesarean section	
Chronic renal disease	1		Major congenital anomaly	
With diminished renal disease	3		Infant > 10 lb (> 4.5 kg)	
With increased BUN	3		One instance of above	1
Hypertension (pre-existing)			Two or more instances in different	2
> 140 / > 90	1		pregnancies	
> 160 / > 110	2		Rh isoimmunized mother	
SCORE (circle one)	0 1 2 3		+ Homozygous father	2
			+ History of erythroblastosis	3

Present Pregnancy				
Bleeding, early (< 20 weeks)			Toxemia I	1
Alone	1		Toxemia II	3
With pain	2		Eclampsia	3
Bleeding, late (> 20 weeks)			Hydramnios (single fetus)	3
Ceased	1		Multiple pregnancy	2
Continuous	2		Abnormal glucose tolerance	1
With pain	3		Decreasing insulin requirment	3
With hypotension	3		Maternal acidosis	3
Spontaneous premature rupture	1		Maternal pyrexia	1
of membranes			Pyrexia and FHR > 160 beats/min	2
Latent period > 24 hr	2		RH negative	
Anemia			With rising titer	2
< 10 g	1		With amniotic fluid in zone III	3
< 8 g	2			
No prenatal care	2			
< 3 prenatal visits	1			
SCORE (circle one)	0 1 2 3			

Gestational Age				
≤ 28 wks	4		≤ 37 wks	1
≤ 32 wks	3		≥ 42 wks	1
≤ 35 wkd	2		≥ 43 wks	2
SCORE (circle one)	0 1 2 3			

BUN = blood urea nitrogen; FHR = fetal heart rate.
Courtesy of James W. Goodwin, M.D., F.R.C.S.(C), et al, Department of Obstetrics and Gynecology, University of Toronto and the Women's College Hospital, Toronto, Ontario.

birth weight, Apgar scores, and infant intensive care measures (length of stay). Some outcome measures include gestational age, method of delivery (vaginal vs. cesarean), and hemorrhage.

IV. Practical Application

In practice, the risk assessment system often is dictated by state perinatal organizations, practice partners, or the prenatal form in common use. A comprehensive initial assessment is completed using this form, and risks are placed on a problem list. Plans are made for special care, consultation, or referral if necessary. Ongoing risk assessment by means of an interval history, brief examination, or tests should occur at each visit because the patient's risk status may change as the pregnancy progresses.

V. Summary

Antenatal risk assessment is a standard part of maternity care and ensures a comprehensive evaluation of the patient. When applying a risk-scoring system to their population, providers need to be aware of the statistical and scientific validity of the system, the characteristics of their practice population, and the fact that half of adverse pregnancy outcomes cannot be predicted before labor.

References

1. Brody H, Thompson JR: The maximum strategy in modern obstetrics. J Fam Pract 12:977–986, 1981.
2. Kelly RB, Acheson LS, Zyzanski SJ: Comparison of three prenatal risk scores in a series of low-risk pregnancies. Fam Med 20:122–127, 1988.
3. Lefevre M, Williamson HA, Hector M: Obstetric risk assessment in rural practice. J Fam Pract 28:691–695, 1989.
4. Lindmark G: Assessing the scientific basis of antenatal care. Intl J Tech Assess Health Care 8(Suppl 1): 2–7, 1992.
5. Rosenberg SN, Albertsen PC, Jones EE, et al: Complications of labor and delivery following uncomplicated pregnancy. Med Care 19:68–79, 1981.
6. Scherger JE: Commentary. J Fam Pract 27:162–163, 1988.
7. Wall E: Assessing obstetric risk. A review of obstetric risk-scoring systems. J Fam Pract 27:153–163, 1988.
8. Wilson RW, Schifrin BS: Is any pregnancy low risk? Obstet Gynecol 55:653–656, 1980.

CHAPTER 2

Content of Prenatal Care

SECTION A.
HISTORY OF PRENATAL CARE

Janis E. Byrd, M.D.

Prevention is a primary tenet of family medicine, and in no area is it considered as important as in prenatal care. The routines of prenatal care were credited for improved perinatal outcomes without much investigation of their scientific basis. These routines were established prior to understanding the epidemiology of pregnancy complications. They have remained remarkably unchanged over time and have been applied broadly to many populations.[12] As the British Social Security Committee report stated in 1980: "While we unhesitatingly accept the often reiterated claim of antenatal care as a means of reducing perinatal and neonatal mortality, what exactly antenatal care consists of, and how it works, has been less clear to us."[13]

I. Difficulty of Change
The difficulty of changing routine is underscored by studies showing poor compliance with new recommendations. In 1979, the Swedish Committee for Maternal and Child Health Care recommended broader attention to social and environmental factors and preparation for parenthood. Little hard data on the value of standard procedures was offered, however, and the structure of prenatal care remained essentially the same as defined in the British Ministry of Health Memorandum in 1929.

In 1989, the U.S. Public Health Service Expert Panel on the Content of Prenatal Care evaluated and rated the scientific basis of many components of prenatal care and published recommendations based on their findings.[15] Follow-up studies found that only 10.4% of mothers reported receiving all the health behavior advice recommended by the Expert Panel.[17] Peoples-Sheps et al.[14] found that at the initial prenatal visit the history and physical examination (long-standing routines) were completed 95% to 100% of the time. Compliance with recommended laboratory tests was achieved 72% to 92% of the time. Only 50% of patients received routine counseling on health behaviors. Only 11% of women had a preconceptual visit.

II. Current Research Directions
Despite widespread agreement on the importance of prenatal care and adherence to many long-standing components, lack of progress on major problems such as low birth weight (LBW)[2] and racial disparity in infant mortality[16] is causing many researchers to examine more critically the scientific basis of antenatal care routines. Although randomized controlled trials of standard versus alternative antenatal care can be outlined,[3] it may not be realistic to offer some women services they do not need or to withhold services from others. Multiple confounding factors influence outcomes, such as race, ethnicity, socioeconomic status, education, age, marital status, smoking and other substance

abuse, and stress.[2] Much basic work still needs to be done in defining the appropriate content, interventions (high-risk medical versus population-based)[16] and outcomes of prenatal care (birth weight and mortality versus family planning, immunizations, or acute care visits).[18] In the following sections, evidence from the Public Health Service Expert Panel and other work is given, where available. Many of the recommendations simply reflect current standard of practice.

III. Definition

To accomplish its broad objectives, basic prenatal care must include ongoing risk assessment, education and counseling to promote health, and intervention and follow-up when problems are identified. Attention to psychosocial risks must be as assiduous as attention to medical risks. A comprehensive flow chart such as those available from the American Academy of Family Physicians, Management of Maternity (MOM) program, or the American College of Obstetricians and Gynecologists (ACOG) documents completion of activities by all who are caring for the patient and efficiently transfers information to other providers, consultants, and hospital staff. Such a flow chart may prevent oversights and improve the quality of care.

SECTION B.
DIAGNOSIS AND DATING OF PREGNANCY

I. Diagnosis

A diagnosis of pregnancy usually is made by the patient history of missed menses and a confirmatory positive urine pregnancy test. Often the patient performs a home pregnancy test. This test result should be confirmed by an office test for urinary human chorionic gonadotropin (hCG) to rule out false-negative or false-positive results. These tests are highly sensitive and specific as well as inexpensive. Urinary tests generally are positive at about the time of the first missed menses and detect levels of 25 mIU/ml of hCG. Quantitative serum hCG tests can detect levels of 10 to 15 mIU/ml but are more expensive, are invasive, and are not necessary for diagnosis in uncomplicated cases.[6]

II. Dating

Once the diagnosis of pregnancy is made, additional data are necessary to determine the age of the pregnancy. A clinical estimated date of confinement (EDC), the date that will be used for management of the pregnancy, should be established by 20 weeks of gestation because dating becomes increasingly more inaccurate after this time. If the last menstrual period (LMP) is known with certainty, this is still the most accurate piece of data for establishing gestational age. Only 25% of patients, however, are certain of the date of their LMP. Another 71% have an approximate date, and 4% have an unknown LMP.[11] Additional menstrual historical factors that are important in assigning an EDC are the regularity and length of the cycle, ovulation or conception information, and whether or not the LMP was the first one after discontinuing oral contraceptives.

A. Uncertain LMP

If the LMP is uncertain, the last menses was a pill period, there is a size-date discrepancy, or any other uncertainty exists about the EDC, a first-trimester ultrasound scan can confirm a gestational age within ± 4 days.[10] A single ultrasound scan at 18 weeks of gestation can be used for confirmation of dating to within ± 1.5 weeks, in addition to scanning for anomalies.

B. Clinical Indicators of Gestational Age

Bimanual palpation of uterine size at 8 to 10 weeks of gestation is a helpful adjunct for dating in that the uterine fundus generally is not palpable on transabdominal examination. Fetal heart tones (FHTs) usually can be detected with a hand-held

Doppler at 11 to 13 weeks of gestation. At 15 to 16 weeks of gestation, the uterine fundus is in a midposition between the symphysis pubis and the umbilicus. Quickening (perception of fetal movement) usually is detected by the multiparous patient at 16 to 18 weeks and by the nulliparous patient at 19 to 20 weeks.

SECTION C.
PRENATAL VISITS

I. Preconceptual Care

The advocacy of early prenatal care has extended retrograde with recommendations for a first visit to occur in the preconceptual period.[15] This visit allows assessment and modification of risk before the critical period of early organogenesis preceding the earliest prenatal visits, which typically are not scheduled until 6 to 8 weeks of gestation (see Chapter 1, section A). Preconceptual visits are most appropriate for risk factor identification, delivery of health behavior advice, treatment of substance abuse, management of chronic illnesses, family planning for optimal spacing or timing of high-risk pregnancy, and arranging services for pyschosocial risks. Of women ages 18 to 64 years, 20% lack health insurance until after conception occurs and become ineligible again soon after delivery.[9,19] Minorities, women younger than age 30, unmarried women, and women with low educational and economic attainment are at greatest risk of being uninsured. These are the same groups that are independently at risk for adverse pregnancy outcomes.

II. Prenatal Care

A. Initial Prenatal Assessment

A first prenatal visit for all women should occur at 6 to 8 weeks of gestation. If there has been a recent preconceptual visit, this visit can be abbreviated, but it should include a thorough history of the patient's LMP, assessment of current problems or symptoms, and a bimanual examination to assess the size of the uterus for early pregnancy dating. After an initial evaluation that includes risk assessment and health promotion counseling (Table 1), the U.S. Public Health Service Expert Panel recommended fewer visits for healthy women than is current practice.[15] These recommendations were based on expert judgment of the panelists, and supportive data on outcomes are lacking.

B. Cost-Effective Prenatal Care

There is potential risk that increased attention in normal pregnancy may lead to unnecessary interventions and increased risk from procedures as well as adverse psychological consequences. Economic pressures also exist that encourage the best use of limited resources.[4,12] Medicaid finances one quarter of the nation's births. Medicaid managed care programs are growing rapidly in an attempt to control spiraling costs. Many other women are covered under other managed care programs. Savings from appropriate reduction in use of unnecessary costly procedures and specialists could be channeled into strategies addressing health behaviors and access problems as well as more intensive care for high-risk patients.[1] More frequent prenatal visits early in pregnancy for women with modifiable risk factors, such as smoking, substance abuse, or mental health problems, could reduce risk and improve pregnancy outcome.

C. Schedule of Prenatal Visits

The traditional schedule is monthly visits until 32 weeks, then biweekly visits at 32 and 34 weeks, and weekly visits through delivery. This schedule originally was set for the detection of hypertension and preeclampsia. Newer data suggest that the risk of developing preeclampsia decreases after 33 weeks in women who have not developed hypertension before this time. These data suggest that an increased frequency of

TABLE 1.   First Pregnancy Visit: Health Promotion Activities

Content	Studied by Panel	Evidence of Association	Recommended Population	Research*
Counseling to Promote and Support Healthful Behavior				
Nutrition counseling	Yes	Good	Some†	H
Avoidance of teratogens	Yes	Poor	All	H
Safer sex	No	NA	All	H
General Knowledge of Pregnancy and Parenting				
Physiologic and emotional changes in pregnancy	No	NA	All	H
Sexually	No	NA	All	H
Fetal growth and development	Yes	Poor	All	H
Self-help strategies for discomfort	Yes	Poor	Some	H
Early pregnancy classes on nutrition physiologic changes, psychological adaption, exercise, and fitness	Yes	Poor	All	H
Information on Proposed Care				
Preparation for screening and diagnostic tests	Yes	Good	All	H
Content and timing of prenatal visits	No	NA	All	H
Need to report danger signs	No	NA	All	H

* Indication of the need for research and priority ranking. H = high.
† Panel was unable to reach agreement on whether counseling should be recommended for some or all women.

prenatal visits in the second trimester would be more likely to detect women at risk for preeclampsia at an earlier time. Studies on whether earlier detection would improve outcomes are lacking.

SECTION D.
INITIAL ASSESSMENT

I. Risk Scoring (see Chapter 1)
Identifying patients at risk and obtaining early consultation and referral are key components of regionalization of care, which attempts to improve outcomes. This improvement is more likely to occur if prenatal care is readily available locally at level 1 centers. For family physicians and nurse-midwives who provide maternity services in larger centers, risk assessment facilitates guiding patients to the appropriate level of care. Although data on risk assessment and referral do not exist for every condition in relation to place of delivery, there is clear evidence that premature and low-birth-weight infants have better outcomes when delivered at level 3 centers.

II. Nutritional Risks, Medication, Alcohol, Tobacco, and Other Drug History
A patient's nutritional, medication, alcohol, tobacco, and other drug history should be obtained, including the use of oral contraceptives. If this history is obtained during a preconceptual visit, oral contraceptives should be discontinued for 1 to 3 months before conception and an alternate method of birth control used. This practice allows more accurate dating of the pregnancy as well as eradication of any possible risks of the contraceptive itself. Over-the-counter medications, diet foods, and vitamin and mineral supplements should be investigated. All nonessential medication should be discontinued, and abstinence from alcohol, tobacco, and street drugs should be advised. The family physician should offer patients assistance and timely referral for counseling services (see Chapters 3 and 4).

III. Occupational Risks

Occupational risks, such as toxic or radiation exposure, excessive hours, or excessive levels of strenuous activity, should be assessed, and appropriate recommendations should be provided (see Chapter 4, section B).

IV. The Living Situation

The living situation, family support, partner support, and adequacy of financial resources are important areas of inquiry. Attention has focused on the importance of inquiring about family violence because it may be directed toward the pregnant woman with increased frequency (see Chapter 4, section C)

The U.S. Public Health Service Expert Panel evaluated the literature on the efficacy of all the previously mentioned activities and judged the evidence for their association with outcome of pregnancy to be good for all except stress levels, social support, and extremes of physical activity.[15] The quality of evidence for these latter factors was judged to be fair.

V. Reproductive History

Reproductive history, including contraceptive and sexual history, is recommended by the U.S. Public Health Service Expert Panel. A sexual history may identify risks for sexually transmitted diseases or ectopic pregnancy. Obstetric and gynecologic history identifies women with previous adverse events, such as fetal demise, intrauterine growth restriction, abruption, postpartum hemorrhage, or more than three spontaneous abortions, that place them at high risk for recurrence of these events. Previous preterm birth is a strong predictor of preterm delivery for the current pregnancy.[8] Multiple prior therapeutic abortions or other cervical procedures or abnormalities place the patient at risk for an incompetent or, conversely, a stenotic cervix, depending on the type or extent of the procedure. Previous infants weighing greater than 4000 to 4500 g, difficult labor or delivery, and uterine anomalies place the patient at increased risk for intrapartum problems. Short interpregnancy intervals place the pregnancy at nutritional risk.

VI. Family History

Family history may suggest genetic or medical risks, such as diabetes mellitus, hypertension, hemoglobinopathies, congenital disorders or anomalies, or a propensity for multiple births (maternal history only).

VII. Current and Past Medical History

The patient's current and past medical history identifies additional medical risks, such as heart disease, blood dyscrasias, hyperthyroidism or hypothyroidism, allergies or asthma, gastrointestinal disorders, renal disease, recurrent urinary tract infection, phlebitis, or seizure disorders.

VIII. Complete Physical Examination

A complete physical examination should be performed, but the evidence of association with improved outcomes is superior with other items (Table 2).

XI. Papanicolaou Smear Testing

Papanicolaou (Pap) smear testing is increasingly important because the incidence of human papillomavirus infection of the cervix and cervical dysplasia continues to increase (see Chapter 8, section F). All women with cervical dysplasia should have colposcopy. Biopsies may be done during pregnancy, but many clinicians prefer to wait until after pregnancy in the case of mild disease. Patients can be followed with repeat

TABLE 2.   Preconception Risk Assessment: Physical Examination

Content	Studied by Panel	Evidence of Association	Recommended Population	Research*
General physical examination	No	NA	All	N
Blood pressure/pulse	Yes	Good	All	N
Height	Yes	Good	All	N
Weight	Yes	Good	All	H
Height/Weight	Yes	Fair	All	H
Pelvic examination and clinical pelvimetry	Yes	Poor	All	M
Breast examination	No	NA	All	N

* Indication of the need for research and priority ranking. H = high; M = medium; N = not recommended for research or placed at lower priority for study.

colposcopies at 3-month intervals. Treatment of noninvasive disease usually is deferred until completion of the pregnancy.

SECTION E.
MONITORING THE PROGRESS OF PREGNANCY

I. Ongoing Risk Assessment
History taking after the initial complete evaluation should focus on continuous risk assessment. If prior risks, such as substance abuse, poor nutrition, teratogen exposure, or social problems, have been identified, these should be investigated further. Counseling or referral should be encouraged if not already completed. Symptoms commonly encountered in pregnancy or suggestive of medical problems, including nausea, bleeding, discharge, contractions, and dysuria, should be elicited at each visit. Fetal movement and preterm labor symptoms are important parts of the history as the pregnancy progresses. In the third trimester, symptoms of edema, headache, visual disturbance, and abdominal pain assume increased importance in screening for hypertensive disorders.[5]

II. Physical Examination
Physical examination usually is limited to maternal weight, blood pressure, edema, fundal height in centimeters, and fetal heart tones, unless other symptoms are present. If the patient's blood pressure, urinalysis, or symptom complex suggests a possible diagnosis of preeclampsia, a careful neurologic assessment, including examination of the deep tendon reflexes and presence of clonus should be done.

III. Laboratory Testing
The evidence and rationale for routine and selective laboratory testing in pregnancy are presented in the following section and are addressed in Chapter 4, section A and Chapter 8, section A.

IV. Health Promotion Activities
Health promotion efforts should be directed at educating the woman and her family about physiologic changes of pregnancy, sexuality, and common discomforts that most women experience, along with corresponding comfort measures. Exercise and fitness and the benefits of breast-feeding should be encouraged beginning early and continuing throughout normal pregnancy. Advice on seatbelts and travel precautions should be given. In the third trimester, more information on fetal development, anticipated family adjustments, childbirth (normal and possible complications), and parenting classes is appropriate. Beginning at 32 to 36 weeks of gestation, information regarding the signs and symptoms of labor, logistics of contacting the primary care provider, circumcision,

and postpartum family planning should be covered. All patient education should be documented in the record.[5]

References

1. Armstead RC, Gorman JK: Baby love and budget relief: some promising practices in prenatal managed care in Medicaid. JAMA 50:178–181, 1995.
2. Atrash HK: Not all prenatal care is appropriate care. JAMA 50:144–146, 1995.
3. Bakketeig LS: Methodological problems and possible endpoints in the evaluation of antenatal care. Int J Technol Assess Health Care 8(suppl 1):33–39, 1992.
4. Brody H, Thompson JR: The maximum strategy in modern obstetrics. J Fam Pract 12:977–982, 1981.
5. Byrd JE, Larimore WL, Reed M: Normal Pregnancy: Reference Guide, 7th ed. ABFP, 1999.
6. Deutchman M: Advances in the diagnosis of first-trimester pregnancy problem. Am Fam Physician, 44(5 Suppl):15S–30S, 1991.
7. Enkin MW: Randomized controlled trials in the evaluation of antenatal care. Int J Technol Assess Health Care 8(suppl 1):40–45, 1992.
8. Hoffman HJ, Bakketeig LS: Risk factors associated with the occurrence of preterm birth. Clin Obstet Gynecol 27:539–551, 1984.
9. Hughes DC: Prenatal care and public policy: Lessons for promoting women's health. JAMA 50:156–159, 1995.
10. Kramer MS, McLean FH, Boyd ME, et al: The validity of gestational age estimation by menstrual dating in term, preterm, and postterm gestations. JAMA 260:3306–3308, 1988.
11. Lagrew DC, Freeman RK: Management of postdate pregnancies. Am J Obstet Gynecol 154:8–13, 1986.
12. Lindmark G: Assessing the scientific basis of antenatal care. Int J Technol Assess Health Care 8(suppl 1):2–7, 1995.
13. Lindmark G: The scientific basis of antenatal care routines. Introduction. Int J Technol Assessment Health Care 8(suppl 1):1, 1992.
14. Peoples-Sheps MD, Hogan VK, Ng'andu N: Content of prenatal care during the initial workup. Am J Obstet Gynecol 174:220–226, 1996.
15. Public Health Service Expert Panel on the Content of Prenatal Care: Caring for Our Future: The Content of Prenatal Care. Washington, D.C., Public Health Service, Department of Health and Human Services, 1989.
16. Rowley DL: Framing the debate: Can prenatal care help to reduce the black-white disparity in infant mortality? JAMA 50:187–193, 1992.
17. Sable MR, Herman AA: The relationship between prenatal health behavior advice and low birth weight. Public Health Rep 112:332–339, 1997.
18. Stringer M: Issues in determining and measuring adequacy of prenatal care. J Perinatol 18:68–73, 1998.
19. Wise PH, Wampler N, Barfield W: The importance of extreme prematurity and low birthweight to U.S. neonatal mortality patterns: Implications for prenatal care and women's health. JAMA 50:152–155, 1995.

SECTION F.
SCREENING IN PREGNANCY AND PREDICTIVE VALUE

Matthew K. Cline, M.D.

I. Appropriate Settings and Criteria for Screening Tests

For screening of medical conditions in pregnancy to be of value, the condition and the screening test have to satisfy several criteria:

• The condition has a significant impact on care or outcomes.
• The incidence of the problem is sufficient to support the costs of screening.
• Acceptable treatment exists.
• There is an asymptomatic window during which the screening test can detect the condition.
• Treatment during the asymptomatic phase yields superior results.
• The screening test needs to be:

Available	Acceptable to patients
Accurate (sensitive and specific)	Affordable

One test that meets these criteria is the screening of all prenatal patients for syphilis at the first prenatal visit. Congenital syphilis can have a significant impact on prenatal outcomes because it may cause stillbirth, miscarriage, or newborn disease as well as cardiac or neurologic infection in the mother. The incidence, although low, has been increasing slowly in the United States since the mid-1980s. Injectable penicillin is an effective and acceptable treatment, and treatment during early pregnancy can cure the mother and prevent neonatal complications. The screening test is widely available, has good accuracy except in very early or late disease, is generally acceptable to patients in that it is a simple blood test, and is affordable. With all of these factors, cost analysis has shown that prenatal screening for syphilis is cost-effective when the prevalence of disease is as low as 1 in 20,000 patients (0.005%).[18]

II. U.S. Preventive Services Task Force and Prenatal Screening

Specific tests to be offered to all women during the course of prenatal care, based on the recommendations of the U.S. Preventive Services Task Force (1996),[16] are listed in Table 3. Additional tests are recommended for high-risk patients (e.g., screening for gonorrhea in patients with multiple sexual partners), whereas others are not recommended based on existing literature (e.g., universal screening for gestational diabetes; routine group B streptococcal cultures; routine screening ultrasound; or screening titers for toxoplasmosis, cytomegalovirus, or varicella).

Rather than quoting information from numerous studies, the U.S. Preventive Services Task Force grades recommendations based on the *quality* of evidence supporting a specific test. These levels—A, B, C, D, and E—are defined in Table 4. In practical terms, tests with a level A or B recommendation are those that have solid support for inclusion into standard prenatal care. Tests with a level C recommendation generally lack evidence to support universal use but may be recommended by experts in the field. Tests that receive a level D or E recommendation generally should not be used for screening, unless the specific case in question mandates it.

III. Use of the Number Needed to Diagnose

The evaluation of screening tests is affected by the varying prevalence in different populations. This variation leads to changing positive and negative predictive value depending on the disease prevalence of the screened population. Positive predictive value is the likelihood that a positive test result reflects the presence of the target condition or disease, whereas negative predictive value is the likelihood that a negative test result reflects the absence of a target condition or disease.

TABLE 3.   USPSTF Recommended Screening Tests for Prenatal Evaluation*

- Blood pressure (Chapter 14, section G)
- Hemoglobin and hematocrit (Chapter 7, section E)
- Hepatitis B surface antigen
- RPR or VDRL
- Chlamydia
- Consider HIV
- Rubella serology
- Blood type, Rh, and antibody screening
- Offer hemoglobinopathy screening
- Offer amniocentesis or chorionic villus sampling for maternal age ≥ 35 y
- Urine culture at 12–16 wk or first prenatal visit
- Offer serum α-fetoprotein at 15–20 wk
- Offer multiple marker testing for Down syndrome

* Universal screening for diabetes using a one-hour glucola is not currently recommended by the USPSTF but is discussed in Chapter 6, section A. Universal screening for group B streptococcus currently is not recommended by the USPSTF but is discussed in Chapter 8, section A.
RPR = rapid plasma reagin; VDRL = Venereal Disease Research Laboratory; HIV = human immunodeficiency virus.
From U.S. Preventive Services Task Force: Guide to Clinical Preventive Services, 2nd ed. Baltimore, William & Wilkins, 1996, pp lxx–lxxi, with permission.

TABLE 4. USPSTF Strength of Recommendations for Screening Tests

Level A
   There is good evidence to support the recommendation that the condition be specifically considered in a periodic health evaluation.
Level B
   There is fair evidence to support the recommendation that the condition be specifically considered in a periodic health examination.
Level C
   There is insufficient evidence to recommend for or against the inclusion of the condition in a periodic health examination, but recommendations may be made on other grounds.
Level D
   There is fair evidence to support the recommendation that the condition be excluded from consideration in a periodic health examination.
Level E
   There is good evidence to support the recommendation that the condition be excluded from consideration in a periodic health examination.

From U.S. Preventive Services Task Force: Guide to Clinical Preventive Services, 2nd ed. Baltimore, Williams & Wilkins, 1996, pp 347–359, with permission.

Evidence-based medicine has led to widespread use of the concept of *number needed to treat.* One method of evaluating screening tests that is less dependent on population details is the *number needed to diagnose* (NND), which is defined as the number of patients with the condition in question who need to be screened to detect a single case.[11] In this construct, a perfect test would have a NND of 1.00, whereas most screening tests in use vary from NNDs of just above 1.00 to 1.5. The larger the NND, the greater the number of patients (with the target condition) that would have to be screened to detect a single case. The NND would allow each clinician to determine the usefulness of any screening test in a local population based on local prevalence of a known condition.

As an example of the use of the NND, consider the alternatives to urine culture for diagnosis of asymptomatic bacteriuria (for further details, see section I later): dipstick tests (presence of leukocyte esterase or nitrite) or microscopic evaluation of the sediment for white blood cells and bacteria. For each of these alternative tests, the average sensitivity, specificity, and NND would be as follows:

Test	Sensitivity (%)	Specificity (%)	NND
Leukocyte esterase	85%	73%	1.72
Nitrite	60%	96%	1.78
Microscopic evaluation	83%	59%	2.38

Given this information, the dipstick tests would be viewed as superior to a microscopic evaluation of the urinary sediment as a screening test for asymptomatic bacteriuria, with the leukocyte esterase having a slightly better NND. With a NND higher than 1.5, however, none of these tests would serve as a good screening test because they require 1.72 to 2.38 patients with asymptomatic bacteriuria to be screened to detect 1 patient with the condition. Because of this limitation, culture remains the recommended screening test.

IV. Specific Screening Tests
A. Hepatitis B Surface Antigen
More than 20,000 births occur each year in women who have active hepatitis B infection. Women who are positive for hepatitis B e antigen at the time of delivery have a 70% to 90% risk of infecting their offspring. Vaccination plus a single dose of hepatitis B immune globulin given within 12 hours of birth is at least 75% effective in preventing hepatitis B infection in the newborn.[13]

Risk factors for maternal hepatitis B infection include multiple sexual partners and intravenous drug abuse, but population studies have failed to find a known risk factor in greater than 30% of cases.[14] Targeted screening in urban and minority populations has been able to detect only 35% to 65% of pregnant women who are positive for hepatitis B surface antigen. The U.S. Preventive Services Task Force states that universal screening at the first prenatal visit is a level A recommendation, indicating that all pregnant women should be screened at the initial prenatal visit with a hepatitis B surface antigen assay.

Presence of hepatitis B surface antigen is detected by an immunoassay that has a reported sensitivity and specificity exceeding 98%.[15] Using 0.98 for each, the NND for this test is 1.04, which is excellent (i.e., to detect 1 patient with the presence of hepatitis B surface antigen using this immunoassay would require screening 1.04 patients who actually have this condition).

B. Syphilis

Congenital syphilis is spread in a transplacental fashion during pregnancy from an infected mother to the fetus and can result in perinatal or fetal death in 40% of cases as well as abnormalities of the newborn resulting from infection. In 1998, the reported rate of congenital infection was 20.6 cases per 100,000 live births, or 1 per 4854 live births.[3]

Early detection allows use of antibiotics that can cure infection and prevent future sequelae or congenital infection of the newborn. Cost-effectiveness studies show benefit for prenatal screening when the prevalence of disease is 1 in 20,000 births (0.005%). The U.S. Preventive Services Task Force recommends (level A) routine serologic testing of all pregnant women for syphilis at the onset of prenatal care,[16] and the Centers for Disease Control and Prevention suggests repeat serologic testing in the third trimester for patients at high risk, such as those with multiple sexual partners or intravenous drug users.[4]

Testing for syphilis is done using a serologic (nontreponemal test) such as the rapid plasma reagin (RPR) or Venereal Disease Research Laboratory (VDRL). These tests are sensitive to the anticardiolipin antibody that occurs during the primary stage of syphilis, and during secondary syphilis, sensitivity is nearly 100%. During the first few weeks of the infection, sensitivity is 62% to 76%, and during late tertiary syphilis, sensitivity is 70%. False-positive results are common because similar antibodies can occur during other medical illnesses such as systemic lupus erythematosus. Specificity is reported as 75% to 85%.[10] Because of this lower specificity, a positive serologic test always should be confirmed by a specific treponemal test, such as the fluorescent treponemal antibody absorption (FTA-ABS) or micro-hemagglutination–*Treponema pallidum* (MHA-TP). These tests have a specificity of about 96% but remain positive for life (as compared with serologic tests, which decline in titer or revert to negative with successful treatment).

With the aforementioned sensitivity and specificity, serologic tests of syphilis have a range of NND based on the stage of the illness. For early primary and late tertiary syphilis, the NND is 2.1 to 2.7. For late primary and secondary syphilis, the NND is 1.18 to 1.33.

C. Chlamydia

Chlamydia is the most common nonviral sexually transmitted disease in the United States, with more than 2.4 million cases reported annually. Greater than 70% of women are asymptomatic. About 155,000 mothers each year are infected at the time of delivery, and more than half of their offspring develop infection (either a conjunctivitis or pneumonitis).

Detection early in pregnancy allows for treatment with oral antibiotics, such as erythromycin or azithromycin. This treatment has been linked with significantly lower rates of preterm delivery, preterm rupture of membranes, and low birth weight compared with infected women who are not treated. The incidence in pregnant populations is considerably lower in women older than age 25 and women who are married, however, leading the U.S. Preventive Services Task Force to recommend only targeted screening (level B). Pregnant women at high risk of infection, including those younger than age 25, should be tested. Universal screening in pregnancy carries a recommendation with level C evidence.[16]

Although culture has been quoted as the gold standard for detection of chlamydia, it requires special handling and has a lower sensitivity than other methods of detection (with a NND of 1.11 to 1.42). Currently, enzyme immunoassay (EIA), direct fluorescent antibody, and DNA probe are used on specimens collected from the cervix. EIA and direct fluorescent antibody have sensitivity of 70% to 90% and specificity of 97% to 99%, giving these tests a NND of 1.12 to 1.49. The DNA probe has sensitivity and specificity of at least 95%, giving it a maximum NND of 1.11. Although considerably more expensive (currently > $100), the polymerase chain reaction test can be done on a first-voided urine sample and has a sensitivity of 95% to 99% and specificity of at least 99%, giving it a NND of 1.01 to 1.06. The ease of obtaining the voided urine specimen for polymerase chain reaction may give it advantages in a screening setting over tests that require a direct swab specimen from the cervix once its cost becomes lower.

D. Human Immunodeficiency Virus

With studies showing decreased perinatal transmission (from a transmission rate of 22.6% to 7.6%) when antiretroviral therapy is given during the third trimester and throughout labor, prenatal human immunodeficiency virus (HIV) screening can now offer benefit to the fetus as well as the mother and care team.[6] Risk factors for HIV infection include use of intravenous drugs, receipt of a blood transfusion between 1978 and 1985, and high-risk sexual practices or sexual partners with high-risk behaviors. Pregnant women infected with HIV who have CD4 counts less than 200 are appropriate candidates for prophylaxis against *Pneumocystis* and other infections (see Chapter 8, section 12).

Although the U.S. Public Health Service and ACOG recommend universal screening, the U.S. Preventive Services Task Force rates HIV testing for all pregnant women as a level C recommendation. Screening of patients who are at increased risk or who come from a community where the prevalence of seropositive newborns is greater than 1 per 1000 should occur at the beginning of prenatal care (level A).

Testing is done using an EIA for specific antibodies against HIV; these occur 3 weeks to 6 months after infection, leaving a window period during which the patient can be infected and transmit the disease but have a negative test. Outside this window period, sensitivity approaches 100%, and specificity is 99.7% or better (NND of 1.003), but false-positive results can occur with immunologic disease (such as lupus or rheumatoid arthritis) and have been reported to occur after many routine vaccinations. Because of these false-positive results, each positive EIA is followed by a Western blot for confirmation, which has a sensitivity greater than 98% and specificity nearly 100%. The NND of the Western blot is 1.031, which is higher than that of the EIA because of the decreased sensitivity and supports the use of EIA rather than Western blot for population screening.

E. Maternal Rubella Serology

Congenital rubella syndrome is a constellation of findings in newborns who were infected with the rubella virus before the 16th week of gestation and includes hearing loss, developmental delay, and ocular and cardiac defects. Intrauterine infection can lead to miscarriage and stillbirth. The incidence has declined dramatically since the introduction of rubella vaccination in 1969. Because of low levels of immunity in certain racial and ethnic groups (Amish, Hispanics, and Asians), 31 cases of congenital rubella syndrome were reported in 1991, giving a rate of 0.8 per 100,000.[16]

Detection of lack of immunity during preconceptual visits can allow for appropriate immunization before pregnancy because vaccination provides long-lasting immunity in greater than 90% of healthy recipients. The vaccine is contraindicated during pregnancy because of possible concerns over teratogenicity but can be given at least 3 months before conception or during the postpartum period.[1]

Testing for immunity to rubella is done using EIA or latex agglutination testing. Sensitivity is 92% to 100%, and specificity is 71% to 100%, giving a NND of 1.00 to 1.58. Testing has its shortcomings. In 1990, when the records of mothers with 21 cases of congenital rubella syndrome were evaluated, 71% had a previous positive serologic test for immunity.[12]

F. Maternal Blood Type, Rh, and Antibody Screening

Since the introduction of anti-D (RhoGAM) immune globulin injections during and after pregnancy in women who are D antigen negative, the incidence of isoimmunization has fallen from 10 cases to 1.3 cases per 1000 live births. Currently the U.S. Preventive Services Task Force recommends blood type, Rh, and antibody screen at the first prenatal visit, with a full dose of 300 mg of RhoGAM to be given to all D-negative women who deliver a D-positive infant (level A). A repeat antibody screen at 24 to 28 weeks, followed by a full dose of RhoGAM to help prevent sensitization from small hemorrhages that can occur in the third trimester carries a level B recommendation.[16]

G. Hemoglobinopathy Screening

Sickle cell disease occurs in 1 in 375 African-Americans in the United States and 1 in 3000 Native Americans. α-Thalassemias are common in Southeast Asians, with 1% having the 3 gene deletion of the α-hemoglobin gene known as *hemoglobin H* associated with significant anemia. The U.S. Preventive Services Task Force recommends offering screening for hemoglobinopathy to all pregnant women at the first prenatal visit (level B). Maternal carriers identified through screening should have the father tested and should receive information on the availability of prenatal diagnosis if the father also is a carrier and the fetus is at risk for a clinically significant hemoglobinopathy.[16] Preconceptual screening can play an important role in appropriate counseling of patients at risk for having a child with a hemoglobinopathy.

Screening is done by hemoglobin electrophoresis with thin-layer isoelectric focusing, which has a sensitivity of 96%, a specificity of nearly 100%, and a NND of 1.05. The positive predictive value of this test is 73%, but the negative predictive value exceeds 99.9%.[8]

H. Amniocentesis or Chorionic Villus Sampling for Maternal Age of 35 or Older (see Chapter 4, section D)

Risk of specific genetic abnormalities of the fetus increases with maternal age, including trisomy 21 (Down syndrome). When a mother reaches the age of 35, the risk of genetic defect in the offspring reaches 1 in 204 (with a risk of Down syndrome of 1 in 385). Because of this increased risk, the U.S. Preventive Services Task Force recommends offering amniocentesis at 15 to 18 weeks to women of advanced maternal age (level B).[16] Other organizations, including ACOG, the Canadian Task Force, and the American College of Medical Genetics (ACMG), also recommend amniocentesis for advanced maternal age or presence of other risk factors (most importantly a positive family history) that would increase suspicion for a genetic defect.

Because cytogenetic analysis requires growth of fetal cells (or placental cells, in the case of chorionic villus sampling [CVS]) in culture, the possibility for an inaccurate diagnosis based on genetic mosaicism or through contamination with maternal

TABLE 5.   Comparison of Chorionic Villus Sampling and Amniocentesis

	Chorionic Villus Sampling	Amniocentesis
Technique	Transabdominal or transcervical biopsy of placental cells	Transabdominal removal of amniotic fluid
Gestational age	10–12 wk	15–18 wk (may now be done < 15 weeks)
Abnormalities detected (studies done)	Fetal aneuploidy DNA-based diagnosis of certain genetic conditions Cannot detect NTD	Fetal aneuploidy DNA-based diagnosis of genetic conditions AFP testing for NTD
Advantages	Earlier detection of genetic abnormalities than amniocentesis	Ability to test amniotic fluid for AFP and acetylcholinesterase
Risks	Miscarriage 0.5–1% Limb deficiency 0.03-0.1%	Miscarriage 0.25 – 0.5%

AFP = α-fetoprotein; NTD = neural tube defects.
From Centers for Disease Control and Prevention: Chorionic villus sampling and amniocentesis: Recommendations for prenatal counseling. MMWR Morb Mortal Wkly Rep 44(RR-9):1–12, 1995.

cell lines exists. Despite these theoretic shortcomings, amniocentesis has a sensitivity for trisomy 21 (and similar genetic translocations) of 97%, with specificity of 100%, giving it a NND of 1.03.

When evaluating these tests as part of the screening tests of pregnancy, there is a unique aspect that should be considered: risk to the fetus caused by the test itself. The generally reported risk of miscarriage after amniocentesis is 0.5% and after CVS is 1% to 1.5%. CVS has a currently reported risk of transverse limb defects of 0.03% to 0.1%, with the risk being higher before 10 weeks. After 10 weeks, most of the limb defects associated with CVS have been limited to the digits.[5] Table 5 compares CVS and amniocentesis.

I. Urine Culture at 12 to 16 Weeks for Asymptomatic Bacteriuria

Asymptomatic bacteriuria occurs in 2% to 7% of all pregnant women. If untreated, 13% to 27% of these patients develop pyelonephritis, which is associated with an increase in the risk of preterm labor and delivery. The gold standard for diagnosis is culture, with growth of 100,000 organisms per milliliter or greater of a single species on a clean-catch specimen considered a positive result. A single culture at 12 to 16 weeks identifies 80% of patients who have asymptomatic bacteriuria during the pregnancy, with repeated monthly screening only adding about 2% more per month. Screening with a single culture in early pregnancy is cost-effective as long as the prevalence of asymptomatic bacteriuria is greater than 2%.[17]

Despite its accuracy for asymptomatic bacteriuria and urinary tract infection, culture has its drawbacks: It is labor intensive, is more expensive than rapid tests, and involves some delay before the results are known. Alternatives that have been evaluated include dipstick tests for leukocyte esterase or nitrites and microscopic examination of urinary sediment. When compared with culture, leukocyte esterase has sensitivity of 72% to 97%, with specificity 64% to 82%, giving a NND of 1.27 to 2.78. A positive nitrite on the dipstick test has a lower sensitivity of 35% to 85% but a higher specificity of 92% to 100%, yielding a NND of 1.17 to 3.70. During pregnancy, microscopic evaluation of the urinary sediment for bacteriuria or pyuria had a sensitivity of 83% but a specificity of 59%,[2] resulting in a NND of 2.38. As noted earlier, these tests are not accurate enough to fit the criteria of a good screening test, especially with a NND greater than 1.5. The U.S. Preventive Services Task Force recommends routine urine culture at the first visit in all patients (level A), with routine screening using dipstick testing to be avoided (level D).[16]

J. Serum α-Fetoprotein Screening

Neural tube defects occur in about 7.2 to 15.6 cases per 10,000 live-born infants, and vary from small asymptomatic cases of spina bifida to open myelomeningoceles to anencephaly (which is incompatible with prolonged life after birth). Maternal serum levels of α-fetoprotein are elevated in greater than 80% of pregnancies in which the fetus has an open neural tube defect; other anomalies, such as open ventral wall defects of the abdomen, also can lead to increased levels. Folate supplementation of at least 0.4 mg started at least 4 weeks before conception and continued through the first 6 weeks of pregnancy is associated with a decreased incidence of neural tube defects. Larger doses (4 mg) are associated with a lower incidence of recurrence among mothers with a previous infant affected by a neural tube defect.

An elevated maternal serum α-fetoprotein (MSAFP) generally is defined as greater than 2.5 MoM (multiples of the median). In one study, sensitivity of MSAFP was reported as 85%, with specificity of 96%, positive predictive value of 4.8%, and negative predictive value of 99.9%; these numbers result in a NND of 1.23.

Elevated MSAFP values can be caused by factors other than a neural tube defect. Inaccurate gestational age is the most common cause of a falsely elevated result, but this also can occur with multiple gestation, intrauterine growth restriction (IUGR), or fetal demise. An ultrasound can be used to differentiate these possibilities. In high-risk prenatal populations and centers with special expertise, ultrasound has been shown to have a sensitivity of 79% to 96% and a specificity of 90% to 100% at detecting open neural tube defects; this results in a NND of 1.04 to 1.45.[16]

Patients who have an unexplained elevation after ultrasound are offered an amniocentesis, by which an amniotic fluid α-fetoprotein and amniotic fluid acetylcholinesterase can be determined. Even if the amniocentesis studies are normal, an unexplained elevated MSAFP has been associated with an increased risk of stillbirth, congenital anomalies, and low birth weight.

K. Multiple Marker Testing for Down Syndrome

In high-risk women (e.g., those > 35 years old or who have had a prior pregnancy complicated by chromosomal abnormalities), the definitive test for chromosomal abnormalities is CVS or amniocentesis with karyotype determination because the possibility of genetic abnormality is thought to exceed the potential risk of fetal loss (Table 6). In low-risk patients, the risk of miscarriage resulting from amniocentesis is significantly greater than the chance of detecting a chromosomal abnormality. In early studies of MSAFP testing, there were associations between low values and chromosomal abnormalities. The addition of hCG levels and (in some centers) maternal serum estriol has been used to reduce the false-positive rate of this multiple marker testing (MMT) to less than 5%.

Reported sensitivity of MMT varies from 48% to 91%, with specificity of 96% (positive predictive value of 1.2% to 1.8% and negative predictive value of 99.9%).

TABLE 6. Age Specific Rates of Trisomy 21 and Chromosomal Abnormalities

Maternal Age	Risk for Trisomy 21	Risk for Any Chromosomal Abnormalities
20	1/1667	1/526
25	1/1250	1/476
30	1/952	1/384
35	1/385	1/204
40	1/106	1/65
45	1/30	1/20

Adapted from Gabbe SG, Niebyl JR, Simpson JL (eds): Obstetrics: Normal and Problem Pregnancies, 3rd ed. New York, Churchill Livingstone, 1996, p 221.

This gives a range of NND from 1.15 to 2.27, which is considerably higher than the MSAFP test for NTD. Similar to MSAFP testing, MMT can be falsely abnormal with inaccurate gestational age, twin gestation, and IUGR, necessitating an ultrasound for determination of accurate dates and other information as part of the evaluation of an abnormal test. Should the ultrasound confirm gestational age in an apparently normal singleton pregnancy, amniocentesis should be considered for karyotyping.

One alternative is the use of MMT to decrease the need for widespread amniocentesis or CVS in patients older than age 35. In one cohort study of 5385 women older than age 35 with no other risk factors, all patients had MMT along with amniocentesis for karyotyping. If the MMT testing cutoff of 1 in 200 had been used as the level for amniocentesis, 75% of the amniocenteses could have been avoided while missing 11% of the fetuses with Down syndrome.[9] Multiple marker testing with follow-up ultrasound and possible amniocentesis is a level B recommendation by the U.S. Preventive Services Task Force.

The possibility of screening for Down syndrome and other chromosomal defects using ultrasound, using such markers as increased nuchal fold thickness, currently is not recommended but may become appropriate as equipment and expertise continue to improve (see section H in this chapter).

References

1. American Academy of Pediatrics: Rubella. In Peter G (ed): 1997 Red Book: Report of the Committee on Infectious Diseases. 24th ed. Elk Grove Village, IL, American Academy of Pediatrics, 1997, pp 456–462.
2. Bachman JW, Heise RH, Naessens JM, et al: A study of various tests to detect asymptomatic urinary tract infection in an obstetric population. JAMA 270:1971–1974, 1993.
3. Centers for Disease Control and Prevention: Congenital syphilis—United States, 1998. MMWR Morb Mortal Wkly Rep 48:757–761, 1999.
4. Centers for Disease Control and Prevention: 1998 Guidelines for treatment of sexually transmitted diseases. MMWR Morb Mortal Wkly Rep 47(no. RR-1):40–41, 1998.
5. Centers for Disease Control and Prevention: Chorionic villus sampling and amniocentesis: Recommendations for prenatal counseling. MMWR Morb Mortal Wkly Rep 44(no. RR-9):1–12, 1995.
6. Connor EM, Sperling RS, Gelbar R et al: Reduction of maternal-infant transmission of HIV-1 with zidovudine treatment. N Engl J Med 331:1173–1180, 1994.
7. Gabbe SG, Niebyl JR, Simpson JL (eds): Obstetrics: Normal and problem pregnancies, 3rd ed. New York, Churchill Livingstone, 1996, p 221.
8. Githens JH, Lane PA, McCurdy RS, et al: Newborn screening in Colorado: The first ten years. Am J Dis Child 144:466–470, 1990.
9. Haddow JE, Palomaki GE, Knight GJ, et al: Reducing the need for amniocentesis in women 35 years of age or older with serum markers for screening. N Engl J Med 330:1114–1118, 1994.
10. Hart G: Syphilis tests in diagnostic and therapeutic decision making. Ann Intern Med 104:368–376, 1986.
11. How good is that test? II. Bandolier (on-line version) May 1996; 27-2. http://www.jr2.ox.ac.uk/bandolier/band27/b27-2.html
12. Lee SH, Ewert DP, Frederick PD, et al: Resurgence of congenital rubella syndrome in the 1990s: Report on missed opportunities and failed prevention policies among women of childbearing age. JAMA 267:2616–2620, 1992.
13. Lo K-J, Tsai Y-T, Lee S-D, et al: Immunoprophylaxis of infection with hepatitis B virus in infants born to hepatitis B surface antigen-positive carrier mothers. J Infect Dis 152:817–822, 1985.
14. Margolis HS, Alter MJ, Hadler SC: Hepatitis B: Evolving epidemiology and implications for control. Semin Liver Dis 11:84–92, 1991.
15. McCready JA, Morens D, Fields HA, et al: Evaluation of enzyme immunoassay (EIA) as a screening method for hepatitis B markers in an open population. Epidemiol Infect 107:673–684, 1991.
16. U.S. Preventive Services Task Force: Guide to Clinical Preventive Services, 2nd ed. Baltimore, Williams & Wilkins, 1996.
17. Wadland WC, Plante DA: Screening for asymptomatic bacteriuria in pregnancy. A decision and cost analysis. J Fam Pract 29:372–376, 1989.
18. Williams K: Screening for syphilis in pregnancy: An assessment of the costs and benefits. Commun Med 7:37–42, 1985.

SECTION G.
MEDICATIONS IN PREGNANCY

Kent Petrie, M.D.

I. History
Until the beginning of the 20th century, most physicians believed that the uterus provided a protective environment for the fetus and served as a barricade against harm from the external environment. The fetal anomalies caused by thalidomide use in the 1960s shattered this concept, bringing increased public awareness to the potential harmful effects of medications on the developing fetus. Administered as an antianxiety and antinausea agent in the first trimester, thalidomide caused limb reduction defects in one third of infants exposed. The drug had been determined safe in animal studies, so it took several years and many thousands of grossly malformed infants before the cause-effect relationship was recognized. The thalidomide experience prompted the first drug regulations in the United States, requiring a drug to be proved safe and effective for the conditions of use prescribed in its labeling.[3]

II. Medication Use in Pregnancy
A. Extent of Medication Use in Pregnancy
The World Health Organization International Survey of Drug Utilization in Pregnancy in 1991 (22 countries on four continents) showed that 86% of the women surveyed took medication during pregnancy, receiving an average of 2.9 prescriptions (range 1 to 15); this did not include over-the-counter medications taken without the advice of a physician.[3]
B. Drug Exposure in Early Pregnancy
At least half of the pregnancies in North America are unplanned, placing hundreds of thousands of fetuses at risk of exposure to drugs before the pregnancy is known.[5]
C. Use of Medically Indicated Medications
Women may require drug therapy during pregnancy for chronic conditions diagnosed before pregnancy (e.g., epilepsy, asthma), pregnancy-induced conditions (hypertension, gestational diabetes), or acute conditions that develop during pregnancy (e.g., infections, nausea and vomiting).
D. Prescribing Imperatives During Pregnancy
The two imperatives for the family physician prescribing medications in pregnancy are to alleviate maternal suffering and illness, while causing no harm to the fetus.

III. Teratogens
A. Classic Teratogens
Thalidomide was the classic teratogen, which had its effect in the *classic teratogenic period*. If one considers a 280-day gestation, this teratogenic period is 31 to 71 days from the LMP (or about the 5th to 10th week of gestation). This is the period during which maternal-fetal transport of substances is established and organogenesis occurs. During this time, chemicals can affect target organs at their time of greatest development.[2]
B. Broadened Definition of Teratogen
In the past, a teratogen was simply considered to be an agent that caused a physical malformation. The definition of teratogen[2] has been extended to include a broader range of abnormal development, including complete pregnancy loss, structural anomalies, abnormal growth in utero, and long-term functional defects.

C. Latency Period
It now is recognized that drug effects can be subtle, unexpected, and delayed (i.e., manifest changes after a latency period). Diethylstilbestrol (DES) is the classic example of the long latency period that can exist between fetal exposure and drug effect. Between 1940 and 1971, 6 million mothers and their fetuses were exposed to this estrogenic hormone to prevent a variety of reproductive problems ranging from miscarriage to premature delivery. By the late 1960s, it was clear that as adults, these exposed offspring were at significant increased risk of adenocarcinoma of the cervix and vagina and male reproductive anomalies.[3]

D. Background Incidence of Malformations
1. Malformations as structural abnormalities

The risk of drug or chemical exposures in pregnancy must be assessed against the background incidence of malformations.[3] If congenital malformations or anomalies are defined as structural abnormalities of prenatal origin, present at birth, that interfere with viability or physical well-being, the incidence of such malformations is as follows:
   a. Major malformations—3% (e.g., cleft palate, congenital heart defect)
   b. Minor malformations—4% (e.g., accessory digit, external ear tag)

E. Causes of Congenital Malformations
Drugs account for only 3% of congenital malformations. Infections and maternal diseases account for 7%, and genetic causes account for 20%. Unknown causes account for most anomalies (70%).

IV. Classification of Medications in Pregnancy
A. Known Teratogens
Although there are more than 1000 chemicals that are known teratogens in animals, the number of medications proven to pose teratogenic risk in humans is relatively small (Table 7).[2]

B. Methods of Identifying Teratogens
1. Animal studies

Animal studies may fail or may not be helpful.
   a. Interspecies variation: Thalidomide was shown safe in rats and mice but later was reported to cause anomalies in monkeys and rabbits.
   b. Animal defect data: These data may be so conclusive that warnings are issued before U.S. Food and Drug Administration (FDA) approval. For example, isotretinoin (Accutane) animal studies showed craniofacial, cardiac, and central nervous system anomalies, prompting a category X rating and strict product labeling before release.[3]
2. Case reports

Case reports identify rare events, often implicating drugs as teratogens that are exonerated by further studies. For example, Bendectin (pyridoxine 10 mg plus

TABLE 7. Medications with Known Teratogenic Effects

Alcohol	Chemotherapeutic agents (antimetabolites
Androgens	and alkylating agents)
Angiotensin-converting enzyme	Iodides
inhibitors	Isotretinoin
Angiotensin II receptor blockers	Lithium
Anticonvulsants (trimethadione,	Tetracyclines
valproic acid, phenytoin,	Thalidomide and diethylstilbestrol*
carbamazepine)	Warfarin

* Of historic interest.

TABLE 8.   U.S. Food and Drug Administration Use in Pregnancy Classification

Category	Description of Risk
A	*Controlled studies show no risk* Well-controlled human studies have failed to demonstrate risk to the fetus
B	*No evidence of risk in humans* Either animal studies show no fetal risk and no human data are available, or animal studies show a risk but human studies do not show fetal risk
C	*Risk cannot be ruled out* Either animal studies indicate a fetal risk and there are no controlled studies in humans, or there are no available studies in humans or animals
D	*Positive human evidence of fetal risk* Studies show fetal risk in humans, but potential benefits may outweigh the potential risk in certain situations
X	*Contraindicated in pregnancy* Studies in animals or humans, or based on human experience show definite fetal risk

Adapted from Fed Reg 44:37434–37467, 1979.

doxylamine 10 mg) was useful in the 1970s for treatment of morning sickness. Implication of associated anomalies was never proved in careful epidemiologic studies. Excessive litigation, however, prompted Merrill-Dow to remove the drug voluntarily from the marketplace in 1982.[3]

3. Epidemiologic studies

Epidemiologic studies are the best and most difficult means of linking drugs to birth defects. Case-controlled studies and cohort studies require prohibitively large numbers to be statistically significant.

C. FDA Classification of Drugs in Pregnancy

1. Pregnancy precaution categories

Based on animal and human data, the FDA rates drugs into five pregnancy precaution categories: A, B, C, D, and X (Table 8). The safest drugs are those in category A, in which no fetal risk has been shown in well-controlled human studies. The relative risk of teratogenic effects increases through categories B, C, D, and X. Drugs in category X are known teratogens and should be avoided during pregnancy.

2. Criticisms of current system

The FDA has been criticized for the ambiguous statements used in the classification system and for not modifying ratings when new data are made available. The Teratology Society has proposed that the FDA abandon the system in favor of a more evidence-based classification.[8]

3. New pregnancy labeling system

In an attempt to address these concerns, the FDA's Reproductive Health Drugs Advisory Committee has proposed a new system of pregnancy labeling.[4] The new format includes a clinical management statement, a summary risk statement, and a section discussing the available data for each drug (Table 9).

V. Patient Counseling

Every day in practice the family physician is faced with the important task of counseling patients during their preconception and prenatal periods[1] and must be prepared to address several questions.

A. "Is this medication safe to take during my pregnancy?"

Patients need to know that using medications during pregnancy entails acceptance of some small degree of risk. Failure to treat illness may jeopardize the health of the mother and child. Patients should be informed of known indications,

TABLE 9. New U.S. Food and Drug Administration Pregnancy Labeling System

For each medication, the following information will be listed:
1. Clinical Management
   Discussion of the appropriate clinical use of the medication during pregnancy
2. Summary Risk Assessment
   Review of the known risks of the medication's use during pregnancy
3. Discussion of Data
   Review of the specific animal and human data used to make the above recommendations

risks, and benefits of any drug therapy and be involved in decisions regarding medications as much as possible.

B. "Since I took this drug before I knew I was pregnant, will my baby be born with a birth defect?"

The clinician should gather as much information as possible to share with patients regarding risks of drug exposures. High-resolution ultrasound to detect major anomalies before 20 weeks may be offered to those for whom termination of pregnancy is an option or to prepare the parents for the birth of an infant with special needs.

C. "Did any of the medications I took cause this birth defect?"

Open and direct discussion is important, showing an understanding of the patient's disbelief, anger, and guilt. The physician should describe basic teratology and the small window of vulnerability of the fetus, emphasizing that second and third trimester exposure is unlikely to cause a major defect. Consultation with a specialist in dysmorphology may give insight into the problem. Autopsy is helpful in the case of intrauterine fetal death. Family counseling is essential in the event of loss or the challenge of raising a child with special needs.

VI. Table of Common Medications in Pregnancy

Most drugs fall into FDA category C, and descriptions of drugs that appear in the *Physicians' Desk Reference*[7] and similar sources often contain statements such as "Use in pregnancy is not recommended unless the potential benefits justify the potential risks to the fetus." Such disclaimers, although understandable from a medicolegal standpoint, are of little help to the practicing physician.[5]

To provide a useful tool for the busy family physician, Table 10 lists common medications used in pregnancy and classifies them as *acceptable*, to be used with *caution*, or to *avoid*. The table is compiled based on the best available data from large cohort studies or meta-analyses and the FDA ratings as published in references 1, 3, 5, and 6. Where they exist, current controversies are listed under "Comments."

TABLE 10. Drugs for Common Conditions in Pregnancy

	Caution/Avoid	Acceptable	Comments
Vitamins and nutritionals	Alcohol Caffeine Saccharin Excessive vitamin A	Prenatal vitamins Aspartame (Nutrasweet) Sucralose (Splenda)	Caffeine use in moderation (< 300 mg/d) is considered safe by most authorities. Saccharin has not been shown to be teratogenic in humans, but second-generation animal studies show increased incidence of bladder tumors. Vitamin A at doses >10,000 IU/d has been associated with craniofacial, CNS, and cardiac defects.

(Table continued on next page.)

TABLE 10.   Drugs for Common Conditions in Pregnancy *(Continued)*

	Caution/Avoid	Acceptable	Comments
Coughs and colds	Phenylpropanolamine Phenylephrine Iodide preparations Pseudoephedrine	Dextromethorphan Guaifenesin Codeine (caution near term) Hydrocodone (caution near term)	Rare malformations have been reported with the sympatho-mimetic amines phenylpropanolamine and phenylephrine. Prolonged exposure to iodides may cause fetal hypothyroidism and goiter. Narcotic cough suppressant use near term may cause neonatal withdrawal. Gastroschisis after first trimester exposure to pseudoephedrine has been reported.
Allergic rhinitis	Brompheniramine	Chlorpheniramine Diphenhydramine Triprolidine Loratadine (Claritin) Cetirizine (Zyrtec) Astemizole (Hismanal) Fexofenadine (Allegra) Nasal steroids Nasal cromolyn	Antihistamines are generally considered safe. Case reports do exist for malformations associated with Brompheniramine use, and long-term studies are limited on newer antihistamines.
Asthma		Inhaled bronchodilators Epinephrine Theophylline Terbutaline (Brethine) Cromolyn (Intal) Leukotriene receptor antagonists Inhaled steroids Prednisone Prednisolone	Pregnancy need not change the drug regimen for asthma. The newest class of drugs, leukotriene receptor antagonists, are listed as FDA category B and appear safe in pregnancy.
Nausea and vomiting Motion sickness	Scopolamine (transdermal) (avoid at term)	Meclizine (Bonine, Antivert) Dimenhydrinate (Dramamine) Doxylamine (Unisom) Phosphorated carbohydrate solution (Emetrol) Trimethobenzamide (Tigan) Pyridoxine (vitamin B6) Prochlorperazine (Compazine) Promethazine (Phenergan) Metoclopramide (Reglan) Ondansetron (Zofran)	Antihistamines and phenothiazines at usual doses are considered safe. Because of reports of CNS symptoms in nonpregnant adults taking high doses of pyridoxine, vitamin B_6 doses should not exceed 75 mg/d during pregnancy. Neonatal effects may occur with use of the anticholinergic scopolamine at term.
Acid peptic disorders	Misoprostol (Cytotec)	Antacids H_2 antagonists Sucralfate (Carafate) Omeprazole (Prilosec) Lansoprazole (Prevacid)	Misoprostol has been used increasingly at term for labor induction, but should be otherwise avoided. *H. pylori* infection may be treated during pregnancy with proton-pump inhibitors and antibiotics (see below)
Constipation	Aloe vera laxatives	Psyllium Senna Milk of magnesia Docusate sodium (Colace) Docusate calcium (Surfak)	Aloe vera laxatives have been associated with fetal meconium passage

(Table continued on next page.)

TABLE 10. Drugs for Common Conditions in Pregnancy *(Continued)*

	Caution/Avoid	Acceptable	Comments
Diarrhea/in-flammatory bowel disease	Bismuth subsalicylate (Pepto-Bismol)	Kaolin/pectin Diphenoxylate (Lomotil) Loperamide (Imodium) Sulfasalazine (Azulfidine) Mesalamine (Rowasa, Asacol)	Bismuth in bismuth subsalicylate may bind to fetal bone. Prolonged chronic use of kaolin/pectin may cause maternal iron deficiency. Avoid sulfasalazine at term due to risk of neonatal jaundice.
Headache (tension) and analgesia	NSAIDs (caution near term)	Acetaminophen Aspirin (caution near term) Ibuprofen (caution near term) Codeine and other nar-cotics (caution near term) Tramadol (Ultram)	Avoid narcotics near term because of potential neonatal withdrawal. Avoid aspirin and NSAIDs near term because of constriction of the fetal ductus arteriosus and risk of persistent pulmonary hypertension in the newborn.
Headache, migraine	Ergotamines	Triptans Butalbital Isometheptene/ dichloralphenazone (Midrin)	Avoid ergotamines because of oxy-tocic properties. Triptans have not been associated with increased malformations. Data are accumu-lating to evaluate other side effects. Prophylactic medications for migraine (β-blockers, TCAs, and calcium channel blockers) may be used (see other categories).
Depression/ psycho-tropics	Lithium Benzodiazepines Meprobamate (Miltown)	TCAs (tricyclics) Chloral hydrate SSRIs Bupropion (Wellbutrin) Buspirone (BuSpar) Trazodone (Desyrel) Mirtazapine (Remeron) Zolpidem (Ambien) Zaleplon (Sonata)	Despite their listing as category D by the FDA, TCAs have not been shown consistently to cause mal-formations after first trimester ex-posure and are considered safe by most authorities. Case reports do exist suggesting neonatal with-drawal to TCAs, warranting obser-vation of the neoborn. SSRIs have shown no teratogenic effects but may affect the miscarriage rate and fetal growth rate and have been associated with prematurity. Early reports of diazepam's association with oral clefts have not been con-firmed. Concern still exists with benzodiazepines about neonatal withdrawal when used near term.
Hypertension and cardio-vascular disease	ACE inhibitors Angiotensin II receptor blockers Diuretics Reserpine HMG-CoA reductase inhibitors	Methyldopa Hydralazine β-blockers (caution near term) Labetalol (caution near term) Calcium channel blockers Prazosin (Minipress) Digoxin Nitroglycerin	ACE inhibitors cause fetal renal failure and oligohydramnios. β-blockers and combined α/β-blockers may cause IUGR, and neonates should be ob-served for 48 h for bradycardia, hypotension, and hypoglycemia. Diuretics may decrease maternal plasma volume when admin-istered in the second and third trimester. Reserpine near term can cause nasal discharge and respira-tory distress in the newborn. Case reports of fetal malformations as-sociated with in utero exposure to HMG-CoA reductase inhibitor, lo-vastatin, warrant avoidance of this class of drugs during pregnancy.

(Table continued on next page.)

TABLE 10.   Drugs for Common Conditions in Pregnancy *(Continued)*

	Caution/Avoid	Acceptable	Comments
Thrombo-phlebitis/ anticoagu-lation	Warfarin (Coumadin) Streptokinase/ urokinase	Heparin Enoxaparin (Lovenox)	Warfarin teratogenicity includes skeletal and CNS defects and the Dandy-Walker syndrome (cystic expansion of the fourth ventricle with hydrocephalus). Small amounts of streptokinase cross the placenta. Heparin and low-molecular-weight heparin do not cross the placenta.
Epilepsy	Phenytoin (Dilantin) Phenobarbital Valproic acid (Depakene) Carbamazepine (Tegretol) Trimethadione Lamotrigine (Lamictal) Gabapentin (Neurontin)	Ethosuximide (Zarontin)	Carbamazepine has long been considered the drug of choice for epilepsy in pregnancy, but reports exist of a fetal hydantoin-like syndrome associated with its use in the first trimester. Although animal studies have not shown teratogenicity with lamotrigine and gabapentin, few human studies involving these newer agents exist. Ethosuximide appears to have a lower terato-genic potential than other anticonvulsants.
Hormonal medications	Oral contraceptives Medroxyprogesterone (Depo-Provera) Androgenic steroids Danocrine (Danazol) Clomiphene (Clomid) Tamoxifen (Nolvadex) Raloxifene (Evista)	Prednisone Prednisolone Parenteral steroids	Patients can be reassured about inadvertent first-trimester expo-sure to oral contraceptives, medroxyprogesterone, and clomiphene. Meta-analyses of existing data show no relation-ship between exposure and malformations in particular.
Diabetes	Oral sulfonylureas Metformin (Glucophage) Acarbose (Precose) Miglitol (Glyset) Repaglinide (Prandin) Pioglitazone (Actos) Rosiglitazone (Avandia)	Insulin	The known risk of hypoglycemia with the sulfonylureas and the presumed risk with newer oral agents make insulin the drug of choice for the treatment of diabetes in pregnancy.
Thyroid medications	Radioactive iodine Propylthiouracil (PTU) Methimazole (Tapazole)	Thyroxine (T$_4$) (Synthroid) Triiodothyronine (T$_3$) (Cytomel)	Propylthiouracil is preferred over methimazole because of higher placental transfer of methima-zole and its association with aplasia cutis of the scalp. β-blockers may be used for symptomatic hyperthyroidism.
Bacterial infections	Tetracyclines Erythromycin estolate (Ilosone) Quinolones (ciprofloxacin) Aminoglycosides Nalidixic acid Clarithromycin (Biaxin)	Penicillins ± clavulanate Erythromycin base Sulfonamides (avoid near term) Trimethoprim (avoid first trimester) Nitrofurantoin (avoid near term) Vancomycin Azithromycin (Zithromax)	Tetracycline chelates to developing teeth after the fifth month of pregnancy, causing intense yellow staining. Aminoglycosides are potentially ototoxic to the developing fetus. Quinolone fetal arthropathy in animal studies has prompted warnings in human pregnancy. Erythro-mycin estolate is associated with maternal hepatotoxicity. Animal teratogenenicity data have *(Table continued on next page.)*

TABLE 10. Drugs for Common Conditions in Pregnancy *(Continued)*

	Caution/Avoid	Acceptable	Comments
Bacterial infections *(cont.)*		Cephalosporins Loracarbef (Lorabid) Clindamycin (Cleocin) Metronidazole (Flagyl) Chloramphenacol (avoid at term)	warranted caution with clarithromycin use despite FDA Category C listing. Trimethoprim is a folic acid antagonist and should be avoided preconception and in the first trimester. Sulfonamides at term can cause fetal hemolytic anemia and neonatal jaundice. Nitrofurantoin at term may cause hemolytic anemia in the rare fetus with G6PD deficiency. Oral metronidazole, previously considered teratogenic and carcinogenic in the first trimester, is now believed to be safe in all trimesters. Chloramphenicol at term has been associated with newborn cardiovascular collapse (gray baby syndrome).
Viral infections	Ribavirin	Acyclovir (Zovirax) Amantadine (Symmetrel) Rimantadine (Flumadine) Zidovudine (AZT) Zanamivir (Relenza) Oseltamivir (Tamiflu)	Ribavirin has been shown to be teratogenic in nearly all animal species studied. No adverse outcomes have been reported with newer antiherpetic agents (famciclovir, valacyclovir), but acyclovir is preferred because of the quantity of data available. Among the newer anti-influenza drugs, inhaled zanamivir (Cat. B) is preferred over oral oseltamivir (Cat. C).
Fungal infections	Fluconazole (Diflucan) (caution first trimester) Ketoconazole (Nizoral) (caution first trimester) Itraconazole (Sporanox) (caution first trimester) Terbinafine (Lamisil) (caution first trimester) Griseofulvin	Nystatin (Mycostatin) Miconazole (Monistat) Clotrimazole (Lotrimin) Terconazole (Terazole)	Griseofulvin is contraindicated in pregnancy. Systemic triazole and imidazole antifungal therapy in the first trimester may induce fetal malformations.
Tuberculosis infections	Streptomycin Pyrazinamide	Isoniazid (INH) Para-aminosalicylic acid (PAS) Rifampin (Rifadin) Ethambutol (Myambutol)	Streptomycin ototoxicity warrants avoidance in pregnancy. Other standard antituberculous drugs may be given alone or in combination. Lack of clinical studies warrants caution with use of pyrazinamide.
Parasitic infections	Lindane (Kwell) Primaquine Quinine	Permethrin (Nix, Elimite) Pyrethrins and piperonyl butoxide (RID) Pyrantel pamoate (Antiminth) Chloroquine	Lindane's potential neurotoxicity warrants avoidance in pregnancy. Primaquine and furazolidone may cause hemolytic anemia in the rare retus with G6PD deficiency. Quinine *(Table continued on next page.)*

TABLE 10.   Drugs for Common Conditions in Pregnancy *(Continued)*

	Caution/Avoid	Acceptable	Comments
Parasitic infections *(cont.)*		Hydroxychloroquine Quinacrine Mefloquine (Lariam) (caution first trimester) Crotamiton (Eurax) Furazolidone (Furoxone) (avoid at term) Mebendazole (Vermox)	teratogenicity has been reported. Concern exists about mefloquine fetal toxicity in the first trimester.
Dermato- logic agents	Isotretinoin (Accutane) Etretinate (Tegison) Podophyllum Podophilox (Condylox) Imiquimod (Aldara)	Topical tretinoin (Retin-A, Renova) Topical antibiotics Topical antifungals Topical steroids Calcipotriene (Dovonex) Benzoyl peroxide Hydroquinone bleaching agents	Isotretinoin and etretinate are potent teratogens. Topical retinoids are minimally absorbed and appear safe. ACOG recommends cryo-therapy for genital warts in preg-nancy and considers the use of topical agents contraindicated. Small doses of topical dermato-logic agents are safe during pregnancy.

CNS = central nervous system; NSAIDs = nonsteroidal anti-inflammatory drugs; TCAs = tricyclic anti-depressants; SSRIs = selective serotonin reuptake inhibitors; ACE = angiotensin-converting enzyme; G6PD = glucose-6-phosphate dehydrogenase.

References

1. Abrams RS: Will It Hurt the Baby? Reading, MA, Addison-Wesley Publishing, 1990.
2. American College of Obstetricians and Gynecologists: Teratology. ACOG Educational Bulletin, no. 233, 1997.
3. Briggs GG, Freeman RK, Yaffe SJ: Drugs in Pregnancy and Lactation, 5th ed. Baltimore, Williams and Wilkins, 1998.
4. Fed Reg 44:37434–37467, 1979.
5. Koren G, Pastuszak A, Ito S: Drugs in pregnancy. N Engl J Med 338:1128–1137, 1998.
6. Niebyl JR: Drugs in pregnancy and lactation. In Gabbe SG, et al (eds): Obstetrics, Normal and Problem Pregnancies, 3rd ed. New York, Churchill Livingstone, 1996, p 249–277.
7. Physicians' Desk Reference. Montvale, NJ, Medical Economics Company, 1999.
8. Teratology Society Public Affairs Committee: FDA classification of drugs for teratogenic risk. Teratology 49:446–447, 1994.

SECTION H.
ALTERNATIVE MEDICINE IN MATERNITY CARE

Kent A. Petrie, M.D.

Family physicians are confronted daily with questions from their patients about alterna-tive medicine. When maternity care patients seek information about such therapies, careful attention must be paid to issues of safety and efficacy for the mother and her unborn child.

I. Alternative Medicine Use in the United States

The growth of alternative medicine in the United States was striking in the 1990s. In a landmark study[8] and a follow-up report,[7] Eisenberg et al. investigated the prevalence and costs of alternative medicine use between 1990 and 1997. Americans' annual use of at least one form of alternative medicine grew from 34% to 42% during that time. Visits to alternative therapists increased from 427 million to 629 million per year, exceeding annual visits to all primary care physicians. Although greater than 80% of patients using alternative medicine also sought treatment for the same condition from a physician, only

TABLE 11. NIH Offce of Alternative Medicine Categories of Complementary and Alternative Medicine

Mind-Body Interventions
  Biofeedback, relaxation therapies, meditation, hypnosis, imagery, aerobic exercise, yoga, tai chi, therapeutic support groups, prayer and spiritual healing, hydrotherapy

Bioelectromagnetic Therapies
  TENS, pulsed electromagnetic fields, fixed magnets

Alternative Systems of Medical Practice
  Chinese Medicine (acupuncture/acupressure), Indian Ayurveda, homeopathy

Manual Healing Methods
  Osteopathy, chiropractic, physical therapy, massage therapy, therapeutic touch, reflexology

Pharmacologic and Biologic Treatments
  Chelation therapy, shark cartilage, ozone therapy

Herbal Medicine
  Medicinal herbs, essential oils (aromatherapy)

Diet and Nutrition Therapies
  Vitamin therapy, lifestyle modification (macrobiotics, Gerson diet)

TENS = transcutaneous electrical nerve stimulation.

39% informed their physician they were doing so. By 1997, Americans spent $21.2 billion on this care, $12.2 billion of which was out-of-pocket expense.

II. Categories of Alternative Medicine
In response to growing consumer interest in and use of alternative medicines, the National Institutes of Health (NIH) established its Office of Alternative Medicine in 1992 to investigate the safety and efficacy of such therapies. For purposes of further study, the NIH created seven categories of Complementary and Alternative Medicine (Table 11).[1,22] Many of the NIH categories are familiar and have been accepted into mainstream practice by primary care physicians.

III. Selected Alternative Therapies and Their Applications in Maternity Care
Many alternative medicine therapies have found application in the care of the maternity patient. Alternative therapies with the most evidence-based literature supporting their use include acupuncture, herbal medicine, and chiropractic and other manipulative therapies. Although not supported by a significant body of evidence, homeopathy also is growing in popularity and is discussed.
A. Acupuncture and Traditional Chinese Medicine
1. Acupuncture overview
Acupuncture (from Latin, *acus* = needle, *punctura* = puncture) involves the insertion of hair-thin needles into specific points in the body to prevent or treat disease. It is one component of the system of Traditional Chinese Medicine that has been in use for more than 2000 years.[17]

Acupuncture stimulates channels of energy, *Qi* (pronounced *chee* in Chinese, *key* in Japanese), that are said to flow through 12 major meridians under the surface of the skin, each of which is connected to a specific organ.[17] Classic acupuncture describes 365 points along these meridians.[17] Over time, this number of points has increased to more than 2000, as a result of localized versions of acupuncture of the ear and hand.[29] Each point is given a number and often a name (e.g., P6 Neiguan). Chinese acupuncture points also may be stimulated by firm finger or mechanical pressure (acupressure), electric stimulation, or smoldering cones of the herb artemesia vulgaris or mugwort (moxybustion).[17] Acupuncture points commonly used in maternity care are diagrammed in Figure 1.

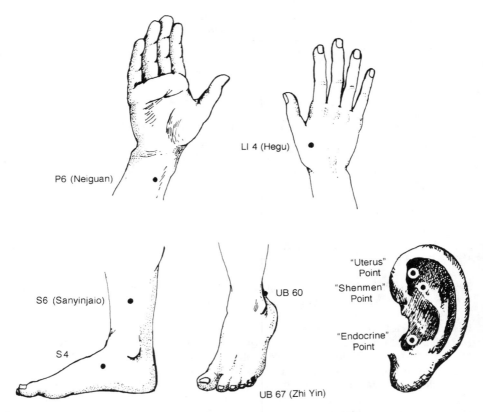

FIGURE 1. Common acupuncture points in maternity care. (Courtesy Charmayne Bernhardt, Vail, CO.)

P6 (pericardium 6, *Neiguan*): reduces nausea and vomiting
LI4 (large intestine 4, *Hegu*): stimulates labor and reduces pain
S6 (spleen 6, *Sanyinjaio*): stimulates labor and reduces pain
S4 (spleen 4): reduces premature labor
UB 60 (urinary bladder 60): relieves low back pain
UB 67 (urinary bladder 67, *Zhi-Yin*): facilitates version of breech
Uterus ear point: reduces labor pain and promotes relaxation
Shenmen ear point: reduces labor pain and promotes relaxation
Endocrine ear point: stimulates labor

Complications of acupuncture are rare. There have been only 10 case reports of injury to internal organs since 1965 in the United States, and disposable needles have reduced the risk of infection.[10] Acupuncture and acupressure are safe in pregnancy.[29] In early pregnancy, it is recommended to avoid stimulation of points associated with uterine contractions (e.g., S6 and LI 4).[6]

2. Acupuncture Applications in Maternity Care

a. Nausea and vomiting in pregnancy: Stimulation of P6, or Neiguan point (3 fingerbreadths proximal to the distal wrist crease and between the two central flexor tendons of the forearm), by acupuncture needles, acupressure (purposeful stimulation for 5 minutes every 4 hours while awake), or continuous pressure with seasickness wrist bands has been shown in multiple trials[18] to be effective in reducing nausea and vomiting.

b. Version of the breech presentation: Moxybustion has been studied when applied at acupuncture point UB 67 on the lateral aspect of the fifth toe. When performed bilaterally for 15 minutes each day beginning at 33 weeks of gestation, a 75% version rate by 35 weeks was shown compared to 47% in matched controls.[4] It is postulated that this stimulation causes increased maternal adrenocortical activity, increasing uterine tone and fetal activity, which stimulates spontaneous version.

c. Premature labor: Acupuncture point Spleen 4 (S4), located at the base of the first metatarsal, has been reported in nonrandomized trials to treat premature labor successfully. Bilateral stimulation daily for 1 week at the onset of premature labor then weekly thereafter has been demonstrated to delay the onset of labor.[30]

d. Induction and augmentation of labor: Two small nonrandomized studies of multiple-point acupuncture have shown significant increases in contraction onset, frequency, and intensity.[16,30] Acupuncture points most commonly used to stimulate contractions are LI 4 (Hegu), on the back of the hand in the web space between the thumb and index finger, and S6 (Sanyinjaio), 4 fingerbreadths above the medial malleolus of the ankle. Acupressure may be applied to these points in 6 or more equal on-off cycles of 10 to 60 seconds, repeated as needed. Such stimulation has been suggested for outpatient cervical ripening.[29] Transcutaneous electrical nerve stimulation of these points has been reported to induce labor successfully in a series of postterm pregnancies.[6] The ear acupuncture point Endocrine also may be stimulated to increase contraction strength.[29]

e. Pain relief in labor: Stimulation of LI 4 and S6 have been shown to relieve pain as well as stimulate labor.[13] Acupressure may be applied to these points for 10 to 60 seconds, repeated as needed.[13] Two ear acupuncture points, Uterus and Shenmen, may be stimulated to reduce pain and promote general relaxation during labor.[29] Self-adhesive acupressure beads may be applied to one or both of these points and periodically pressed during labor by the patient or her birth attendant.

B. Herbal Medicine

1. Overview

Late 20th century dissatisfaction with the cost and side effects of synthetic pharmaceuticals has fostered a renewed interest in herbal remedies.[2] In 1997, U.S. sales of herbal products reached $3.24 billion, and herbal remedies were the top pharmacy growth category in drugstores.[2,20]

Various forms of herbal medicines are available. Teas, steeped from delicate fresh or dried leaves or flowers, can be taken as hot or cold liquids. Tinctures or extracts are concentrated solutions, which can be taken by drops or teaspoon. Capsules or tablets are prepared from powdered herbs. Essential oils are highly concentrated oils naturally present in a plant. They have distinct aromas and are used for massage and aromatherapy.

Safety and efficacy testing of herbal preparations is not as strictly controlled as for testing of pharmaceuticals.[2] Under the 1994 FDA Dietary Supplement Health and Education Act, herbal products are considered *nutritional supplements*, not drugs. Although the FDA has forbidden placement of therapeutic information on labels, they are now tightening the restrictions on herbal remedy claims.[2] English translation of the *German Commission E Monographs*[3] documents the European experience and has increased greatly the availability of credible information regarding herbal remedies. The *PDR for Herbal Medicines* was first published in 1998.[21] Controlled trials of many remedies are being sponsored

TABLE 12.   Herbs to Avoid in Pregnancy

Common Name (Latin Name)	Side Effects in Pregnancy
Aloe (*Aloe vera*)	Stimulates fetal meconium passage
Arbor vitae (*Thuja occidentalis*)	Induces menses
Beth root (*Trillium erectum*)	Reduces uterine blood flow
Black cohosh (*Cimicifuga racemosa*)*	Stimulates uterine contraction
Blue cohosh (*Caulophyllum thalictroides*)*	Stimulates uterine contraction
Cascara (*Rhamnus purshianus*)	Stimulates uterine contraction
Chinese angelica, dong quai (*Angelica sinensis*)	Coumarin-like effect
Cinchona (*Cinchona* sp.)	Quinine-like effect
Cotton root bark (*Gossypium hebaceum*)	Stimulates uterine contraction
Evening primrose oil (*Oenothera biennis*)*	Stimulates uterine contraction
Feverfew (*Tanacetum parthenium*)	Stimulates uterine contraction and induces menses
Ginseng (*Panax ginseng*)	Stimulates uterine contraction
Golden seal (*Hydrastis canadensis*)	Stimulates uterine contraction
Hawthorne (*Crataegus oxacantha*)	ACE inhibitor activity
Juniper (*Juniperus communis*)	Stimulates uterine contraction and potent diuretic
Kava kava (*Piper methysticum*)	Fetal and maternal sedative
Licorice (*Glycyrrhiza glabra*)	Hypertension and cholestasis
Ma-huang (*Ephedra sinica*)	Hypertension
Meadow saffron (*Crocus sativus*)	Abortifacient
Pennyroyal (*Mentha pulegium*)	Abortifacient
Poke root (*Phytolacca americana*)	Diarrhea and hypotension
Rue (*Ruta graveolens*)	Abortifacient
Sage (*Salvia officinalis*)**	Stimulates uterine contraction
Senna (*Cassia senna*)	Stimulates uterine contraction and fetal cathartic
Tansy (*Tanacetum vulgare*)	Abortifacient
Tea tree oil (*Melaleuca alternifolia*)	May be applied externally
White peony (*Paeonia lactiflora*)	Abortifacient and induces menses
Wormwood (*Artemisia absinthium*)	Stimulates uterine contraction
Yarrow (*Achillea millefolium*)	Induces menses
Yellow dock (*Rumex crispus*)	Stimulates uterine contraction
Herbs to Avoid while Nursing	**Herbs That Appear Safe in Pregnancy and Nursing**
Black cohash (*Cimicifuga racemosa*)	Echinacea (*Echinacea* sp.)
Cascara (*Rhamnus purshiana*)	Ginkgo (*Ginkgo biloba*)
Chinese rhubarb (*Rheum palmatum*)	Milk thistle (*Silybum marianum*)
Comfrey (*Symphytum officinale*)	St. John's wort (*Hypericum perforatum*)
Garlic (*Allium sativum*)	Valerian (*Valeriana officinalis*)
Kava kava (*Piper methysticum*)	
Parsley (*Petroselinum crispum*)	
Sage (*Salvia officinalis*)	
Senna (*Cassia senna*)	

 * May be used for labor augmentation or pain
 ** May be used to suppress lactation

by the NIH, and more evidence-based articles on herbal remedies are beginning to appear in the primary care literature.[20,23] Often, however, patients think, "If it's natural, it must be safe." Herbs are potent chemicals. Many are emmenagogues (stimulate menses), and others stimulate uterine contractions. Table 12 lists herbal remedies to avoid, particularly in early pregnancy.

2. Applications of herbal medicine in maternity care
  a. Nausea and vomiting
    i. Powdered gingerroot capsules (*Zingiber officinale*): Gingerroot at an oral dose of 250 to 500 mg four times a day has been shown to reduce nausea and emesis significantly in patients hospitalized with hyperemesis

gravidarum.[9] Ginger's efficacy is believed to be due to its antispasmodic properties as well as enhancing salivary secretions and increasing gastric motility.[5] A systematic review of the literature,[31] however, has cast some doubt on its absolute safety in pregnancy. Concerns have been raised because of ginger's effect on thromboxane synthetase activity and testosterone binding, which theoretically could increase bleeding in early pregnancy. The author concludes that ginger should be used with caution in pregnancy and should be avoided if the patient has a history of bleeding disorders or miscarriage.[31]

    ii. Vitamin B_6 (pyridoxine): Studies of pyridoxine in pregnancy show safety and efficacy in oral doses of 25 mg two to three times per day.[18] Because high doses of vitamin B_6 have been associated with neurologic problems in nonpregnant adults, questions have been raised about what constitutes excessive dosing for a developing embryo. Until further information is available, it is recommended that doses in pregnancy not exceed 75 mg/d.[18]

b. Induction and augmentation of labor

    i. Blue cohosh (*Caulophyllum thalictroides*): Blue cohosh tincture taken orally has been anecdotally reported to ripen the cervix and induce and augment labor.[5] Also known as squaw root and papoose root, blue cohosh is a traditional Native American herb used by various tribes to facilitate childbirth.[5] It contains steroidal saponins, which are known to stimulate the uterus.

    ii. Oil of evening primrose (*Oenothera biennis*): Oil of evening primrose by mouth or by placement of a capsule on the cervix has been reported for labor augmentation. The component of oil of evening primrose thought to stimulate uterine activity is the essential fatty acid gammalinoleic acid, a precursor of prostaglandin E_1.[5]

c. Lactation suppression and prevention of engorgement

    i. Jasmine flowers: Jasmine flowers taped to the breast have been shown to be as effective as bromocriptine mesylate in suppression of lactation.[25]

    ii. Sage and parsley: Sage and parsley capsules taken by mouth have been reported to decrease the flow of milk.[29]

    iii. Cabbage leaves: Application of cold cabbage leaves, with holes cut to allow the nipples to remain dry, has been shown in randomized trials to prevent engorgement and has been associated with greater long term breastfeeding success.[19]

d. Increase breast milk production: Fenugreek, fennel seed, nettle, blessed thistle, and raspberry leaf have been described to increase milk flow when taken individually as capsules or combined in a tea.[29]

C. Homeopathy

1. Overview

Dr. Samuel Hahnemann (1755–1843) of Germany founded the practice of homeopathy (from Greek, *homois* = similar, *pathos* = suffering).[10] In the 5th century B.C., Hippocrates claimed that there were two ways of healing, by *opposites* and *similars*.[10] Hahnemann founded homeopathy on the "law of similars" (i.e., like cures like"); for example, for diarrhea, a dilute medicine is given that in high doses could cause diarrhea. Orthodox medicine, which Hahnemann named *allopathy*[10] (from Greek, *allo* = other, different), focuses on opposites; for example, for constipation, a medicine is given that could cause diarrhea.

In addition to the law of similars, the principles of homeopathy include "potentization by dilution and succussion" (vigorous shaking). This claim, that

homeopathic remedies become stronger by successive dilution, has caused much skepticism among allopathic physicians, who claim that homeopathic remedies work by placebo effect only.[10] Potency scales of homeopathic remedies are noted as follows:
- Decimal scale (i.e., 6X = 6 dilutions of 10 [1:9])
- Centissimal scale (i.e., 30C = 30 dilutions of 100 [1:99])
- M scale (i.e., 50M or LM = 50 dilutions of 1000 [1:999])

Homeopathic remedies generally are considered safe for administration during pregnancy because of their minimal concentrations.[29]

Randomized controlled trials of homeopathic remedies for a variety of illnesses are beginning to appear in the literature to investigate their safety and efficacy.[10] There has been significant criticism of both the randomized controlled trials and the meta-analyses of these studies, however.[14]

2. Applications of homeopathy in maternity care
   a. Nausea and vomiting: Case reports of homeopathic remedies that purport to be effective include 30X to 30C dilutions of nux vomica (poison nut), *Pulsitilla* (windflower), *Cephaelis ipecacuanha* (ipecac), *Silicea* (silica), *Sepia* (cuttlefish), *Colchicum* (yellow saffron), and *Symphoricarpos racemosa* (snowberry).[29]
   b. Stimulation of labor: Homeopathic remedies have been studied prospectively to prepare the uterus for labor. A study group given *Pulsitilla nigrans*, *Secale cornutum*, *Caulophyllum thalictroides*, *Aceta racemosa*, and *Arnica montana* daily for 1 to 2 weeks before their due date had less false labor, fewer protracted first stages, and less postpartum blood loss than a control group.[32] Homeopathy remedies given during labor to stimulate progress include *Caulophyllum* (blue cohosh) and *Pulsitilla* (windflower) 30C administered hourly.[29]
   c. Perineal care: The homeopathic remedy frequently used in the postpartum period is *Arnica montana* 30C every 2 to 4 hours as a liquid or tablet. It is reported to reduce bruising of the perineum, to prevent bleeding, and to reduce pain.[12] Witch hazel cleansings and lavender oil baths are reported to reduce perineal infection and pain.[29]

D. Chiropractic and Other Manipulative Medicine
1. Manipulative therapy overview

Chiropractic and osteopathy are two systems of manipulation that differ in theory and practice. In the simplest terms, osteopaths use arms and legs as fulcrums for bending and twisting the body (long-lever manipulation), whereas chiropractors generally manipulate only the protruding parts of the spinal vertebrae (short-lever manipulation).[10]

In the 20th century, osteopathy has evolved in the direction of conventional medicine and is no longer considered alternative. Chiropractic has continued its focus on spinal manipulation and today chiropractors provide 94% of all manipulative therapy in the United States[24]; however, many primary care physicians (M.D. and D.O. trained) now are learning and applying techniques of spinal manipulation and mobilization in their practices.[11] Chiropractic care and other forms of spinal manipulation and mobilization are safe in pregnancy if treatments avoid direct pressure on the abdomen and uterus and avoid prolonged supine positioning.[29] Manipulative therapy should be delivered gently, respecting the increased laxity of spinal and pelvic ligaments during pregnancy.

2. Applications of manipulative therapy in maternity care
   a. Back pain: During pregnancy, the hormone relaxin causes laxity of the anterior and posterior longitudinal ligaments of the spine as well as the

TABLE 13. An Office Library on Alternative Medicine

Balch JF, Balch PA: Prescription for Nutritional Healing. Garden City Park, NY, Avery Publishing Group, 1997.
Blumenthal M, Gruenwald J, Hall T, et al: German Commission E Monographs: Medicinal Plants for Human Use. Austin, TX, American Botanical Council, 1998.
Chevallier A: The Encyclopedia of Medicinal Plants. New York, DK Publishing, 1996.
Duke JA: The Green Pharmacy. Emmaus, PA, Trondal Press, 1997.
Fugh-Berman A: Alternative Medicine: What Works. Baltimore, Williams & Wilkins, 1997.
Gordon JS: Manifesto for a New Medicine: Your Guide to Healing Partnerships and the Wise Use of Alternative Therapies. Reading, MA, Addison-Wesley, 1996.
PDR for Herbal Medicines. Montvale, NJ, Medical Economics Company, 1998.
Tiran D, Mack S: Complementary Therapies for Pregnancy and Childbirth. London, Bailliere Tindall, 1995.

symphysis pubis and sacroiliac joints. These changes, along with the body's altered center of gravity, contribute to back pain.[15] Chiropractic care has been proved effective in treatment of acute low back pain and can be administered safely during pregnancy.[29]

  b. Pain in labor: Counterpressure techniques applied during contractions and any time pain develops have been shown to reduce pain in the lumbar and sacroiliac areas effectively.[28] Techniques described in the literature include:
    • Back counterpressure[26]—steady direct manual pressure applied to the low back while the patient is standing, kneeling, sitting, or side-lying
    • Knee counterpressure[26]—longitudinal pressure applied along the axis of the femur with hip and knee flexed while the patient is sitting in a chair or a birthing bed
    • Hip squeeze[26]—firm pressure applied to both hips.

  A variety of massage techniques have been shown to be safe and effective during labor.[27] It is important to encourage patient feedback on which of many massage techniques are helpful.

IV. Incorporating Alternative Medicine into Maternity Care

Incorporating alternative medicine into family practice maternity care is a challenge for the busy family physician. Table 13 lists reliable references for an office library. Ongoing research information can be obtained from the NIH Office of Alternative Medicine at the internet website, http://altmed.od.nih.gov. Adding alternative medicines to maternity care requires that physicians adopt a *low-tech* approach in a *high-tech* world. Evidence is accumulating, however, on the safety, efficacy, and improved outcomes when low-tech and alternative therapies are applied to the care of the maternity patient.

References
1. Alternative Medicine: Expanding Medical Horizons: A report to the National Institutes of Health on Alternative Medical Systems and Practices in the United States. Washington, D.C., U.S. Government Printing Office, 1994.
2. Bartels CL, Miller SJ: Herbal and related remedies. Nutr Clin Pract 12:5–19, 1998.
3. Blumenthal M, Gruenwald J, Hall T, et al: German Commission E Monographs: Medicinal Plants for Human Use. Austin, TX, American Botanical Council, 1998.
4. Cardini F, Weixin H: Moxibustion for correction of breech presentation: A randomized controlled trial. JAMA 280:1580–1584, 1998.
5. Chevallier A: The Encyclopedia of Medicinal Plants. New York, DK Publishing, 1996.
6. Dunn DA, Rogers D, Halford K: Transcutaneous electrical nerve stimulation at acupuncture points in the induction of uterine contractions. Obstet Gynecol 73:286–290,1989.
7. Eisenberg DM, Davis RB, Ettner SL, et al: Trends in alternative medicine use in the United States, 1990–1997. Results of a follow-up national survey. JAMA 280:1569–1575, 1998.

8. Eisenberg DM, Kessler RC, Foster C, et al: Unconventional medicine in the United States. Prevalence, costs, and patterns of use. N Engl J Med 328:246–252, 1993.
9. Fischer-Rasmussen W, Kjaer SK, Dahl C, et al: Ginger treatment of hyperemesis gravidarum. Eur J Obstet Gynaecol Reprod Biol 38:19–24, 1990.
10. Fugh-Berman A: Alternative Medicine: What Works. Baltimore, MD, Williams & Wilkins, 1997.
11. Gordon JS: Alternative medicine and the family physician. Am Fam Physician 54:2205–2212, 1996.
12. Hofmeyr GJ, Piccioni V, Blauhof P: Postpartum homeopathic arnica montana: A potency-finding pilot study. Br J Clin Pract 44:619–621, 1990.
13. Jimenez SLM: Acupuncture: Pain relief at your fingertips. Int J Childbirth Ed 10:7–10, 1995.
14. Kleijnen J, Knipschild P, terRiet G: Clinical trials of homeopathy. BMJ 302:316–323, 1992.
15. Kristiansson K, Svardsudd K, von Schoultz B: Serum relaxin, symphyseal pain, and back pain during pregnancy. Am J Obstet Gynecol 175:1342–1347, 1996.
16. Kudista E, Kucera H, Muller-Tyl E: Initiation contractions of the gravid uterus through electroacupuncture. Am J Chin Med 3:343–346, 1975.
17. Macipocia G: The Foundations of Chinese Medicine. Edinburgh, Churchill Livingstone. 1998.
18. Murphy PA: Alternative therapies for nausea and vomiting of pregnancy. Obstet Gynecol 91:149–155, 1998.
19. Nikodem VC, Danziger D, Gebka N, et al: Do cabbage leaves prevent breast engorgement? A randomized controlled study. Birth 20:61–64, 1993.
20. O'Hara MA, Kiefer D, Farrell K, et al: A review of 12 commonly used medicinal herbs. Arch Fam Med 7:523–536, 1998.
21. PDR for Herbal Medicines. Montvale, NJ, Medical Economics Company, 1998.
22. Practice and Policy Guidelines Panel, NIH Office of Alternative Medicine: Clinical practice guidelines in complementary and alternative medicine. Arch Fam Med 6:149–154, 1997.
23. Shaughnessy AF: Weeds and seeds: The evidence behind natural products. FP Recert 19:53–56, 1997.
24. Shekelle PG, Brook RH: A community based study of the use of chiropractic services. Am J Public Health 81:439–442, 1991.
25. Shrivastav P, George K, Balasubramanium N, et al: Suppression of puerperal lactation using jasmine flowers (jasminum sambac). Aust N Z J Obstet Gynaecol 28:68–72, 1998.
26. Simkin P: Simkin's Ratings of Comfort Measures for Childbirth. Waco, TX, Childbirth Graphics, 1997.
27. Simkin P: Psychological and other non-pharmacologic techniques. In Principles and Practice of Obstetric Analgesia and Anesthesia, 2nd ed. Baltimore, Williams & Wilkins, 1995.
28. Simkin P: Reducing pain and enhancing progress in labor: A guide to non-pharmacologic methods for maternity caregivers. Birth 22:161–171, 1995.
29. Tiran D, Mack S: Complementary Therapies for Pregnancy and Childbirth. London, Bailliere Tindall, 1995.
30. Tsuei JJ, Lai Y-F, Sharma SD: The influence of acupuncture stimulation during pregnancy: The induction and inhibition of labor. Obstet Gynecol 50:479–488, 1997.
31. Udani J, Hardy M: Ginger for motion sickness, hyperemesis gravidarum, chemotherapy, and anesthesia. Altern Med Alert 1:133–137, 1998.
32. Ventoslovsky BM, Popov AV: Homeopathy as a practical alternative to traditional obstetric methods. Br Homeopath J 79:201–205, 1990.

SECTION I.
DIAGNOSTIC ULTRASOUND
IN PREGNANCY

Ellen L. Sakornbut, M.D.

I. Common Indications
- Dating of pregnancy, management of preterm labor, preterm rupture of membranes, postdates, assessment of growth, and timing and interpretation of the maternal serum α-fetoprotein level
- Vaginal bleeding, including first-trimester bleeding, placenta previa, vasa previa, and abruptio placentae
- Growth assessment for diagnosis of intrauterine growth restriction, macrosomia, and fetal abnormalities
- Fetal well-being assessment, including amniotic fluid assessment and biophysical profile
- Evaluation of preterm labor, preterm rupture of membranes, and incompetent cervix
- Diagnosis of malpresentation or malposition

- Evaluation of multiple gestation
- Maternal pelvic masses, uterine abnormalities, and pelvic pain, including possible ectopic pregnancy
- Guidance during amniocentesis (genetic and third-trimester uses), chorionic villus sampling, external version, intrapartum use in delivery of multiple gestation, fetal procedures

II. Clinical Standards for Obstetric Ultrasound Examinations
A. Content of the Standard Examination
The American Institute of Ultrasound in Medicine (AIUM), the American College of Radiology, and ACOG are in agreement regarding the content of the standard ultrasound examination. This agreement replaces concepts regarding level 1 and level 2 examinations, previously developed by the British MSAFP screening program.
  1. First-trimester scan
     a. Location of gestational sac, identification of embryo, and measurement of crown-rump length
     b. Documentation of fetal life
     c. Documentation of fetal number
     d. Evaluation of uterus, cervix, and adnexa
  2. Second- or third-trimester scan
     a. Fetal presentation, fetal number, and fetal life
     b. Placental location, appearance, and relationship to internal cervical os
     c. Biometric measurement: Biparietal diameter, head circumference, abdominal circumference, and femur length are measured for gestational age assessment. Abdominal diameters or circumferences are more reflective of the nutritional status of the fetus in the third trimester. Gestational age determination is less accurate in the third trimester (+3 weeks), but fetal weight determination may be of clinical value. Whenever possible, appropriateness of interval change from other measurements should be recorded. Biometric measurements should be recorded as actual measurements and not solely as the corresponding average gestational age on a chart.
     d. Evaluation of uterus and adnexa
     e. Fetal anatomic survey: The anatomic survey includes, but is not limited to, the lateral ventricles, a four-chamber view of the heart, spine, stomach, kidneys, urinary bladder, and umbilical cord insertion on the abdominal wall. Other areas of interest include the shape of the skull, right and left ventricular outflow tracts, determination of a three-vessel cord, and the posterior fossa. Routine ultrasound examination in the second and third trimester should include documentation of organ survey to the greatest extent possible. Clear visualization of anatomic structures varies with position of the fetus and gestational age.
B. Role of Limited Ultrasound
Ultrasound should not be performed as a limited study except in special clinical circumstances (e.g., determination of breech presentation in labor, inability to find fetal heart tones, assessment of fluid in a patient with variable decelerations during monitoring). Otherwise, all initial studies should contain full assessment and documentation as listed. It is clinically advisable to perform complete ultrasound examinations in any patient, whether or not she has had previous scans, unless there is a clinical reason to perform a limited study.
C. Targeted Scans
Ultrasound examinations that seek to address possible fetal abnormality or a specific question by more extensive examination of the fetus are designated as targeted, referral, or consultative scans, rather than level 2.

III. Clinical Applications
A. Routine Screening
1. Randomized controlled trials

Randomized controlled trials have shown that routine ultrasound results in an earlier diagnosis of twin gestation and a decrease in the incidence of induction for postdates pregnancy indications. The largest randomized controlled trial, the (Routine Antenatal Diagnostic Imaging with Ultrasound) RADIUS study, failed to show clinical benefit associated with *routine* ultrasound[6] and failed to detect a change in outcome associated with the diagnosis of congenital malformations, despite a greater than threefold increase in detection of malformations between the screened and control group.[3] European trials looking at the issue of routine ultrasound found that perinatal mortality rates were reduced because of more frequent pregnancy terminations when serious malformations were diagnosed before 24 weeks of gestation.[3,6]

Criticisms of the RADIUS trial include a relatively low rate of malformations detected before 24 weeks, but this rate appears to be consistent with another large trial with a similar number of patients.[6] The large group of women randomized in the RADIUS study excluded approximately 60% of pregnant women from randomization to routine ultrasound or the control group because of identified indications.

2. Use in clinical practice

Because of the differing prevalence of complications in different populations, some physicians may use ultrasound routinely in their practice. Others obtain scans only to address specific indications or risk factors (e.g., gestational dating in patients at increased risk for preterm delivery). Regardless of the strategy chosen, ultrasound should not be trivialized as a procedure, and its limits as a diagnostic tool must be understood. A normal ultrasound scan does not guarantee a normal fetal outcome or the absence of congenital defects.

Any time an ultrasound examination is done, it should be performed methodically and with adherence to recognized guidelines for biometric measurement and organ survey.[10] Ultrasound should not be used for routine establishment of fetal sex because this is not a biomedical concern in most patients.

B. Dating of Pregnancy
1. First trimester

First-trimester transabdominal scans can establish the gestational age of a pregnancy within 3 to 5 days using the crown-rump length. Transvaginal scanning uses a higher frequency transducer with improvement of resolution, enabling small structures to be seen earlier. A fetal pole can be measured by approximately 6 weeks' menstrual age (42 days) by transvaginal scanning, whereas it is not visualized until 7 to 8 weeks by transabdominal scanning.

Measurement of a gestational sac before appearance of an embryo produces less certain results with respect to dating of pregnancy. Crown-rump length measurements after 12 weeks are unreliable because of fetal spine flexion.

2. Second trimester

A second-trimester ultrasound scan (before 22 weeks of gestation) is probably the most useful for confirmation of dates for patients with average risk status. Multiple parameter dating, including biparietal diameter, head and abdominal circumference, and femur length, produces an accurate gestational age within ± 1.4 weeks. Fetal anatomy should also be evaluated with performance of an organ survey.

3. Third trimester

Ultrasound performed late in the second trimester and throughout the third trimester of pregnancy is increasingly less accurate in establishing gestational age, with a variance of 2.6 to 3 weeks in patients who have technically satisfactory scans. Generally, gestational age established by reliable ultrasound or ultrasound plus clinical data in early pregnancy (before 22 weeks of gestation) should not be altered by findings from a third-trimester ultrasound.

C. Growth Assessment

IUGR is divided into two types (see Chapter 6, section F): Symmetric IUGR comprises 30% and asymmetric IUGR comprises 70% of fetuses with inadequate growth.

1. Symmetric intrauterine growth restriction

Symmetric IUGR, such as occurs in fetuses with intrauterine infection or trisomy, can be established as a reliable diagnosis only with serial ultrasound examinations, unless menstrual dates are unequivocal, and a follow-up scan shows abnormal growth velocity.

2. Asymmetric intrauterine growth restriction

Asymmetric IUGR can be suspected on a single ultrasound scan that shows a proportionately small abdominal circumference relative to head and long bone measurements. This appearance occurs most commonly late in the second trimester or in the third trimester. A patient thought to be at risk for IUGR should have gestational age established firmly before 20 weeks of gestation. Screening for IUGR can be pursued with follow-up scans between 32 and 34 weeks of gestation, or sooner if there is poor fundal height progression or suggested compromise to uterine blood flow (e.g., preeclampsia).

3. Fetal macrosomia

A diagnosis of fetal macrosomia may be established if the gestational age has been established previously. Fetal weight estimates in the early third trimester can be plotted on a growth curve to obtain a percentile rank. If the estimated fetal weight is above the 90th percentile, the diagnosis of macrosomia is suspected. Fetal weight estimates close to term are no more accurate than ± 10% to 15%, limiting the use of this information in management decisions. Ultrasound assessment of macrosomia is most beneficial in conjunction with assessment of the diabetic patient. For further information regarding the use of ultrasound at term in patients with suspected macrosomia, see Chapter 16, section A.

D. Assessment of Bleeding

1. First-trimester bleeding

First-trimester bleeding is discussed more fully in Chapter 5. Ultrasound can be used to determine fetal viability and the presence or absence of an intrauterine pregnancy to rule out ectopic pregnancy.

2. Late pregnancy

Later in pregnancy, ultrasound is helpful to assess for placenta previa and abruption (discussed in more detail in Chapter 16, section A). Placenta previa, marginal previa, or low-lying placenta are frequent incidental findings during early dating scans (1:20). The accuracy of establishing the exact relationship of the placenta to the cervical os is better with transvaginal ultrasound than with transabdominal ultrasound. Two choices of management are acceptable, as follows.

    a. Repeat scanning: Because approximately 9 of 10 patients with suspected placenta previa (by ultrasound done at < 20 weeks of gestation) do not have a placenta previa in late pregnancy, a scan may be repeated after 30 weeks. Patients who have a placenta previa may present before this time, however, with vaginal bleeding

    b. Transvaginal confirmation: Patients with suspected placenta previa may be evaluated at the time of the initial diagnostic scan with transvaginal ultrasound to eliminate the possibility of placenta covering the internal cervical os. In one series of patients evaluated by transabdominal scanning and transvaginal scanning for low-lying or suspected placenta previa, a change in diagnosis was established by transvaginal scanning in approximately 25% of cases.[12] In another study of more than 3600 patients, the placenta extended to or over the internal cervical os in 1.5% of women evaluated by transabdominal and transvaginal ultrasound scans. Use of a cutoff of placental extension 15 mm or more over the internal os leads to 19% positive predictive value for placenta previa at delivery with 100% sensitivity.[13] This finding occurred in only 0.7% of women. Although the positive predictive value of this finding was low, follow-up ultrasound examinations were needed in only a small percentage of women scanned. Use of this strategy should reduce the need for follow-up scans by fivefold (1:20 scans, or 5% reduced to < 1%).

E. Assessment of Fetal Well-Being

For use of ultrasound in assessment of fetal well-being, see Chapter 10, section B.

F. Assessment for Possible Fetal Abnormality

Screening for fetal aneuploidy with the aim of decreasing need for genetic amniocentesis has been the target of many investigations. Minor malformations associated with trisomies include shortened femur length, renal pyelectasis, nuchal skin fold greater than 6 mm, echogenic intracardiac foci, and widened fetal iliac angle. Sonographic scoring systems in some studies have been successful in identifying 60% to 80% of fetuses with trisomy 21,[2,14] whereas using low MSAFP or advanced maternal age as the sole criterion for amniocentesis detects only about 40% of fetuses with trisomy 21.[1] Ultrasound studies for identification of trisomies have been conducted in tertiary facilities. A large, population-based study in Scotland was successful in detecting nearly 60% of trisomy 21 combining ultrasound and biochemical screening methods.[11] This study of more than 200,000 pregnancies found an overall detection rate of fetal abnormalities of 62%; when ultrasound was performed at 18 to 22 weeks of gestation, the detection rate increased to 92%.

Other studies have used fetal nuchal translucency measured at 10 to 14 weeks of gestation, with detection of 85% of trisomy 21 when combined with low free β-hCG and low pregnancy-associated plasma protein levels.[4] Such methods have not been compared with the current practices in the United States, such as offering MMT screening to all patients between 15 and 20 weeks and incorporation of standard risk assessment methods.[5]

IV. Terminology and Abbreviations

Table 14 lists terminology and abbreviations pertinent to ultrasound scanning.

TABLE 14. Terminology and Abbreviations Used in Diagnostic Ultrasound

AC—Abdominal circumference
AD—Abdominal diameter
AFI—amniotic fluid index, using the sum of measurements of the deepest pocket of amniotic fluid in each quadrant (see antenatal testing)
APD—anterior-posterior diameter
BPD—biparietal diameter
CI—cephalic index, used to assess whether the fetal skull shape is normal and to validate inclusion of the BPD in gestational age calculations
CRL—crown-rump length
EFW—estimated fetal weight, usually calculated using a formula or charts that use head, abdominal, and femur measurements
FL—femur length
FL/AC—femur length/abdominal circumference ratio, used in assessment of fetal growth

Table continued on next page.

TABLE 14. Terminology and Abbreviations Used in Diagnostic Ultrasound *(Continued)*

FL/BPD—femur length/biparietal diameter ratio, used to determine limb abnormalities, microcephaly, and other cranial abnormalities
GS—gestational sac
HC—head circumference
HC/AC—head/abdomen ratio, also used in growth assessment
MSD—mean sac diameter
Placental grade—using a system that includes the presence of echogenic densities, lobulation, and other characteristics. The placenta may be graded from 0 to 3. Although grade 3 placentas are characterized as mature, they do not correlate fully with fetal lung maturity. Many patients reach term without demonstration of a grade 3 placenta.
TAD—transverse abdominal diameter
TAS—transabdominal scanning
TLU—translabial ultrasound (see intrapartum use)
TPS—transperineal scanning (same as TLU)
TTD—transverse trunk diameter
TVS—transvaginal scanning
YS—yolk sac

References

1. Benacerraf B: The second trimester fetus with Down's syndrome: Detection using sonographic features. Ultrasound Obstet Gynecol 7:147–55, 1996.
2. Bromley G, Shipp T, Benacerraf B: Genetic sonogram scoring index: Accuracy and clinical utility. J Ultrasound Med 18:523–528, 1999.
3. Crane J, Lefevre M, Winborn R, et al: A randomized trial of prenatal ultrasonographic screening: Impact on the detection, management, and outcome of anomalous fetuses. The RADIUS Study Group. Am J Obstet Gynecol 171:392–399, 1994.
4. De Graaf I, Pajkrt E, Bilardo C, et al: Early pregnancy screening for fetal aneuploidy with serum markers and nuchal translucency. Prenat Diagn 19:458–462, 1999.
5. Jackson M, Rose N: Diagnosis and management of fetal nuchal translucency. Semin Roentgenol 33:333–338, 1998.
6. Lefevre M, Bain R, Ewigman B, et al: A randomized trial of prenatal ultrasonographic screening: Impact on maternal management and outcome. RADIUS (Routine Antenatal Diagnostic Imaging with Ultrasound) Study Group. Am J Obstet Gynecol 169:483–489, 1993.
7. Queisser-Lluft A, Stopfkuchen H, Stolz G, et al: Prenatal diagnosis of major malformations: Quality control of routine ultrasound examinations based on a five-year study of 20,238 newborn fetuses and infants. Prenat Diagn 18:567–576, 1998.
8. Saari-Kemppainen A, Karjalainen O, Ylostalo P, et al: Ultrasound screening and perinatal mortality: Controlled trial of systematic one-stage screening in pregnancy. Lancet 336:337–391, 1990.
9. Saari-Kemppainen A, Karjalainen O, Ylostalo P, et al: Fetal anomalies in a controlled one-stage ultrasound screening trial: A report from the Helsinki Ultrasound Group. J Perinat Med 22:279–289, 1994.
10. Seeds J: The routine or screening obstetrical ultrasound examination. Clin Obstet Gynecol 39:814–830, 1996.
11. Smith N, Hau C: A six year study of the antenatal detection of fetal abnormality in six Scottish health boards. Br J Obstet Gynaecol 106:206–212, 1999.
12. Smith R, Lauria M, Comstock C, et al: Transvaginal ultrasonography for all placentas that appear to be low-lying or over the internal cervical os. Ultasound Obstet Gynecol 9:22–24, 1997.
13. Taipale P, Hiilesmaa V, Ylostalo P: Transvaginal ultrasonography at 18–23 weeks in predicting placental previa at delivery. Ultrasound Obstet Gynecol 12:422–425, 1998.
14. Vergani P, Locatelli A, Piccoli M, et al: Best second trimester sonographic markers for the detection of trisomy 21. J Ultrasound Med 18:469–473, 1999.

CHAPTER 3

Patient and Family Education

SECTION A.
NUTRITION IN PREGNANCY AND LACTATION

Elizabeth G. Baxley, M.D.

During pregnancy, energy is necessary to support the physiologic, metabolic, and biochemical changes that occur in response to the growth and development of a healthy and appropriate-for-gestational-age weight fetus. The pregnant woman's diet is the main source of this necessary energy.[2] One of the earliest purposes of prenatal care was to counsel patients regarding nutrition.[4] Pregnant women benefit from instruction on basic dietary adequacy and the extra nutritional requirements of pregnancy. Sound nutritional and weight gain advice by prenatal care providers, along with maternal compliance with these recommendations, has a positive effect on birth outcomes.[14] Early in the course of prenatal care, an assessment of maternal nutritional risk should be made, and a goal for total weight gain should be set jointly with the patient. This plan should be monitored subsequently throughout the pregnancy.

I. Nutritional Status
A. Nutritional Evaluation
1. History and dietary recall

Assessment of nutritional adequacy may be achieved by use of a dietary recall, which provides information about balance of food groupings as well as improper habits, such as fasting and meal skipping. Questions should be asked in a nonthreatening manner and should cover several days of dietary recall. Weekly food charts have been recommended but may suffer from poor patient compliance.[2]

The dietary history may alert the provider to patients at potential risk secondary to their nutritional habits, such as food faddists, women who practice pica, or women with low intake of dairy products. Women of high parity and women with previous low-birth-weight infants or short interconceptual periods also are at risk. These women need special counseling and follow-up during their pregnancies. Beliefs and preferences regarding foods should be discussed, acknowledging the importance of ethnic, cultural, and family eating patterns. Financial stability and ability to purchase food should be determined, and women who lack financial resources to purchase sufficient amounts of nutritious foods should be referred to Women, Infants and Children (WIC), a federal supplemental food program for pregnant women and their children. The dietary history should include some estimate of energy expenditure.

2. Physical examination and laboratory evaluation

One way of categorizing patients as underweight, normal weight, overweight, or obese is through use of the body mass index:

$$\frac{\text{Weight (kg)}}{\text{Height (cm)}} \times 100$$

TABLE 1.   Recommended Weight Gain During Pregnancy

Maternal Classification	Weight gain (kg)		Weight gain (lb)	
	Total (kg)	*Rate (kg/4 wk)**	*Total (lb)*	*Rate (lb/4 wk)**
Prepregnant BMI[†]				
Underweight (< 19.8)	12.7–18.2	2.3	28–40	5.0
Normal weight (19.8–28.0)	11.4–15.9	1.8	25–35	4.0
Overweight (28.1–29.0)	6.8–11.4	1.2	16–25	2.6
Obese (> 29.0)	6.8	0.9	15	2.0
Twin gestation	15.9–20.4	2.7	35–45	6.0

* Rate applies to the second and third trimesters.
† Body mass index (BMI) is derived from metric units.
Adapted from National Academy of Sciences: Nutrition During Pregnancy. Washington, DC, National Academy Press, 1990.

Recommended weight gain can be estimated based on measurement of the body mass index (Table 1). In the absence of other hematologic abnormalities, the hemoglobin is a useful test of nutritional status.[2] Values of less than 11.0 g/dl in the first and third trimesters and less than 10.5 g/dl in the second trimester may indicate inadequate nutrition, and a ferritin level less than 20 mg/dl indicates deficient iron stores.

B. Caloric Needs and Weight Gain

1. Calories

The average pregnant woman should consume an average increase of 300 kcal/d depending on gestational age, with an additional 150 kcal/d needed during the first trimester and an additional 300 to 500 kcal/d during the second and third trimesters. An estimated total caloric intake for most pregnant women in the range of 1900 to 2750 kcal/d is recommended. Maternal weight gain is the best index for the adequacy of caloric intake.

2. Calorie sources

Carbohydrates are necessary for normal energy production and provision of glucose for the fetus. A diet deficient in carbohydrates leads to decreased fetal growth and may contribute to neurologic defects.[3] Carbohydrates should comprise 50% to 60% of the total caloric intake, which may be achieved with a minimum of four servings of breads and cereals and two servings of fruits and vegetables. The best sources of carbohydrates include whole-grain foods, fresh fruits and vegetables, and milk.

Proteins should comprise 20% of the total calories of the pregnant woman's diet, with an additional 30 g/d required over nonpregnant needs (75–80 g/d). Protein is needed for fetal growth and development, placental growth, increased maternal blood volume, growth of the uterus and breasts, and colostrum production.[3] The enhanced requirements of pregnancy can be achieved by 8 oz of a meat or meat substitute, plus three to four milk servings per day. Additional protein supplementation beyond this level has not been shown to improve pregnancy outcomes. Some evidence suggests that high-protein nutritional supplementation has been associated with impaired fetal growth and may increase the risk of neonatal death.[8]

Prepregnancy, high daily intake of total fat increases the risk of severe hyperemesis gravidarum.[15] During pregnancy, fats should contribute no more than 30% of total daily calories in the diet, although they are necessary for maternal energy production. They also provide fatty acids for myelination of nerve cells and absorption of fat-soluble vitamins as well as being stored for lactation.

TABLE 2. Components of Weight Gain in Normal Pregnancy

Organ, Tissue, or Fluid	Weight (g)
Maternal	
Uterus	970
Breasts	405
Blood	1250
Water	1680
Fat	3345
Subtotal	7650
Fetal	
Fetus	3400
Placenta	650
Amniotic fluid	800
Subtotal	4850
Total	12,500

Adapted from Hymen FE, Leitch L (eds): The Physiology of Human Pregnancy, 2nd ed. Oxford, Blackwell Scientific Publications, 1971.

3. Weight gain

Maternal weight gain during pregnancy is a major determinant of birth weight and is a primary indicator of infant mortality and morbidity.[1] Numerous studies have confirmed the observation that weight gain during pregnancy and prepregnancy weight are related directly to the weight of the infant. There is a linear relationship between maternal weight gain and infant birth weight at all levels of prepregnancy body mass, age, parity, and mother's level of education.[14] The components of weight gain during pregnancy are listed in Table 2.

The pattern of weight accumulation is an important factor in the overall picture of weight gain during pregnancy. The maternal component begins in the first trimester and is greatest during the first half of the pregnancy. Fetal growth is most rapid in the second half of pregnancy, with the fetus more than tripling its weight in the last trimester.[2] The remainder of weight gained represents interstitial fluid. In addition to the body mass index, recommendations for weight gain must consider other individual characteristics, such as maternal age (especially in adolescent pregnancies), parity, singleton versus multiple gestation, smoking, medical conditions, and special dietary needs.

    a. Normal prepregnancy weight: If a woman is at a desirable weight at the time of conception, a 25- to 35-lb weight gain for the pregnancy is recommended. Only 2 to 5 lb of this should be gained during the first trimester. For the second and third trimesters, an average gain of 0.5 to 1 lb per week is desirable.

    b. Underweight women: Women at less than 90% of desired body weight at the beginning of pregnancy are at risk of delivering a low-birth-weight infant. When possible, women should be encouraged to gain weight before pregnancy. During pregnancy, a 30- to 35-lb weight gain is recommended for underweight women, with special attention placed on initial and ongoing dietary counseling and education to minimize the complications associated with low-birth-weight infants.

    c. Overweight women: Women at greater than 120% of their desirable body weight at the time of conception have a greater risk of developing gestational diabetes, pregnancy-related hypertension, and thromboembolic complications. The impact of weight gain on the birth weight of the infant is diminished as compared with normal-weight or underweight women. Weight loss is not recommended, but lower rates of weight gains may be appropriate, with a weight gain of 18 to 20 lb recommended. Adherence to these parameters may reduce the rate of macrosomia and facilitate subsequent maternal weight loss after delivery.[14]

   d. Management of nonstandard weight gain patterns

      i. Excessive gain: Excessive weight gain is defined as greater than 6.5 lb/mo. In cases of excessive weight gain, the patient's diet should be reviewed for sources of excess calories. Medical complications should be excluded, including pregnancy-associated edema, diabetes, and preeclampsia. Weight loss should not be promoted, but slowing the rate of weight gain may be accomplished by reducing portion sizes and decreasing fat content. Excessive fat deposited during pregnancy contributes to chronic obesity, but fat stores can be reduced postpartum by breastfeeding.[3]

      ii. Inadequate gain: Careful evaluation is needed for the pregnant woman who has gained less than 2.2 lb/mo at the end of the first trimester or less than 10 lb at 20 weeks' gestation.[3] Inadequate gain is associated with low maternal prepregnancy weight, smoking during pregnancy, low family income, low educational level, unmarried status, and age younger than 20 or older than 35.[14] Vigorous nutritional intervention is indicated because low weight gain is associated with reduced expansion of plasma volume and development of intrauterine growth restriction (IUGR). Patients should be cautioned against dieting and meal skipping. Increasing the fat content in the diet and adding high-calorie dietary supplements three times per day should be recommended.

C. Vitamin and Mineral Needs

Blood levels for most vitamins and minerals are lower during pregnancy than at other times in a woman's life. All nutrients except for iron usually are supplied by a well-balanced diet, however. Routine multivitamin supplementation in women following a well-balanced diet may not be necessary but is common practice. Medical indications for supplementation include patient inability to eat the required diet or demonstration of high nutritional risk (Table 3).[2]

   1. Iron

   Requirements for iron are increased during pregnancy because of maternal blood volume expansion, fetal blood volume requirements, fetal iron storage, and blood loss during delivery. During the second trimester, red cell synthesis falls behind the expanding blood volume, resulting in the well-known physiologic anemia of pregnancy. Most often, these increased requirements can be met through dietary intake of iron-containing foods.

   Although routine iron supplementation may improve hematologic indices, a report published by the U.S. Preventive Services Task Force[16] failed to show that these changes translate into improved clinical outcomes. In healthy, well-nourished women, routine iron supplementation is of unproven benefit. High doses of iron are more likely to cause unpleasant gastrointestinal symptoms and have been associated with an increased risk of neonatal seizures in the first year of life. Selective supplementation for women with a hematocrit less than 30% before 33 weeks' gestation and less than 32% after 33 weeks' gestation is appropriate.[5] Routine low-dose iron supplementation may be warranted in populations in which iron deficiency is common.[11]

TABLE 3. Recommended Daily Allowances

Nutrient	Nonpregnant			Pregnant	Lactating (First 6 mo)
	15–18 y	*19–24 y*	*25–50 y*		
Protein (g)	44	48	50	60	65
Calcium (mg)	1200	1200	800	1200	1200
Phosphorus (mg)	1200	1200	800	1200	1200
Magnesium (mg)	300	280	280	300	355
Iron (mg)	15	15	15	30	15
Zinc (mg)	12	12	12	15	19
Vitamin A (µg RE)	8000	800	800	800	1300
Vitamin D (µg)	10	10	5	10	10
Vitamin E (mg α-TE)	8	8	8	10	12
Vitamin C (mg)	80	80	60	70	95
Thiamine (mg)	1.1	1.1	1.1	1.5	1.6
Riboflavin (mg)	1.3	1.3	1.3	1.6	1.8
Niacin (mg NE)	15	15	15	17	20
Vitamin B_4 (mg)	1.5	1.6	1.8	2.2	2.1
Folic acid (µg)	180	180	180	400	280
Vitamin B_{12} (µg)	2	2	2	2.2	2.6

From National Academy of Sciences: Recommended Dietary Allowances, 10th ed. Washington, DC, National Academy Press, 1989.

Iron-rich foods include liver, legumes, dried fruits, whole-grain enriched breads, and iron-fortified cereals. When supplements are needed, 30 to 60 g of elemental iron should be added to the diet. This level can be found in 150 mg of ferrous sulfate, 300 mg of ferrous gluconate, or 100 mg of ferrous fumarate.[4] Supplementation should continue 2 to 3 months postpartum to replenish maternal stores.

Gastrointestinal side effects of iron supplementation are common and include nausea and constipation. Nausea can be minimized by waiting until the second trimester to begin supplementation and by taking iron after a meal, although this results in decreased absorption. Aluminum-containing and magnesium-containing antacids can be used concomitantly without adversely affecting absorption. Increasing dietary fiber and fluid intake may reduce constipation associated with iron supplementation.

2. Folic acid

One of the most common vitamin deficiencies in pregnancy is folic acid. In addition to the prevention of megaloblastic anemia, most evidence shows a reduction in incidence of neural tube defects with increased folic acid consumption.[9] Women of reproductive age should be advised to take multivitamin supplements containing 0.4 mg of folic acid daily. Most multivitamin preparations formulated for pregnancy contain 0.5 to 1.0 mg of folic acid.

In women who have previously had or aborted an infant with a neural tube defect, high-dose supplementation (4 mg/d) preconceptually and during the first 4 to 6 weeks of pregnancy results in substantial reduction ($> \frac{2}{3}$) in the frequency of neural tube defects.[10] Neural tube closure is complete by 4 weeks after conception; supplementation beyond this time is of no added value.

Additional folate supplementation is necessary in women with multiple gestations, women who had used oral contraceptives before conception, and women who are taking anticonvulsant medication. Folate supplementation is important in women who had a short interconceptual period (< 2 years) and women whose diet was inadequate before pregnancy.[3] Good food sources of folic acid include dark green leafy vegetables, whole grains, and seeds.

3. Calcium

For the developing fetal skeleton, 1200 mg of calcium is needed daily, an increase of 400 mg over the allowance for the nonpregnant adult. Almost all of the skeletal accumulation occurs during the third trimester. Calcium supplementation below this rate may result in maternal demineralization because fetal needs are met by taking from the mother.[3] Three to four milk servings per day (equivalent to 1 quart of milk) are sufficient to achieve this additional need. In patients who are lactose intolerant, a supplement is needed.[3]

4. Vitamin C

The increased requirement for vitamin C during pregnancy is necessary for collagen synthesis. Food sources for vitamin C include citrus fruits and juices and fresh vegetables.

5. B vitamins

Additional B vitamins are needed for fetal amino acid and protein synthesis and can be derived from whole grains, nuts, seeds, beans, some meats, and fish.

6. Vitamin D

Vitamin D is obtained from the maternal diet as well as sun exposure on the skin. In some vegetarians or women who have little or no sun exposure, deficiency may occur. Vitamin D requirements are elevated moderately in pregnancy, and the frequency of neonatal hypocalcemia (hyperirritability) is lower in women who take vitamin D supplements.[11] Vitamin D supplementation at the end of pregnancy should be considered in vulnerable groups, such as women taking the anticonvulsant phenytoin, women with a short interconceptual period, and women with low levels of sunlight exposure.[11]

7. Vitamin toxicity

Vitamin excesses can result in fetal or neonatal abnormalities, and overuse of vitamin supplements should be observed for and cautioned against in pregnant patients. Vitamin A in doses greater than 25,000 IU/d may be teratogenic, resulting in urogenital anomalies, ear malformations, cleft palate, and neural tube defects.[2] Megadose vitamin C (> 5 g/d) has been known to cause infantile scurvy, a dependency withdrawal syndrome in neonates.[3] Vitamin D toxicity may result in infantile hypercalcemia syndrome, characterized by supraclavicular aortic stenosis, elfin facies, and mental retardation.[2]

D. Substances to Avoid

1. Alcohol

Alcohol use during pregnancy has been associated with the development of fetal alcohol syndrome, whether with chronic or binge use (see Chapter 4, section F). Safe levels of alcohol use during pregnancy have not been established, and it is best to recommend total avoidance. Alcohol depletes the body of zinc and magnesium, which are necessary for fetal development.

2. Caffeine

The association between maternal caffeine use and pregnancy complications has been controversial, with some studies suggesting that excess intake increases the risk of IUGR, low birth weight, and spontaneous abortion.[3] One prospective cohort study reported that caffeine consumption of less than 300 mg/d (about three cups of coffee) did not increase the risk of spontaneous abortion, IUGR, or microcephaly.[12] A case-control study of caffeine consumption and fetal loss showed a significant twofold increase in the risk of spontaneous abortion associated with caffeine consumption of 163 mg/d during the first trimester.[6] The safety of low levels of caffeine intake (< 5 cups of coffee per day) has been supported through measurement of maternal serum paraxanthine (a metabolite of caffeine) levels and correlation with rates of spontaneous abortion in women who were part of the National Collaborative Perinatal Project.[7] In this study, only very high serum paraxanthine concentrations (equivalent to > 6 cups per day) were associated with an increased abortion risk. Based on available evidence, it is safe to reassure women about low-to-moderate caffeine intake in the first trimester, as it relates to risk for spontaneous abortion.

II. Special Conditions Requiring Dietary Management
A. Diabetes
Pregnant women with diabetes, regardless of the classification, should follow an American Diabetes Association diet modified for the increased nutritional needs during pregnancy.[3] The goal for these patients is adequate weight gain with normalization of blood glucose levels and absence of ketonuria. Caloric and nutrient requirements are the same as in the nondiabetic pregnancy, evenly distributed throughout the day with three meals and two to three snacks. Increasing the soluble fiber content (with fruits, vegetables, nuts, seeds, beans, and oat bran) and regular exercise help to improve glycemic control.

B. Vegetarianism
Plant proteins lack one or more amino acids needed for protein metabolism, but through a combination of different plant foods, pregnant women can achieve complete protein needs.[3] Complementary proteins must be consumed at the same meal for the amino acids to be used effectively for protein synthesis.[3] Lactoovovegetarians, who eat vegetables, dairy products, and eggs, need additional iron, zinc, and vitamin B_{12}, but have no other nutritional problem during pregnancy.[13] Lactovegetarians, who eat only vegetables and dairy products, need additional iron, zinc, iodine, and vitamin B_{12}. Strict vegans who eat no animal food, dairy products, or eggs may be deficient in protein, calcium, vitamin B_{12}, riboflavin, iron, iodine, and zinc. These latter two groups require special supplementation during pregnancy and lactation. With knowledge of these deficiencies, dietary counseling, and special care, the pregnant vegetarian can meet the recommended daily allowances for pregnancy.

C. Adolescent Pregnancy
Pregnant adolescents have unique needs related to the nutritional needs of pregnancy being added to the demands of their own growth (see Chapter 4, section D).[3] Weight gain during pregnancy in teenagers has less effect on infant birth weight of all women studied, likely resulting from a combination of the greater demands for growth and the poor quality of their nutrition.[14] Adolescents often are concerned with their own body image, which may be in conflict with necessary weight gain to support the pregnancy. Providers should be alert to possible eating disorders when caring for pregnant teens. Dietary recommendations should include a daily caloric intake of 2700 kcal and 1600 mg/d of calcium.

D. Hyperemesis
Nausea and vomiting, particularly in early pregnancy, may necessitate specific dietary modifications. Eating dry carbohydrate, soft, low-fat foods and avoiding heavy seasonings and odors may lessen the nausea associated with pregnancy. Other helpful practices include increasing the frequency of meals, eating smaller portions, and avoiding drinking fluids with meals. If nausea and vomiting become severe (defined by dehydration, ketosis, hypochloremia, or hypocalcemia), intravenous fluids and occasionally parenteral nutrition are required to achieve adequate nutrition until symptoms abate. Medications that lessen the severity of pregnancy-related nausea and vomiting are discussed in Chapter 2, section G.

E. Lactose Intolerance

Lactose intolerance is a dose-dependent phenomenon, with 4 to 5 g of milk products or more causing symptoms of gastrointestinal pain and diarrhea.[3] To achieve adequate calcium supplementation in women with lactose intolerance, a reduction in portion size, substitution of cheese or yogurt, or the addition of lactase enzyme tablets may be recommended.

F. Pica and Citta

Pica is the compulsive eating of nonnutritive substances, such as clay, starch, ice, and dirt. These substances bind iron, preventing its absorption. It is unclear whether pica predisposes to iron deficiency or iron deficiency leads to pica because it has been shown that pica can be cured by iron supplementation.[14] An additional risk of intestinal obstruction occurs in patients with this type of eating disorder.

Citta refers to unusual food cravings, which may occur during pregnancy. This condition usually is not problematic, unless women frequently substitute nonnutritious food in responding to their cravings.

G. Multiple Gestation

Nutritional needs in women with multiple gestations are greater because of the demands created by the increased blood volume and larger placental and fetal mass. A dietary consultation is advised when multiple gestation is recognized.

III. Nutritional Requirements for Lactation

The physiology of pregnancy prepares a woman's body to lactate and breast-feed. Preparation for breastfeeding begins during prenatal care and includes evaluation for nutritional risk factors, education, and counseling.[2]

A. Caloric Needs

Production of breast milk requires an additional 640 kcal/d over nonpregnant needs so that optimal milk production requires a minimum of 1800 kcal/d.[2] Individual needs depend on the nutritional status of the mother and her weight gain during pregnancy. A weight gain of 22 to 28 lb lasts the woman 3 months while breastfeeding; for women nursing longer than 3 months, additional calories are needed. The energy source for these calories comes from maternal fat stores and diet. Neither increasing caloric intake above minimum requirements nor purposefully taking in excess fluid significantly increases milk production, and neither practice is recommended. A lactating mother of normal weight can expect to lose approximately 2 lb per month, whereas an obese mother may lose 4 lb per month. Rapid weight reduction is not recommended.

B. Components

Lactation requires a minimum of 20 g of protein over nonpregnant needs, which can be gained by additional milk or meat added to the diet. Calcium needs during lactation are 400 mg/d over the nonpregnant state, achieved through three to four milk servings per day or a calcium supplement.

C. Vitamins and Minerals

The increased daily food requirements necessary to support lactation usually are sufficient to meet minimum vitamin and mineral needs for maternal health and breast milk production. Neither vitamin nor mineral supplementation is required routinely.[2] An associated loss of maternal iron occurs with breastfeeding, but it amounts to approximately one half that of menses. The amenorrhea associated with lactation allows for replenishing of iron stores.

D. Substances to Avoid

Low levels of alcohol intake (1 or 2 drinks per day) may not affect breast milk production, but breast milk levels of alcohol are similar to maternal serum concentrations.

Caffeine also is expressed in breast milk. Two to three cups of coffee per day do not appear to affect infants, but more than three cups of coffee per day may result in an irritable, awake infant and decreased let-down reflex.[2]

References

1. Anderson GD, Bliner IN, McClemont S, et al: Determinants of size at birth in Canadian population. Am J Obstet Gynecol 150:236–244, 1984.
2. ACOG: Nutrition during pregnancy. Technical Bulletin No. 179:1–7, 1993.
3. Campbell MK, Waller L, Andolsek KM: Maternal nutrition. In Andolsek KM (ed): Obstetric Care: Standards of Prenatal, Intrapartum and Postpartum Management. Philadelphia, Lea & Febiger, 1990, pp 51–59.
4. Gabbe SG, Niebyl JR, Simpson JL (eds): Postpartum care. In: Obstetrics: Normal and Problem Pregnancies, 2nd ed. New York, Churchill Livingstone, 1991, pp 222–225.
5. Hemminki E, Merilainen J: Long-term follow-up of mothers and their infants in a randomized trial on iron prophylaxis during pregnancy. Am J Obstet Gynecol 173:205–209, 1995.
6. Infante-Rivard C, Fernandez A, Gauthier R, et al: Fetal loss associated with caffeine intake before and during pregnancy. JAMA 270:2940–2943, 1993.
7. Klebanoff MA, Levine RJ, DerSimonian R: Maternal serum paraxanthine, a caffeine metabolite, and the risk of spontaneous abortion. N Engl J Med 341:1639–1644, 1999.
8. Kramer MS: High protein supplementation in pregnancy. In Enkin MW, Keirse MJNC, Renfrew MJ, Neilson JP (eds): Pregnancy and Childbirth Module of The Cochrane Database of Systematic Reviews, 1995 [updated February 24, 1995]. London, BMJ Publishing Group, 1995.
9. Locksmith GJ, Duff P: Preventing neural tube defects: The importance of periconceptual folic acid supplements. Obstet Gynecol 91:1027–1034, 1998.
10. Lumley J: Periconceptual folate (4 mg/day) vs placebo in high-risk mothers. In Enkin MW, Keirse MJNC, Renfrew MJ, Neilson JP (eds) Pregnancy and Childbirth Module of The Cochrane Database of Systematic Reviews, 1995 [updated February 24, 1995]. London, BMJ Publishing Group, 1995.
11. Mahomed K: Routine iron supplementation in pregnancy. In Enkin MW, Keirse MJNC, Renfrew MJ, Neilson JP (eds): Pregnancy and Childbirth Module of The Cochrane Database of Systematic Reviews, 1995 [updated February 24, 1995]. London, BMJ Publishing Group, 1995.
12. Mills JL, Holmes LB, Aarons JH, et al: Moderate caffeine use and the risk of spontaneous abortion and intrauterine growth retardation. JAMA 269:593–597, 1993.
13. Scott JR, DiSaia PJ, Hammond CB, Spellacy WN (eds): Danforth's Obstetrics and Gynecology. Philadelphia, JB Lippincott, 1990.
14. Seidman DS, Ever-Hadani P, Gale R: The effect of maternal weight gain in pregnancy on birth weight. Obstet Gynecol 74:240–246, 1989.
15. Signorello LB, Harlow BL, Wang S, et al: Saturated fat intake and the risk of severe hyperemesis gravidarum. Epidemiology 9:636–640, 1998.
16. U.S. Preventive Services Task Force: Routine iron supplementation during pregnancy: Policy statement. JAMA 270:2846–2848, 1993.

SECTION B.
CHILDBIRTH EDUCATION

Patricia A. Payne, CNM, MPH

I. History of Prepared Childbirth

In 1952, Dick-Read launched the natural childbirth movement when he published the book *Childbirth without Fear*, ending an era in which physicians aimed at giving women complete amnesia once labor was established.[12] The emphasis in the scientific and lay literature in the early 1950s was on natural childbirth and psychoprophylaxis. Dick-Read argued that labor and delivery could be enjoyable and fulfilling by pointing out that fear and tension, not the contractions themselves, are a major cause of suffering during labor. Since the 1950s, many programs for childbirth preparation have been developed. Initially the primary goal of educating couples was to reduce the fear and anxiety associated with the birth process; however, there now is much greater emphasis on empowerment and developing confidence in the parenting role.

II. Components of Childbirth Education

Prepared childbirth classes are designed to provide information about pregnancy, labor and delivery, breathing and relaxation techniques, nonpharmacologic forms of support for women in labor, and care of the newborn. Traditional Lamaze classes teach mothers to focus their attention during labor on something other than the contractions, usually by use of a rhythmic breathing pattern and a focal point. This practice has the added benefit of helping to relax abdominal, back, leg, and perineal muscles, which lowers the sensation of pain and makes contractions more effective.[12] Mothers are taught to use several patterns of breathing during different stages of labor.[9] The Bradley method, which begins early in the third month of pregnancy, teaches a single type of slow, deep breathing to be used throughout labor. Psychoprophylactic breathing exercises are intended to give the laboring woman control over her pain by developing new conditioned reflexes to overcome the defensive reflexes that cause tension and pain.[12]

The current trend is toward a more eclectic style of classes that promote a variety of options for women to use as their coping tools for labor and birth. There is less emphasis on any one breathing technique with more information about the psychosocial and spiritual aspects of preparing women and their partners for birth.[6] Issues that may affect the childbirth experience, such as sexual abuse,[1] relationship issues, and psychosocial issues, can be addressed in a safe environment by informed, qualified individuals.[2] Many classes include the activity of developing a birth plan for women and their partners to share with providers during an office visit and nursing staff when they are in labor. Birth plans may be in the form of a checklist or may be directed at the individual woman's specific fears and concerns about giving birth, many of which may influence her ability to relax or feel safe. These birth plans often are used as a negotiating tool between patients and providers, with a focus on market demands rather than as an opportunity to explore underlying issues that may have a strong impact on the birth experience.

III. Benefits of Childbirth Education

Women cite several reasons for attending childbirth preparation classes, including improved safety for mother and infant, more humanistic experience, better preparation, reduced fear, and shared childbirth with their partner.[9]

A. Decreased Fear and Anxiety

Being informed about what to expect during the birth process decreases anxiety and dispels fear, resulting in increased relaxation. This information helps women to cope better with the pain of labor and increases maternal confidence significantly.[9] In studies of the relationship of maternal confidence to pain perception, more than one half of the variance in active labor pain may be explained by the mother's confidence in her ability to cope.[8]

B. Reduced Analgesia Requirements

Acquiring knowledge about what to expect in labor and delivery and how to put that knowledge to use is associated with women's desire for an active role during labor and delivery.[2] Prepared childbirth classes may work, in part, by empowering women and their support persons as well as relieving their anxiety, allowing them to cope with the pain of labor with more nonpharmacologic techniques. This approach can reduce the need for analgesia during labor, a finding that has been shown in numerous prospective studies.[4,12]

C. Shorter Stages of Labor

During labor, anxiety can lead to increased plasma cortisol levels, which, in turn, can increase the length of the first stage of labor. Anxiety also can lengthen the second stage of labor by increasing plasma epinephrine, decreasing uterine activity. Prenatal preparation can allay this anxiety, potentially leading to shorter first and second stages of labor, although data conflict in this regard. Continuity of care by supportive laypersons, providers, and nursing staff also has been associated with decreased length of labor, less use of drugs for pain relief in labor, and less need for resuscitation of newborns.[3,5]

IV. Problems with Outcome Studies

Studies of outcomes of prepared childbirth classes have been constrained by the question of whether the positive outcomes measured are related to childbirth education or to specific characteristics of the class attendees.[4] There is some evidence that certain types of individuals feel attracted by birth preparation courses, whereas other, less interested in education, may not attend childbirth classes.[11] Appropriate outcome measures may change over time and are unique to given populations. For example, the frequent use of epidural anesthesia in the United States may speak to a change in the outcomes that women perceive as beneficial. Also, failure to look at outcomes other than use of medication and satisfaction with the birth experience fails to recognize the potential benefit of empowerment for new parents.

A. Adaptive Behaviors

There is little evidence to evaluate a relationship between parenting adaptive behaviors and prenatal education.[3,10] A positive attitude toward the birth experience can be related to support and education.[3] Couples receiving prenatal education about the transition into parenthood have less anxiety and an easier adjustment to parenthood.[10] This situation may translate into an improved ability to deal with the many changes that take place when a new baby joins the family.

V. Obstetric Management

Although outcome studies that attempt to measure the effects of prepared childbirth are difficult to interpret, one thing seems clear: Maternal satisfaction with the birth process is enhanced by prenatal education about the birth process and training on pain-relieving and anxiety-relieving measures. According to Shearer,[11] however, "regardless of how comparable or randomly chosen the class and no-class groups are in a study, obstetric management will completely dominate any effects of teaching. Bedside manner can magnify or render meaningless—or even malignant—any prenatal training." Providers of perinatal care should be aware of the benefits of prepared childbirth as well as their own ability to enhance this training or to render the teachings ineffective by not supporting them during the intrapartum and postpartum periods.

References

1. Courtois CA, Riley CC: Pregnancy and childbirth as triggers for abuse memories: Implications for care. Birth 19:222–223, 1997.
2. Gabbe SG, Niebyl JR, Simpson JL (eds): Postpartum care. In: Obstetrics: Normal and Problem Pregnancies, 2nd ed. New York, Churchill Livingstone, 1991, pp 222–225.
3. Gjerdingen DK, Froberg DG, Fontaine P: The effects of social support on women's health during pregnancy labor and delivery and the postpartum period. Fam Med 23:370–375, 1991.
4. Hetherington SE: A controlled study of the effect of prepared childbirth classes on obstetric outcomes. Birth 17:86–90, 1990.
5. Hodnett ED: Continuity of caregivers for care during pregnancy and childbirth. In Enkin MW, Keirse MJNC, Renfrew MJ, Neilson JP (eds): Pregnancy and Childbirth Module. Cochrane Database of Systematic Reviews, Cochrane Updates on Disk. Oxford, Update Software, 1999.
6. Kane A: The Biopsychosociospiritual approach to birth care. IJCE 14:34–37, 1999.
7. Langer M, Czermak B, Ringler M: Couple relationship, birth preparation and pregnancy outcome: A prospective controlled study. J Perinat Med 18:201–208, 1990.
8. Lowe NK: Maternal confidence in coping with labor: A self-efficacy concept. J Obstet Gynecol Neonatal Nurs 20:457–463, 1991.
9. Mackey MC: Women's preparation for the childbirth experience. Matern Child Nurs J 19:143–173, 1990.
10. Midmer D, Wilson L, Cummings S: A randomized, controlled trial of the influence of prenatal parenting education on postpartum anxiety and marital adjustment. Fam Med 27:200–205, 1995.

11. Shearer MH: Effects of prenatal education depend on the attitudes and practices of obstetric caregivers. Birth 17:73–74, 1990.
12. Sturrock WA, Johnson JA: The relationship between childbirth education classes and obstetric outcome. Birth 17:82–90, 1990.

SECTION C.
PREPARATION FOR PARENTING AND FAMILY ISSUES

Elizabeth G. Baxley, M.D.

I. Prenatal Counseling

Prenatal counseling regarding parenting issues is a clinical practice that has been recommended widely for physicians who care for newborns.[5] Although most physicians do conduct prenatal counseling visits, they do so with few of their patients. In reality, these visits are scheduled infrequently.[1,6] There are numerous reasons to discuss pediatric issues before the birth of a newborn. Doing so fosters an ongoing relationship with the expectant family and helps to build the foundation for a strong physician, parent, and child interaction, which, in turn, helps facilitate adequate health care supervision for the family. In follow-up interviews, the educational resource rated highest by new parents was prenatal discussion with their physician.[4]

II. Prenatal Pediatric Visit

The term *prenatal pediatric visit* refers to a visit in which emphasis is placed on discussion of preparation for the birth and parenting of a newborn. In addition to reviewing pertinent aspects of the prenatal history, this visit allows the provider to identify psychosocial factors that may affect a family's adjustment to the newborn, answer parents' questions and relieve anxieties about the upcoming birth and hospital care, and discuss practical aspects of infant care. This visit also provides the physician with an opportunity to discuss issues of anticipatory guidance to promote child health and safety.[1]

A. Format

The ideal timing for the prenatal pediatric visit is in the latter part of the third trimester.[2] This visit should be scheduled with both parents present, and 30 to 45 minutes should be set aside for the session. A physician's private office may be a more desirable location to conduct this visit than an examination room. When time for scheduling and reimbursement systems are problematic, the provider may consider holding this type of visit with a group of parents in their third trimester, held in the evening so as not to interfere with busy office schedules and to allow more partners to attend. This approach has the advantage of group interaction among expectant couples, but it may hinder individuals or couples from sharing important psychosocial information. Another alternative to conserve time is to incorporate components of this visit into several routine prenatal visits.

B. Content

The provider should show concern for the entire family and a willingness to discuss psychosocial and parenting-readiness issues. Open-ended questions are best to encourage more open discussion by the parents. Questions should be encouraged and answered. An important goal of this visit is for the couple to leave feeling empowered in their new role as parents.

  1. Psychosocial history
  The psychosocial history should include information about previous family function and experiences, including, when applicable, information about the new parents' families of origin. Feelings about this pregnancy should be ascertained: Was the pregnancy planned or unplanned? What has been the reaction of both

partners to the pregnancy? Is the expected infant seen as a solution to marital turmoil? Has either parent experienced depression before or during the pregnancy? If this is not their first pregnancy, inquiring about prior parenting problems is appropriate, and a discussion of how these may be solved is appropriate.

Information about planned living arrangements should be ascertained, and expectant parents should identify support systems to call on after delivery. Discussion about the father's role is important, including identifying the occupational status of both parents and their individual plans for time out of work after the birth. Inquiring about psychosocial issues requires careful interviewing skills coupled with the ability to observe interactions between the parents or between parents and other children, if applicable.[1]

2. Hospital concerns

Newborn feeding plans should be inquired about and counseling regarding the benefits of breastfeeding is appropriate because most women make a decision about breastfeeding versus bottle-feeding in the third trimester. Questions about circumcision may be answered, and specific religious restrictions or preferences should be documented.[1] Rooming-in and sibling visitation protocols for the hospital of delivery may be discussed, and referral to hospital programs for siblings should be made when available.

3. Home concerns

Issues of home safety, sleeping arrangements, and further questions about feeding may be discussed during this visit as well as in the hospital after delivery. The couple should identify, in advance, additional help for their first days at home, to provide the mother with opportunities for rest.[3]

4. Family adaptation

With the birth of a baby, a new family is formed, often with changes in the way that family members have responded to each other previously. This new situation typically requires some adaptation for new parents as well as any siblings that might be involved in the transformation. The physician should discuss expectations that parents may have about potential impact that the newborn may have on family function (see Chapter 20). When applicable, the involvement of grandparent or other extended family members in newborn care should be discussed.

5. Schedule of infant well-child visits

At the conclusion of a prenatal pediatric visit, it is helpful to leave parents with a schedule for follow-up well-child visits and timing of immunizations. This visit can serve to review night-coverage arrangements and schedule of hospital visits as well as fee arrangements for inpatient and outpatient care.

III. Hospital Care and Counseling

The care of the mother and her newborn during their postpartum hospitalization allows new parents and their provider another chance to review pertinent aspects of newborn care and family adjustment as well as to answer any questions that may have arisen since the prenatal visit. It is also an opportunity to review events that occurred during or surrounding the birth, assess maternal satisfaction with the birth process, and address any new problems or concerns related to the hospital course.

References

1. Becker PG, Mendel SG: A family practice approach to the pediatric prenatal visit. Am Fam Physician 40:181–186, 1989.
2. Berger LR, Rose E: The prenatal pediatric visit revisited. Clin Pediatr 22:287–289, 1983.
3. Gruis M: Beyond maternity: Postpartum concerns of mothers. MCN Am J Matern Child Nurs 2:182–188, 1977.
4. Pridham KF, Schutz ME: Preparation of parents for birthing and infant care. J Fam Pract 13:181–188, 1981.

5. Sprunger LW, Preece EW: Characteristics of prenatal interviews provided by pediatricians. Clin Pediatr 20:778–782, 1981.
6. Sprunger LW, Preece EW: Use of pediatric prenatal visits by family physicians. J Fam Pract 13:1007–1012, 1981.

SECTION D.
BREASTFEEDING PROMOTION

Patricia A. Payne, CNM, MPH

Breastfeeding in the United States, as in many other industrialized countries, witnessed a renaissance in popularity between the early 1970s and the mid-1980s. This resurgence spawned breastfeeding support groups as well as a growing appreciation for more education and advocacy for breastfeeding by health care workers.[2,3,6,14] Although there has been an increasing trend in the incidence and duration of breastfeeding among middle-income, upper-income, and well-educated women, breastfeeding among minority and economically disadvantaged women continues to lag far behind.[2,10,17] Overall rates declined after the early 1990s.

The American Academy of Pediatrics stated that "exclusive breastfeeding is ideal nutrition and sufficient to support optimal growth and development for approximately the first 6 months after birth."[2] Many health professionals lack accurate information about breastfeeding trends and practices and knowledge about how best to promote breastfeeding. Often, there is a lack of commitment to promoting breastfeeding, or inappropriate advice is given to patients. In fact, women usually receive little, if any, breastfeeding information or encouragement from health care workers if they initially express a preference for bottle-feeding. Of bottle-feeders, 78% reported they had been given no encouragement to breast-feed; among breast-feeders, 42% said they had been encouraged to do so.[4]

Women's experiences and education from earliest childhood influence their attitudes and performance in relation to breastfeeding in later life.[7] A positive attitude toward breastfeeding is imperative to helping women be successful in their attempts to breast-feed.[12] Health care workers should be not only knowledgeable about the health, nutritional, and physiologic and psychological aspects of breastfeeding, but also they should be familiar with the mechanics of breastfeeding and how best to support the normal physiologic process for mothers in a hospital or birth center as well as at home (see Chapter 18, section C).

I. Benefits of Breastfeeding

The superiority of breastfeeding has been well established for nutritional, immunologic, psychological, and contraceptive issues.[2,16] Colostrum, the first milk produced after delivery, has a high content of proteins, fat-soluble vitamins, and anti-infective properties, sometimes leading to its being referred to as the infant's *first immunization*.[12] Immunologic benefits of breast milk protect infants against acute infections during the first year of life and offer protection against childhood lymphoma, childhood-onset insulin-dependent diabetes, Crohn's disease, and allergy-related symptoms such as eczema and asthma. Breast-feeding provides women with protection against future development of breast cancer, ovarian cancer, and osteoporosis.[2,5] Studies have shown that these benefits translate into lower medical costs.[8,22] In addition to medical benefits, breastfeeding offers the most convenient and economical method for feeding and, by enhancing the mother's attachment to her child, empowers mothers and plays a crucial role in the transition to motherhood and the formation of strong family bonds.[10]

II. Interventions to Promote Breast-Feeding

Despite the advantages of breastfeeding and the fact that almost all women are physically able to breast-feed, many choose not to breast-feed or discontinue breastfeeding early. Breast-feeding promotion programs often exist in environments in which bottle-feeding is treated as an appropriate feeding method and in which infant formula is given free to hospital nurseries, is readily available on grocery store shelves, and is advertised on television. A more subtle influence comes from free educational materials provided by formula manufacturers on breastfeeding. These materials often include a clear message related to bottle-feeding. Breast-feeding is a complex interaction between mother and infant that can be enhanced or inhibited by a wide range of social, psychological, and physiologic factors. An enlightened medical practice can increase the prevalence and length of successful lactation.[15,24] Medical personnel have the responsibility and the opportunity to increase the status of breastfeeding within the profession and within the community.[6]

A. Information and Support

Many women decide on a preferred method of feeding before pregnancy, and almost all have decided before the third trimester.[12] Children may develop an unconscious decision about breastfeeding as they develop their sexual identity around age 5. Numerous children's books are available about breastfeeding. These may be made available to children in waiting rooms, libraries, and at home, to model breastfeeding as the best form of infant nutrition. Researchers have addressed the impact of breastfeeding promotion education before pregnancy during family planning visits, using incentives such as gift bags, tickets to sporting events, and coupons and providing support with counseling sessions, home visits, and follow-up phone calls for postpartum mothers.[11,15,23] Implementation of the WHO Baby Friendly Initiative in an outpatient setting creates a breastfeeding–friendly environment for all family members (Table 4).

Two significant factors in a mother's decision to breast-feed are her intent in early pregnancy and the support from her partner and family, with little influence by health care providers.[20] Reasons why women choose to breast-feed include health benefits for the infant, closeness between mother and child, and the belief that it is the natural thing to do. For multiparous women, there is a strong correlation between how previous children were fed and how subsequent children are fed, making an argument for the importance of supporting a primiparous patient for successful breastfeeding because it influences feeding patterns for later children as well.[26]

TABLE 4. Ten Steps to Successful Breast-Feeding

1. Have a written breastfeeding policy that is communicated routinely to all health care staff
2. Train all health care staff in skills necessary to implement this policy
3. Inform all pregnant women about the benefits and management of breastfeeding
4. Help mothers initiate breastfeeding within 30 minutes of birth
5. Show mothers how to breast-feed and how to maintain lactation even if they should be separated from their infants
6. Give newborn infants no food or drink other than breast milk, unless medically indicated
7. Practice rooming-in to allow mothers and infants to remain together 24 hours a day
8. Encourage breastfeeding on demand
9. Give no artificial teats or pacifiers to breastfeeding infants
10. Foster the establishment of breastfeeding support groups and refer mothers to them on discharge from the hospital or clinic

From World Health Organization: Protecting, Promoting and Supporting Breast-feeding: The Special Role of Maternity Services. A Joint WHO/UNICEF statement. Geneva, WHO, 1989.

Reasons why women choose not to breast-feed may include a history of family violence in mothers or their children and a desire not to breast-feed in public.[1,19]

The key to counseling women on breastfeeding is to tailor a personal approach to specific needs identified from knowledge of the individual and her social environment.[12] A series of specific manageable steps may increase the incidence and duration of breastfeeding. First, a careful assessment should be made regarding attitudes, beliefs, knowledge, and experience a woman has about breastfeeding. Anxiety associated with unfounded fears of lactation failure and milk insufficiency are among the most common reasons cited for mothers' failing to initiate breastfeeding, interrupting it prematurely, or beginning supplementary feedings before they are nutritionally necessary.[12] A wide variety of studies point to reliable information and support by health care workers as significant predictors of breastfeeding success. Women who are given support after delivery and discharge from the hospital or birth center by someone knowledgeable in breastfeeding are more likely to be nursing exclusively at 2 months of age.[9,15,24]

B. Hospital Routines

In many cases, routine hospital procedures for healthy infants work in ways that interfere with normal physical and psychological processes of the immediate postpartum period. As such, they decrease the likelihood of successful initiation and maintenance of breastfeeding. Anything that restricts feeding contact during the first 14 days of life is associated with less successful breastfeeding. The International Lactation Consultant Association[9] has published *Evidence-Based Guidelines for Breastfeeding Management during the First Fourteen Days* that promote new thinking about the following common routines that have become a standard of practice.

1. Immediate skin-to-skin contact

An infant's rooting and sucking reflexes are particularly strong immediately after delivery. Encouraging skin-to-skin contact between mother and infant at this time and allowing the infant to suck at the breast help strengthen bonding and stimulate breast milk secretion. Oxytocin release occurs as a result of suckling and facilitates uterine contractions and the expulsion of the placenta during the third stage of labor. Early skin-to-skin contact is related to greater likelihood of prolonged breastfeeding.[25] Early contact may be a simple way of promoting breastfeeding for some mother-infant pairs in the highly technologic delivery units of hospitals today.

2. Rooming-in

Keeping the infant within easy reach of the mother 24 hours a day has been shown to increase the likelihood of successful breastfeeding.[18] When mothers have unlimited access to their newborns, breastfeeding on demand is facilitated more easily, and the risk of neonatal infection is lower than in a closed nursery environment. Rooming-in allows for closer contact with the father and other family members, while increasing staff availability because mothers care for their own infants. Mothers who have rooming-in have been shown to have more self-confidence in the management of their infants and have sought advice less often in the first postpartum month.[19] Many women consider rooming-in if it is discussed as part of a prenatal discussion and not a decision made at the time of birth, when they are tired and may not appreciate the benefit of contact with their infant.

3. Demand feeding

Demand feeding means allowing the infant to nurse whenever he or she desires, without any fixed time schedule. This type of feeding favors better, faster establishment of lactation because sucking is a potent stimulus for secretion of oxytocin and prolactin, which stimulate milk let-down and initiate milk secretion.

Breast-feeding is found more likely to be successful among infants on demand feedings.[25] Crying is a late cue for hunger[2,9]; mothers who room-in and demand feed their infants are able to identify early signs of hunger that can be missed if infants are on scheduled feedings. This approach also works to accelerate postpartum involution of the uterus.[2]

4. Supplements

Exclusive breastfeeding should be the norm. Under normal circumstances, the neonate requires no water or other supplement during the first 2 to 4 days after birth while lactation is being established. Routine administration of formula before nursing or complementary supplements reduce the infant's sucking on the breast and the secretion of milk. Additionally, supplementing carries an implicit message to the new mother that she cannot meet the infant's needs by herself. Infants should be given nothing orally but breast milk during their hospital stay. Bottle-feeding serves as a potent force against the successful initiation and maintenance of lactation by reducing the frequency and strength of sucking by the infant.[12] Alternating between an artificial nipple and natural breast confuses the infant's oral response and may make the infant's sucking motions inappropriate for breastfeeding. Less work is required to suck at a rubber nipple, causing the infant's cheek muscles to weaken, and the desire for the breast becomes extinct.

5. Pacifiers

Studies have shown that infants using pacifiers are more likely to be weaned early.[9] This situation may reflect a combination of problems caused by the nipple itself and by the motivation of the mother or the nursing staff to use a pacifier to comfort an infant.

6. Medications and surgical interventions

Anesthesia, strong sedation, prolonged labor, surgical interventions, and other sources of stress, discomfort, and fatigue for mothers and infants may impede the initiation of lactation. Central nervous system depressants given during labor reduce nutritive sucking by the infant and, in the case of barbiturates, may take 5 to 6 days for the effects to disappear.[26] Ergonovine maleate interferes with prolactin secretion and may decrease milk production. Mothers giving birth by cesarean section have later first breastfeeding, but if the cultural and hospital environments generally promote breastfeeding, cesarean birth has little impact on breastfeeding outcome.[13] Milk production is not affected by postpartum sterilization if done within the first 24 hours after delivery but is reduced if done on days 4 to 6 after delivery during the crucial period for establishment of milk production and lactation.

C. Discharge Planning

With early hospital discharge (12 to 24 hours), lactation usually is not well established and may not have started. In many cases, however, breastfeeding is more successful when women are discharged early from the hospital.[21] This finding may be a reflection of more home visiting associated with mothers discharged early, a difference in the mothers' support at home, and less time to expose mothers and infants to hospital routines that inhibit a positive lactation experience. It is important that mothers leave the hospital clear and confident about what they should do to breastfeed successfully and who will provide support for them. Lactation consultants and breastfeeding support groups, such as the local LaLeche League, should be members of the health care team who provide information and support for the nursing mother once she and her infant go home. Employment often is a barrier to continued breastfeeding; efforts should be made to assist women in planning to return to work.[15] Combining information and support with sensible hospital routines and postpartum follow-up should act as a powerful promoter of breastfeeding success.

References

1. Acheson L: Family violence and breast-feeding. Arch Fam Med 4:650–652, 1995.
2. American Academy of Pediatrics: Breastfeeding and the use of human milk. Policy statement. Pediatrics 100:1035–1039, 1997.
3. Barnett E, Sienkiewicz M, Roholt S: Beliefs about breastfeeding: A statewide survey of health professionals. Birth 22:15–20, 1995.
4. Bryant C, Lazarov M, Light R, et al: Best start: Breastfeeding for healthy mothers, babies—a new model for breast-feeding promotion. J Tenn Med Assoc 82:642–643, 1989.
5. Dermer AL: Breastfeeding and women's health. J Womens Health 2, 1998.
6. Freed G, Clark SJ, Curtis P, Sorenson JR: Breast-feeding education and practice in family medicine. J Fam Pract 40:263–269, 1995.
7. Friel JK, Hudson NI, Banour S, Ross A: The effect of a promotion campaign on attitudes of adolescent females towards breast-feeding. Can J Public Health 80:195–199, 1989.
8. Hoey C, Ware JL: Economic advantages of breastfeeding in an HMO setting: A pilot study. Am J Manag Care 3:861–865, 1997.
9. International Lactation Consultant Association: Evidence-Based Guidelines for Breastfeeding Management during the First Fourteen Days. 1999.
10. Iowa Department of Public Health: Promoting breast-feeding. Iowa Med 81:352, 1991.
11. Jennings VH: Breastfeeding promotion in family planning programs. Int J Gynecol Obstet 3l(suppl L):131–133, 1990.
12. Joint WHO/UNICEF: Appendix 3: Protecting, promoting and supporting breast-feeding: The special role of maternity services. Int J Gynecol Obstet 31(suppl 1):171–183, 1990.
13. Kearney MH, Cronenwett LR, Reinhardt R: Cesarean delivery and breast-feeding outcomes. Birth 17:97–105, 1990.
14. Kramer MS: Poverty, WIC, and promotion of breast-feeding. Pediatrics 87:399–400, 1991.
15. Krishna VR, Plichta SB: The role of social support in breastfeeding promotion: A literature review. J Hum Lact 14:41–45, 1998.
16. Lawrence RA: A Review of the Medical Benefits and Contraindications to Breastfeeding in the United States. Washington, DC, U.S. Department of Health and Human Services Public Health Services Health Resources and Services Administration Maternal and Child Health Bureau, Maternal and Child Health Technical Information Bulletin, 1997.
17. Lazarov M, Fleshood L, Light R, et al: Innovative approaches to the promotion of breast-feeding. J Tenn Med Assoc 82:486–487, 1989.
18. Lindenberg CS, Artola RC, Jimenez V: The effect of early post-partum mother-infant contact and breast-feeding promotion on the incidence and continuation of breast-feeding. Int J Nurs Stud 27:179–186, 1990.
19. Marchand L, Morrow MH: Infant feeding practices: Understanding the decision-making process. Fam Med 26:319–324, 1994.
20. Piper S, Parks PL: Predicting the duration of lactation: Evidence from a national survey. Birth 23:7–12, 1996.
21. Renfrew MJ, Lang S: Early versus late discharge from hospital after childbirth. In: The Cochrane Library, Issue 1. Oxford, Update Software, 2000.
22. Riordan JM: The cost of not breastfeeding: A commentary. J Hum Lact 13:93–97, 1997.
23. Sciacca JP, Phipps BL, Dube DA, Ratliff MI: Influences on breast-feeding by lower-income women: Incentive-based, partner-supported educational program. J Am Diet Assoc 95:323–328, 1995.
24. Silorski J, Renfrew MJ: Support for breastfeeding mothers. In Enkin MW, Keirse MJNC, Renfrew MJ, Neilson JP (eds): Pregnancy and Childbirth Module. Cochrane Database of Systematic Reviews, Review No. 04173 Cochrane Updates on Disk. Oxford, Update Software, 2000.
25. WHO: Evidence for the Ten Steps to Successful Breastfeeding. Geneva, WHO, 1998.
26. Winikoff B, Baer EC: The obstetrician's opportunity: Translating "breast is best" from theory to practice. Am J Obstet Gynecol 138:105–115, 1980.

SECTION E.
PHYSIOLOGIC CHANGES AND COMMON DISCOMFORTS OF PREGNANCY

Elizabeth G. Baxley, M.D.

Most pregnant women experience a variety of symptoms related to the normal physiologic changes of the pregnancy. Most symptoms are merely inconvenient, others may cause moderate discomfort, and some may represent real or potential danger. It is important for physicians who provide prenatal care to be familiar with the common discomforts of pregnancy to differentiate warning signs (see section F) from benign conditions and to provide advice regarding comfort measures.

I. Gastrointestinal Complaints
A. Nausea and Vomiting and Morning Sickness
Nausea and vomiting are common, occurring in 70% of pregnancies.[3] Typically, these symptoms begin early (6 to 8 weeks) and continue until 13 to 16 weeks' gestation, although occasionally, nausea with or without vomiting may continue throughout the entire pregnancy. This condition is known to occur more commonly in primigravidas, younger women, women with less than 12 years' education, nonsmokers, and women weighing greater than 77 kg (170 lb).[11] Although data to support a clear cause are lacking, hyperemesis frequently is more severe in women with higher human chorionic gonadotropin levels, such as those with multiple gestation and hydatidiform mole.[15] Emotional factors appear to play an important role but are thought to be contributory rather than causative. Concomitant thyroid disease should be ruled out when nausea and vomiting are persistent or severe because this may be an early manifestation of hyperthyroidism.

Although distressing, nausea and vomiting of pregnancy rarely is prolonged or severe enough that nutrition suffers. It is a significant problem, however, in that 50% of employed women believe that their work efficiency is reduced because of these symptoms, and 24% report requiring time off from work because nausea and vomiting were disabling.[21]

Symptoms often are alleviated by dietary measures, such as keeping food in the stomach with frequent, small meals. Other nonpharmacologic measures include avoidance of greasy and spicy foods, eating a protein snack at bedtime, and keeping dry crackers at the bedside to eat before rising in the morning. Patients who are nauseated should avoid sudden movements. Beneficial effects have also been found with the use of ginger (250 mg capsule four times per day) and vitamin B_6 (25 mg three times per day), both of which have been shown to reduce the amount and severity of nausea and vomiting in women with severe symptoms. Women with only mild symptoms experience less of a beneficial response. Acupressure at the P-6 (pericardium 6, or *Neiguan*) point on the volar surface of the forearm just above the wrist has been shown to be the most helpful complementary method of dealing with these symptoms.[1,2,6,7,14,22] Hypnosis has been studied with insufficient evidence found for its benefits (see Chapter 2, section H).[1,4,12,20]

Antiemetics occasionally are needed when vomiting does not respond to conservative measures or when dehydration, ketosis, or electrolyte abnormalities are present. Women suffering from morning sickness that is not controlled by nonpharmacologic methods can use antihistamines safely because H_1-blockers in the first trimester do not increase the teratogenic potential.[16] Meclizine (Antivert, category B) is an H_1-blocker that is effective in relieving symptoms of nausea in doses of 12.5 to 25 mg every 8 hours as needed. Often, symptoms that are clustered in the morning respond to a single nightly dose of meclizine. Diphenhydramine (Benadryl, category B) and metoclopramide (Reglan, category B) have been found to be safe and effective antiemetics for use during pregnancy. Prospective studies have produced conflicting results regarding the use of phenothiazines (promethazine [Phenergan], prochlorperazine [Compazine], both category C) during early pregnancy. Use of this class of drugs is best reserved when nausea and vomiting threaten maternal nutrition.[6-8] Ondansetron (Zofran, a serotonin receptor antagonist, category B) has been studied and used in the treatment of hyperemesis gravidarum.[17,19,23] This drug appears to be safe and effective for use in pregnancy but should be reserved for situations in which nutritional or hydration status of the mother is compromised. In these cases, a dose of 10 mg intravenously every 8 hours as needed has been used, although it has not been found to be superior to promethazine in controlling symptoms and costs considerably more.[17]

Management of this common condition should include reassurance that symptoms usually are self-limited and that they may represent higher circulating levels of maternal estrogen, which have been associated with improved pregnancy outcome.[3,10,18] Women who experience nausea and vomiting are more likely to have recurrences in subsequent pregnancies than those who did not have symptoms in the first pregnancy.[10]

B. Heartburn

Reflux of gastric acid is common during pregnancy, causing the gravid woman to feel epigastric burning followed by a sense of fullness. The cause for this increased frequency in pregnancy is twofold. The predominant contributor to early pregnancy heartburn is reduced smooth muscle motility–related relaxation of the lower esophageal sphincter, which is mediated by high levels of circulating progesterone in the first trimester. Later in pregnancy, typically during the third trimester, the expanding uterus displaces the stomach upward, compounding the reflux.[15]

Overeating and eating spicy foods exacerbate heartburn. Pregnant women should be advised to eat frequent small meals and to avoid lying recumbent soon after eating. Fried and gas-producing foods, such as cabbage, brussel sprouts, and onions, should be avoided. Sleeping on stacked pillows or raising the head of the bed on blocks may help prevent reflux. When reflux does occur, antacids have been shown to relieve heartburn symptoms.[8] Antacids containing magnesium hydroxide or magnesium trisalicylate are safe and effective for use, but pregnant women should be advised to avoid use of baking soda or antacids with a high sodium content, which can cause water retention and alkalosis. Aluminum-containing antacids may worsen constipation.[3]

C. Constipation

Another common problem during early and late pregnancy is constipation. Similar to heartburn, this physiologic discomfort is due to steroid-induced decreased bowel transit time (first trimester) and is aggravated by displacement and compression of the intestine by the enlarging uterus (third trimester). Iron supplementation may exacerbate constipation.

Liberal consumption of fluids (at least 2 quarts/d) and the addition of bulk fiber (with fresh fruit, vegetables, or whole grains) help prevent this problem.[9] Regular exercise provides additional benefit in the prevention and treatment of constipation. Mild laxatives, such as milk of magnesia and stool softeners, or bulk producers (methylcellulose, psyllium hydrophilic mucilloid) are safe and effective for use. Cathartic laxatives and enemas are needed rarely and should not be used without physician consultation, because they may stimulate premature uterine contractions.

D. Hemorrhoids

Hemorrhoids are varicose veins of the rectum and are exacerbated by the increases in venous pressure that accompany advancing pregnancy. They are usually only mildly irritating but are made worse by untreated constipation. Pregnant women should be advised to alert their physician if hemorrhoids become hard and tender (indicating potential thrombosis) or cause bleeding. Prevention is aimed at avoidance of constipation and prolonged sitting.

Kegel exercises improve muscle tone in the rectal area and should be recommended routinely, including after bowel movements. Although hemorrhoids often regress after delivery, they often do not disappear completely, and sometimes they become worse immediately after delivery when there has been a long second stage of labor and excessive pushing. Commonly used therapies, such as Proctofoam, Anusol, and Preparation H, are safe and effective for use during pregnancy. Thrombosed external hemorrhoids may be able to be treated conservatively but often require incision and evacuation under local anesthesia.[3]

II. Urinary Complaints
A. Frequency
Urinary frequency and stress incontinence occur most commonly during the first and third trimesters of pregnancy. In early gestation, the uterus places increased pressure on the bladder, limiting its ability to fill and resulting in urinary urgency. As the uterus rises out of the pelvis in the second trimester, symptoms may improve transiently, only to worsen again late in pregnancy when engagement of the presenting part exerts pressure on the urinary bladder. Glomerular filtration rate is increased throughout pregnancy, contributing to urinary frequency. A pregnant woman who experiences burning or pain with urination should be evaluated to rule out urinary tract or vaginal infection, either of which may increase the risk for premature labor, fetal loss, or acute and chronic pyelonephritis. Decreasing fluid intake close to bedtime may help symptoms of frequency and urgency, although women should be cautioned not to restrict overall fluid intake.
B. Incontinence
Urinary incontinence during pregnancy usually is of the stress type, occurring when coughing, sneezing, or laughing increases pressure on the bladder. It is a common problem of late pregnancy and at times may be confused with premature rupture of membranes. Multigravidas, secondary to poor muscle tone in the perineal muscles supporting the bladder, experience this symptom more often. Symptoms may be reduced or alleviated by doing Kegel exercises, although they may not resolve completely until after delivery.

III. Abdominal Pain
The most common abdominal pain experienced during pregnancy is the sharp pain caused by spasm of the round ligaments. As the uterus enlarges, more stretch is placed on these ligaments, which then become susceptible to strain. Often, this pain is associated with abrupt movements and is seen more often on the right side because of the normal dextrorotation of the uterus.[5] Improved physical fitness and abdominal wall muscle tone through regular exercise provides added support for the uterus and helps reduce round ligament strain. Patients should be advised to rise and sit gradually, avoiding sudden movements. Rest, accompanied by local heat application (e.g., heating pad, warm bath), is the best treatment for this condition. Analgesia is necessary occasionally and can be achieved safely and effectively with acetaminophen.

Abdominal pain in a pregnant woman in her second or third trimester should be evaluated to rule out premature contractions or other serious medical or obstetric complications (see Chapter 6, section D, and Chapter 15, section D). Providers should be alert to the possibility of abdominal problems that are unrelated to the pregnancy, such as gastroenteritis, appendicitis, and renal or biliary colic.

IV. Backache
As the uterus enlarges during pregnancy, a woman's center of gravity is altered, and abdominal muscles are stretched. To maintain balance, her shoulders are shifted backward, and her head is angled forward, causing a compensatory lumbar lordosis that predisposes to low back pain.[3] During the latter half of pregnancy, ligaments and joints of the back and pelvis are more lax, further promoting back injury or pain. Women with

poor abdominal muscle tone or poor posture are more prone to back problems during pregnancy.

Prevention is aimed at avoidance of excessive weight gain, improving posture, proper bending with a straight back, and wearing flat or low-heeled shoes. A firm bed mattress may help, and local heat, with or without massage, may relax back muscles. If unilateral leg pain or weakness in one or both legs accompanies the back pain, patients should be evaluated for lumbar disk disease.

V. Respiratory Complaints

A. Shortness of Breath

In early pregnancy, increased circulating progesterone contributes to an increase in minute ventilation, often referred to as *pregnancy-induced hyperventilation*. Late in pregnancy, the growing uterus creates a mechanical limitation in the excursion of the diaphragm, bringing about a reduction in residual volume and functional residual capacity. These changes often cause a pregnant woman to experience dyspnea. Measures that may help improve or alleviate this dyspnea include having the woman stand, sit erect, or when lying, prop her shoulders and head up on one or more pillows. The woman should be advised to breathe slowly and deeply and to pace herself to accommodate the added demand pregnancy places on pulmonary function.

B. Nasal Congestion

Increased perivascular edema and enlargement of the nasal turbinates occurs in early pregnancy, mediated by estrogen and progesterone. This occurrence often results in bothersome nasal stuffiness, which may exacerbate preexisting allergy or sinus problems. Nosebleeds also are common and can be reduced or prevented by application of petroleum jelly to the nasal mucosa with a cotton-tipped applicator. Use of a room humidifier may alleviate some of the nasal congestion associated with pregnancy. Saline nose drops are safe and effective to use, as are topical nasal decongestants when indicated, as long as their use is limited to 2 to 3 days at a time to avoid rebound rhinitis medicamentosus. Nasal steroids are best used continuously and have a 3- to 7-day delay in their onset of action but may be the most appropriate agents for patients with more chronic symptoms.

VI. Headaches

Headaches are common during pregnancy. Some headaches are related to sinus congestion from the increased blood flow and nasal edema. Other common explanations cited for headache during pregnancy include fatigue, tension, eyestrain, and migraines, although in most cases no demonstrable cause is found.[3]

Relaxation and use of warm compresses may help with symptom relief, and acetaminophen may be necessary for analgesia. Health care providers should be alert to headaches that are accompanied by dizziness, blurred vision, or scotomata and evaluate the patient for preeclampsia if these symptoms are reported.

VII. Circulatory Problems

A. Dizziness and Syncope

Venous pooling results from compression of lower extremity and pelvic veins that occurs with advancing uterine size. This pooling may cause pregnant women to experience dizziness or syncope. This problem is potentiated in warmer weather when peripheral vessels are dilated to dissipate body heat.[3] In late pregnancy, women may experience similar symptoms on lying recumbent, secondary to pressure of the gravid uterus on the vena cava and resulting supine hypotension. Calf exercises and use of full-length support stockings may help the former, whereas positioning in the left lateral tilt position improves the latter.

B. Edema

Slowed venous return from uterine pressure on the vena cava contributes to lower extremity edema commonly seen in the third trimester. Women should avoid sitting or standing for long periods and should perform daily leg exercises to prevent swelling. Support stockings are helpful in this situation, but tight waistbands or elastic leg bands may make the situation worse. Uncomplicated pregnancy-associated lower extremity edema usually responds to rest and leg elevation. Patients and providers should be alert for edema that progresses rapidly or does not lessen overnight, particularly in the third trimester, when it may herald early preeclampsia.

C. Varicose Veins

Increased venous pressure in the pelvis and lower extremities accompanies advancing pregnancy and may result in superficial varicosities of the legs and vulva. This impairment of circulation also leads to leg fatigue and painful nighttime leg cramps. As with dependent edema, rest, elevation, and elastic stockings with good support may help relieve symptoms. Vulvar varicosities respond to added support, which may be achieved by wearing several perineal pads.[13] Varicose veins that become warm, hard, and painful suggest phlebitis and should be evaluated (see Chapter 7, section D).

VIII. Dental Problems

Gum hypertrophy and bleeding are common during pregnancy, when estrogen can cause the gums to become hyperemic and softened.[3] Tooth decay often progresses more rapidly. Use of a soft toothbrush, mild toothpaste, and daily flossing is recommended. Dental work can be done during pregnancy with local anesthesia, but general anesthesia should be avoided.

IX. Skin and Hair Changes

Several characteristic skin changes occur during pregnancy, primarily owing to stimulation of the melanocytes by estrogen and progesterone. The areolae of the breasts become darker, and a line of increased pigmentation develops from the xiphoid to the symphysis, termed the *linea nigra*. Moles that were present before pregnancy may darken. A reddish brown color over the bridge of the nose and under the eyes is called the *mask of pregnancy*. All of these changes are benign and reversible and can be minimized initially by avoidance of direct sun and use of appropriate sunscreen.

Striae (stretch marks) develop over the abdomen, breasts, and hips in 65% of pregnant women.[3] Although striae typically remain after delivery, they usually fade in color to a pink or silver color. There is no proven method for preventing stretch marks, which are genetically predisposed, although cocoa butter, vitamin E, and lotions may help with the itching that often accompanies striae formation.

X. Breast Changes

Early in pregnancy, women normally experience breast tenderness. This pain may be mild to severe and usually is transient, abating by the end of the first trimester. Breasts also increase in size and become more nodular during early pregnancy, and nipples become darker and more erectile. During the third trimester, colostrum may be produced. A good support bra should be worn throughout pregnancy and typically needs to be one size larger than that worn before pregnancy. When symptoms are severe, acetaminophen and cold compresses may help alleviate pain.

XI. Leukorrhea

Vaginal discharge typically is increased in amount because of higher estrogen levels and greater vaginal blood flow. Whitish in color and variable in consistency, this leukorrhea of pregnancy is not indicative of a problem, unless the discharge is accompanied by itching, burning, foul odor, or labial swelling. A change in the quality or quantity of discharge in the third trimester should be differentiated from leaking or ruptured membranes or from cervical dilation if accompanied by cramping or pressure.

Patients should be advised to bathe daily and wear cotton underwear. Tub bathing is safe because water does not enter the vagina under normal conditions. Douching rarely is indicated and should be used only if advised by a physician.[15] Use of a bulb syringe for douching is contraindicated owing to the risk of air embolism.[3]

References

1. Aikins MP: Alternative therapies for nausea and vomiting of pregnancy. Obstet Gynecol 91:149–155, 1998.
2. Belluomini J, Litt RC, Lee KA, et al: Acupressure for nausea and vomiting of pregnancy: A randomized, blinded study. Obstet Gynecol 84:245–248, 1994.
3. Carroll J, Biringer A: Prenatal Care. Monograph, Edition No. 165, Home Study Self-Assessment Program. Kansas City, MO, American Academy of Family Physicians, 1993.
4. Fuchs K, Paldi E, Abramovici H, et al: Treatment of hyperemesis by hypnosis. Int J Clin Exp Hypn 28:313–323, 1980.
5. Gabbe SG, Niebyl JR, Simpson JL (eds): Postpartum care. In: Obstetrics: Normal and Problem Pregnancies, 2nd ed. New York, Churchill Livingstone, 1991, pp 222–225.
6. Jewell MD: Benzylamine and dramamine for nausea in pregnancy. In Enkin MW, Keirse MJNC, Renfrew MJ, Neilson JP (eds): Pregnancy and Childbirth Module of the Cochrane Database of Systematic Reviews. Oxford, Oxford University Press, 1995.
7. Jewell MD: Phenothiazines for nausea in pregnancy. In Enkin MW, Keirse MJNC, Renfrew MJ, Neilson JP (eds): Pregnancy and Childbirth Module of the Cochrane Database of Systematic Reviews. Oxford, Oxford University Press, 1995.
8. Jewell MD: Antacid therapy for heartburn in pregnancy. In Enkin MW, Keirse MJNC, Renfrew MJ, Neilson JP (eds): Pregnancy and Childbirth Module of the Cochrane Database of Systematic Reviews. Oxford, Oxford University Press, 1995.
9. Jewell MD: Treatments for constipation in pregnancy. In Enkin MW, Keirse MJNC, Renfrew MJ, Neilson JP (eds): Pregnancy and Childbirth Module of the Cochrane Database of Systematic Reviews. Oxford, Oxford University Press, 1995.
10. Klebanoff MA, Koslowe PA, Kaslow R, Rhoads GG: Epidemiology of vomiting in early pregnancy. Obstet Gynecol 66:612–616, 1985.
11. Kramer MS: High protein supplementation in pregnancy. In Enkin MW, Keirse MJNC, Renfrew MJ, Neilson JP (eds): Pregnancy and Childbirth Module of the Cochrane Database of Systematic Reviews, 1995 [updated February 24, 1995]. London, BMJ Publishing Group, 1995.
12. Murphy PA: Alternative therapies for nausea and vomiting of pregnancy. Obstet Gynecol 91:149–155, 1998.
13. Pridham KF, Schutz ME: Preparation of parents for birthing and infant care. J Fam Pract 13:181–188, 1981.
14. Sahakian V, Rouse D, Sipes S, et al: Vitamin B6 is effective therapy for nausea and vomiting of pregnancy: A randomized, double-blind placebo-controlled study. Obstet Gynecol 78:33–36, 1991.
15. Scott JR, DiSaia PJ, Hammond CB, Spellacy WN (eds): Danforth's Obstetrics and Gynecology. Philadelphia, JB Lippincott, 1990.
16. Seto A, Einarson T, Koren G: Pregnancy outcome following first trimester exposure to antihistamines: A meta-analysis. Am J Perinatol 14:119–124, 1997.
17. Sullivan CA, Johnson CA, Roach H, et al: A pilot study of intravenous ondansetron for hyperemesis gravidarum. Am J Obstet Gynecol 174:1565–1568, 1996.
18. Tierson FD, Olsen CL, Hook EB: Nausea and vomiting of pregnancy and association with pregnancy outcome. Am J Obstet Gynecol 155:1017–1022, 1986.
19. Tincello DG, Johnstone MJ: Treatment of hyperemesis gravidarum with the 5-HT3 antagonist ondansetron (Zofran). Postgrad Med J 72:688–689, 1996.
20. Torem MS: Hypnotherapeutic techniques in the treatment of hyperemesis gravidarum. Am J Clin Hypn 37:1–11, 1994.
21. Vellacott ID, Cooke EJ, James CE: Nausea and vomiting in early pregnancy. Int J Obstet Gynecol 27:57–62, 1988.
22. Vutyavanich T, Wongtra-ngan S, Ruangsri R: Pyridoxine for nausea and vomiting of pregnancy: A randomized, double-blind, placebo-controlled trial. Am J Obstet Gynecol 173:881–884, 1995.
23. World MJ: Ondansetron and hyperemesis gravidarum. Lancet 341:185–188, 1993.

SECTION F.
GENERAL PRECAUTIONS

Elizabeth G. Baxley, M.D.

I. Danger Signs
As part of routine prenatal patient education, signs and symptoms that might warn of possible serious threats to the pregnancy should be discussed.

A. Vaginal Bleeding
Vaginal bleeding enough to soak a sanitary pad could signify bleeding from a placenta previa or abruptio placentae and should be reported to the physician immediately.

B. Leakage of Fluid
Any significant leakage of fluid from the vagina necessitates an examination for premature rupture of the amniotic membranes.

C. Abdominal Pain
Abdominal pain that is severe or persistent might signify premature labor or placental abruption, preeclampsia, acute fatty liver, or other medical or surgical complication and requires that the patient have a clinical examination and a period of fetal monitoring.

D. Reduction in Fetal Movement
A marked reduction in fetal movement should be reported because this may be an indication of a stressed fetus. Fetal surveillance testing may called for, depending on the clinical situation; if reassuring, the patient should be given instructions to perform fetal kick counts at home. Serial testing is not indicated unless an underlying abnormality is discovered.

E. Other Ominous Symptoms
Severe or persistent headache, dizziness, or blurred vision; sharp right upper quadrant pain; and swelling of the face or fingers may be warning signs of pregnancy-induced hypertension.

F. Dysuria
Dysuria, particularly if accompanied by low back or costovertebral angle pain, fever, or nausea and vomiting, should be evaluated to rule out acute pyelonephritis or nephrolithiasis. Upper and lower tract disease has been associated with an increased risk of preterm labor.

II. Patient Education and Premature Labor
Early in the third trimester, women should be educated about the signs and symptoms of labor and given instructions about how to contact the physician. The presence of bloody show, rupture of membranes, or consistently regular uterine contractions helps guide patients in deciding when their labor has begun.

SECTION G.
EXERCISE AND PREGNANCY

Elizabeth Joy, M.D.

Physical activity and maintenance of physical fitness are essential to the health of women in their childbearing years. Pregnancy is a normal condition for women, and exercise can be part of a normal pregnancy. In the absence of medical or obstetric complications, women should be encouraged by their obstetric care provider to exercise regularly throughout pregnancy. Physicians and midwives need to be knowledgeable about the American College of Obstetricians and Gynecologists (ACOG) guidelines[1] for exercise during pregnancy and the postpartum period as well as contraindications to exercise during pregnancy and the signals to stop exercising. Providers should be able to counsel women on the maternal and fetal benefits of regular exercise during pregnancy and know how to write an appropriate exercise prescription based on a woman's fitness level, interests, and exercise goals.

Nearly half of 10,000 women surveyed[29] report exercising during pregnancy. Research to date supports the decision to continue or initiate an exercise program during pregnancy. The literature dealing with exercise during pregnancy has shown no deleterious effects of exercise on the mother or developing fetus.[26] Women are able not only to maintain, but also to improve their fitness levels during pregnancy,[11,18] and a report suggests that infants of exercising mothers may be healthier than those of sedentary mothers.[12] Exercising women also report fewer discomforts of pregnancy than their sedentary counterparts.[16] For most pregnant women, exercise is not only safe, but also beneficial to the health of the mother and the infant.

I. Guidelines for Exercise During Pregnancy

In 1985, the ACOG[1] published its first guidelines for exercise during pregnancy. These guidelines were based on limited scientific data and were criticized.[14,20] After numerous studies showed maternal benefits and no fetal or neonatal risks from regular maternal exercise, the ACOG[2] revised and liberalized their guidelines for exercise during pregnancy and the postpartum period in 1994. Table 5 lists the guidelines from 1985 and 1994. The most striking changes from the earlier guidelines included *removal* of the recommendations not to exceed a heart rate of 140 beats/min or exercise beyond 15 minutes' duration and the recommendation to avoid exercises employing the Valsalva maneuver (specifically weight lifting). These recommendations are only a *guide*. Each pregnant woman has a different experience with pregnancy and exercise. Exercise guidelines must be tailored to each individual woman.

TABLE 5.   American College of Obstetricians and Gynecologists Guidelines for Exercise During Pregnancy and the Postpartum Period

1. Regular activity (3 times/week) is preferable to intermittent activity.

2. Pregnant women who exercise in the first trimester should augment heat dissipation by ensuring adequate hydration, appropriate clothing, and optimal environmental surroundings

3. Morphologic changes in pregnancy should serve as a relative contraindication to types of exercise in which balance could be detrimental to maternal or fetal well-being, especially in the third trimester. Any type of exercise involving the potential for mild abdominal trauma should be avoided

4. Women should be aware of the decreased oxygen available for aerobic exercise during pregnancy. They should be encouraged to modify the intensity of exercise according to maternal symptoms. Pregnant women should stop exercising when fatigued and not exercise to exhaustion. Weight-bearing exercises may be continued under some circumstances at intensities similar to those before pregnancy throughout pregnancy. Non–weight-bearing exercises, such as cycling or swimming, minimize the risk of injury and facilitate the continuation of exercise during pregnancy

5. Women should avoid exercise in the supine position after the first trimester. Such a position is associated with decreased cardiac output in most pregnant women. Prolonged periods of motionless standing also should be avoided

6. Pregnancy requires an additional 300 kcal/d to maintain metabolic homeostasis. Women who exercise during pregnancy should be particularly careful to ensure adequate diet

7. Many of the physiologic and morphologic changes of pregnancy persist 4–6 weeks postpartum. Prepregnancy exercise routines should be resumed gradually

Data from ACOG: Exercise during pregnancy and the postnatal period. In: ACOG Home Exercise Programs. Washington, DC, ACOG, 1985, pp 1–5; ACOG: Exercise during pregnancy and the postpartum period. ACOG Technical Bulletin No. 189. Washington, DC, ACOG, 1994.

II. Contraindications to Exercise During Pregnancy

The ACOG guidelines apply to healthy women having normal pregnancies. There are absolute and relative obstetric and medical contraindications to exercise during pregnancy.

A. Absolute Obstetric Contraindications

Absolute obstetric contraindications include pregnancy-induced hypertension, premature rupture of membranes, incompetent cervix or cerclage, persistent second- or third-trimester bleeding, and IUGR. The ACOG also lists preterm labor during the prior or current pregnancy or both as an absolute contraindication. One could argue that if a definitive cause for preterm labor (e.g., multiple gestations, pyelonephritis) in the prior pregnancy could be identified and was not evident in the present pregnancy, one could exercise safely.

B. Absolute Medical Contraindications

Absolute medical contraindications include hemodynamically significant heart disease, uncontrolled hypertension, uncontrolled renal disease, hemodynamically significant anemia, and uncontrolled diabetes mellitus.

C. Relative Obstetric Contraindications

Relative obstetric contraindications include multiple gestation, breech position in the third trimester, and a history of precipitous labor and delivery. If any evidence suggests fetal compromise, maternal complication, or preterm labor, exercise activities would need to be changed or eliminated.

D. Relative Medical Contraindications

Relative medical contraindications may include but are not limited to malnutrition, certain cardiac arrhythmias, symptomatic anemia, active thyroid disease, and extreme obesity. Women with conditions such as these need to participate in a closely monitored exercise program.

III. Benefits of Exercise During Pregnancy

The many maternal benefits of exercise during pregnancy include improved cardiovascular fitness[11,18]; control of maternal weight gain[19]; reduction of some discomforts of pregnancy, such as swelling, leg cramps, fatigue, and shortness of breath[16]; and a positive influence on labor and delivery. Clapp[7] found that compared with women who discontinued exercise in the first trimester, women who exercised regularly at 50% of preconceptional levels throughout pregnancy had a lower incidence of vaginal or abdominal operative delivery, shorter active labor, and increased fetal tolerance of labor and delivery. Clinical evidence of fetal stress (e.g., meconium, fetal heart rate pattern, and Apgar score) was less frequent in the exercising group compared with the control group (see Table 6).[7]

Regular exercise does not appear to affect early pregnancy outcome negatively. Clapp[4] prospectively followed 47 recreational runners, 40 aerobic dancers, and 28 physically active, fit controls. Spontaneous abortion occurred in 17% of the runners and 18% of the aerobic dancers compared with 25% in the control group. These results should be reassuring to obstetric care providers and their patients who exercise regularly.

The greatest benefits of exercise during pregnancy may be psychological. In one study, women reported that the chief benefits of exercise during pregnancy were related to improved mental outlook, self-image, and sense of control and a relief of tension.[19]

There appear to be neonatal and childhood benefits to regular exercise during pregnancy as well. Clapp[10] reported on the offspring of 20 women who exercised and compared them with those of 20 physically active control subjects. He found that at birth, head circumference and length were similar, but the offspring of exercising women weighed less (3400 g vs. 3640 g) and had less body fat (10.5 % vs. 15.1 %). At 5 years of age, head circumference and length were similar, but the offspring of exercising women still weighed less (18.0 kg vs. 19.5 kg) and had a lower sum of five skin-folds (37 mm vs. 44 mm). Motor, integrative, and academic readiness skills were evaluated

TABLE 6. Course of Labor after Endurance Exercise During Pregnancy

	Exercise group (n = 87)*	Control group (n = 44)†
Incidence of preterm labor	9%	9%
Length of gestation	277 d	282 d
Incidence of abdominal operative delivery	6%	30%
Incidence of vaginal operative delivery	6%	20%
Duration of labor	264 min	382 min
Clinical evidence of fetal stress‡	26%	50%

Note. Study comprised 113 well-conditioned recreational athletes.
* Women who continued regular exercise at 50% of their preconceptional level throughout pregnancy.
† Women who discontinued exercise before the end of the first trimester.
‡ Meconium, fetal heart rate pattern, Apgar score.
From Clapp JF: The course of labor after endurance exercise during pregnancy. Am J Obstet Gynecol 163:1799–1805, 1990.

by developmental psychologists blinded to maternal exercise status and were found to be similar in the two groups. The exercise offspring performed significantly better on Wechsler scales and tests of oral language skills, however.

IV. Physiologic Adaptations to Pregnancy and Their Interaction With Exercise
A. Cardiovascular
Many cardiovascular adaptations throughout pregnancy influence and interact with a woman's ability to exercise. Cardiac output increases substantially during pregnancy as a result of increased venous return, which increases ventricular filling, and an increase in myocardial contractility. Heart rate is thought to increase as a result of decreased vagal tone or an increase in sympathetic drive to the sinoatrial node. During pregnancy, a woman's systemic vascular resistance decreases during aerobic exercise, resulting in larger increases in the cardiac output response to exercise.

Exercise and pregnancy have opposing effects on one another with respect to regional blood flow distribution. During exercise, splanchnic blood flow is diminished as blood flow is redistributed to skin and exercising muscles. During pregnancy, blood flow is shunted preferentially to uterine, renal, and cutaneous circulations. Increases in cardiac output, blood volume, and resting venous capacitance may negate any relative decline in uteroplacental blood flow during exercise, however. Placental adaptations to exercise may aid in fetal acquisition of oxygen and substrate. Clapp found that placental volumes were significantly greater in women who maintained a regular exercise regimen through the midtrimester of pregnancy. It seems safe to conclude that this increase in placental volume would result in enhanced extraction of oxygen and substrate from the uteroplacental circulation and diminish further any relative decrease in uteroplacental circulation resulting from exercise.
B. Pulmonary
During pregnancy and exercise, minute ventilation and oxygen consumption increase. The 50% increase in minute ventilation during pregnancy largely is due to an increase in tidal volume. This increase results in an increase in arterial oxygen tension to 106 to 108 mmHg in the first trimester, declining to 101 to 106 mmHg in the third trimester.[2] Despite this increase in oxygen tension, the increased resting oxygen requirements of pregnancy and the increased work of breathing for any given workload result in decreased oxygen available for aerobic exercise. Most women appreciate a subjective increase in workload and a decline in maximal exercise performance.[2,6]

C. Thermoregulatory

Pregnancy and exercise result in an increase in maternal heat production. Exercise can result in significant increases in core temperature. During exercise, heat dissipation occurs as a result of increased blood flow to the skin, resulting in sweating. Fetal core temperature is approximately 0.5° to 1.0° C higher than maternal core temperature. This higher temperature normally is dissipated through umbilical and uterine circulations. Healthy, fit pregnant women tolerate thermal stress better than in the nonpregnant state as a result of maternal adaptations that eliminate the gradient between maternal and fetal circulation. Clapp[8] studied 18 recreational athletes before, during, and after 20 minutes of continuous exercise at 64% of maximum oxygen consumption. He found that peak rectal temperature reached during exercise decreased by 0.3° C at 8 weeks, then fell at a rate of 0.1° C per month through the 37th week. These changes were related to a decrease in rectal temperature at rest and a decrease in temperature when sweating occurred. The thermal stress for a given task is decreased by 20% in early pregnancy and 50% by the third trimester. No studies have shown fetal teratogenesis attributed to thermal stress in women participating in vigorous exercise during early pregnancy.[6]

D. Endocrine and Metabolic

Endocrine response and substrate use of pregnancy and exercise generally are in opposition to one another. This situation raises a concern that substrate may be diverted from the fetus to exercising muscles, resulting in lower fetal birth weights. In women who exercise at moderate levels, however, there appears to be no adverse effect on fetal birth weight.[23] Studies show lower blood glucose levels after a period of exercise in pregnant women.[25] It is prudent to remind women who exercise that they need to meet not only the extra energy demands of pregnancy, but also the energy demands of their exercise program. On average, a pregnant woman requires an extra 300 kcal of energy intake per day.[2] One can estimate safely that each 1 mile walked or run, every 3 miles on a bike, or 15 to 20 minutes of moderate-level aerobic dance requires an additional 100 kcal of energy.

Theoretic concerns regarding the conflicting endocrine responses during exercise and pregnancy relate primarily to whether the excess catecholamines and prostaglandins liberated during exercise result in uterine stimulation and subsequent preterm birth. No studies to date have shown any increase in the incidence of preterm delivery as a result of maternal exercise programs in otherwise healthy normal pregnancies.[28]

V. Exercise Prescription

The goal of exercise during pregnancy should be to maintain maternal fitness levels, while minimizing risk to the developing fetus. Exercise guidelines should be tailored to each individual woman. The key to maintaining a safe, comfortable exercise program is flexibility of thought. As a woman's pregnancy changes, so must her exercise program. She should be prepared to stop or change her exercise regimen in response to changes in her pregnancy. When discussing or designing an exercise program, one must take into account a woman's fitness level, goals of exercise (maintain fitness, stress relief, weight management, competitive activities), work activities and job requirements, and gestational age. Exercise intensity, duration, and frequency should be kept at a level that does not result in excessive fatigue, pain, or extreme shortness of breath. For most women, over the course of their pregnancy, overall exercise performance decreases considerably as a result of pregnancy-related fatigue, nausea, vomiting, weight gain, and other morphologic changes.[2] Switching to non–weight-bearing forms of exercise, such as swimming or bicycling, may allow some women to continue with moderate to vigorous intensity exercise programs throughout their

TABLE 7. Guide to Exercise Prescription During Pregnancy

Sedentary Women	
Mode	Walking, bicycling, stair climbing, aerobic dance, water aerobics, swimming
Intensity	65–75% maximum heart rate; perceived exertion = moderately hard
Duration	30 min
Frequency	Minimum of 3 times/wk
Recreational Athletes/RegularFitness Exercisers	
Mode	Same as above plus running/jogging, dance, tennis *Depending on skill level and gestational age:* cross country skiing, downhill skiing, water skiing (recommend wearing a wet suit), horseback riding
Intensity	65–85% maximum heart rate; perceived exertion = moderately hard to hard
Duration	30–60 min
Frequency	3–5 times/wk
Elite Athletes	
Mode	Same as above plus some competitive activities, *depending on gestational age*
Intensity	75–85% maximum heart rate; perceived exertion = hard
Duration	60–90 min
Frequency	4–6 times/wk

pregnancy.[3] Women whose job requires certain physical stresses (quiet standing, long hours, protracted ambulation, or heavy lifting) may be at increased risk for premature birth and low birth weight.[9] In addition to making appropriate changes in the work environment to avoid this risk, one must take these activities into account when discussing any exercise regimen.

Although there is no generally agreed on formula for determining an appropriate exercise prescription, one can recommend safely most exercise activities that women were doing before becoming pregnant. For women initiating an exercise program, there are many fitness activities that can be started safely during early pregnancy. Table 7 lists exercise modalities and their intensity, duration, and frequency appropriate for three levels of maternal fitness: previously sedentary women, recreational athletes and regular fitness exercisers, and elite athletes.

Women should be counseled regarding environmental conditions and their impact on maternal and fetal stress; this is especially true in regard to heat. Women should be cautioned to avoid exercise outdoors during the heat of the day. Women should dress appropriately to avoid excessive thermal stress and drink appropriate amounts of fluid before, during, and after exercise to counteract sweat losses. Recommendations regarding physical activity at altitude during pregnancy are based on few scientific studies, and providers should err on the side of caution when advising women facing short-term exposure to high altitude (> 8000 ft above sea level) during pregnancy. Women who reside at higher altitudes and have higher levels of fitness tolerate altitude stress better than women who do not. Altitude in excess of 8000 ft should be avoided in the first 4 to 5 days of short-term exposure, and if exercise is to be performed at altitude, acclimatization should take place by exercising at lower altitudes for a few days.[17]

TABLE 8. Signals to Stop Exercising

Fatigue	Excessive nausea	Decreased fetal movement
Breathlessness	Chest pain or tightness	Uterine contractions
Dizziness	Palpitations or racing heart	Vaginal bleeding
Headache	Difficulty walking	Leakage of amniotic fluid
Muscle weakness	Significant swelling in feet or legs	Pain—back, hips, or pubic bone

From Paisley JE, Mellion MB: Exercise during pregnancy. Am Fam Physician 38:143–150, 1988.

TABLE 9. Exercises to Avoid During Pregnancy
Contact/collision sports   Boxing, field hockey, football, rugby, ice hockey, martial arts, rodeo, soccer, wrestling

High-risk activities
  Deep-sea diving, hang-gliding, parachute jumping, rock climbing, springboard diving, fencing,
  power weightlifting

Other at-risk activities*   Competitive distance running, competitive bodybuilding, professional dance, ballet

* Participation limited to women with high fitness and skill levels and under close medical supervision.

VI. Signals to Stop Exercising

Providers and patients need to be aware of the signals to stop exercising when pregnant. Table 8 lists symptoms that should elicit prompt evaluation and appropriate modification in activity to avoid further risk to either mother or fetus.

VII. Exercises to Avoid

Table 9 lists activities that one should in most cases avoid during pregnancy and activities that should prompt more frequent monitoring. Although there are no generally agreed on sports or activities that pregnant women can or cannot do, most practitioners take a commonsense approach in advising against activities that pose a threat of abdominal trauma. A woman's fitness level, skill level, and her own assumption of personal risk need to be taken into consideration when decisions are made regarding sports participation. Scuba diving during pregnancy is discouraged because the fetus is not protected from decompression problems and is at risk of malformation and gas embolism after decompression disease.[13] Maximal weight-lifting has been shown to result in dramatic increases in blood pressure and probably should be avoided. Moderate strength training has not been shown to cause any deleterious effects among pregnant women, however.[18] The issue of high-intensity endurance training among elite athletes continues to be investigated. There is some evidence that vigorous training performed throughout pregnancy results in lower birth weight infants, but there is no evidence of preterm birth.[15] Although there are no definitive guidelines for monitoring the high-intensity athlete during pregnancy, one should take a commonsense approach to this and look for signs of fetal stress.

VIII. Conclusion

In the 1990s, exercise during pregnancy has been found to be not only safe, but also beneficial in most cases to the mother and the developing fetus. Obstetric care providers should encourage patients to continue or initiate exercise programs during pregnancy and work with them on a regular basis to modify exercise regimens in response to changes in the pregnancy.

References

1. ACOG: Exercise during pregnancy and the postnatal period. In: ACOG Home Exercise Programs. Washington, DC, ACOG, 1985, pp 1–5.
2. ACOG: Exercise during pregnancy and the postpartum period. ACOG Technical Bulletin No. 189. Washington, DC, ACOG, 1994.
3. Artal R, Masaki DI, et al: Exercise prescription during pregnancy: Weight-bearing versus non-weight-bearing exercise. Am J Obstet Gynecol 161:1464–1469, 1989.
4. Clapp JF: The effects of maternal exercise on early pregnancy outcome. Am J Obstet Gynecol 161:1453–1457, 1989.
5. Clapp JF: Oxygen consumption during treadmill exercise before, during and after pregnancy. Am J Obstet Gynecol 161:1458–1464, 1989.
6. Clapp JF: Exercise in pregnancy: A brief clinical review. Fetal Med Rev 2:89–101, 1990.

7. Clapp JF: The course of labor after endurance exercise during pregnancy. Am J Obstet Gynecol 163:1799–1805, 1990.
8. Clapp JF: The changing thermal response to endurance exercise during pregnancy. Am J Obstet Gynecol 165:1684–1689, 1991.
9. Clapp JF: Pregnancy outcome: Physical activities inside versus outside the workplace. Semin Perinatol 20:70–76, 1996.
10. Clapp JF: Morphometric and neurodevelopmental outcome at age five years of the offspring of women who continued to exercise regularly throughout pregnancy. J Pediatr 129:856–863, 1996.
11. Clapp JF, Capeless E: The VO_{2max} of recreational athletes before and after pregnancy. Med Sci Sports Exerc 23:1128–1133, 1991.
12. Clapp JF, Rizk KH: Effect of recreational exercise on midtrimester placental growth. Am J Obstet Gynecol 167:1518–1521, 1992.
13. Camporesi EM: Diving and pregnancy. Semin Perinatol 20:292–302, 1996.
14. Gauthier MM: Guidelines for exercise during pregnancy: Too little or too much? Physician Sportsmed 14:162–169, 1986.
15. Hale RW, Milne L: The elite athlete and exercise in pregnancy. Semin Perinatol 20:277–284, 1996.
16. Horns PN, Ratcliffe LP, Leggett JC, et al: Pregnancy outcomes among active and sedentary primiparous women. J Obstet Gynecol Neonat Nurs 25:49–54, 1996.
17. Huch R: Physical activity at altitude in pregnancy. Semin Perinatol 20:303–314, 1996.
18. Kulpa PJ, White BM, Visscher R: Aerobic exercise in pregnancy. Am J Obstet Gynecol 156:139–143, 1987.
19. Lee VC, Lutter JM: Exercise and pregnancy: Choices, concerns, and recommendations. In: Obstetric and Gynecologic Physical Therapy. New York, Churchill Livingstone.
20. Monahan T: Should women go easy on exercise? Physician Sportsmed 14:188–197, 1986.
21. Paisley JE, Mellion MB: Exercise during pregnancy. Am Fam Physician 38:143–150, 1988.
22. Pivarnik JM: Cardiovascular responses to aerobic exercise during pregnancy and postpartum. Semin Perinatol 20:242–249, 1996.
23. Pivarnik JM: Potential effects of maternal physical activity on birth weight: Brief review. Med Sci Sports Exerc 30:400–406, 1998.
24. Pivarnik JM, et al: Effects of maternal aerobic fitness on cardiorespiratory responses to exercise. Med Sci Sports Exerc 25:993–998, 1993.
25. Soultanakis HN, Artal R, Wiswell RA: Prolonged exercise in pregnancy: Glucose homeostasis, ventilatory and cardiovascular responses. Semin Perinatol 20:315–327, 1996.
26. Sternfield B: Physical activity and pregnancy outcome: Review and recommendations. Sports Med 23:33–47, 1997.
27. Veille JC: Maternal and fetal cardiovascular response to exercise during pregnancy. Semin Perinatol 20:250–262, 1996.
28. Veille JC, Hohimer AR, Burry K, et al: The effect of exercise on uterine activity in the last 8 weeks of pregnancy. Am J Obstet Gynecol 151:727–730, 1985.
29. Zhang J, Savitz DA: Exercise during pregnancy among US women. Ann Epidemiol 6:53–59, 1996.

CHAPTER 4

Pregnancy Interventions

SECTION A.
OCCUPATIONAL INTERVENTIONS

Roger Kimber, M.D.

Many women need or desire to work during pregnancy. The clinician's task is to advise women and their employers whether any special precautions or change in role or task is necessary or if a job change is indicated. The quality of the evidence that exists about risks of various occupational exposures varies greatly and does not necessarily include randomized controlled trials (RCTs). Therefore, the clinician's judgment is required, and patients' preferences need to be taken into account.

I. Potential Reproductive Risks from Occupational Exposure
Potential reproductive risks are summarized in Table 1.

II. Known or Suspected Occupational Hazards
Tables 2 and 3 list common well-documented occupational hazards.[1] This is a changing field. A comprehensive list is beyond the scope of this chapter.[3] Table 4 lists sources of timely, detailed information and assistance.

III. Evaluation
A detailed occupational history is key (Table 5). Past occupational, home, and avocational exposures and the father's occupational and avocational exposures may need to be evaluated. A knowledgeable, interested local/regional occupational medicine specialist may be of help. Interpretation of the literature with respect to causation must be approached with caution in the individual patient because the quality of data regarding occupational exposures is variable.

A. Preconceptual Planning
1. During the preconceptual planning process, patients may initiate inquiries. Health maintenance visits and premarital testing provide additional opportunities to evaluate occupational risks.
2. Inquiries and advice should be limited to known reproductive hazards in the workplace that affect women and men (see Tables 2 and 3).
3. Prior reproductive problems, such as recurrent spontaneous abortions or infertility, should be assessed. The physician should eliminate known occupational reproductive hazards and intrinsic problems of both partners and then consider suspected occupational hazards as possible causes (see Tables 2 and 3).

B. Approaches
Once a hazard has been identified, several approaches to eliminating or minimizing the risk to the current or future pregnancy exist.

89

TABLE 1. Potential Reproductive Risks from Occupational Exposure

Risk	Comment
Infertility	Father's occupational exposure may also be relevant
Pregnancy loss	Father's occupational exposure may also be relevant; early or late; multiple mechanisms
Vertical transmission of occupationally acquired pathogens	Health care settings and elsewhere; father's occupational exposure may be relevant
Chromosomal/congenital anomalies secondary to workplace chemical, physical, biologic exposures	
Neurodevelopmental injury secondary to workplace chemical, physical, biologic exposures	
Preterm delivery associated with physical or psychological stress of job	Controversial
Maternal exhaustion/nutritional depletion leading to small-for-gestational age infant	Probably relevant in extreme circumstances/complicating maternal conditions
Maternal occupational injuries	As a result of changes in maternal body habitus or physiology

1. Job/task modification

This may occur through redesigning the process, engineering controls of the worker's environment, or eliminating use of the offending agent. This is the ideal approach, but it is not always possible or economic.

2. Limitation of hours/duties

This may be all that is needed for some occupations involving prolonged standing or extremes of exertion or for complicated pregnancies; this is not always compatible with the job requirements.

3. Special shielding/equipment

Personal protective gear, although relatively inexpensive, is often inconvenient to use and either not consistently used or interferes with job performance.

4. Job leave

Some companies allow compensated or uncompensated leave for the duration of pregnancy or that part of pregnancy when there is significant risk.

5. Job change

Some situations are not amenable to the aforementioned approaches.

C. Negotiating Changes in the Work Environment

Occupational health physicians may be helpful to the practitioner in advising or negotiating with employers on behalf of the pregnant woman. Phone contacts with employers, insurance carriers, or union representatives before written communication (if needed) may help in developing an optimal solution.

D. Pregnancy Leave Guidelines

The 1984 American Medical Association guidelines (Table 6) are not supported by well-done studies,[2] and there is no consensus in practice as to how long an otherwise healthy woman should work at a given job during an uncomplicated pregnancy.[2]

E. Breastfeeding and Occupational Exposure

The benefits of breast milk over formula feeding make it unnecessary to formula-feed an infant with most chemical exposures. Most chemicals to which women are environmentally or occupationally exposed probably pass to breast milk to some degree. There are few data to substantiate risk to the infant in usual occupational settings. See Table 7 for guidelines on the limited number of chemicals for which they exist.

TABLE 2. Some Agents Associated with Adverse Female Reproductive Capacity or Developmental Effects in Human and Animal Studies

Agent	Human Outcomes	Strength of Association in Humans*	Animal Outcomes	Strength of Association in Animals*
Anesthetic gases[†]	Reduced fertility, spontaneous abortion	1,3	Birth defects	1,3
Arsenic	Spontaneous abortion, low birth weight	1	Birth defects, fetal loss	2
Benzo[a]pyrene	None	NA[‡]	Birth defects	1
Cadmium	None	NA	Fetal loss, birth defects	2
Carbon disulfide	Menstrual disorders, spontaneous abortion	1	Birth defects	1
Carbon monoxide	Low birth weight, fetal death (high doses)	1	Birth defects, neonatal mortality	2
Chlordecone	None	NA	Fetal loss	2,3
Chloroform	None	NA	Fetal loss	1
Chloroprene	None	NA	Birth defects	2,3
Ethylene glycol ethers	Spontaneous abortion	1	Birth defects	2
Ethylene oxide	Spontaneous abortion	1	Fetal loss	1
Formamides	None	NA	Fetal loss, birth defects	1
Inorganic mercury[†]	Menstrual disorders, spontaneous abortion	1	Fetal loss, birth defects	1
Lead[†]	Spontaneous abortion, prematurity, neurologic dysfunction in child	2	Birth defects, fetal loss	2
Organic mercury	CNS malformation, cerebral palsy	2	Birth defects, fetal loss	2
Physical stress	Prematurity	2	None	NA
Polybrominated biphenyls (PBBs)	None	NA	Fetal loss	2
Polychlorinated biphenyls (PCBs)	Neonatal PCB syndrome (low birth weight, hyperpigmentation, eye abnormalities)	2	Low birth weight, fetal loss	2
Radiation, ionizing	Menstrual disorders, CNS defects, skeletal and eye anomalies, mental retardation, childhood cancer	2	Fetal loss, birth defects	2
Selenium	Spontaneous abortion	3	Low birth weight, birth defects	2
Tellurium	None	NA	Birth defects	2
2,4-Dichlorophenoxyacetic acid (2,4-D)	Skeletal defects	4	Birth defects	1
2,4,5-Trichlorophenoxyacetic acid (2,4,5-T)	Skeletal defects	4	Birth defects	1
Video display terminals	Spontaneous abortion	4	Birth defects	1
Vinyl chloride[†]	CNS defects	1	Birth defects	1,4
Xylene	Menstrual disorders, fetal loss	1	Fetal loss, birth defects	1

* 1 = Limited positive data; 2 = strong positive data; 3 = limited negative data; 4 = strong negative data.
[†] Agents that may have male-mediated effects.
[‡] Not applicable because no adverse outcomes were observed.
CNS, central nervous system.
From Agency for Toxic Substances and Disease Registry: Exposure to hazardous substances and reproductive health. Am Fam Physician 48:1442, 1993, with permission.

TABLE 3.   Some Agents Associated with Male Reproductive Dysfunction

Agent	Human Outcomes	Strength of Association in Humans*	Animal Outcomes	Strength of Association in Animals*
Boron	Decreased sperm count	1	Testicular damage	2
Benzene	None	NA[†]	Decreased sperm motility, testicular damage	1
Benzo[a]pyrene	None	NA	Testicular damage	1
Cadmium	Reduced fertility	1	Testicular damage	2
Carbon disulfide	Decreased sperm count, decreased sperm motility	2,3	Testicular damage	1
Carbon monoxide	None	NA	Testicular damage	1
Carbon tetrachloride	None	NA	Testicular damage	1
Carbaryl	Abnormal sperm morphology	1	Testicular damage	1
Chlordecone	Decreased sperm count, decreased sperm motility	2	Testicular damage	2
Chloroprene	Decreased sperm motility, abnormal morphology, decreased libido	2	Testicular damage	1
Dibromochloropropane (DBCP)	Decreased sperm count, azoospermia, hormonal changes	2	Testicular damage	2
Dimethyl dichlorovinyl phosphate (DDVP)	None	NA	Decreased sperm count	2
Epichlorohydrin	None	NA	Testicular damage	1
Estrogens	Decreased sperm count	2	Decreased sperm count	2
Ethylene oxide	None	NA	Testicular damage	1
Ethylene dibromide (EDB)	Abnormal sperm motility	1	Testicular damage	2,3
Ethylene glycol ethers	Decreased sperm count	1	Testicular damage	2
Heat	Decreased sperm count	2	Decreased sperm count	2
Lead	Decreased sperm count	2	Testicular damage, decreased sperm count, decreased sperm motility, abnormal morphology	2
Manganese	Decreased libido, impotence	1	Testicular damage	1,3
Polybrominated biphenyls (PBBs)	None	NA	Testicular damage	1
Polychlorinated biphenyls (PCBs)	None	NA	Testicular damage	1
Radiation, ionizing	Decreased sperm count	2	Testicular damage	2

* 1 = Limited positive data; 2 = strong positive data; 3 = limited negative data; 4 = strong negative data.
[†] Not applicable because no adverse outcomes were observed.
From Agency for Toxic Substances and Disease Registry: Exposure to hazardous substances and reproductive health. Am Fam Physician 49:1442, 1993, with permission.

TABLE 4. Occupational Reproductive Hazards Resources

Computer data bases

MEDLINE: National Library of Medicine (Bethesda, MD)—contains references from 3000 biomedical journals

TOXLINE: National Library of Medicine (Bethesda, MD)—contains more than 400,000 references to published human and animal toxicologic studies

TOXNET: National Library of Medicine (Bethesda, MD)—toxicology-oriented data bank

REPROTOX: Reproductive Toxicology Center (Washington, DC)—contains referenced summaries of reproductive data for over 800 physical and chemical agents

ON-LINE CATALOG OF TERATOGENIC AGENTS: Central Laboratory for Human Embryology (Seattle, WA)—free data base on teratogenic effects of nearly 2000 substances

Hotlines

Pregnancy/Environmental Hotline (serves primarily Massachusetts, but will accept calls from practitioners nationally)—(800) 322–5014 (MA only); (617) 787–4957. National Birth Defects Center, Kennedy Memorial Hospital (Boston, MA)

Pregnancy Exposure Information Service (serves Connecticut)—(800) 325–5391 (CT only). University of Connecticut Health Center (Farmington, CT)

Washington State Poison Control Network—(800) 732–6985 (WA only); (206) 526–2121. University of Washington, Seattle, WA

Regulatory and related agencies

Occcupational Safety and Health Administration (OSHA) (Washington, DC, regional and local state offices)—responsible for promulgation and enforcement of standards for workplace hazards; performs workplace inspections at request of employee, union, or health care provider

National Institute of Occupational Safety and Health (NIOSH) (Atlanta, GA and local state offices)— develops scientific documents for use in standard settings; investigates health and safety hazards in workplaces on request

Agency for Toxic Substances and Disease Registry (ATSDR) (E33), Division of Health Education, Office of the Director, 1600 Clifton Rd. NE, Atlanta, GA 30333; (404) 639-6204.

Written reference materials

American College of Obstetricians and Gynecologists/National Institute for Occupational Safety and Health: Guidelines on Pregnancy and Work. Washington, DC, U.S. Government Printing Office, 1977

Barlow SM, Sullivan F: Reproductive Hazards of Industrial Chemicals. New York, Academic Press, 1982

Brown NA, Scialli AR (eds): Reproductive Toxicology: A Medical Letter on Environmental Hazards to Reproduction. Published bimonthly by the Reproductive Toxicology Center, 2425 L Street NW, Washington, DC

Clarkson TW, Nordberg G, Sager PR (eds): Reproductive and Developmental Toxicity of Metals. New York, Plenum Press, 1983

National Institute for Occupational Safety and Health: Registry of Toxic Effects of Chemical Substances, September 1980, with Supplement 1983–84. Washington, DC, U.S. Government Printing Office, DHHS-86-103, November 1985

Shepard TH: Catalog of Teratogenic Agents. Baltimore, The Johns Hopkins University Press, 1986

U.S. Congress, Office of Technology Assessment: Reproductive Hazards in the Workplace. Washington, DC, U.S. Government Printing Office, OTA-BA-266, December 1985

From Paul M, Himmelstein J: Reproductive hazards in the workplace: What the practitioner needs to know about chemical exposures. Obstet Gynecol 71:921–938, 1988, with permission.

TABLE 5.   Occupational History

Current work
  Job title
  Employer
  Duration of employment
  Description of job tasks
  Potential exposures
    Chemical (vapors, fumes, dusts)
    Physical (noise, prolonged standing, heavy lifting)
    Biologic (cytomegalovirus)
    Psychological (stress)
  Protective measures used to minimize exposures, e.g., personal protective equipment (gloves, respirator), engineering controls (ventilation, lifting devices)
  If symptomatic, temporal relationship of symptoms to work exposures

Previous work: details as for current work may be relevant for chemical exposures with prolonged biologic half-lives (e.g., lead, lipid-soluble substances)

Nonoccupational exposures
  Personal habits (e.g., smoking, drug use)
  Community exposures (via air or water contamination)
  Exposure to hazardous substances owing to occupational exposure of family members (e.g., lead or asbestos dust)
  Hobbies

From Paul M, Himmelstein J: Reproductive hazards in the workplace: What the practitioner needs to know about chemical exposures. Obstet Gynecol 71:928, 1988, with permission.

TABLE 6.   Guidelines for Continuation of Various Levels of Work During Pregnancy*

Job Function		Week of Gestation
Secretarial and light clerical		40
Professional and managerial		40
Sitting with light tasks		
Prolonged	(>4 hr)	40
Intermittent		40
Standing		
Prolonged	(>4 hr)	24
Intermittent	(>30 min/hr)	32
	(<30 min/hr)	40
Stooping and bending below knee level		
Repetitive	(>10 times/hr)	20
Intermittent	(<10 >2 times/hr)	28
	(<2 times/hr)	40
Climbing		
Vertical ladders and poles		
Repetitive	(≥4 times/8-hr shift)	20
Intermittent	(<4 times/8-hr shift)	28
Stairs		
Repetitive	(≥4 times/8-hr shift)	28
Intermittent	(<4 times/8-hr shift)	40
Lifting		
Repetitive	>23 kg	20
	<23 >11 kg	24
	<11 kg	40
Intermittent	>23 kg	30
	<14 >11 kg	40
	>11 kg	40

* Note: These guidelines are based on opinions of experts and not on well-done studies evaluating risks and benefits (which do not exist).
From AMA Council on Scientific Affairs: Effects of pregnancy on work performance. JAMA 251: 1996, 1984, with permission.

TABLE 7. Suggested Breast-Feeding Guidelines for Occupational Exposures

Substance	Guidelines	Comments
Mercury	OK to breastfeed if milk mercury <4 mg/L	Only chemical for which the FDA has set clear guidelines in milk
PCBs and related compounds	Acute effects unlikely at any tolerated maternal blood level	Unless large ingestion, breast-feeding can continue in most cases
Organic solvents	Avoid maternal exposure; temporarily stop breastfeeding for acute exposure (express and discard)	Most are excreted relatively rapidly; breastfeeding may resume several days after exposure
Lead	Women with lead exposure should have blood and breast milk lead levels determined as should their newborn infants. Lead levels >10 mg/dL in infants are associated with adverse outcomes	Ratio of breast milk to blood lead is reported to be approximately 1 but is highly variable. Breast-feeding may be done if breast milk and infant lead levels are monitored. Maternal lead exposure should be terminated

From Paul M, Himmelstein J: Reproductive hazards in the workplace: What the practitioner needs to know about chemical exposures. Obstet Gynecol 71:921–938, 1988, with permission.

References

1. Agency for Toxic Substances and Disease Registry: Exposure to hazardous substances and reproductive health. Am Fam Physician 48:1442–1448, 1993.
2. Barman MR: Guidelines on time off work. Contemp Obstet Gynecol, April, 81–82, 1984.
3. Paul M, Himmelstein J: Reproductive hazards in the workplace: What the practitioner needs to know about chemical exposures. Obstet Gynecol 71:921–938, 1988.

SECTION B.
PSYCHOSOCIAL INTERVENTIONS

Elizabeth G. Baxley, M.D.

The relationship between psychosocial risk factors and birth outcomes is well-established, with specific maternal behaviors and experiences demonstrated to relate to adverse pregnancy outcomes.[11] Sociocultural factors that have been shown to directly influence the quality of prenatal care include unstable income, insurance status, and negative attitudes toward health care providers. Additionally, denial of the pregnancy, negative attitudes toward being pregnant, and the perception that prenatal care is not important may cause women to delay seeking prenatal care.[14,17]

Late entry into prenatal care, or not seeking prenatal care, is most common among women with unplanned pregnancy or those who perceive the pregnancy negatively. According to data collected by the CDC in their ongoing Pregnancy Risk Assessment Monitoring System (PRAMS), the prevalence of unintended pregnancy resulting in a live-born infant ranged from 33.9% to 50% depending on geographic location of the women studied.[11] In most states, women who were younger, had less than a high-school education, were African-American, and received Medicaid were more likely to report an unintended pregnancy and were less likely to seek prenatal care early in the pregnancy, or not at all.

Psychosocial risk factors during the antenatal period may also herald *postpartum* morbidity. Child abuse and postpartum abuse of the mother by her partner were more strongly correlated with a history of lack of social support, recent life stressors, psychiatric disturbance in the mother, and an unwanted pregnancy.[31]

I. Interventions

A. Aid to Families with Dependent Children (AFDC) / Medicaid

These programs provide reimbursement for physician services and prenatal care. SOBRA legislation has expanded eligibility for maternity services, up to 185% of poverty level, to provide coverage for the "working poor" and married women of low socioeconomic status. In many cases, this expanded eligibility removed historical barriers to care, although in some settings limited access still exists owing to a limited number of providers who accept Medicaid. Medicaid also provides retroactive coverage for treatment of potentially life-threatening conditions, such as childbirth, to nonresidents. This emergency Medicaid (E-Med) program is a needed source of funding for patients and clinicians serving a large number of immigrants.

Medicaid programs for maternity care vary in their comprehensiveness. An evaluation of expanded Medicaid coverage in Tennessee showed more targeted women covered by Medicaid but no improvement in early prenatal care, birth weight, or neonatal mortality, although the power of the study was insufficient to exclude differences in the last two outcomes.[27] The bulk of the poor outcomes continue to occur in women who have been traditionally eligible for Medicaid.[4] Historical evaluations have suggested that Medicaid has produced some incremental improvement in outcome in those populations.[4,5]

B. WIC/Food Stamps

WIC is a supplemental feeding program that provides nutritional supplementation for low-income women and their children. It should be offered to all eligible pregnant women where available. The program's effectiveness in improving pregnancy outcomes has been questioned, but some statewide programs have demonstrated improvement.[18,22] It is important to provide strong educational support for breastfeeding in conjunction with the WIC program because the financial incentive of the program has historically favored bottle-feeding over breastfeeding. However, new mothers can receive supplemental WIC vouchers to ensure the adequacy of their own nutrition throughout breastfeeding, and the WIC program now actively promotes breast milk as the ideal nutrition for newborns.

C. Social Service

A team approach to prenatal care involves effective use of other health care providers. Licensed medical social workers (LMSWs) provide evaluation and referral for patients, linking them to resources such as parenting classes, housing assistance, financial aid, domestic violence shelters, and child care facilities. Social workers also may serve an important role as effective family and individual counselors or case managers. Many of the needs addressed by social workers cannot be adequately met by prenatal providers alone in the context of the traditional prenatal visit. These services are often reimbursable through the Medicaid system.

D. Psychosocial Support

Adverse psychosocial conditions that are known to negatively affect pregnancy and childbearing outcomes include poverty, single parenthood, teenage pregnancy, lack of social support, family dysfunction, substance abuse, and physical or sexual abuse. Higher rates of low-birth-weight infants, medical complications of pregnancy, and postpartum depression are seen in women with these risk factors (Table 8).[13,17] Psychosocial risk factors during the antenatal period may also herald *postpartum* morbidity. Even for high-risk neonates (newborn intensive care unit graduates), the most powerful predictor of functioning in later life is quality of family function and structure rather than complications in the neonatal period.[2]

The prevalence of adverse perinatal outcomes also varies among ethnic groups. African-American infants are 4.5 times more likely than white infants to die as a result of low birth weight, and African-American and Hispanic women are less

TABLE 8. Adverse Pregnancy and Parenting Outcomes Associated with Adverse Psychosocial Conditions

Maternal	Adolescent/adult
Increased maternal stress	Physical/sexual abuse
Medical complications of pregnancy and childbirth	Substance use/abuse
Postpartum depression	Poor school performance/limited
Infant	educational achievement
Low birth weight (and associated neonatal morbidity	Premature sexual activity
and mortality)	Second-generation teen pregnancy
Poor attendance at well-child visits	Single parenthood
Delayed or absent immunization	Poor attachment to the labor force
Increased infant morbidity and mortality	Limited earning potential
Growth (failure to thrive) and development delay	Criminality
Child	
Decreased immunization rates	
Increased childhood morbidity	
Child abuse	
Poor school performance	

likely than white women to obtain prenatal care in the first trimester.[14] Specific interventions aimed at providing social support, facilitating access to care, health education, and encouragement to verbalize feelings about problems have been shown to be significantly associated with the number of problems that pregnant African-American women have been able to resolve during prenatal care.[17]

It has been postulated that providing psychosocial services beyond basic medical care may ameliorate some of these adverse outcomes. Yet, interventions for psychosocial problems remain an area of investigational interest. RCTs of psychosocial support (including emotional support, tangible assistance, and information/instruction) in the home, clinic, or over the phone have not been shown to improve rates of low birth weight or any other important medical outcome of pregnancy.[20] While some improvement in immediate psychosocial outcomes has been demonstrated, longer follow-up is needed to provide real evidence for an overall significant enhancement in pregnancy outcomes.

Provider attention to psychosocial risks and interventions may play a significant role in the ultimate success or failure of these interventions to positively influence pregnancy outcomes. In one study, half of couples interviewed considered the information and instruction they received prenatally to be inadequate in the areas of marital adjustment, changing sexual life, adjustment of siblings, father's preparation for parenthood, and postpartum fatigue.[21] In caring for pregnant women, the family physician's role should extend beyond routine medical care of the pregnancy to include a focus on each expectant parent and the new family relationship that is developing. Socially high-risk prenatal patients and their families should be identified early and monitored closely throughout, to help increase compliance with recommendations and foster improved pregnancy outcomes.

E. Comprehensive Prenatal Care

Comprehensive prenatal care has been defined as care that includes medical, nutritional, and psychosocial components on site, with outreach services as needed, to enhance delivery and compliance. Federal funding for prenatal care for indigent women encourages states to provide funding mechanisms for systems of comprehensive prenatal care.

Cohort-based studies of comprehensive prenatal care versus routine medical model prenatal care have shown a decreased rate of low birth weight and adverse short-term pregnancy outcomes, but populations studied were not comparable.[4,5] A greater percentage of the patients in the routine care cohorts were of low socioeconomic status or increased medical risk, making interpretation of these studies difficult to apply to all patients. Many state and community agencies are currently engaged in joint ventures with medical care providers to provide systems of comprehensive care and study their outcomes in patients of varying medical and psychosocial risk.

II. Domestic Violence

Physical and sexual abuse are commonly encountered in women of childbearing age, with 4–17% reporting domestic violence or battering during the current pregnancy.[7,8,15,16,24] Approximately 40–45% of all battered women are victims of sexual abuse by their partners.[9,12,14] Despite this prevalence, a history of abuse is frequently not elicited, either because providers may be uncomfortable in asking questions about violence or because some women are reluctant to discuss the abuse they suffer. The single most important thing a physician can do for a battered woman is to ask about violence.[1,6]

There is often an increase in domestic violence in the postpartum period. Child abuse and postpartum abuse of the mother by her partner have been strongly correlated with lack of social support, recent life stressors, psychiatric disturbance in the mother, and unwanted pregnancy.[31] Intervening to prevent domestic violence has been said to be the single best way to combat child abuse.[12]

A. Risk Factors

Risk factors for physical or sexual abuse include substance abuse in the patient, partner, or other family members; unmarried status; and history of abuse in the patient's family of origin.

B. Clinical Clues

Abused pregnant women often postpone prenatal care or have a complete lack of prenatal care. For those who do seek prenatal care, a variety of signs and symptoms are associated with physical or sexual abuse, and may afford the provider with clinical clues to domestic violence prior to the recognition of obvious immediate sequelae (Table 9).

C. Possible Obstetric Consequences

Injuries resulting from abuse in pregnant women may be more directed at the pregnancy. The face and abdomen are struck more frequently, the latter presumed to be in an attempt to induce pregnancy loss.[3,10,19,30] Victims of domestic abuse are often concomitantly the victims of sexual abuse, with injury directed toward the breasts and genitals.[25]

Few good-quality studies exist that measure perinatal outcomes in women who have been victims of abuse. Two studies do suggest an increased incidence of low birth weight as a result of physical abuse.[26] Clinical impressions suggest numerous possible consequences, including either resistance to caregivers or late prenatal care versus overcompliance and frequent calls or visits that may herald a patient's cry for help. Appearance of dissociation or withdrawal, difficulty tolerating vaginal examinations and other invasive procedures, perception of difficult labor, and failure to progress in labor are other findings associated with perinatal violence.[24,25]

TABLE 9.   Clinical Clues to a History of Physical or Sexual Abuse

Physical Abuse	Early onset of consensual sexual activity
Anxiety	Gynecologic problems, including chronic pelvic pain
Depression	Multiple medical problems
Posttraumatic stress syndrome	Obesity
Sleeping and eating disorders	Poor self-esteem
Substance use and abuse	Promiscuity
Recurrent vaginal infections	Prostitution
Sexual abuse	Recurrent surgeries (possibly unnecessary)
Abdominal pain, chronic and recurrent	Somatization and dissociation
Depression	Substance use and abuse

TABLE 10. Abuse Assessment Screen

1. Have you ever been emotionally or physically abused by your partner or someone important to you (someone in your family)?
2. As a child, have you been hit, slapped, kicked, or otherwise physically hurt by someone?
3. Within the last year, have you been hit, slapped, kicked, or otherwise physically hurt by someone?
4. Since you have been pregnant, have you been hit, slapped, kicked, or otherwise physically hurt by someone?
    Score the most severe incident according to the following scale:
    1 = Threats of abuse, including use of a weapon
    2 = Slapping, pushing; no injuries and/or lasting pain
    3 = Punching, kicking, bruises, cuts, and/or continuing pain
    4 = Beaten up, severe contusions, burns, broken bones
    5 = Head, internal, and/or permanent injury
    6 = Use of weapon, wound from weapon
5. As a child, did anyone force you to have sexual activities?
6. Within the last year, has anyone forced you to have sexual activities?
7. Since you have been pregnant, has anyone forced you to have sexual activities?
8. Are you afraid of your partner or anyone you listed above?
9. If you were forced to have sex as a child or adult or physically hurt as an adult or child, did you tell any one about it? If so, who?
10. If you did tell someone about your abuse, how well supported did you feel?
11. Have you received counseling for either the abuse that you have experienced or the aftereffects of the abuse?
12. Who is your primary source of emotional support?
13. Do you feel well (or poorly) supported by that person (those people)?

D. Identification

Case finding or screening for abuse has been established as a standard of care and is consistent with the goals of family-centered perinatal care. McFarlane has developed and validated a simple Abuse Assessment Screen for identifying current abuse in pregnant women.[24] A modified McFarlane's Abuse Assessment Screen helps to identify women who have been victimized as children as well (Table 10). Improved surveillance and inquiry will foster earlier and higher rates of recognition, providing opportunities for intervention prior to an adverse pregnancy outcome.

E. Acute Interventions During Routine Prenatal Visits

Often, much encouragement and support are needed before a woman who is a victim of abuse gains the necessary self-esteem to seek help. Pregnancy may provide an opportunity to intervene that would have been rejected previously, as women may be more willing to leave an abusive situation if they believe their children are at risk. For those women not ready to accept help from the health care team, questions regarding abuse should be asked in a nonjudgmental manner at each subsequent visit. It may be helpful to find out if these women have ever confided in anyone else about their victimization and what the response was, or if they have ever had counseling or participated in support groups for abused women.

Counseling for women who are victims of abuse should be directed at providing the following:

1. Reassurance that they are not at fault and are not alone.
2. Knowledge regarding the recurrent and progressive nature of abuse, including information about how repetitive patterns of abuse may affect families and children.
3. Encouragement to find a safe living situation immediately, either with friends, relatives, or a local women's shelter.

4. Encouragement to undergo counseling or join support groups of women in similar situations.

F. Intrapartum

Active labor is a difficult time to inquire about abuse. However, some clues exist that may suggest abuse in cases in which the provider was previously unaware of a pattern of violence. One of the first indications may be difficulty tolerating vaginal examinations out of proportion to that which results from the pain of labor. If abuse is discovered in this case, an attempt should be made to minimize vaginal examinations, have a female companion or nursing staff member present for all vaginal examinations, consider alternatives (e.g., ultrasound to rule out breech), and speak in a reassuring manner during the examination. If it is early in the labor, it may be appropriate to raise the issue of abuse in a confidential manner. Normalizing the problem ("Many women have trouble with vaginal examinations"), identifying abuse as a possible cause for their difficulty with the examination ("Some of them have been physically or sexually abused in the past"), commenting on the frequency of abuse in pregnant women, and giving them an opportunity to respond may facilitate discovery of domestic violence that has occurred during the pregnancy. Simply raising the issue in a sensitive, supportive manner may enable labor to proceed more smoothly.

Making suggestions to relax or using visual imagery of opening or letting go may make the abused woman more anxious in labor. Women who have been abused often have been told to relax while being abused and are afraid to let go or lose control. Distraction techniques (such as Lamaze) are probably better methods for psychoprophylaxis during labor for these women.[29]

Lack of progress or arrest of progress in labor without apparent physiologic or anatomic cause may relate to a history of abuse.[29] Sedation in early labor or an epidural in active labor may help. Exploration of the issue at a later time, such as during routine postpartum care in the hospital, or at an outpatient postpartum checkup or well-child visit, is warranted. In-hospital assessment and timely intervention may be indicated when level of suspicion or family circumstances dictate.

G. Postpartum

Poor bonding or postpartum depression may suggest a past or current abuse. Inquiring about symptoms and identifying abuse as a possible factor may encourage a woman to confide about abuse to her health care provider. She should be informed that children in the family are at risk for abuse, and that help is available for her, her newborn, and any other children in the household. Social service agencies and caregivers should be alert to the potential for child abuse.

References

1. Ambuel B, Brownell EE, Hamberger LK: Implementing a community model for training medical students and physicians to diagnose, treat, and prevent family violence. In Program of the Society of Teachers of Family Medicine Conference on Violence Education. Albuquerque, NM, November 1994.
2. Barnard KE: Caring for high-risk infants and their families. Presented at Symposium on Psychosocial Aspects of the Family: The New Pediatrics, cosponsored by the Department of Pediatrics, Indiana University School of Medicine and the Institute for Pediatric Service, Johnson & Johnson Co., Chicago, 1984.
3. Bereson AB, Stiglich NJ, Wilkinson GS, et al: Drug abuse and other risk factors for physical abuse in pregnancy among white, non-Hispanic, black, and Hispanic women. Am J Obstet Gynecol 164:1491, 1991.
4. Buescher PA, Smith C, Holliday, JL, et al: Source of prenatal care and infant birth weight: The case of a North Carolina county. Am J Obstet Gynecol 156:204–210, 1987.
5. Buescher PA, Ward NI: A comparison of low birth weight among Medicaid patients of public health departments and other providers of prenatal care in North Carolina and Kentucky. Pub Health Rep 107:54–59, 1992.
6. Burge SK: Violence against women. Prim Clin Office Pract 24:67–81, 1997.
7. Campbell J, Poland M, Waller J, et al. Correlates of battering during pregnancy. Res Nurs Health 15:219-226, 1992.

8. Campbell JC, Lewandowski LA: Mental and physical health effects of intimate partner violence on women and children. Psychiatric Clin North Am 20:353–374, 1997.
9. Campbell JC, Oliver C, Bullock L: Why battering during pregnancy? AWHONN 4:343, 1993.
10. Campbell JC, Alford P: The dark consequences of marital rape. Am J Nurs 89:946–949, 1989.
11. Colley Gilbert BJ, Johnson CH, Morrow B, et al: I. Prevalence of selected maternal and infant characteristics, Pregnancy Risk Assessment Monitoring System (PRAMS), 1997. Mor Mortal Wkly Rep CDC Surveill Summ 48:1–37, 1999.
12. Datner EM, Ferroggiaro AA: Violence during pregnancy. Emerg Med Clin North Am 17:646–656, 1999.
13. Dowling PT, Fisher M: Maternal factors and low birthweight infants: A comparison of African Americans with Mexican-Americans. J Fam Pract 25:153–158, 1987.
14. Fields, S. Family-centered maternity care. In JW Saultz (ed): Textbook of Family Medicine: Defining and Examining the Discipline. McGraw-Hill, 2000, pp 455–471.
15. Gazmararian JA, Lazorick MD, Spitz A, et al: Prevalence of violence against pregnant women. Am J Public Health 275:1915–1920, 1996.
16. Gielen AC, O'Campo P, Faden R, et al: Interpersonal conflict and physical violence during the childbearing years. Soc Sci Med 39:781–787, 1994.
17. Gonzalez-Calvo J, Jackson J, Hansford C, et al: Psychosocial factors and birth outcome: African-American women in case management. J Health Care Poor Underserved 9:395–419, 1998.
18. Graham GE: WIC: A food program that fails. The Public Interest, Spring, 1991.
19. Helton A, McFarlane J, Anderson ET: Battered and pregnant: A prevalence study. Am J Public Health 77:1337–1339, 1987.
20. Hodnett ED: Support from caregivers during at-risk pregnancy. In Enkin MJ, Keirse MJNC, Renfrew MJ, Neilson JP (eds): Pregnancy and Childbirth Module. Cochrane Database of Systematic Reviews: Review No. 04169. Published through Cochrane Updates on Disk, Oxford, Update Software, 1993.
21. Hostetter H, Andolsek KM: Psychosocial issues in pregnancy. In Andolsek KM (ed): Obstetric Care: Standards of Prenatal, Intrapartum, and Postpartum Management. Philadelphia, Lea & Febiger, 1990.
22. Kotelchuck M, Schwartz JB, Anderka MT, et al: WIC participation and pregnancy outcomes: Massachusetts statewide evaluation project. Am J Pub Health 74:1086–1092, 1984.
23. McFarlane J: Battering during pregnancy: Tip of an iceberg revealed. Women Health 15:69–84, 1989.
24. McFarlane J, Parker B, Soken K, et al: Assessing for abuse during pregnancy: Severity and frequency of injuries and associated entry into prenatal care. JAMA 267:3176–3178, 1992.
25. Newberger EH, et al: Abuse of pregnant women and adverse birth outcome: Current knowledge and implications for practice. JAMA 267:2370–2372, 1992.
26. Parker B, McFarlane J, Soken K: Abuse during pregnancy: Effect on maternal complications and birth weight in adult and teenage women. Obstet Gynecol 84:323–328, 1994.
27. Piper JM, Ray WA, Griffin MR: The effects of Medicaid eligibility expansion on prenatal care and pregnancy outcome in Tennessee. JAMA 264:2219–2223, 1990.
28. Russell DE: The incidence and prevalence of intrafamilial and extrafamilial sexual abuse of female children. Child Abuse Negl 7:133–146, 1983.
30. Simpkins P: Childhood sexual abuse and its effects on pregnant women: Treating survivors of childhood sexual abuse. Presentation at the 1992 Birth Conference, Boston, 1992.
31. Stewart DE, Cecutti A: Physical abuse in pregnancy. Can Med Assoc J 149:1257, 1993.
32. Wilson LM, Reid AJ, Midmer DK, et al: Antenatal psychosocial risk factors associated with adverse postpartum family outcomes. CMAJ 154:785–799, 1996.

SECTION C.
ADOLESCENT PREGNANCY INTERVENTIONS

V. Leigh Beasley, M.D.

The pregnant adolescent often presents to her primary care provider with both psychosocial needs and biomedical risks. While these needs are often formidable for the individual maternity care provider, family physicians are well suited to care for pregnant adolescents and assist them in preparation for parenthood. Coordinating adolescent prenatal care with social workers, drug and alcohol counselors, nutritionists, family counselors, child birth educators, breastfeeding counselors, clergy and the school system will assist the individual practitioner in caring for these challenging patients and optimize the outcome for both mother and child.

I. Historical Perspective/Incidence

Historically, adolescent fertility rates have tended to follow trends in pregnancy rates for all women of childbearing age except for young women 10–14 years old, a group for whom the fertility rate has been steadily increasing. Birth rates to all adolescents increased sharply in the late 1980s, but subsequently declined for American teenagers from 1991–1997, falling to 16% for age group 15–17 and 11% for age group 18–19.[13] Despite these decreases, pregnancy and birth rates for adolescents in the U.S remain among the highest in industrialized countries. In 1995, 101.1 per 1000 teenagers age 15–19 became pregnant, and 54.4 per 1000 young women gave birth.

A. Increasing Importance of Adolescent Pregnancy

Several factors explain why adolescent pregnancy is perceived to be an increasing problem.

1. Over the last 20 years, total birth rates have fallen much more than adolescent birth rates. Therefore, births to adolescents make up a larger proportion of all births.
2. An increasing proportion of adolescent pregnancies occur in unmarried young women, resulting in a rising birth rate for single teens (Table 11). This coupled with a falling marriage rate (both preconception and postconception) for this age group makes teen pregnancy part of the larger social problem of single parenthood.[1]
3. Adoption is less common.
4. Employment opportunities for adolescents are generally limited by the fact that more pregnant teens do not complete high school.
5. Adolescent pregnancy costs American taxpayers $16.6 billion dollars per year in Aid to Families with Dependent Children (AFDC), Medicaid, and food stamps.[14]

B. Contributing Factors to Adolescent Pregnancy

Many single adolescents who are at risk for pregnancy may be identified in advance through a careful history (Table 12). Most adolescent sexual activity is not planned or anticipated. It is more the result of age-appropriate lack of anticipation of future consequences. In some cases the pregnancy is actually planned, hoped for, or desired. In these situations, the single adolescent may have unrealistic expectations of what a baby will do for her (e.g., love her, get her out of a bad home situation, cause her boyfriend to marry her, make her feel good about herself). These young mothers-to-be are often not knowledgeable about the demands of parenthood or realistic about their ability to meet them.

The pregnant adolescent may also be cognitively ill-prepared to consider long-term consequences for herself and her baby, a skill that is helpful in dealing with the challenges of pregnancy and parenthood. One intervention, known as previewing, helps

TABLE 11. Birth Rates (per 1000) for Unmarried and Married Women Ages 15–19, 1940–1988

Year	Unmarried	Married
1940	7.4	—
1950	12.6	410
1960	15.1	530
1970	22.4	443
1980	27.5	350
1988	36.8	378

U.S. Department HEW, PHS, National Office of Vital Statistics: Vital Statistics of the U.S. 1990, Vol. 1. Washington, DC, GPO, 1994.

TABLE 12. Factors Associated with Adolescent Pregnancy

Personal Characteristics	Family Characteristics
Smoking	Divorced or single parent
Drinking alcohol	Alcoholic or substance-abusing parent
Using drugs	Other family dysfunction
Victim of physical or sexual abuse	Domestic violence
Few religious ties	History of sexual abuse
Regularly unsupervised after school	
Poor or no relationship with father	

pregnant teens to think about future events with their child and gives them an opportunity to "practice" their responses to certain situations. Use of this technique may assist the teen parent and health care provider in together identifying potential problems involving pregnancy and parenting, so that positive solutions can be developed.[12]

II. Developmental Concerns

The pregnant adolescent must face the challenges of her own age-specific developmental tasks (e.g., individuation, autonomy, and vocational choices) while at the same time taking on the demands of parenting and guiding her child's development. As the age of menarche has become younger, there is a larger "gap" between the physical development of most teens and their cognitive and emotional development. Inquiring about the reason(s) that a teen patient gives for becoming pregnant may help identify some of her own developmental needs that have not been met. By identifying these needs, health care professionals can design interventions that address patient-specific developmental needs.[7]

III. Increased Risks of Adolescent Pregnancy
A. Adolescent

The incidence of sexually transmitted diseases (particularly among single adolescents), late onset of prenatal care, preterm labor, cephalopelvic disproportion, and possibly pregnancy-induced hypertension (especially in women < 16, although this may be related to race and primigravid state, rather than age) is increased in pregnant adolescents.

Pregnancy often results in curtailed educational achievement and poverty for many single teenage mothers. It also typically results in single parenthood for at least part of their childrearing years.

B. Infant/Child

Pregnant adolescents have higher rates of prematurity and deliver more low-birthweight infants than older women. Many of their children grow up in poverty. Multiple factors converge to cause higher rates of poor school performance, child abuse and neglect, poor work history, single parenthood, and, for boys in particular, criminal behavior among offspring of adolescent mothers.

IV. Management Principles
A. Family Considerations

Adolescent pregnancy may represent a family crisis or may be considered a cultural norm, with variation in responses among different families. As such, it presents an opportunity for the physician to identify latent family problems that may have increased the likelihood of the pregnancy occurring. In doing so, attitudes of blame should be avoided, as they hinder the necessary acceptance of responsibility and ability to change dysfunctional patterns.

B. Concurrent Psychosocial Risks

The presence of other psychosocial risk factors such as substance abuse and domestic violence should be assessed, with interventions as indicated. One in five pregnant adolescents report physical or sexual abuse. Abused teens tend to enter prenatal care later, often in the third trimester. Abuse during pregnancy has been shown to be a significant risk factor for low birth weight, low maternal weight gain, first- or second-trimester bleeding, smoking and the use of drugs and alcohol.[6]

Health care providers need to be aware of the risk of increased interpersonal violence in the pregnant teen's life and actively screen patients for this. Short abuse assessment screens are available (Table 10). When issues of abuse are identified, the health care provider must be familiar with referral sources, such as individual and family counselors and "safe houses."

C. Extended Family

Involvement of the extended family, especially grandparents, may be an essential contributor to the well-being of both the adolescent parent and child. Data suggest improved short-term to intermediate-term outcome for high-risk children if living with a grandmother.[8]

D. Social Isolation

Teenagers who are living alone or with friends typically have poor social support. Pregnant teens often face difficulty in locating appropriate housing and reliable transportation. Maternity care providers and other members of the health care team should conduct ongoing assessments of patient support systems and provide referral and individualized help as indicated. The Friends and Family Apgar is one validated tool that has been applied to a variety of ethnic groups and measures a woman's perception of support for her family and friends (Table 13).[9,10]

E. Role of Education

All pregnant adolescents should be asked about their educational and vocational plans, and should be encouraged to complete at least secondary education in order to enhance their employability in the future. Most pregnant teens recognize the importance of education and remaining in school. One study found school dropout

TABLE 13. Friends and Family Apgar Scoring System

Please fill out the following section to help us understand your family/friend support. "Family" means the person with whom you usually live. If you live alone your "family" means the person whom you feel closest to emotionally.

For each question, check only one box:

	Never	Hardly Ever	Some of the Time	Almost Always	Always
I am satisfied that I can turn to my family for help when something is troubling me					
I am satisfied with the way that my family talks over things with me and shares problems with me					
I am satisfied that my family accepts and supports my wishes to take on new activities and directions					
I am satisfied with the way my family expresses affection and responds to my feelings, such as anger, sadness, and love					
I am satisfied with the way my family and I share time together					
I have a close friend to whom I can turn for help					
I am satisfied with the support I receive from family and friends					

rates to be more strongly related to sociocultural factors than individual characteristics (such as emotional support or psychological well-being). Dropouts in this study tended to be white and had lower family incomes.[11] Many teen parents are eligible to participate in night school or adult educational programs to earn their GED or high school diploma.

Childbirth education, nutritional assessment and counseling (particularly looking for evidence of eating disorders), parenting classes, and encouragement and education for breastfeeding are also important for both the pregnant adolescent and her partner.

F. Continuity of Care

Adolescents, in particular, benefit from continuity of prenatal care providers. Teenagers may fail to get early and continuous prenatal care for many reasons: fear of informing family members about the pregnancy, denial of the pregnancy itself, lack of knowledge about the availability and importance of prenatal care, economic concerns, or transportation problems. Pregnant teens typically experience a range of emotions during the course of prenatal care, including fear, denial, anger, and excitement.

Prenatal care of the teen must address medical, social, and emotional concerns. Scheduling appointments every 2–3 weeks instead of the traditional monthly visits may be beneficial in addressing all the various needs of the pregnant teen and her family. Pregnant adolescents may also benefit from seeing one or two trusted providers who can better coordinate the variety of services the teen may need. A team approach among the family physician and a social worker, registered nurse, or other allied health care provider can be helpful in addressing *all* aspects of caring for the pregnant teen.

Teen mothers should be followed closely in the immediate postpartum period. The traditional 6-week postpartum visit may be too late to address issues such as resumed sexual activity, the need for birth control, breastfeeding problems, postpartum stress or depression, and infant care. Ideally, teens should be seen within 2 weeks of delivery to address these concerns. Studies have shown improved maternal and infant outcomes by using home health nursing visits during the immediate postpartum period.[3,4] An intensive early intervention program in which teens received 4 prenatal classes and approximately 17 home visits during the prenatal and postpartum period demonstrated a reduction in premature births to teens and a reduction in infant hospitalization during the first 6 weeks postpartum.[4]

G. Decision Making

Adolescents have often made decisions regarding the fate of their pregnancy before seeking medical care. Nonetheless, many benefit from the opportunity to discuss their feelings about adoption, child rearing, or abortion. A sensitive and nonjudgmental approach is most appropriate when discussing short-term and long-term consequences for the mother and her child. Providing a pregnant teen with accurate information regarding all available medical options will help guide her decisions. In order to establish a trusting, therapeutic relationship, the physician should explain the confidential nature of any of their interactions.

Close follow-up is necessary regardless of the teen's final decision regarding the pregnancy, as she may face coercion, blame, or anger from her family or her partner. Counseling issues often cannot be adequately addressed in the constraints of prenatal office scheduling; referring the woman for more intensive supportive or crisis counseling in these situations is appropriate.

H. Parenting Skills

Family physicians should coordinate ongoing efforts (classes, one-on-one counseling) of the health care team in order to help prepare the adolescent and her partner for the responsibilities of parenthood. These efforts should extend throughout the first several years after childbirth.

I. Breastfeeding

Breastfeeding should be encouraged for adolescents even though they are historically less inclined to breastfeed. There is evidence of improved bonding between mother and child for breastfed infants. Breastfeeding also helps to teach and reinforce good nutritional concepts for the adolescent mother, causing her to focus on her own nutrition and that of her baby. Adolescent mothers who breastfeed may derive some personal developmental benefit from having successfully accomplished this task. This enhanced self-esteem and sense of competency may subsequently provide long-term benefits for the entire family unit.

Issues surrounding breastfeeding and returning to work or school are important to address. A teen mother may need to schedule classes so she can have breaks to "pump" or feed her baby. Ensuring a comfortable and private place for nursing or pumping may be difficult for the teen; family physicians should advocate for young mothers with the local school system in order to support higher breastfeeding rates. Educating school administrators about the superiority of breastfeeding as a feeding choice will often help break down barriers that young mothers are unable to accomplish.

J. Role of Father

It is essential to ascertain the current and intended level of involvement and commitment demonstrated by father of the child. Although long-term benefits of involving the father in prenatal care and education have not been demonstrated, doing so is often beneficial in individual cases. Many young fathers are intimidated by the clinic or office setting and may not feel welcome. Fathers who desire involvement in prenatal visits should be strongly encouraged to do so. The opportunity to "hear the baby's heartbeat" using the Doppler and "see the baby" during an ultrasound examination may help the father to bond more closely with the unborn child. Pregnant adolescents should be asked if they are comfortable with the involvement of the baby's father in the exam room. During each visit the adolescent should have time alone with a health care provider when she can voice any concerns or problems relating to an abusive situation.

K. Labor Support

Labor support is important for the adolescent patient. Experienced supportive family members or friends, doulas, trained labor and delivery nurses, and the physician in attendance during the labor may all function in this role. Attendance at childbirth preparation classes will facilitate the teen mother's effective use of labor support persons.

L. Postpartum

During the postpartum period, strategies for caring for teen parents should include the following.

1. Home visits

Regular home visits by health professionals over a 2-year period have demonstrated improved child health and development outcomes.[3,4]

2. Follow-up

Initiating follow-up 2–3 days after hospital discharge instead of the traditional 2-week infant visit or 6-week postpartum visit. Adolescents are at increased risk to discontinue breastfeeding prematurely and need increased levels of nursing and medical support to sustain this activity, as well as to screen for postpartum emotional disorders and possible child abuse. This may take the form of home health care nursing follow-up or a short office visit to check for jaundice, breastfeeding problems, etc.

3. Teens who select adoption

For teen mothers who have selected adoption, there is increasing recognition of the grief process that accompanies this process. Many adoption agencies provide postadoption counseling to help deal with the grief response. Physicians should play an important role in facilitating this process.

4. Family planning

The risks and benefits of abstinence and other methods of birth control must be fully explored with each patient and every effort should be made to promote follow-up and compliance with the plan. From 1991–1997 there has been a 21% decrease in the rate of second births to teens. Discussion of future contraceptive use should be initiated during the prenatal visits so that the patient can be familiar with her options following delivery. Inquiring about past difficulty in remembering to take prenatal vitamins may predict success or failure in using birth control pills and lead the patient and physician to consider other contraceptive methods. New long-term contraceptive methods may be appropriate for the adolescent mother.

5. Rapid repeat pregnancy

Rapid repeat pregnancy, defined as a pregnancy occurring within 12–24 months of the previous pregnancy, has been associated with physical or sexual abuse and higher rates of low-birth-weight infants among low-income adolescents.[2] Information gained from such studies emphasizes the need for close follow-up and continued care of the pregnant adolescent after delivery.

References

1. Fredrick, I: Teenage Pregnancy. Presentation at Scientific Assembly, New York State Academy of Family Physicians, Sarasota Springs, 1989.
2. Jacoby M, Gorenflo D, Black E, et al: Rapid repeat pregnancy and experiences of interpersonal violence among low-income adolescents. Am J Prev Med 16:318–321, 1999.
3. Kahn JR, Anderson KE: Intergenerational patterns of teenage fertility. Demography 29:39–57, 1992.
4. Koniak-Griffin D, Mathenge C, Anderson NL, et al: An early intervention program for adolescent mothers: A nursing demonstration project. J Obstet Gynecol Neonatal Nurs 28:51–59, 1999.
5. Olds DL, Henderson CR, Chamberlin R, et al: Preventing child abuse and neglect: A randomized trial of nurse home visitation. Pediatrics 78:65–78, 1986.
6. O'Sullivan AL, Jacobson BS: A randomized trial of a health care program for first-time adolescent mothers and their infants. Nurs Res 41:210–215, 1992.
7. Parker B, McFarlane J, Soeken K: Abuse during pregnancy: Effects on maternal complications and birth weight in adult and teenage women. Obstet Gynecol 84(3):323–328, 1994.
8. Poole C. Adolescent pregnancy and unfinished developmental tasks of childhood. J Sch Health 57:271–273, 1987.
9. Pope SK, Whiteside MS, Brooks-Gunn J, et al: Low-birth-weight infants born to adolescent mothers: Effects of coresidency with grandmother on child development. JAMA 269:1369–1400, 1993.
10. Smilkstein G, Ashworth C: Validity and reliability of the Family APGAR as a test of family function. J Fam Pract 15:303–311, 1982.
11. Smilkstein G: The family APGAR: a proposal for a family function test and its use by physicians. J Fam Pract 6:1231–1239, 1978.
12. Stevenson W, Maton KI, Teti DM; School importance and drop-out among pregnant adolescents. J Adolesc Health 22:376–382, 1998.
13. Trad PV: Adolescent pregnancy: An intervention challenge. Child Psychiatry Hum Dev 24:99–113, 1993.
14. Ventura SJ, Mathews TJ, Curtin SC: Declines in teenage birth rates, 1991–97: National and state patterns. Natl Vital Stat Rep 47:1–17, 1998.

SECTION D.
GENETIC INTERVENTIONS

Louise Acheson, M.D.

This section presents a brief overview of a rapidly changing field: prenatal genetic diagnosis. Birth defects, many of which have a genetic basis, occur in 3% of live births and account for 20% of neonatal mortality.[1]

Many patients, when confronted with the likelihood of having a child who is seriously afflicted with a major defect, may choose to terminate the pregnancy. Other patients, for personal or religious reasons, may not want to consider this option. Practitioners must respect the wishes of their patients while striving to ascertain who is at increased risk for serious inherited disorders or major birth defects. This information should be communicated to patients in a clear, nonjudgmental manner.

I. Types of Genetic Disorders
A. Single-Gene Disorders[2,6]
1. Autosomal dominant
These include some forms of polycystic kidney disease, Marfan syndrome, etc.
2. Autosomal recessive
Examples of this disorder include cystic fibrosis and sickle cell anemia.
3. X-linked abnormalities
These disorders, such as hemophilia, are seen almost exclusively among males who inherit the abnormal X chromosome from carrier females, who are usually phenotypically normal.
4. Triplet repeat disorders
These may be X-linked, like fragile X syndrome, or autosomal dominant, like Huntington's chorea. These are disorders caused by an abnormally increased number of repetitions of a particular three base-pair DNA sequence (e.g., [CGG CGG CGG] x 300 repetitions) affecting the function of a particular gene. Most repeated DNA sequences are between genes and do not affect function; individual variation in the number of repeats does not matter, although it can be used to uniquely identify an individual by his or her DNA. A few, mostly neurologic conditions, such as fragile X syndrome of mental retardation, Huntington's chorea, and myotonic dystrophy, are inherited when a greatly expanded repeated sequence occurs in or near a functioning gene.[4]

When the repeated sequence becomes abnormally long, it becomes "unstable;" the strands of DNA tend to "slip" during replication, causing expansion of the repeated sequence and worsening clinical manifestations from one generation to the next. The genetic abnormality for fragile X mental retardation is on the X chromosome. Affected individuals are usually males who inherited an abnormal X chromosome from their mothers. Mothers are usually phenotypically normal because they have one normal copy of the gene, although some females with a large number of triplet repeats may have mild abnormalities.[2]
5. Mitochondrial disorders
Rarely, mutations in mitochondrial genes can cause diseases related to abnormal oxidative metabolism (usually affecting muscle, eye, and nervous system). All mitochondria are inherited from one's mother, but either sex of offspring may be affected.[6]
B. Chromosomal Abnormalities
1. Extra chromosomes
These include disorders such as trisomy disorders (21, 18, 13) or Klinefelter's syndrome (XXY).
2. Missing chromosomes
An example of this is Turner's syndrome (X0).
3. Structural chromosomal abnormalities
Examples of chromosomal abnormalities include deletions such as Prader-Willi syndrome, or balanced translocations in infants whose parents are normal but whose offspring have increased incidence of chromosomal abnormalities
C. Genetic and Environmental Interactions[2,6]
The majority of congenital abnormalities resulting in live births—e.g., congenital hip dysplasia, neural tube defects, or congenital cardiac defects—are linked to many

genes (polygenic) as well as to environmental factors; the combination results in a variable incidence of defects at birth or later in life.

II. Genetic Counseling: Who Should Be Screened?
Genetic counseling, preconceptually and prenatally, is discussed in Chapters 1 and 2.

III. Techniques for Prenatal Diagnosis
A. Amniocentesis[1]
Amniocentesis is a well-established and technically simple method of obtaining fetal cells and amniotic fluid for prenatal genetic diagnosis. The clinician should know which patients are at increased risk of chromosomal defects as well as of the following characteristics associated with this procedure.
1. Fetal/pregnancy risks
   a. Risk of fetal loss: 0.5–1.0%
   b. Amnionitis in 1 per 1000.
   c. Maternal isoimmunization: Incidence of 1% in Rh-negative women if Rh immune globulin is not given. 300 µg of Rh immune globulin should be given to Rh-negative women at the time of amniocentesis.
   d. Increased risk of neonatal respiratory distress.
2. Disadvantages of procedure
   a. Procedure usually not performed until 16 weeks' gestation, although some centers may perform it as early as 13–15 weeks. Early amniocentesis poses a greater risk of pregnancy loss (2–3%).
   b. Results are not available for 10–14 days.
   c. Cell culture failure rates are about 1%.
3. Indication for amniocentesis
   a. The most common indication for genetic amniocentesis is maternal age > 35 years. These patients can be offered combined maternal serum alpha-fetoprotein (MSAFP), unconjugated estriol, and maternal serum hCG testing as a screen for Down syndrome. These tests, if normal, greatly reduce the probability of having a fetus with a chromosomal defect, but will fail to detect 15% of cases of Down syndrome in women over 35, whereas amniocentesis should detect > 99%.[5]

B. Chorionic Villus Sampling (CVS)
Chorionic villus sampling (CVS) involves the biopsy of chorionic villi using ultrasound guidance through either a transcervical or transabdominal approach.[8]
1. Advantage of chorionic villus sampling over amniocentesis
Chorionic villus sampling is performed between 9 and 12 weeks' gestation. When abnormal results are obtained, termination of pregnancy can occur at an earlier time with less maternal morbidity.
2. Risks associated with chorionic villus sampling
Alfirevic has performed a meta-analysis of the three large RCTs in Europe and Canada (n = 5600), which has resulted in the following conclusions regarding risk of chorionic villus sampling compared to amniocentesis.[1]
   a. Chorionic villus sampling resulted in a higher false-positive rate such that 10% of the women in the Canadian trial had repeat chorionic villus sampling. However, in the United States collaborative trial, only 1% required repeat sampling.[1,8]
   b. Fetal loss, stillbirth, and neonatal death rates were increased in groups allocated to CVS compared to amniocentesis. The procedure-associated excess of pregnancy losses with CVS compared to amniocentesis ranged from 0.6% to 3.6%. Complication rates of CVS, unlike amniocentesis, are

dependent on operator experience. Up to 400 procedures may be required to achieve the lowest complication rates.[8] CVS is best obtained in high-volume, experienced centers.

    c. There is a possible association with limb reduction defects with CVS earlier than 10 weeks gestation.[1,8]

3. Transabdominal versus transcervical chorionic villus sampling

It appears that the safety of transabdominal chorionic villus sampling may be greater than for the transcervical approach and may approach that of amniocentesis.[1,8]

4. Summary

Clinicians should inform patients who are considering CVS that they should balance the benefit of earlier diagnosis with increased risks of fetal loss and other adverse pregnancy outcomes.

C. Ultrasonography

In some settings, ultrasonography has become an important tool in making prenatal genetic diagnoses. Patterns of fetal anomalies visualized using ultrasound can correspond to specific chromosomal abnormalities.[3]

    Pregnancies at increased risk for structural anomalies because of genetic, teratogenic, or infectious factors can undergo detailed ultrasound surveys of fetal anatomy to provide either reassurance if normal or perinatal preparedness if abnormal.

    A detailed ultrasound scan may be an acceptable follow-up test after an elevated MSAFP in lieu of proceeding with an amniocentesis. (See Chapter 6, section J)

D. Fetal Blood Sampling

This is carried out beginning at 18 weeks' gestation with the insertion of a 20- or 22-gauge spinal needle, using ultrasound guidance, into the umbilical cord. Fetal blood sampling can be used to make hematologic, infectious, metabolic, and cytogenetic diagnoses. Fetal loss rates are approximately 2%. Hence, this procedure should be carried out by specialists, and only when rapid diagnosis of these disorders is essential.[3]

E. Fetoscopy

Fetoscopy and fetal tissue sampling are associated with fetal loss rates of 2–5%. This technique has largely been superseded by high-resolution ultrasound and molecular genetic testing.[6]

F. Embryo Biopsy in Conjunction with In Vitro Fertilization

By this technique, which is still in experimental stages, a single cell of a 6–10-cell cultured embryo is removed by suction micropipette, its DNA analyzed by oligonucleotide probes or potentially by fluorescence in situ hybridization for a specific genetic defect, prior to implantation. "Healthy" embryos free of the specific defect would be selected for implantation.[6]

G. Recovery of Fetal Cells from the Maternal Circulation

DNA isolated from nucleated fetal red cells in the maternal circulation has been amplified by PCR and analyzed for specific genetic mutations. This technique is still experimental and not in clinical use.[4,6]

IV. Analysis of Fetal Genetic Material
A. Cytogenetic Analysis

1. Fetal karyotype

This technique stains for chromosome bands in dividing cells and shows the number of each chromosome. It can detect large deletions or rearrangements of chromosomal material.

2. Fluorescence in situ hybridization (FISH)

FISH is a recently developed molecular cytogenetic technique. A fluorescently labeled segment of DNA (probe) is hybridized to the DNA of chromosomes on a microscope slide. It can be used to detect the presence or absence of specific DNA sequences, diagnosing deletions and rearrangements of small or large bits of chromosomal material. This technique can also be applied to nondividing nuclei for rapid detection of trisomies, for example, without waiting for amniocyte culture.[6]

B. Molecular Genetic (DNA) Analysis

1. Restriction endonuclease analysis

Fetal DNA is cut into fragments at specific sequences recognized by specific enzymes. The pattern of fragments differs for mutant and wild-type ("normal") alleles.[2,4]

2. Allele-specific oligonucleotide probe analysis

The binding of specific, short sequences of synthetic DNA (called probes) to the patient's DNA is tested. If the sequences do not match, they will not bind and replicate that stretch of DNA. Thus, the presence or absence of a specific, wild-type or mutant sequence can be ascertained.[2,4]

C. Biochemical Analysis of Gene Products

In some cases, when the gene has not been cloned, it is possible to test for the protein produced by that gene, which may be abnormal or absent in affected individuals.

D. Conditions for Which Different Types of Prenatal Diagnosis Can Be Used

DNA testing is currently available for at least 300 of the 5700 known genetic disorders; this number will continually grow. These tests are not done for screening, but to identify a particular genetic disorder for which the fetus is considered to be at high risk (usually because of family history). Detailed consideration of prenatal diagnosis of each genetic disorder is beyond the scope of this book. Comprehensive information about genetic disorders can be found in On-line Mendelian Inheritance in Man (OMIM) at http://www.ncbi.nlm.nih.gov/Omim/.

1. Direct testing for a mutation

This can be done when the gene causing the disorder is known and when the disease-causing mutation in the patient's family has been characterized. Examples of diseases currently diagnosed by direct DNA analysis include: cystic fibrosis, sickle cell anemia, Duchenne muscular dystrophy, Tay-Sachs disease, alpha-1-antitrypsin deficiency, thalassemias, familial adenomatous polyposis, Gaucher's disease, and spinal muscular atrophy.[4] Diseases diagnosed by analyzing the number of triplet repeats in the gene include: fragile X syndrome, Huntington's chorea, Friedreich's ataxia, and myotonic dystrophy.[4]

2. Indirect testing through linkage analysis

This involves testing several affected and unaffected family members, using a genetic marker that is so close to the disease-causing gene that they are inherited together. Diseases currently diagnosed by linkage analysis include Marfan syndrome, neurofibromatosis, and von Willebrand's disease.[4]

References

1. Alfirevic Z, Gosden C, Neilson JP: Chorionic villous sampling versus amniocentesis for prenatal diagnosis (Cochrane Review). In The Cochrane Library, Issue 1, 2000. Oxford: Update Software.
2. Acheson LS, Root S, Tyler CV: Clinical Genetics. Monograph, Edition No. 240, Home Study Self-Assessment Program. Kansas City, MO, American Academy of Family Physicians, May 1999, pp 15–31.
3. D'Alton M, DeCherney A: Prenatal diagnosis. N Engl J Med 328:114–120, 1993.
4. Gupta GK, Bianchi DW: DNA diagnosis for the practicing obstetrician. Ob Gyn Clin North Am 24:123–142, 1997.
5. Haddow J, Palomake G, et al: Reducing the need for amniocentesis in women 35 years of age or older with serum markers for screening. N Engl J Med 330:1114–1118, 1994.
6. Kingston HM: ABC of Clinical Genetics, 2nd ed. London, BMJ Publishing Group, 1997, pp 4–11, 22–30, 41–49.
7. Reece EA: Early and midtrimester amniocentesis: Safety and outcomes. Ob Gyn Clin North Am 24:71–81, 1997.
8. Wapner RJ: Chorionic villus sampling. Ob Gyn Clin North Am 24:83–110, 1997.

SECTION E.
SUBSTANCE ABUSE IN PREGNANCY

V. Leigh Beasley, M.D.

Three major areas of substance abuse—cocaine, opiates, and alcohol—are particularly problematic when encountered in pregnant women. Short-term and long-term effects on both maternal and infant health are significant. Clinicians in all practice settings commonly encounter these problems, particularly if they screen for them regularly. Effective strategies for intervention and treatment exist and should be offered to any pregnant woman who has a diagnosis of substance abuse.

I. Crack and Cocaine Abuse in Pregnancy
A. Pharmacology
Cocaine is available in two forms: cocaine hydrochloride and the more purified cocaine alkaloid, known as crack. The former is water-soluble and is administered orally, intravenously, or nasally; the latter is not soluble in water and is smoked.[37] Cocaine exerts profound effects on the central and peripheral nervous systems by stimulating the adrenergic receptors thorough buildup of neurotransmitters at nerve synapses. Chronic use of cocaine results in a depletion of dopamine, which, in turn, leads to marked dysphoria and accompanying cravings.

B. Prevalence in Groups at Increased Risk
The estimated prevalence of cocaine use in pregnancy is between 10% and 15% among women in at-risk groups.[32] Although certain subgroups have higher usage rates, cocaine use among pregnant women occurs within *every* income and ethnic group. Of women delivering at a private suburban hospital, 6% tested positive for cocaine use by neonatal meconium analysis.[31] Statewide drug abuse screening in public health clinics in Alabama failed to demonstrate any difference in the incidence of positive drug screenings between high-risk and low-risk populations.[16] Women with higher prevalence rates of cocaine use include those living in urban settings, particularly those of lower socioeconomic status.

C. Adverse Obstetric Outcomes
Numerous adverse outcomes are associated with maternal cocaine use. Causation is more difficult to ascertain because of multiple confounding factors, such as coexisting higher rates of smoking and poor nutritional status in substance-abusing mothers.[30]

    1. Low-birth-weight infants

Of 14 studies reviewed, 11 demonstrated a significant association between cocaine use in pregnancy and low-birth-weight (LBW) outcomes.[33] Many of these LBW babies experienced much higher rates of morbidity and mortality.

        a. Prematurity. Some of the LBW is attributable to increased rates of preterm labor and delivery, particularly among cocaine-using women who receive little prenatal care. Many of these women also have concurrent conditions (e.g., sexually transmitted diseases and urinary tract infections) that have been associated with prematurity and LBW and must be identified and effectively treated.

        b. Intrauterine growth restriction (IUGR). Multiple studies reviewed showed an independent association between cocaine use and IUGR, regardless of gestational age.[17,33]

    2. Placental abruption

Increased rates of placental abruption are associated with cocaine use, particularly if the use is continued throughout the pregnancy.[33]

3. Spontaneous abortion

In a study of 400 pregnant women presenting to an emergency department in Philadelphia with spontaneous abortion, 29% tested positive for cocaine compared to 21% among 570 women who had ongoing pregnancies followed through 22 weeks' gestation. Based on risk estimate, cocaine use accounted for 8% of spontaneous abortions in this population.[28]

4. Physical and sexual abuse

Pregnant women diagnosed with substance abuse are more often victims of violence, as compared to mothers who do not use drugs.[1] Studies also suggest that one third to one half of substance-abusing women have experienced some sort of sexual abuse as a child.[19]

5. Comorbid mental health disorders

Epidemiologic studies reveal that a majority of women with substance abuse have coexisting mental disorders, with depression being the most common co-diagnosis.[19]

D. Adverse Neonatal Outcomes

The increased rate of low birth weight is the most significant medical complication of cocaine use in pregnancy when cost, morbidity, and mortality are considered. Additional adverse neonatal effects include the following:

1. Neonatal withdrawal

Neonatal withdrawal symptoms may occur among infants whose mothers used cocaine. The withdrawal syndrome is characterized by irritability, hypertonicity, hyperactivity, tachypnea, decreased sleep, and loose stools.[30]

2. Teratogenic effects

Microcephaly and deficiencies of cerebral midline neuronal development, such as optic atrophy have been associated with maternal cocaine use.[37] Genito-urinary and renal anomalies secondary to cocaine ingestion have also been suggested by one large case-control study.

3. Central nervous system effects

Destructive effects to the fetal central nervous system, such as cerebral infarcts, may occur in utero as a result of vasospasm and hypoxemia related to placental insufficiency.[37]

E. Adverse Post-neonatal Outcomes

1. Increased incidence of sudden infant death syndrome (SIDS)

The risk of SIDS may be somewhat increased in infants of substance-abusing mothers, but the association is not enough to justify home apnea monitoring of all of these newborns. Parental neglect may, at times, play an associated role.[2]

2. Long-term effect on neurobehavioral development

Although suspected, an effect of substance abuse on subsequent neurobehavioral development has been difficult to determine because few instruments can assess subtle neurobehavioral differences. Additionally, many confounding variables that often coexist with substance abuse have a deleterious effect on development (e.g., nutritional and environmental factors).[32,39]

F. Diagnostic Options

1. Self-reporting

This is the most commonly used method of assessing substance abuse in pregnant women. Underreporting of the true incidence of this problem occurs, however, because of patient reluctance to divulge sensitive information and clinician reluctance to inquire about substance abuse.

2. Administering a structured questionnaire

By administering a questionnaire that asked for detailed information about past or current substance abuse, Christmas and associates identified twice as many substance-abusing women than would have been identified with intermittent drug screenings alone.[9]

3. Prenatal drug screening

Prenatal drug screening is most frequently accomplished by urine drug testing. However, because testing occurs sporadically, up to 47% of exposed infants are still missed.[37]

4. Neonatal drug screening

Neonatal urine testing identifies maternal cocaine use that occurred within the week before delivery. Testing of infant meconium for cocaine metabolites can document maternal use of cocaine that occurred up to 20 weeks before delivery.[29] Neonatal hair analysis may also be conducted to assess remote maternal cocaine use.[18]

Waiting to test the neonate, instead of screening the mother prenatally, misses the opportunity to refer the drug-using mother for counseling and structured substance abuse treatment programs. This results in several more months of drug exposure for the fetus and potentially worse birth outcomes.

G. Ethical and Medicolegal Concerns

Although a thorough discussion of these issues is beyond the scope of this book, some of the more controversial issues include:

1. Involuntary versus voluntary drug screening

Voluntary consent for urine drug testing is preferred. Most successful prenatal substance abuse programs employ voluntary screening, with consequences of a positive drug test explained to the patient prior to screening. Experience in a rural public health clinic in South Carolina shows that nearly all patients consented to voluntary drug testing, when screening and follow-up of positive drug screens is presented in a nonthreatening manner.[4]

2. Maternal versus fetal rights

There is little disagreement that drug use is harmful for both mother and fetus. What is often more difficult is to determine whether or not a specific court, or state, will see maternal or fetal rights as primary, and at what gestational age. This issue has been decided in one state in favor of the rights of a viable fetus over the mother, in the case of Whitner vs. The State of South Carolina. In the maternal use of illegal substance(s) the South Carolina Supreme Court wrote: "…during her pregnancy after the fetus attained viability, Whitner enjoyed the same freedom to use cocaine that she enjoyed earlier in and predating her pregnancy—none whatsoever." They went on to say that the "issue of maternal rights [over the fetus] to use illegal substances is indeed not an issue."[Whitner v. State of S.C., p 38]

3. Involvement of law enforcement

Threat of criminal or civil sanctions with mandatory reporting is often applied inequitably to different socioeconomic or ethnic groups.[7] In South Carolina, reporting maternal drug use to the child protection agency (DSS) after 24 weeks' gestation is mandated under the child abuse and neglect statutes.[4] Despite numerous concerns that were raised when this mandate was enacted, evidence has shown that more women now receive substance abuse treatment than prior to the law. Only if a women displays resistance or noncompliance with treatment are criminal or civil sanctions employed. The focus of the program is on treatment for the substance-abusing pregnant mother, a belief that is shared by health care providers, social service agencies, and law enforcement.

The threat of losing custody of her children has been noted as a strong motivator for a pregnant woman to receive treatment.[20] Failing to screen during pregnancy may lead to a missed "window of opportunity" for the patient at a time when her motivation to seek help is typically higher. A concern raised in association with the South Carolina mandate was that substance-abusing pregnant women would fear screening and avoid prenatal care. This concern has not held true as there has been no increase in the number of mothers with no prenatal care in several of the programs where universal voluntary testing was in place before and after the mandate.[4]

4. Preservation of patient confidentiality[30]

The clinician faces a major challenge in attempting to respect patient confidentiality while needing to adhere to state laws and trying to attain the best possible neonatal outcome.

H. Treatment

Maternity care providers must acknowledge that substance abuse occurs in every practice setting. Early screening and accurate diagnosis are essential. It is recommended that clinicians consider using both a detailed questionnaire and intermittent toxicology screenings to identify the substance-abusing prenatal patient. The risk of a cocaine-abusing patient having a premature infant has been estimated to be reduced twofold to threefold if the patient remains in a system of adequate prenatal care.[14]

The following are important components of successful prenatal substance abuse treatment programs.

1. Coordination of care

Family physicians and their staff often need to coordinate the care of these women with government agencies (such as child protective services), high-risk prenatal care providers, substance abuse counselors, agencies, and in-hospital treatment programs.

2. Systems for identifying pregnant substance abusers

These systems are important so that intervention is started as early as possible in the pregnancy.

3. Intensive case management

This is often a critical component of prenatal care to link substance abusing pregnant women with the services they need, such as child care, job training, transportation, and housing.[20]

II. Abuse of Opiates During Pregnancy
A. Pathophysiology

Opiates are derived from naturally occurring opium alkaloids and chemically related derivatives. Opiates work within the central nervous system affecting mood, sensorium, pain tolerance, alertness, and many other factors. Physiologic addiction and tolerance, the need for ever-increasing amounts of drug ingestion, occur commonly.[39]

B. Prevalence

An estimated 10,000 infants a year are born to women who use opiates during pregnancy. Every family physician in urban, suburban, or rural settings can be expected to encounter opiate-addicted women during pregnancy, although this problem is difficult to detect on a routine prenatal visit.

C. Associated Perinatal Effects[23]

Several associations and complications have been reported in opiate-using mothers and their infants.

1. Concurrent use of other substances

Opiate-using mothers have a higher consumption of alcohol, cigarettes, and other street drugs.

2. Increased incidence of preterm deliveries and IUGR

3. Increased incidence of intrauterine hypoxia and fetal distress[38]

D. Long-Term Sequelae

Infants and children of opiate-addicted mothers are at increased risk for growth and developmental disorders. The degree, however, to which these disorders can be ascribed to intrauterine exposure to opiates versus multiple associated environmental risks remains difficult to measure.[39]

E. Diagnostic Options

Screening options for opiates are virtually the same as those discussed in the previous section dealing with cocaine abuse.

F. Treatment

Similar to programs geared toward the cocaine-using pregnant woman, treatment for opiate users must be comprehensive in scope and must address many of the areas listed in the treatment summary section.[36]

III. Abuse of Alcohol During Pregnancy

A. Perinatal Associations

Alcohol use during pregnancy has been strongly associated with birth defects in the offspring of drinking mothers. One third of pregnant women who ingest six or more drinks per day during pregnancy have offspring with signs of fetal alcohol syndrome (FAS), the leading cause of preventable mental retardation.[11] While maternal alcohol consumption of less than two drinks (1 ounce of alcohol) per day has not been associated with an increase in birth defects, it is possible that unmeasured deleterious effects do occur.[27] As such, abstinence should be recommended for all pregnant women. Patients who refuse or are unable to comply with this recommendation should be considered at risk for alcohol-related maternal and infant complications.

Even if regular, daily use is not discovered in alcohol use screening during pregnancy, clinicians should specifically ask about the presence of binge drinking, defined as intake of five or more alcoholic drinks on any one occasion. Data from the CDC's Behavioral Risk Factor Surveillance System estimated the prevalence of binge drinking among pregnant women to be 2.9% in 1995 (compared to 11% in nonpregnant women), up from 0.7% in 1991. Risk factors for binge drinking during pregnancy include being unmarried, being employed, and currently smoking.[12] Half of all pregnancies in the U.S. are unintended and many women are not aware of their pregnancy status until 6–8 weeks' gestation. Therefore, women may unknowingly expose their fetuses to large amounts of alcohol concentration if they have a drinking binge during this critical time. Clinicians need to inquire about binge drinking in both pregnant and nonpregnant patients and inform patients of the risks associated with binge drinking.

Physician advice to avoid alcohol during pregnancy has been shown to be influential in patients' decision-making process. Women receiving advice not to drink during routine health maintenance care self-report a lower risk of alcohol use during pregnancy.[21]

B. Prevalence of Alcohol Abuse (Risk Drinking)

The prevalence of alcohol abuse in prenatal populations ranges from 4–14% (depending on the characteristics of the practice population), as compared to 7% in the general female population. Although this problem may be more prevalent in certain low socioeconomic settings, all patient groups have a substantial percentage of alcohol-abusing women.

C. Adverse Perinatal Outcomes

1. Prenatal

Alcoholism during pregnancy may serve as a proximate marker for other risk factors, such as smoking, domestic abuse, depression, and poor social support. When some or all of these conditions contribute to the pregnant woman receiving sporadic or nonexistent prenatal care, the risk of adverse perinatal outcomes, such as prematurity and IUGR, is even greater.

TABLE 14. Principal Features of the Fetal Alcohol Syndrome Observed in 245 Persons Affected

Feature	Manifestation
Central Nervous System Dysfunction	
Intellectual	Mild-to-moderate mental retardation*
Neurologic	Microcephaly*
	Poor coordination, hypotonia[†]
Behavioral	Irritability in infancy*
	Hyperactivity in childhood
Growth Deficiency	
Prenatal	<2 SD for length and weight*
Postnatal	<2 SD for length and weight*
	Disproportionately diminished adipose tissue[†]
Facial Characteristics	
Eyes	Short palpebral fissures*
Nose	Short, upturned[†]
	Hypoplastic philtrum*
Maxilla	Hypoplastic[†]
Mouth	Thinned upper vermilion*
Retrognathia in infancy*	
Micrognathia or relative prognathia in adolescence[†]	

* Feature seen in >80% of patients.
[†] Feature seen in >50% of patients.
From Clarren S, Smith D: The fetal alcohol syndrome. N Engl J Med 298:1063–1067, 1978, with permission.

  2. Neonatal
  Alcohol risk-taking (> 1 ounce of alcohol or two drinks per day) during pregnancy has well-defined teratogenic effects that may result in central nervous system dysfunction, growth deficiencies, a cluster of facial abnormalities, and other major and minor malformations. An infant has FAS when all of these categories of effects are present (Table 14).[10] When a subset of these effects are present, they are termed fetal alcohol effects (FAE). Clinicians should be adept at recognizing this syndrome (Fig. 1).[23]

D. Long-Term Sequelae
Infants born with FAS have long-term sequelae, most notably mild to moderate mental retardation. Even infants born of alcoholic mothers with no apparent stigmata of FAS are at increased risk of delayed-onset fetal alcohol effects, including hyperactivity and mental retardation.[18] Long-term studies into adolescence indicate that intellectual and behavioral deficits in these children often widen, in part mediated by unstable family environments.[35]

E. Diagnostic Options
  1. Self-reporting
  This method of screening often carries the risk of underreporting referred to previously.
  2. Application of systematic screening tools
    a. CAGE questionnaire. The CAGE questionnaire (Table 15) was developed in 1970 and remains one of the most reliable and easy screening instruments for the detection of alcoholism.[13] A single affirmative answer on this screening should alert the provider to the possibility of alcohol abuse, although most studies using the CAGE survey have used two positive

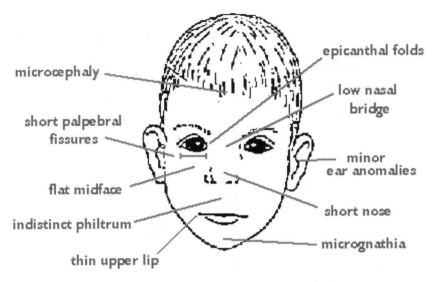

microcephaly

short palpebral fissures

flat midface

indistinct philtrum

thin upper lip

epicanthal folds

low nasal bridge

minor ear anomalies

short nose

micrognathia

FIGURE 1.   Appearance of fetal alcohol syndrome.

answers as the threshold for further evaluation.[27] The validity of this instrument has not been determined within a prenatal population.

    b. T-ACE questionnaire.[34] This modified version of the CAGE questionnaire has proven to be a sensitive, reliable screening instrument for excessive alcohol intake in a study involving women initiating prenatal care at Brigham and Women's Hospital in Boston, MA.[6] The questionnaire requires only 1 minute to administer and the tolerance question is considered the strongest predictor of excessive alcohol consumption. As a screening tool, the T-ACE has a sensitivity of 69%, specificity of 89%, and positive predictive value of 23% in a population that has a 4.3% incidence of consuming two or more drinks per day. The T-ACE is scored by assigning two points to an affirmative response on the tolerance (T) question and one point each to the others. A score of 2 or greater qualifies as a positive screening test (Table 16).

F. Treatment

    1. Preconceptual diagnosis and intervention

The primary prevention of fetal alcohol syndrome can be accomplished with proper identification and treatment of women with alcohol abuse prior to conception. Family planning counseling and encouragement of contraceptive use should be included in early treatment efforts until the woman is sober and regularly participating in an outpatient recovery program.

TABLE 15.   The CAGE Questions

C	Ever felt need to **C**ut down drinking?
A	Ever felt **A**nnoyed by criticism of drinking?
G	Had **G**uilty feelings about drinking?
E	Ever take morning **E**ye-opener?

From Ewing J: Detecting alcoholism: The CAGE questionnaire. JAMA 252:1905–1907, 1984, with permission.

TABLE 16. T-ACE Questions*

T	How many drinks does it take to make you feel high (**T**olerance)?
A	Have people **A**nnoyed you by criticizing your drinking?
C	Have you felt you ought to **C**ut down on your drinking?
E	Have you ever had a drink first thing in the morning to steady your nerves or get rid of a hangover (**E**ye-opener)?

* Found to be significant identifiers of risk drinking, i.e., alcohol intake sufficient to potentially damage the embryo/fetus.
From Sokol R, Martier S, Ager J: The T-ACE questions. Am J Obstet Gynecol 160:863–870, 1989, with permission.

   2. Treatment options
      a. Provision of referral to freestanding alcohol treatment programs.
      b. Establishment of on-site treatment capabilities in high-risk settings that have direct tie-ins to other social support services.
      c. Participation with community-based coalitions that provide additional outreach, education, and intensive case management. These programs have been developed to address special populations in which the incidence of fetal alcohol syndrome is markedly increased.[25]
      d. Recognition that for some patients, especially adolescents, pregnancy may provide an opportunity to intervene in order to decrease current or future substance abuse use.[15]

IV. Summary Recommendations
Intervention strategies dealing with substance abuse and pregnancy have not been studied in a prospective fashion. The following recommendations are based on successful demonstration projects.[36]

A. Screening
Assess for the past or current use of potentially harmful drugs in a systematic fashion, both in the preconceptual and prenatal periods. Screening instruments, such as the T-ACE, can be incorporated into a larger questionnaire that asks for detailed information on past or current use of substances when the initial screen is indicative of a problem. Intermittent use of toxicology screening during pregnancy should be considered.

B. Treatment
Develop a treatment plan that incorporates office staff and community resources to assist with both substance abuse counseling and unmet social service needs, such as housing, nutrition, and education. Optimal prenatal care for the substance-abusing patient can be provided when a mechanism exists to track progress and compliance with recommended care. Lay or professional staff can be used for this purpose.

C. Outcomes
Recognize that these patients have, in general, higher behavioral risks profile, which may contribute to adverse perinatal outcomes. Ongoing risk assessment of the pregnancy is necessary and appropriate interventions should be offered when available.

D. Postpartum and Early Childhood Care
All of the supportive services provided for substance-abusing pregnant women during the prenatal period should be continued and strengthened during the year following childbirth. With the stress of a new baby, a new mother may revert to previous "coping patterns" (i.e., drug use) unless new coping skills are presented and

developed in the prenatal visits. Close follow-up with continued counseling and support may prevent relapse.

E. Prevention

Physicians can and should play a role in the primary, secondary, and tertiary prevention of this major public health epidemic, both in the office and community settings.

References

1. Amaro H, Fried L, Cabral H, et al: Violence during pregnancy and substance use. Am J Public Health 80:575–579, 1990.
2. Bass M, Kravath R, Glass L: Death-scene investigation in sudden infant death. N Engl J Med 315:100–105, 1986.
3. Bauchner H: Cocaine, sudden infant death syndrome, and home monitoring. J Pediatr 117:904–906, 1990.
4. Beasley VL. Personal communication.
5. Campbell D, Fleischman A: Ethical challenges in medical care for the pregnant substance abuser. Clin Obstet Gynecol 35:803–812, 1992.
6. Chang G, Goetz MA, Wilkins-Haug L, et al: Identifying prenatal alcohol use: Screening instruments versus clinical predictors. Am J Addict 8:87–93, 1999.
7. Chasnoff I, Landress H, Barrett M: The prevalence of illicit-drug or alcohol use during pregnancy and discrepancies in mandatory reporting in Pinellas County, Florida. N Engl J Med 322:1202–1206, 1990.
8. Chavey G, Mulinare J, Cordero J: Maternal cocaine use during early pregnancy as a risk factor for congenital urogenital anomalies. JAMA 262:795–798, 1989.
9. Christmas J, Knisely J, et al: Comparison of questionnaire screening and urine toxicology for detection of pregnancy complicated by substance use. Obstet Gynecol 80:750–754, 1992.
10. Clarren S, Smith D: The fetal alcohol syndrome. N Engl J Med 298:1063–1067, 1978.
11. Cyr M, Moulton A, et al: Substance abuse in women. Obstet Gynecol Clin North Am 17:905–922, 1990.
12. Ebrahim SH, Diekman ST, Floyd RL, et al: Comparison of binge drinking among pregnant and nonpregnant women, United States, 1991–1995. Am J Obstet Gynecol 180:1–7, 1999.
13. Ewing J: Detecting alcoholism: The CAGE questionnaire. JAMA 252:1905–1907, 1984.
14. Feldman J, Minkoff H, et al: A cohort study of the impact of perinatal drug use on prematurity in an inner-city population. Am J Public Health 82:726–728, 1992.
15. Flanagan P, Kokotailo P: Adolescent pregnancy and substance abuse. Clin Perinatol 26:55–74, 1999.
16. George S, Price J, et al: Drug abuse screening of childbearing-age women in Alabama public health clinics. Am J Obstet Gynecol 165:924–927, 1991.
17. Gillogley K, Evans A, et al: The perinatal impact of cocaine, amphetamine and opiate use detected by universal intrapartum screening. Am J Obstet Gynecol 163:1535–1542, 1990.
18. Graham K, Koren G, et al: Determination of gestational cocaine exposure by hair analysis. JAMA 262:3328–3330, 1989.
19. Hans SL: Demographic and psychosocial characteristics of substance-abusing pregnant women. Clin Perinatol 26(1):55–74, 1999.
20. Howell EM, Chasnoff IJ: Perinatal substance abuse treatment: Findings from focus groups with clients and providers. J Subst Abuse Treat 17:139–148, 1999.
21. Jones-Webb R, McKiver M, Pirie P, et al: Relationships between advice and tobacco and alcohol use during pregnancy. Am J Prev Med 16(3):244–247, 1999.
22. Lindenberg C, Alexander E, et al: A review of the literature on cocaine abuse in pregnancy. Nurs Res 40:69–75, 1991.
23. Little B, Snell L, et al: Maternal and fetal effects of heroin addiction during pregnancy. J Reprod Med 35:159–162, 1990.
24. Little B, Snell L, et al: Failure to recognize fetal alcohol syndrome in newborn infants. Am J Dis Child 144:1142–1146, 1990.
25. Masis K, May P: A comprehensive local program for the prevention of fetal alcohol syndrome. Pub Health Rep 106:484–489, 1991.
26. Mayfield D, McLeod G, Hall P: The CAGE questionnaire: Validation of a new alcoholism screening instrument. Am J Psychiatry 131:1121–1123, 1974.
27. Mills J, Graubard B: Is moderate drinking during pregnancy associated with an increased risk for malformations? Pediatrics 80:309–314, 1987.
28. Ness RB: Cocaine and tobacco use and the risk of spontaneous abortion. N Engl J Med 340:333–339, 1999.

29. Ostrea E, Brady M, et al: Drug screening of newborns by meconium analysis: A large-scale, prospective epidemiologic study. Pediatrics 89:107–113, 1992.
30. Robins L, Mills J: Effects of in utero exposure to street drugs. Am J Public Health 83(Suppl):3–32, 1993.
31. Schutzman D, Frankenfield M, et al: Incidence of intrauterine cocaine exposure in a suburban setting. Pediatrics 88:825–827, 1991.
32. Singer L, Garber R, Kliegman R: Neurobehavioral sequelae of fetal cocaine exposure. J Pediatr 119:667–672, 1991.
33. Slutsker L: Risks associated with cocaine use during pregnancy. Obstet Gynecol 79:778–789, 1992.
34. Sokol R, Martier S, Ager J: The T-ACE questions: Practical prenatal detection of risk-drinking. Am J Obstet Gynecol 160:863–870, 1989.
35. Streissguth A, Aase J, et al: Fetal alcohol syndrome in adolescents and adults. JAMA 265:1961–1967, 1991.
36. Suffet F, Brotman R: A comprehensive care program for pregnant addicts: Obstetrical, neonatal and child development outcomes. Int J Addict 19:199–219, 1984.
37. Volpe J: Effect of cocaine use on the fetus. N Engl J Med 327:399–405, 1992.
38. Wolmen I, Niv D, et al: Opioid-addicted parturient, labor, and outcome: A reappraisal. Obstet Gynecol Surv 44:592–596, 1989.
39. Zuckerman B, Bresnahan K: Developmental and behavioral consequences of prenatal drug and alcohol exposure. Pediatr Clin North Am 38:1387–1405, 1991.

SECTION F.
SMOKING IN PREGNANCY

Elizabeth G. Baxley, M.D.

Smoking during pregnancy continues to be one of the major causes of preventable perinatal morbidity and mortality.

I. Magnitude of the Problem
A. Prevalence
Despite extensive publicity regarding its dangers, use of tobacco continues in approximately 25% of all pregnancies in the U.S. In the period between 1990 and 1996, a decline in the overall rate of smoking has occurred.[10,34] However, rates for pregnant adolescents remain high. Women 15–19 years of age now have the highest smoking rates of all age groups, decreasing from 59% before pregnancy to 51% in the first trimester and rising again to 62% in the third trimester.[2,8,21] Among race and ethnic groups, American Indian, non-Hispanic white, and Hawaiian women have the highest rates of smoking during pregnancy; Chinese women have the lowest rates.[21] Low-income women who receive prenatal care in public health care settings (23% of all women) also smoke more commonly, with a prevalence between 35% and 40%.[15]
B. Smoking-Related Problems in Pregnancy
The adverse effects of maternal smoking can be easily seen in the number of serious complications associated with tobacco abuse. While a direct causal effect is sometimes difficult to demonstrate, in animal models nicotine has been demonstrated to be a neuroteratogen.[10] Women are generally aware of the risks of continued smoking in pregnancy as evidenced by a cessation rate of up to 18% from the time pregnancy is diagnosed until the onset of prenatal care.[12]

    1. Low-birth-weight infants

    Low-birth-weight (LBW) infants, those weighing less than 2500 g at birth, occur as a result of prematurity, IUGR, or both. Mothers of small-for-gestational-age smoke more often and in greater amounts than mothers of AGA infants.[28] Cigarette smoking in the second trimester is significantly associated with fetal growth restriction in both white and African-American women, in a dose-response relationship.[28] Passive exposure to smoke is also associated with

LBW infants, particularly if the exposure is longer than 2 hours a day.[20] Women who smoke have a prematurity rate that is 50% higher than that of nonsmokers; smoking in pregnancy accounts for up to 11–14% of all preterm births.

2. Placental abruption

A meta-analysis of seven case-control and six cohort studies on a total of over 1 million pregnancies revealed a strong relationship between cigarette smoking and placental abruption and hypertensive disorders.[3] Maternal smoking was associated with a 90% increase in the risk of placental abruption (OR 1.9, 95% CI 1.8–2.0). A dose-response effect was demonstrated with increasing number of cigarettes smoked. The population attributable risk percentage of this effect suggests that 15–25% of placental abruption is due to cigarette smoking. The risk of abruption is greater when pregnant smokers also have chronic hypertension, mild or severe pre-eclampsia, or chronic hypertension with superimposed preeclampsia.

3. Other adverse pregnancy outcomes

Smoking during the first trimester is associated with higher miscarriage rates, likely due to the direct adverse effects of nicotine, cadmium, and polyaromatic hydrocarbons on trophoblastic invasion and proliferation.[10,27] In a series of five meta-analyses, smoking was strongly associated with an elevated risk of placenta previa (pooled odds ratio 1.58), ectopic pregnancy (pooled odds ratio 1.77), preterm premature rupture of membranes (PPROM), and a decreased risk of preeclampsia (pooled odds ratio 0.51).[6,7,25] However, this inverse association between cigarette smoking during pregnancy and preeclampsia must be balanced with the other harmful effects that have strong associations with tobacco use.[6,7]

Maternal smoking is a significant predictor of infant nutrition. Mothers who smoke during all or part of their pregnancy are less likely than nonsmokers to initiate breastfeeding, or to continue breastfeeding beyond 12 weeks. Smokers are also more likely than non-smokers to introduce solid food by twelve weeks.[9]

Smoking during pregnancy has also been associated with adverse effects that continue into childhood and young adulthood. A study of nearly 2,000 Danish children reported that children born to mothers who smoked 15 or more cigarettes per day during pregnancy had hospitalization rates (prior to 8 months of age) twice that of children whose mothers who did not smoke, or who smoked < 15 cigarettes per day. This effect of in utero exposure was shown to be independent of postpartum smoking habits of either the mother or father.[36] In children up to 5 years of age, a population attributable risk of 39.4% for acute middle ear infections is related to in utero exposure to cigarette smoke at the first prenatal visit.[29]

Several independent reports have shown an association between maternal smoking during pregnancy and attention-deficit hyperactivity disorder, conduct disorder, and substance abuse in offspring, some of which followed these offspring through adolescence.[33] It is not clear whether these late effects are a function of social and environmental factors or direct effects of smoking on the developing fetus.[30]

II. Assessing Readiness for Change

Successful smoking cessation is largely dependent on patients' ability to make difficult changes in their lives; quitting use of an addictive substance rarely occurs suddenly and without preparation. Motivation for cessation is greatest early in the pregnancy.[16] Effective counseling for pregnant smokers can be enhanced by understanding each woman's readiness for change (Fig. 2). Provider interventions may help the patient move from the precontemplation to contemplation stage, especially women who have enhanced motivation to do so as a result of pregnancy.[13] When pregnant women are at the

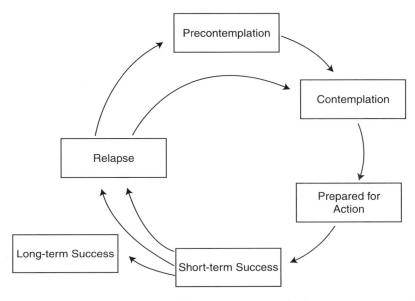

FIGURE 2. The stages of change model. (Adapted from Prochaska JO, Di-Clemente CC: NIH Publication No. 92-3316, 1986, with permission.)

"prepared for action stage" they may elect to cut down on the number of cigarettes smoked in preparation for quitting. Since the effects of tobacco use in pregnancy have been shown to be dose-related, even these efforts at cutting down should be strongly encouraged by the practitioner.

III. Prenatal Smoking Cessation Programs

Smoking cessation programs have been attempted in numerous prenatal programs with varying effectiveness and limited long-term success. In order to assess the effectiveness of specific smoking cessation programs, the Cochrane Pregnancy and Childbirth Group reviewed 44 trials conducted between 1975 and 1998 comprising over 17,000 women, with a principal outcome measure of continued smoking in pregnancy.[14] Interventions commonly included in these programs were provision of information on the risks of smoking to the fetus and infant, and the benefits of quitting; recommendations to quit; feedback about the fetus; and teaching cognitive behavioral strategies for smoking cessation. The interventions varied substantially in their intensity, duration, and people involved in their implementation.

Analyzing subsets of these trials by intervention type demonstrate a significant reduction in the odds of continued smoking in late pregnancy in the intervention group (OR 0.52–0.54, 95% CI 0.42–0.63). The absolute difference in continued smoking ranged from 6.4%-8.1% depending on the intensity of the intervention. Summary conclusions from the Cochrane group suggest that of 100 women still smoking at the time of first antenatal visit, 10 will stop smoking with usual care and a further 6–7 will stop as a result of a formal smoking cessation program. Relapse rates are high, estimated at 25%.

The subset of these trials with information on fetal outcome reveal an actual increase in mean birthweight of 28 g in the intervention group and a non-significant reduction in preterm birth. Based on these findings, it is recommended that smoking cessation programs be implemented in all maternity care settings, including advice to stop smoking, support for smoking cessation, and relapse prevention. Smoking relapse rates are particularly high when there are other smokers in the immediate environment.[17] Intervention strategies need to include offers of help to partners, close family members, and friends.

IV. Pharmacologic Approach to Smoking Cessation in Pregnancy

A. Use of Nicotine Delivery Systems in Pregnancy

Nicotine delivery systems during pregnancy have not been approved by the FDA, although an argument has been made that the potential risks of this therapeutic use in pregnancy are outweighed by the benefits of smoking cessation.[4] In a recent study conducted at the Mayo Clinic, serial measurements of the mother's urinary nicotine and cotinine levels, and indicators of fetal well-being (fetal heart rate and reactivity, systolic/diastolic ratio of blood flow in the umbilical artery, and biophysical profile scores), were made at baseline while the mother was smoking, abstaining from smoking, and using a nicotine patch for 4 days in an inpatient special care unit. Nicotine patch therapy was not found to be associated with indications of fetal compromise during the in-hospital phase of nicotine patch therapy in pregnant smokers who were abstaining.[23] The small sample size and short study period warrant further follow-up studies.

B. Use of Bupropion

The use of the antidepressant bupropion (Wellbutrin, Zyban; pregnancy category B), while widely used in smoking cessation, has never been studied in pregnant women. Rat and rabbit studies using between 3 and 50 times the human dose of bupropion did not find an increase in the incidence of malformations, making this a potential pharmacologic option during pregnancy.[9,31] A registry has been established by Glaxo Wellcome Inc. to assess the safety of bupropion use in pregnancy. Health care providers are encouraged to register patients by calling (800) 722–9292, ext. 39441. Bupropion is excreted in breast milk, although no accumulation of the parent drug or metabolites has been detected in the plasma of the exposed suckling, and no adverse effects have been noted.[5] Because of the potential for serious adverse reactions in nursing infants from bupropion, a risk/benefit decision should be made after careful discussion with the patient.

V. Postpartum Smoking Cessation Efforts

Even if smoking cessation efforts are sustained throughout the pregnancy, many women relapse in the postpartum period.[17] The initial postpartum period is the time of maximum receptiveness to cessation recommendations.[24,32] Providers should focus their continuing patient education efforts on information regarding the significant postnatal effects of secondhand smoke while supporting their cessation efforts.

VI. Cost-Effectiveness

Programs that have demonstrated cessation rates in the 10% range have been shown to be cost-effective by saving $3–6 for every dollar spent on the program.[26] This is particularly true in centers serving high-risk populations, where the break-even point in the prevention of a low-birth-weight outcome is $237. Petersen and colleagues demonstrated an approach that used self-help materials, brief counseling, and a simple charting system that resulted in lower postpartum relapse rates at a cost of $50–111 per patient.[24]

VII. Summary

Numerous medical complications of pregnancy have been associated with smoking during pregnancy. Continued smoking is also a sentinel marker for other important concurrent conditions (e.g., drug use, low income, high parity, living without a partner, depression, poor maternal support, and increased maternal stress) that are themselves risk factors for poor pregnancy outcomes.[19]

Maternity care providers should ensure that smoking cessation programs are available and accessible to all women in their care.[14] High-risk groups (adolescents, women with underlying hypertension, etc.) should receive enhanced targeted education and incentives for quitting. According to AHCPR Clinical Guidelines, prenatal care interventions should consist of the following elements.

A. Identify All Smokers
Strive to understand the perspectives and life circumstances of patients.

B. Deliver Cessation Advice
Encourage members within the same household who also smoke to join in the effort to quit smoking.

C. Assess Motivation and Readiness for Change

D. Provide Detailed Assistance for Those Who Desire to Quit
Obtain or develop education level-appropriate self-help materials for patients that use behavioral strategies. Form linkages with existing health educators or smoking cessation programs to serve as a referral site for interested patients or develop on-site programs.

E. Develop Time-Efficient Patient Counseling Skills
The skills should reinforce the behavioral changes found in the self-help materials (Table 17).

F. Perform Follow-Up
Clinicians are in an ideal place to monitor how their smoking mothers are faring in their attempts to stop smoking, due to the established frequency of prenatal visits.

G. Support Population-Based Strategies to Reduce Smoking
Since even the most effective strategies attempted in pregnancy have a limited effect, supporting population strategies that progressively reduce cigarette smoking in all of society is important for physicians and other members of the health care team.

TABLE 17.   Resources for Smoking Cessation

Organization	Materials Available	Phone Number or Address	Cost
American Academy of Family Physicians	"Stop Smoking Kit" (educational materials, audio tapes, chart stickers, progress cards, signs and waiting room materials)	(800) 274–2237	$50 members $80 nonmembers
American Cancer Society	"The Most Often Asked Questions About Smoking, Tobacco, and Health . . . and the Answers" (a motivational guide for precontemplators and contemplators)	(404) 320–3333 or contact local chapters	Free
	"Smart Move" (an excellent quit-smoking techniques pamphlet)		
American Lung Association	"21-Day Personal Smoking Reduction Program" (a guide and handbook obtained through local chapters)	(212) 315–8700 or contact local chapters	Free

(Table continued on next page.)

TABLE 17.   Resources for Smoking Cessation *(Continued)*

Organization	Materials Available	Phone Number or Address	Cost
American Lung Association *(cont.)*	"Freedom from Smoking in 20 Days" and "A Lifetime of Freedom from Smoking" (two manuals with a plan to quit and stay off cigarettes)	$5/Set	
	"Freedom from Smoking for You and Your Baby" (material specifically for pregnant patients)		
National Institutes of Health, National Cancer Institute	"Clearing the Air" (an excellent quit-smoking techniques pamphlet)	(800) 422–6237	Free
	"How to Help Patients Stop Smoking" (an instructional manual for clinicians, filled with resources and strategies to assist with smoking cessation)		
National Center for Health Promotions	Smoking Cessation literature and self-help programs	(800) 843–6247	Free

References

1. Albrecht SA, Cornelius MD, Braxter B, et al: An assessment of nicotine dependence among pregnant adolescents. J Subst Abuse Treat 16:337–344, 1999.
2. Albrecht S, Cassidy B, Reynolds MD, et al: Developing guidelines for smoking cessation programs interventions for pregnant adolescents. J Pediatr Nurs 3:150–156, 1999.
3. Ananth CV, Smulian JC, Vintzileos AM: Incidence of placental abruption in relation to cigarette smoking and hypertensive disorders during pregnancy: A meta-analysis of observational studies. Obstet Gynecol 93:622–628, 1999.
4. Benowitz N: Nicotine replacement therapy during pregnancy. JAMA 226:3174–3177, 1991.
5. Briggs GG, Samson JH, Ambrose PJ, et al: Excretion of bupropion in breast milk. Ann Pharmacother 27:431–433, 1993.
6. Castles A, Adams EK, Melvin CL, et al: Effects of smoking during pregnancy: Five meta-analyses. Am J Prev Med 16:208–215, 1999.
7. Conde-Agudelo A, Althabe F, Belizan JM, et al: Cigarette smoking during pregnancy and the risk of preeclampsia: A systematic review. Am J Obstet Gynecol 181:1026–1035, 1999.
8. Cornelius MD, Taylor PM, Geva D, et al: Prenatal tobacco and marijuana use among adolescents: Effects on offspring, gestational age, growth, and morphology. Pediatrics 95:738–742, 1995.
9. Edwards N, Sims-Jones N, Breithaupt K: Smoking in pregnancy and postpartum: Relationship to mothers' choices concerning infant nutrition. Can J Nurs Res 30:83–98, 1998.
10. Fields, S: Family-centered maternity care. In Saultz JW (ed): Textbook of Family Medicine: Defining and Examining the Discipline. New York, McGraw-Hill, 2000, pp. 455–471.
11. Haslam C, Draper ES, Goyder E: The pregnant smoker: A preliminary investigation of the social and psychological influences. J Public Health Med 19:187–192, 1997.
12. Hellerstein S, Sachs B: Smoking and reproductive health. ACOG Technical Bulletin 180, 1993.
13. Kristeller JL, Johnson TJ: Smoking Effects and Cessation. In Rosenfield JA (ed): Women's Health in Primary Care. Baltimore, Williams & Wilkins, 1997.
14. Lumley J, Oliver S, Waters E: Interventions for promoting smoking cessation during pregnancy (Cochrane Review). In The Cochrane Library, Issue 1, 2000. Oxford, Update Software.
15. Morbidity Mortality Weekly Report: Cigarette smoking during the last 3 months of pregnancy among women who gave birth to live infants—Maine, 1998–1997. MMWR 8:421–425, 1992.
16. McBride CM, Curry SJ, Lando HA, et al: Prevention of relapse in women who quit smoking during pregnancy. Am J Public Health 89:706–711, 1999.
17. McBride C, Pirie P: Postpartum smoking relapse. Addict Behav 15:165–168, 1990.
18. McCormick M, Brooks-Gunn J, et al: Smoking reduction in pregnancy by a program of self-help and clinical support. Obstet Gynecol 79:924–930, 1992.

19. McCormick M, Brooks-Gunn J: Factors associated with smoking in low income pregnant women: Relationship to birth weight, stressful life events, social support, health behaviors, and mental distress. J Clin Epidemiol 43:441–448, 1990.
20. Martin T, Bracken M: Association of low birth weight with passive smoke exposure in pregnancy. Am J Epidemiol 124:633–642, 1986.
21. Mathews TJ: Smoking during pregnancy, 1990–96. Natl Vital Stat Rep 47:1–12, 1998.
22. Moller AM, Tonnesen H: Smoking cessation and pregnancy. Ugeskr Laeger 161:4985–4986, 1999.
23. Ogburn PL Jr, Hurt RD, Croghan IT, et al: Nicotine patch use in pregnant smokers: Nicotine and cotinine levels and fetal effects. Am J Obstet Gynecol 181:736–743, 1999.
24. Petersen L, Handel J, Kotch J, et al: Smoking reduction in pregnancy by a program of self-help and clinical support. Obstet Gynecol 79:924–930, 1992.
25. Salafia C, Shiverick K: Cigarette smoking and pregnancy II: Vascular effects. Placenta 20:273–279, 1999.
26. Shipp M, Croughan-Minihane M, et al: Estimation of the break even point for smoking cessation programs in pregnancy. Am J Public Health 82:383–390, 1992.
27. Shiverick KT, Salafia C: Cigarette smoking and pregnancy I: Ovarian, uterine and placental effects. Placenta 20:265–272, 1999.
28. Sprauve ME, Lindsay MK, Drews-Botsch CD, et al: Racial patterns in the effects of tobacco use on fetal growth. Am J Obstet Gynecol 181:822–827, 1999.
29. Stathis SL, O'Callaghan DM, Williams GM, et al: Maternal smoking during pregnancy is an independent predictor for symptoms of middle ear disease at five years' postdelivery. Pediatrics 104:e16, 1999.
30. Tong S, McMIchael A: Maternal smoking and neuropsychological development in childhood: a review of the evidence. Devel Med Child Neurol 34:191–197, 1992.
31. Tucker WE: Preclinical toxicology of bupropion: An overview. J Clin Psychiatry 44:60-62, 1983.
32. Wadlington WB, Gwinn K, Riley HD: Who is counseling the pregnant women who smoke? J Tenn Med Assoc 88:7–9, 1995.
33. Weissman MM, Warner V, Wickramaratne PJ, et al: Maternal smoking during pregnancy and psychopathology in maternal offspring followed into adulthood. J Am Acad Child Adolesc Psychiatry 38:892–899, 1999.
34. Windsor R, Li C, et al: The dissemination of smoking cessation methods for pregnant women: Achieving the year 2000 objectives. Am J Public Health 83:173–178, 1993.
35. Windsor R, Lowe J, et al: Health education for pregnant smokers: Its behavioral impact and cost benefit. Am J Public Health 83:201–206, 1993.
36. Wisborg K, Henriksen TB, Obel C, et al: Smoking during pregnancy and hospitalization of the child. Pediatrics 104:e46, 1999.

CHAPTER 5

Diagnosis and Management of First-Trimester Complications

Mark Deutchman, M.D.

SECTION A.
DIAGNOSIS

I. Overview

Early pregnancy loss is a common event. As many as half of all pregnancies conceived are miscarried, many even before the patient is aware of being pregnant. One fourth of clinically diagnosed pregnancies are complicated by bleeding, and half of those abort. The incidence of ectopic pregnancy is rising, reaching 1 in 66 pregnancies in 1988 and 1 in 50 in 1992.[28] Family physicians must be prepared to diagnose and manage first-trimester complications. Some conditions, such as ectopic pregnancy, may result in consultation or referral depending on the practice setting and the surgical skills of the family physician.

II. Patient Presentation

Pregnancy and its complications should be considered in any woman of childbearing age who presents with abdominal pain or vaginal bleeding. Qualitative urine and blood pregnancy testing is widely available and inexpensive and should be initiated early in the process of patient evaluation to establish whether pregnancy is in the differential diagnosis. The following features characterize the patient who should be suspected of having a complication of pregnancy during the first trimester:

- **A.** Abdominal pain
- **B.** Vaginal bleeding
- **C.** Uterus smaller than expected for gestational age
- **D.** Uterus larger than expected for gestational age
- **E.** Fetal heartbeat not audible with hand-held Doppler after 10 to 12 menstrual weeks[24]

III. Differential Diagnosis of First-Trimester Pain or Bleeding
A. Pregnancy-Related
  1. Normal, intrauterine pregnancy
  2. Threatened miscarriage (abortion)
  3. Complete, spontaneous miscarriage (abortion)
  4. Incomplete miscarriage (abortion) with retained products of conception
  5. Subchorionic hemorrhage
  6. Missed abortion, embryonic demise, embryonic resorption, blighted ovum
  7. Ectopic pregnancy
  8. Hydatidiform mole

B. Not Pregnancy-Related
Even if the patient is pregnant, many problems not strictly related to the pregnancy itself should be considered.
1. Appendicitis
2. Adnexal torsion
3. Tubo-ovarian abscess or other manifestation of pelvic infection
4. Ureteral stone with colic
5. Cystitis or pyelonephritis
6. Ruptured ovarian cyst
7. Corpus luteum cyst

IV. Initial Patient Evaluation
A prompt diagnosis usually can be made by combining history, physical examination, laboratory tests, and diagnostic ultrasonography. It is extremely important to consider and search for ectopic pregnancy since it is a potentially life-threatening condition.

A. History
Pregnancies are dated from the first day of the last normal menstrual period before conception (menstrual dating), not from the conception date itself. To estimate the age of the pregnancy and obtain other information needed to assess the patient's risk for abnormal pregnancy, the following information should be sought at a minimum:
1. Last menstrual period
   It is important to date the last menstrual period and whether it was normal or not. A light, late period suggests that the patient conceived the previous month.
2. Previous pregnancy history
3. Recent use of contraception
4. Recent medications taken
5. Recent febrile illnesses
6. Recent attempts at abortion
7. Risk factors for ectopic pregnancy
   a. Tubal reconstructive surgery
   b. Tubal ligation
   c. Previous ectopic pregnancy
   d. Pelvic inflammatory disease
   e. Intrauterine device (IUD)
   f. Progesterone-only contraception
8. Onset, duration, and severity of pain and bleeding
   If generalized abdominal pain is present or if pain is referred to the shoulder area, the possibility of ruptured ectopic pregnancy with hemoperitoneum is high.
9. History of any tissue being passed and whether tissue was saved for pathologic examination
10. History of rubella immunization
11. Blood type and Rh if known
12. General health status

B. Physical Examination
1. Vital signs, including supine and standing blood pressure
   Syncopal symptoms or a fall in systolic blood pressure of 20 mmHg suggest hypovolemia caused by excessive vaginal bleeding from miscarriage or intraperitoneal bleeding from ruptured ectopic pregnancy.
2. General physical examination
   This exam should assess for cardiopulmonary health and signs of acute surgical abdomen.

3. Vaginal speculum examination
   a. Note presence and severity of bleeding.
   b. Note condition and appearance of the cervix. Is the os open? Is any tissue being passed?
   c. Appearance of the posterior fornix: Is there bulging caused by fluid or blood in the cul-de-sac (pouch of Douglas)?
   d. Consider obtaining cervical cultures for gonorrhea and chlamydia.
   e. Consider obtaining urine sample by urethral catheterization if needed.
4. Bimanual pelvic examination
This exam should focus on findings that will help diagnose ectopic pregnancy:[10]
   a. Size, position, and texture of the uterus. Ectopic pregnancy is unlikely if the uterus is greater than 8 week's size.
   b. Presence of tenderness. Unilateral or bilateral tenderness and pain with cervical motion is suspicious for ectopic pregnancy. Pain associated with spontaneous miscarriage is more likely to be midline.
   c. Presence of pelvic masses. Any pelvic mass should suggest ectopic pregnancy until proven otherwise.
5. Use of hand-held Doppler to listen for a fetal heartbeat
This is often best done during the bimanual pelvic examination when the fundus can be identified with the vaginal hand and the transducer aimed at the fundus with the abdominal hand. Using this technique, a fetal heartbeat almost always can be detected by 10–12 weeks even in obese patients. If a fetal heartbeat is heard, miscarriage is ruled out for the present, and the likelihood of ectopic pregnancy is extremely low because most ectopic pregnancies become clinically apparent before 9–10 weeks.

C. Choice of Additional Tests

Findings of history and physical examination determine the necessity and urgency of additional testing. All patients must have initial urine or blood pregnancy testing performed. Complete blood count, blood type, and Rh analysis should be obtained routinely.

1. Positive fetal heart sounds
If a fetal heartbeat is heard by Doppler, no additional tests are needed beyond those ordered for routine prenatal care and scheduling of a follow-up visit. Even patients in whom a fetal heartbeat is noted should be counseled that spontaneous miscarriage is still possible.

2. Absent fetal heart sounds
If no fetal heartbeat is heard, the choice of additional testing depends on the severity of the patient's symptoms and the availability of serum hormone testing and ultrasonography. Although serum hormone testing, in the form of human chorionic gonadotropin (hCG) and progesterone levels, can help establish a diagnosis, ultrasonography promptly yields a definitive diagnosis in a high percentage of cases and should be the first-line test if readily available.[4,11]

V. Ultrasonography

Diagnostic ultrasound is the key to prompt, efficient diagnosis of first-trimester pregnancy problems once the history has been taken and the physical examination has been performed. The diagnostic power of scanning by the transvaginal route is significantly greater than by the transabdominal route because higher-frequency transvaginal transducers produce more detailed spatial resolution and the transvaginal approach avoids intervening bowel and subcutaneous tissue.[19] Transvaginal scanning, however, produces a limited field of view and therefore should follow transabdominal scanning.[19]

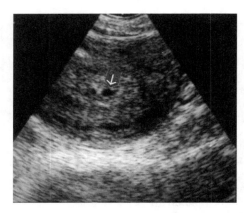

FIGURE 1. The chorionic sac, or gestational sac (arrow), in this case only a few millimeters in diameter. No yolk sac or embryo are yet visible.

A. Normal Landmarks by Menstrual Age

1. Chorionic or gestational sac

The earliest sonographic sign of intrauterine pregnancy is the chorionic sac or gestational sac (Fig. 1). This is a small, lucent area within the uterus surrounded by a brighter, more echogenic ring composed of chorionic villi. The chorionic sac is seen as early as 35–40 menstrual days.[14] The chorionic sac is empty when first seen. It should be rounded in shape and located in the uterine fundus. The chorionic sac grows at 1.1 mm/day up to 80 days.[35]

2. Calculating the menstrual age of the pregnancy

The menstrual age of the pregnancy in days can be calculated by measuring the mean diameter of the chorionic sac in millimeters and adding 30.[35] The mean diameter of the chorionic sac is calculated by adding length plus width plus height and dividing by 3:

menstrual age in days (± 4 days) = mean sac diameter in mm + 30.

3. Yolk sac

The earliest structure of embryonic origin to be seen within the chorionic sac is the yolk sac (Fig. 2). This structure is spherical and appears attached to the chorionic sac wall at one point and should not be larger than 4.5 mm when the mean sac diameter is between 12 and 30 mm (42–60 menstrual days).[22]

4. The embryo

The embryo is first seen as a fetal pole between the yolk sac and chorionic sac wall (Fig 3A). Embryonic cardiac activity often can be seen at the fetal pole

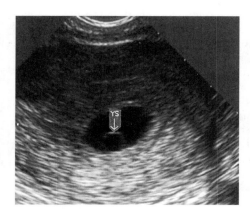

FIGURE 2.   The yolk sac (YS).

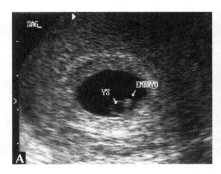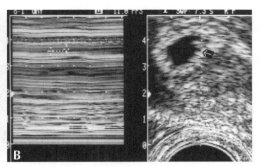

FIGURE 3. **A,** The embryo is first seen as the fetal pole (embryo) between the yolk sac (YS) and chorionic sac wall. **B,** *Left*: Early embryonic cardiac activity documented by M-mode. *Right*, The M-mode beam passes through the fetal pole (arrow) at the edge of the chorionic sac.

before an embryo can easily be measured (Fig. 3B). Embryonic cardiac motion can be documented with an M-mode tracing (Fig. 3B).

5. Calculating the gestational age

The crown-rump length of the embryo provides the most accurate assessment of gestational age and is calculated as follows: Menstrual age in weeks = crown rump length in centimeters + 6.5 (Fig. 4).[48] The yolk sac must *not* be included in the crown-rump measurement.

6. Embryonic cardiac activity

Embryonic cardiac activity is usually seen by the time the crown-rump length is 5–8 mm (7 weeks) but should always be seen by the time the crown-rump length is 14 mm (8 weeks).[5,37,39] When first seen, the embryonic heart rate is about 100.[39] If the heart rate is less than 85 beats/minute, subsequent embryonic demise is highly likely, particularly if the heart rate is under 85 after 8 weeks.[22]

B. Subchorionic Hemorrhage Appearance and Significance[48]

1. Subchorionic hemorrhage

Subchorionic hemorrhage is seen as a wedge-shaped or crescent-shaped lucent area adjacent to the chorionic sac (Fig. 5).

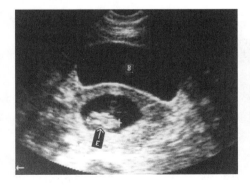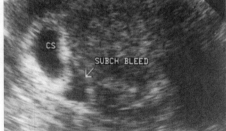

FIGURE 4. Transabdominal transverse image of 9½ week intrauterine pregnancy illustrating the fluid-filled urinary bladder (B) overlying the pregnant uterus. The embryo (E), with a crown rump length of 27 mm, is seen between the calipers.

FIGURE 5. Transvaginal scan of uterus containing a chorionic sac (CS) with an adjacent subchorionic hemorrhage (SUBCH BLEED).

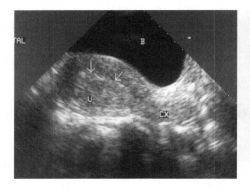

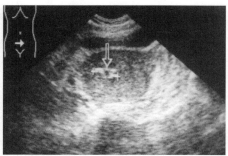

FIGURE 6. A midline sagittal transabdominal scan of the uterus (U) and cervix (CX), with overlying bladder (B) illustrating the endometrial echo (arrows).

FIGURE 7. Transabdominal transverse scan of a uterus containing a 23-mm echogenic area (arrow) indicating retained tissue.

2. Charactreristics of subchorionic hemorrhage

The location is more significant than the size, with hemorrhages that undermine the placental implantation site more often associated with pregnancy loss. Patients with a subchorionic hemorrhage should be counseled to expect additional bleeding. A subchorionic hemorrhage should not be mistaken for a second (twin) chorionic sac. In some studies this finding is associated with a 30% miscarriage rate.

C. Complete, Spontaneous Miscarriage

An empty uterus with a bright endometrial echo is seen in cases of spontaneous complete miscarriage (Fig. 6).

D. Incomplete Miscarriage

Bright echogenic material greater than 5 mm in diameter is characteristic of incomplete miscarriage (Fig. 7).[25] Mixed sonolucent and bright echogenic material also may be seen.

E. Missed Abortion

When the pregnancy dies but is entirely retained with the uterus, a variety of findings are possible.

1. Embryo demise

An embryo is seen with no cardiac motion. In general, embryos that are 5–8 mm in crown-rump length must exhibit a heartbeat during real-time scanning (Fig. 8).[5]

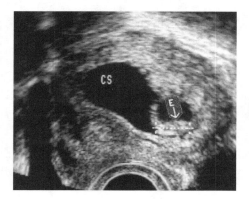

FIGURE 8. Coronal transvaginal scan of a uterus containing a dead embryo (E) between the electronic calipers. No cardiac motion was seen despite the crown rump length of 1.6 cm corresponding to 8+ weeks. (CS = chorionic sac)

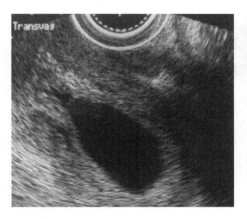

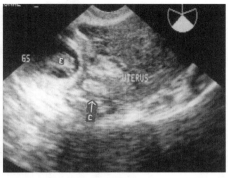

FIGURE 9. Transvaginal scan of an "empty" chorionic sac in a case of embryonic resorption.

FIGURE 10. Coronal transvaginal scan of a confirmed ectopic pregnancy (GS) to the right of the uterus, behind which are blood clots (C). The extrauterine embryo (E) showed cardiac motion.

2. Embryonic resorption or blighted ovum

A sonolucent sac is seen in the uterus with either no embryo or only some echogenic debris (Fig. 9). In general, a chorionic sac of mean diameter 16–20 mm must have an embryo within it to be normal.[35,48]

F. Ectopic Pregnancy

1. Extrauterine embryo

An extrauterine embryo with a heartbeat is positive proof of ectopic pregnancy, but is seen in only 10–24% of cases (Fig. 10).[29,48] The use of transvaginal scanning dramatically improves the likelihood of identifying extrauterine pregnancy.[19]

2. Factors associated with ectopic pregnancy

The presence of adnexal masses and/or free fluid is strongly predictive of ectopic pregnancy (Table 1).[29] The sonographic appearance of free pelvic fluid is shown in Figure 11.

3. Pseudogestational sac

A pseudogestational sac may be seen in some cases of ectopic pregnancy.[33,34] It is a small sonolucent area within the uterus (Fig. 12) that can be confused with a chorionic (gestational) sac. Distinguishing features are the lack of a surrounding echogenic ring of chorionic villi and the lack of a yolk sac or fetal pole within.

4. Simultaneous intrauterine and extrauterine pregnancy

This condition is rare, occurring in 1 in 30,000 pregnancies in the general population or as high as 1 in 6000 patients undergoing ovulation induction.[50] A ruptured corpus luteum cyst, which produces free fluid in the cul-de-sac along with an intrauterine pregnancy, can be confused with simultaneous intrauterine and extrauterine pregnancy.

TABLE 1. Ancillary Findings Predictive of Risk of Ectopic Pregnancy[19]

Finding	Risk of Ectopic Pregnancy (%)
No mass or free fluid	20
Any free fluid	71
Echogenic mass	85
Moderate to large amount of fluid	95
Echogenic mass with fluid	100

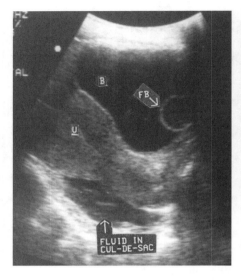

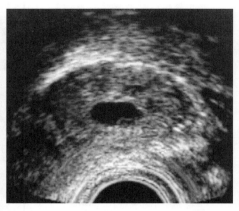

FIGURE 12. Coronal transvaginal scan of a uterus containing a "pseudosac" in an ectopic pregnancy. The pseudosac is not surrounded by an echogenic chorionic ring.

FIGURE 11. A sagittal transabdominal scan showing a large amount of free fluid behind the uterus in a ruptured ectopic pregnancy. The urinary bladder (B) and the Foley catheter balloon (FB) are seen above the uterus (U).

5. Ultrasound of the endometrium

Sonographic measurement of the thickness of the endometrium when no gestational sac is seen has been shown to be helpful in diagnosing abnormal pregnancy including ectopic pregnancy. Pregnancy was abnormal in 97% of cases in which the thickness was ≤ 8 mm.[44]

G. Hydatidiform Mole

This condition is characterized by typical complex echoes filling the uterus (Fig. 13).

H. Twin Intrauterine Pregnancy

A subchorionic hemorrhage should not be mistaken for a second chorionic sac. Avoid making the diagnosis of twin intrauterine pregnancy until two embryos and two heartbeats are seen. The spontaneous loss rate of twin gestation is higher than that of singletons, with combined miscarriage and reduction from twins to singleton reaching 30–40% after initial diagnosis. Even after twins are diagnosed sonographically, the rate of spontaneous reduction to singleton is 20–33%.[16]

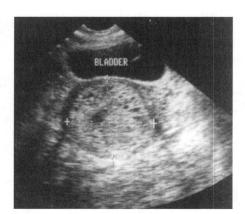

FIGURE 13. Transabdominal transverse scan of a uterus containing typical echoes of hydatidiform mole.

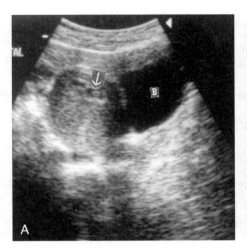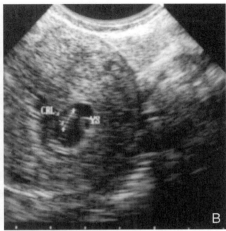

FIGURE 14.   **A**, Transabdominal sagittal scan showing vague intrauterine findings (arrow) (B=bladder). **B**, Transvaginal scan of the same patient on the same day demonstrating an embryo with crown rump length (CRL) measured and yolk sac (YS) visible. Cardiac activity was visible in this 7-mm embryo, corresponding to 7+ weeks.

I. Site and Performance of Ultrasonography
Ultrasonography is most helpful when immediately available and used as an adjunct to complement the physical examination in the office or the emergency department.

J. Types of Scanning
Scanning may be performed by the transabdominal route, the transvaginal route, or both. The transabdominal route provides a wider field of view, whereas the transvaginal route, using higher-frequency transducer, provides more detailed spatial resolution (Fig. 14).

VI. Culdocentesis
Culdocentesis provides a way to sample free fluid seen in the cul-de-sac on ultrasonography. Although ultrasonography can visualize free fluid, culdocentesis is still a useful test in many settings.[49] If non-clotting blood with a hematocrit of 15% or higher is found, an ectopic pregnancy is the diagnosis until proved otherwise.[12] Analysis of pelvic fluid obtained by culdocentesis also can differentiate hemorrhage from the fluid from a ruptured corpus luteum cyst. Culdocentesis is performed as follows:

A. Counsel the patient.

B. Insert a sterile vaginal speculum.

C. Prepare the cervix and posterior fornix with povidone-iodine or other antiseptic solution.

D. Inject a few milliliters of 1% lidocaine (Xylocaine) with epinephrine into the posterior lip of the cervix.

E. Grasp the anesthetized cervix with a tenaculum.

F. Anesthetize the tissue of the posterior fornix with less than 1 ml of 1% Xylocaine with epinephrine.

G. Puncture the posterior fornix with a 20- or 21-gauge needle and aspirate. If ultrasonography is immediately available, the target fluid pocket and needle can be simultaneously imaged, making the procedure faster and less painful for the patient.

VII. Examination of Passed Tissue

If the patient brings in tissue she has passed vaginally, it should be examined for an embryo or chorionic villi. If either is seen, ectopic pregnancy is virtually ruled out (except in the case of simultaneous intrauterine and extrauterine pregnancy). To look for chorionic villi, suspend the tissue in saline and view it either with the naked eye or under low-power magnification using a colposcope. Chorionic villi appear as tiny frond-like structures. Some patients with an ectopic pregnancy pass a decidual cast (Arias-Stella reaction), which may resemble products of conception grossly but contains no chorionic villi.[18]

VIII. Serum Hormone Testing

A. Quantitative hCG Levels

Quantitative hCG levels increase predictably during early pregnancy, doubling every 2 to 3 days during the 4th to 8th weeks of pregnancy.[38] Various reporting standards exist, but most current tests follow the International Reference Preparation (IRP),[36] or third international standard, which are equivalent.[19]

1. The "discriminatory zone"

This is the level of hCG by which a chorionic sac can be seen sonographically. The diagnostic value of this concept is that if an intrauterine chorionic (gestational) sac is not visible by the time the hCG is at or above this threshold, the pregnancy has a high likelihood of being ectopic or otherwise abnormal. Various studies have found this threshold to be about 1800–2000 mIU/ml IRP[14] or even 3000 mIU/ml.[19] The yolk sac should be visible by the time the hCG reaches about 5000 mIU/ml IRP and an embryo with cardiac motion by about 17,000 mIU/ml IRP.

2. Clinical utility

Single or serial quantitative hCG tests can be particularly helpful when transvaginal sonography fails to show an intrauterine pregnancy or definitive signs of ectopic pregnancy. Ectopic pregnancy is virtually assured in such cases if the hCG is above 2000 mIU/ml, particularly if serial testing shows it to be either rising or not falling.[31]

B. Quantitative Serum Progesterone Testing

This has been used to help identify patients with abnormal pregnancies. Living intrauterine pregnancies are associated with quantitative progesterone levels of 25 ng/ml or greater. Values below that level are strongly associated with various forms of pregnancy loss and ectopic pregnancy.[21,46,47,51] Progesterone levels less than 5ng/ml are invariably associated with pregnancy loss including, but not limited to, ectopic pregnancy.[19,32]

C. Serum Hormonal Testing

Results of serum hormone tests are generally not as immediately available as ultrasonography. The cost of multiple serum hormone tests is likely to exceed the cost of a single diagnostic ultrasound examination.[11]

SECTION B.
MANAGEMENT

I. Treatment

A. Threatened Miscarriage (Abortion)

These patients are stable and have bleeding or pain (or both) but have not passed tissue. Even if ultrasonography has demonstrated an embryonic heartbeat, the patient should be cautiously reassured and counseled that miscarriage is still possible with the risk falling from 16% at less than 8 weeks[23] to 2–4% at 12 weeks.[8] Outpatient follow-up should be prompt if bleeding or pain increase. Repeat ultrasonography in about 1 week helps clarify the diagnosis.

    1. Fetal heart tones absent

If a fetal heartbeat is not heard with a hand-held Doppler, hormone treatment with progesterone or hCG has been suggested, mainly for patients who habitually abort as a result of a relative deficiency of progesterone secreted by the corpus luteum. No controlled studies of this treatment exist proving its efficacy.[17,42]

    2. Immunotherapy

Immunotherapy with intravenous immune globulin (IVIg) and a variety of other substances has been proposed for recurrent miscarriage. Benefit over placebo has not been conclusively demonstrated.[43]

B. Complete Miscarriage (Abortion)

Complete, spontaneous expulsion of the products of conception with resolution of bleeding requires no specific medical or surgical intervention.

C. Incomplete or Missed Abortion

This condition may require surgical intervention in the form of a dilatation and curettage (D&C), but medical and expectant management is also reasonable.

    1. There are no absolute criteria for performance of a D&C after pregnancy loss.[2]

    2. Patients with excessive bleeding are most likely to benefit from a D&C.[2]

    3. Complications that early surgical management hopes to avoid are infection, molar degeneration, and excessive bleeding leading to hypovolemia or anemia.

    4. Expectant treatment can avoid surgery (D&C) in over 90% of properly selected patients.[16] Reasonable selection criteria include:

        a. No excessive bleeding

        b. Stable vital signs: blood pressure, pulse, no fever

        c. No excessive pain

        d. Tissue in uterus $\leq$ 5 cm thick by ultrasound

        e. Informed patient, reliable for follow-up

    5. Medical management with prostaglandin has been studied but shows inconsistent results, high failure rates, and requires further study and refinement.[16]

D. Ectopic Pregnancy

Ectopic pregnancy is a potentially life-threatening condition. Patients with a confirmed or strongly suspected ectopic pregnancy should either be hospitalized or followed extremely closely as outpatients. Many choices in treatment are possible depending on clinical factors and expertise of the physician.[26]

    1. Open surgical treatment

This is accomplished with salpingectomy and is most appropriate when a large ectopic pregnancy mass is present or has ruptured, causing hemoperitoneum.[26]

    2. Conservative surgical treatment

This is appropriate for patients who:[45]

        a. Desire future fertility.

        b. Have an unruptured fallopian tube.

        c. Are hemodynamically stable.

    3. Types of conservative surgical treatments

These include the following variants that can be performed by either an open or laparoscopic approach:

        a. Salpingostomy

        b. Salpingotomy

        c. Segmental resection

        d. Fimbrial expression

4. Medical treatment with methotrexate

Methotrexate, a folic acid antagonist, is becoming standard therapy for properly selected patients.[6] This form of treatment has been shown to be safe and effective in randomized trials; it also can be less costly and result in equal or better subsequent fertility than conservative surgical treatment.[41]

5. Patient selection for methotrexate therapy

Not all patients with an ectopic pregnancy are candidates for conservative therapy. A variety of criteria have been proposed,[3] and some controversy exists. This list shows a set of reasonable criteria.

    a. Stable vital signs
    b. No medical contraindication to methotrexate therapy (normal liver enzymes, blood count, platelet count)
    c. Patient reliable for follow-up
    d. Unruptured ectopic pregnancy
    e. Absence of embryonic cardiac motion
    f. Ectopic mass 4 cm or less
    g. Proceed with caution for patients with high starting hCG levels (> 5000 mIU/ml), because it increases the risk of treatment failure and need for additional doses.

6. Methotrexate regimens

A variety of methotrexate regimens have been published, including single or multiple doses given intramuscularly (IM), or by direct injection into the ectopic mass by laparoscopic approach. Single-dosage IM regimens are commonly calculated at 1 mg/kg or 50 mg/m^2. Serum hCG testing is performed on the fourth and seventh post-treatment days and followed until the level reaches 5 mIU/ml, which may take 3–4 weeks. The hCG initially rises slightly, but should fall 15% between days 4 and 7; if not, the dosage should be repeated or surgical therapy performed. Serum progesterone levels may be followed instead of hCG; a drop to 1.5 ng/ml is considered a successful endpoint and usually occurs by about 2–3 weeks.[41]

7. Expectant waiting for spontaneous resolution is based on the fact that some tubal pregnancies undergo spontaneous abortion or resorption. One randomized trial from 1955 showed that about half of expectantly managed patients escaped the need for surgery.[27] Modern reports have focused on identifying patients appropriate for expectant management, including those whose hCG is < 1000 mIU/ml and falling.[1,9,15,30] Patients must be followed with serial hCG, hematocrits, physical exams, and ultrasound as needed until clinical resolution and hCG is less than 5 mIU/ml.

8. Criteria for expectant management of ectopic pregnancy

    a. Minimal pain or bleeding
    b. Patient reliable for follow-up
    c. No evidence of tubal rupture
    d. Starting hCG level less than 1000 mIU/ml
    e. hCG level falling
    f. Ectopic mass less than 3 cm
    g. No embryonic heartbeat

9. Fertility after ectopic pregnancy

Fertility after an ectopic pregnancy is highly variable and depends on pre-existing pelvic abnormalities and the type of surgery performed. Infertility may approach 50%, and recurrent ectopic pregnancy may occur in excess of 25%.[26]

E. Hydatidiform Mole

Hydatidiform mole should lead to prompt suction D&C with serial quantitative hCG testing until the value falls below 5 mIU/ml. Patients must be followed for 6–12 months with serial hCG testing as surveillance for choriocarcinoma. Contraception is essential during the follow-up interval.

II. Summary

First-trimester pregnancy loss is a common presenting problem to family physicians. Discovery of which patients have a potentially life-threatening ectopic pregnancy is a major diagnostic challenge. After the history and physical examination has been performed, diagnostic ultrasonography is the tool most likely to establish a prompt diagnosis. Scanning by the transvaginal route is essential. If the patient is stable and less than 5 weeks have passed from her last normal menstrual period, no diagnostic intrauterine findings are expected on sonography. In such cases, serum hormone testing may be the most appropriate first step until such testing indicates that the hCG has risen to the discriminatory zone in which diagnostic intrauterine findings are expected sonographically. Ectopic pregnancy and hydatidiform mole require prompt intervention. There is an increasing trend to offer medical (methotrexate) therapy and even expectant therapy for properly selected patients with ectopic pregnancy. Other first-trimester complications, such as threatened abortion, incomplete abortion, and missed abortion, may be treated expectantly.

References

1. Adoni A, Milwidsky A, Hurwitz A, Palti Z: Declining β-hCG levels: An indicator for expectant approach in ectopic pregnancy. Int J Fertil 31:40–42, 1986.
2. Ambulatory Sentinel Practice Network: Spontaneous abortion in primary care. J Am Board Fam Pract 1:15–23, 1988.
3. American College of Obstetricians and Gynecologists: Medical management of tubal pregnancy. ACOG Practice Bulletin Number 3, December, 1998. Washington, DC., American College of Obstetricians and Gynecologists.
4. Brennan DF: Ectopic pregnancy—Part II: Diagnostic procedures and imaging. Acad Emerg Med 2:1090–1097, 1995.
5. Brown DJ, Emerson DS, Felker RE, et al: Diagnosis of early embryonic demise by endovaginal sonography. J Ultrasound Med 9:631–636, 1990.
6. Buster JE, Pisarska MD: Medical management of ectopic pregnancy. Clin Obstet Gynecol 42:23–30, 1999.
7. Carroll J, Biringer A, White D, et al: Complications of Pregnancy. AAFP Home Study Self-Assessment Monograph. Kansas City, MO, American Academy of Family Physicians, 1989.
8. Cashner KA, Christopher CR, Dysert GA: Spontaneous fetal loss after demonstration of a live fetus in the first trimester. Obstet Gynecol 70:827–830, 1987.
9. Cohen MA, Sauer MV: Expectant management of ectopic pregnancy. Clin Obstet Gynecol 42:48–54, 1999.
10. Dart RG, Kaplan B, Varaklis K: Predictive value of history and physical examination in patients with suspected ectopic pregnancy. Ann Emerg Med 33:283–290, 1999.
11. Deutchman ME: Advances in the diagnosis of first-trimester pregnancy problems. Am Fam Physician 44:15S–30S, 1991.
12. Droegemueller W: Ectopic pregnancy. In Danforth DN (ed): Obstetrics and Gynecology. Philadelphia, J.B. Lippincott, 1986, pp 403–418.
13. Fernandez H, Yves Vincent SC, Pauthier S: Randomized trial of conservative laparoscopic treatment and methotrexate administration in ectopic pregnancy and subsequent fertility. Human Reproduction 13:339–343, 1998.
14. Fossum GT, Davajan V, Kletzky OA: Early detection of pregnancy with transvaginal ultrasound. Fertil Steril 49:788–791, 1988.
15. Garcia AJ, Aubert JM, Sama J, et al: Expectant management of presumed ectopic pregnancies. Fertil Steril 48:395–400, 1987.
16. Geyman JP, Oliver LM, Sullivan SD: Expectant, medical or surgical treatment of spontaneous abortion in first trimester of pregnancy? A pooled quantitative literature evaluation. J Am Board Fam Pract 12:55–64, 1999.
17. Glass RH, Golbus MS: Pregnancy wastage. In Creasy RK, Resnick R (eds): Maternal Fetal Medicine. Philadelphia, W.B. Saunders, 1989, pp 440–441.
18. Goldstein SR: Endovaginal Ultrasound. New York, A.R. Liss, 1988, p 94.
19. Graczykowski JW, Seifer DB: Diagnosis of acute and persistent ectopic pregnancy. Clin Obstet Gynecol 42:9–22, 1999.

20. Grobman WA, Peaceman AM: What are the rates and mechanisms of first and second trimester pregnancy loss in twins? Clin Obstet Gynecol 41:36–45, 1998.
21. Hahlin M, Wallin JA, Sjoblom P, et al: Single progesterone assay for early recognition of abnormal pregnancy. Hum Reprod 5:622–626, 1990.
22. Harrington C, Lyons EA: Case of the day number 2. J Ultrasound Med 10:3–4, 1991.
23. Howe RS, Isaacson KJ, Alber JL, et al: Embryonic heart rate in human pregnancy. J Ultrasound Med 10:367–371, 1991.
24. Kochenour NK: Course and conduct of normal pregnancy. In Danforth DN (ed): Obstetrics and Gynecology. Philadelphia, J.B. Lippincott, 1986, pp 358–375.
25. Kurtz AB, Shlansky-Goldberg RD, Choi HY, et al: Detection of retained products of conception following spontaneous abortion in the first trimester. J Ultrasound Med 10:387–395, 1991.
26. Leach RE, Ory SJ: Modern management of ectopic pregnancy. J Reprod Med 34:324–338, 1989.
27. Lund J: Early ectopic pregnancy: Comments on conservative treatment. J Obstet Gynaecol Br Emp 62:70–76, 1955.
28. MMWR: Ectopic pregnancy—United states, 1990–1992. JAMA 273:533, 1995.
29. Mahony BS, Filly RA, Nyberg DA, et al: Sonographic evaluation of ectopic pregnancy. J Ultrasound Med 4:221–228, 1985.
30. Mashiach S, Carp JH, Serr DM: Nonoperative management of ectopic pregnancy. J Reprod Med 27:127–132, 1982.
31. Mol BW, Hajenius PJ, Engelsbel S, et al: Serum human chorionic gonadotropin measurement in the diagnosis of ectopic pregnancy when transvaginal sonography is inconclusive. Fertil Steril 70:972–981, 1998.
32. Mol BW, Lijmer JG, Ankum WM, et al: The accuracy of single serum progesterone measurement in the diagnosis of ectopic pregnancy: a meta-analysis. Human Reprod 13:3220–3227, 1998.
33. Nelson P, Bowie JD, Rosenberg ER: Early pregnancy or decidual cast: An anatomic-sonographic approach. J Ultrasound Med 2:543–547, 1983.
34. Nyberg DA, Laing FC, Filly RA, et al: Ultrasonographic differentiation of the gestational sac of early intrauterine pregnancy from the pseudogestational sac of ectopic pregnancy. Radiology 146:755–759, 1983.
35. Nyberg DA, Mack LA, Laing FC, et al: Distinguishing normal from abnormal gestational sac growth in early pregnancy. J Ultrasound Med 6:23–27, 1987.
36. Painter PC: Discordant hCG results in pregnancy: A method in crisis. Diagn Clin Test 27:20–24, 1989.
37. Pennell RG, Baltarowich OH, Kurtz AB, et al: Complicated first-trimester pregnancies: Evaluation with endovaginal ultrasound versus transabdominal technique. Radiology 165:79–83, 1987.
38. Pittaway DE, Reish RL, Wentz AC: Doubling times of human chorionic gonadotropic increase in early viable intrauterine pregnancies. Am J Obstet Gynecol 152:299–302, 1985.
39. Rempen A: Diagnosis of viability in early pregnancy with vaginal sonography. J Ultrasound Med 9:711–716, 1990.
40. Rempen A: Vaginal sonography in ectopic pregnancy: A prospective evaluation. J Ultrasound Med 7:381–387, 1988.
41. Saraj AJ, Wilcox JG, Najmabadi S: Resolution of hormonal markers of ectopic gestation: a randomized trial comparing single-dose intramuscular methotrexate with salpingostomy. Obstet Gynecol 92:989–994, 1998.
42. Scott JR: Human chorionic gonadotrophin (hCG) for recurrent miscarriage (Cochrane Review). In The Cochrane Library, Issue 1, 2000. Oxford, Update Software, 2000.
43. Scott JR: Immunotherapy for recurrent miscarriage (Cochrane Review). In The Cochrane Library, Issue 1, 2000. Oxford, Update Software.
44. Spandorfer SD, Barnhart KT: Endometrial stripe thickness as a predictor of ectopic pregnancy. Fertil Steril 66:474–477, 1996.
45. Stangel JJ, Reyniak JV, Stone ML: Conservative surgical management of tubal pregnancy. Obstet Gynecol 48:241–244, 1976.
46. Stovall TG, Kellermann AL, Ling FW, et al: Emergency department diagnosis of ectopic pregnancy. Ann Emerg Med 19:1098–1103, 1990.
47. Stovall TG, Ling FW, Cope BJ, et al: Preventing ruptured ectopic pregnancy with a single serum progesterone. Am J Obstet Gynecol 160:1425–1431, 1989.
48. Timor-Trisch EL, Rottem S: Pathology of the early intrauterine pregnancy. In Timor-Trisch IE, Rottem S (eds): Transvaginal Sonography. New York, Elsevier, 1991.
49. Vande Krol L. Abbott JT: The current role of culdocentesis. Am J Emerg Med 10:354–358, 1992 .
50. Yaghoobian J, Pinck RL, Ramanthan K, et al: Sonographic demonstration of simultaneous intrauterine and extrauterine gestation. J Ultrasound Med 5:309–312, 1986.
51. Yeko TR, Gorrill MJ, Hughes LH, et al: Timely diagnosis of early ectopic pregnancy using a single blood progesterone measurement. Fertil Steril 48:1048–1050, 1987.

CHAPTER 6

Complications of Pregnancy

SECTION A.
GESTATIONAL DIABETES

Elizabeth G. Baxley, M.D., and Robert Gobbo, M.D.

The diagnosis and management of gestational diabetes is one of the most controversial topics in obstetrics today. Literally thousands of articles have been published on this topic, but extensive research has failed to provide a clear direction for the practicing physician.

Complicating 2–3 % of all pregnancies, gestational diabetes is responsible for the vast majority (90%) of all diabetes cases encountered in gravid women. While generally associated with increased risks of perinatal morbidity and mortality, many of the often-cited complications of impaired glucose intolerance may be attributed to other conditions, such as advanced maternal age and body mass index.[11,21,34,43] It is also likely that the magnitude of this risk has been overestimated, as there are no compelling data to show that detection and treatment of gestational diabetes reduce perinatal mortality rates or rates of significant morbidity to the mother and her newborn.[20]

Gestational diabetes is defined as any degree of glucose intolerance that develops during pregnancy.[25] As such, this diagnosis is applied to a heterogeneous population of women that ranges from undiagnosed pregestational diabetics to women who have only mild elevations in glucose following a glucose challenge test.[39] In an effort to avoid unnecessary labeling and a cascade of costly interventions of questionable benefit, it has recently been recommended that the term gestational diabetes be abandoned. Alternative descriptive terms have been suggested, such as diabetes mellitus diagnosed during pregnancy, impaired fasting glucose diagnosed during pregnancy, gestational carbohydrate intolerance, and impaired glucose tolerance during pregnancy.[17,39] This would allow stratification of women into different groups with markedly different outcomes in terms of perinatal morbidity and mortality and long-term health consequences to the mother.

I. Epidemiology
A. Incidence
The incidence of gestational diabetes ranges from 1% to 5% depending on the population being studied. A major problem contributing to this range in incidence rates is the variation in classification schemes used in different studies; e.g., some include women with pregestational asymptomatic non-insulin-dependent diabetes mellitus and others do not.

Differences in incidence rates of gestational diabetes may not be explained on the basis of race or ethnicity, although rates of pregestational diabetes are disproportionate for some ethnic groups. Sacks et al., in a study of 3505 "unselected" pregnant women, found a mean fasting plasma glucose level difference of < 1 mg/dl among African-Americans, Caucasians, Hispanics, and Asians.[36]

B. Classification
Two systems have historically been used in categorizing diabetes in pregnant women.
  1. The National Diabetes Data Group classification
     a. Type 1—insulin-dependent when not pregnant
     b. Type 2—non-insulin-dependent when not pregnant
     c. Type 3—gestational diabetes (normal hemoglobin A1c before 20 weeks' gestation and reversible hyperglycemia postpartum). Hollingsworth has suggested two distinct subgroups: (1) non-obese—insulin-deficient, sensitive to small doses; (2) obese—hyperinsulinemic and insulin-resistant.[17]
     d. Type 4—impaired glucose tolerance
  2. The White classification (for use during pregnancy)
     a. A1—gestational diabetes not requiring insulin
     b. A2—gestational diabetes requiring insulin
C. Risk Factors for Gestational Diabetes
  1. Personal history
Advanced maternal age, obesity, and a history of gestational diabetes are major risk factors for developing gestational diabetes during the index pregnancy. Women younger than age 25, particularly pregnant adolescents, develop gestational diabetes at much lower rates than older gravidas.
  2. Family history
A family history of diabetes mellitus also places the pregnant patient at risk, but the genetic contribution is much higher with non-insulin-dependent than with insulin-dependent diabetes mellitus.[16]
  3. Obstetric history
Birth of a previous macrosomic infant or unexplained fetal death may be markers for increased risk of gestational diabetes.
  4. Current pregnancy
Polyhydramnios is associated with gestational diabetes.
D. Complications
Interpretation of data regarding maternal and fetal risk is problematic because of the lack of differentiation of gestational diabetes from pre-existing disease. Both the retrospective nature of correct diagnosis and lack of uniform classification and reporting contribute to the problem.
  1. Maternal
Women with gestational diabetes have an increased incidence of pregnancy-induced hypertension, urinary tract infections, and delivery by cesarean section.[42]
  2. Fetal
The probability of perinatal death with a positive glucose tolerance test (all diabetics) has been calculated by Hunter and Keirse to be 4.9%.[20] Hollingsworth notes this has been reduced to 2–3% in some centers.[17] Women with insulin-requiring gestational diabetes have higher rates of perinatal mortality than non-insulin–requiring diabetics.

Congenital anomalies are more often associated with pregestational diabetes, and the rate of major malformations does not appear to increase until the fasting plasma glucose level in pregnancy exceeds 120 mg/dl.[38] Chung and Myrianthopoulos found no increased risk of congenital anomalies with gestational diabetes.[9]
  3. Neonatal
Macrosomia is the most commonly cited neonatal complication of gestational diabetes, occurring in 17% of diabetic women using a birth weight cut-off of ≥ 4000 g and 2.9% using a birth weight cut-off of ≥ 4500 g.[39] Although this rate

is higher than in a non-diabetic population, most macrosomic infants are born to mothers with a normal glucose tolerance test. Associated birth trauma occurs in only 10% of infants weighing ≥ 4000 g, but may also occur in normal-birth-weight infants of diabetic mothers secondary to truncal asymmetry and increased bisacromial diameter. Infants of diabetic mothers have a larger shoulder-to-head ratio, significantly higher body fat, and thicker upper extremity folds.[20,24] Yet, the risk of disproportion and mechanical difficulties during vaginal delivery is low.

Infants born to mothers with gestational diabetes are also at risk for hypoglycemia, which occurs in ≤ 7% of newborns, as well as other transient metabolic abnormalities (e.g. hypocalcemia, hypomagnesemia).[5,42] Evidence for increased risk of jaundice in these newborns is lacking.

II. Pathophysiology

Early in pregnancy, maternal insulin levels are higher and sensitivity to insulin is also increased, resulting in normally lower levels of maternal glucose. Subsequently, in the second half of pregnancy insulin resistance increases and glucose tolerance may occur in susceptible individuals. Glucose freely crosses the placenta, while insulin does not in most cases. The fetus is continuously extracting glucose from the maternal circulation. Therefore, maternal hyperglycemia results in fetal hyperglycemia and a subsequent increase in insulin secretion by the fetal pancreas. Placental hormones also interfere with insulin use by the fetus, and exacerbate the tendency to hyperglycemia.[26]

III. Diagnosis
A. Screening
1. Universal versus selective screening

Universal screening for GDM in pregnancy versus selective screening of those with risk factors is controversial. Ten different guidelines on screening have been critically reviewed by Vogel et al., who found that five recommend screening for all pregnant women, three propose screening based on risk factors, and two did not recommend for or against universal or selective screening[42] (Table 1). Risk factors that were most frequently listed by those who recommended selective screening included:
   a. Advanced maternal age
   b. Obesity
   c. Race (Asian, Hispanic, Native American or African American)
      A recent retrospective cohort study demonstrated that, of 352 women in a Hispanic community who had a normal or negative 1-hour glucola screen, none had a positive screen in a subsequent pregnancy occurring

TABLE 1. Screening Recommendations Based on Published Guidelines[39,42]

Universal Screening	Risk Factor-Based Screening	No Recommendation for Screening
World Health Organization (WHO)	American Diabetes Association (ADA)	U.S. Preventive Services Task Force
Third International Conference on Gestational Diabetes	American College of Obstetricians and Gynecologists (ACOG)	Canadian Task Force on the Periodic Examination
Cousins	Briese et al.	
Kappy	Report of the Expert Committee on the Diagnosis and Classification of Diabetes Mellitus	
ALFEDIAM, Lassmann-Vague	Society of Maternal-Fetal Medicine	

within 4 years.[46] If further studies replicate these findings, it would support a more restrictive approach for screening for GDM in subsequent pregnancies of women with normal testing in a previous pregnancy.
  d. History of macrosomia or previous obstetrical complication
  e. Family history of diabetes

The U.S. Preventive Services Task Force and the Canadian Task Force on the Periodic Examination have both concluded that there is insufficient evidence to recommend for or against universal screening for gestational diabetes. The Cochrane Library concludes that all forms of glucose tolerance testing during pregnancy should be stopped except for research purposes.[43] Adoption of a selective screening approach has been advocated in the report of the Expert Committee on the Diagnosis and Classification of Diabetes Mellitus, and has also been endorsed by the Society of Maternal-Fetal Medicine.[39]

Despite the controversies surrounding the diagnosis and treatment of this condition, universal screening at 28 weeks of gestation is widely practiced, based on the inability to identify 50% of gestational diabetics by risk factors alone.[8,27] However, there is a paucity of evidence that supports the contention that the diagnosis and management of GDM result in improved perinatal mortality, and the impact of this missed identification remains questionable.[7,14,37,44]

2. Timing of screening
  a. Early screening based on risk factors. A first-trimester 50-g glucola test is recommended for patients with a history of prior gestational diabetes, delivery of a previous macrosomic infant, family history of type II diabetes, age > 25 years, in a high-risk ethnic group listed above, or with a maternal pre-pregnancy weight > 200 pounds (or greater than > 120% ideal body weight).
  b. Universal screening. In published guidelines for gestational diabetes screening, large variation is found in testing schedules and gestational age for universal screening, further complicating the controversy and prohibiting proper comparison of outcomes.[42] These range from administering a 50-g glucose load between 24 and 28 weeks' gestation and measuring glucose value 1 hour after administration, measuring a fasting glucose alone, administering a 75-g glucose load between 16 and 20 weeks' gestation and measuring glucose values 1, 2, and 3 hours later, and measuring random blood glucose.[42] The 50-g glucose load (see below) is the most common regimen cited.
  c. Late screening based on complications. Additional screening may be considered later in pregnancy for those patients who develop complications known to be associated with diabetes, such as macrosomia, polyhydramnios, or unexplained fetal death in utero.
3. Method of screening
  a. 50-g glucose challenge test (GCT). For screening purposes, a 50-g oral glucose load is administered to a pregnant woman without regard to fasting state, and a blood sugar measurement is made 1 hour later. Venous blood samples are necessary, as hand-held capillary glucose monitors carry too much variation and have a 3–5% higher reading. Some patients cannot tolerate the 50-g glucola due to gastric irritation. A successful alternative is to have the patient eat 18 Brach's jellie bellies in a five-minute period.

  The 50-gram glucola is a very sensitive test, but an abnormal result will identify many women who do not actually meet diagnostic criteria for gestational diabetes. A value > 140 is an indication for more specific testing with a 3-hour oral glucose tolerance test (sensitivity and specificity of 90%, positive predictive value of 22%, negative predictive value of 99.7%, using underlying population prevalence of 3%). Using a cut-off value of 130 is advocated by some due to a higher sensitivity level of 99%. However, the specificity drops to 75% using this value, as does the positive predictive value (17.3%). Thus, more women are initially "selected out" for further testing, which in many cases is unnecessary. In one analysis, screening 10,000 women would potentially prevent 50 cases of macrosomia, which would only prevent six cases of shoulder dystocia, and only one brachial plexus injury.[4]

Screening values ≥ 190 may obviate the need for further testing and a fasting blood sugar should be checked. If the fasting blood sugar is elevated (95–105 mg/dl, depending on the source cited), the patient is considered to have gestational diabetes and does not need further testing. If it is less than 95 mg/dl, a 3- hour GTT is obtained.

b. 100-g glucose tolerance test (GTT). When screening suggests a need for further diagnostic testing, a 3-hour GTT is administered after an overnight fast for at least 8, but not more than 14, hours. Three days of unrestricted diet and physical activity precede the test. A fasting blood sugar is obtained and a 100-g glucose load is administered. Venous blood sugar samples are then obtained at 1, 2, and 3 hours after the glucose load. Criteria for determining an abnormal result vary depending on the source selected (Table 2). Historically, the criteria most often used have been those of the National Diabetes Data Group, although some centers have adopted a more liberal approach to cut-off values with the Carpenter and Coustan criteria, which leads to a diagnosis of gestational diabetes in 54% more pregnant women than with current standards.[39] Either an elevated FBS or two or more of the 3-hour values being higher than the listed thresholds are diagnostic of gestational diabetes.

IV. Prevention

Women known to be at risk for gestational diabetes can be counseled preconceptually with regard to weight loss, diet, and activity. Fasting and 2-hour postprandial glucose levels and hemoglobin A1c values can be checked before pregnancy to identify women with previously unrecognized type 2 diabetes mellitus. Without this counseling and careful planning of pregnancy, many women with asymptomatic non-insulin-dependent diabetes mellitus present at 6–8 weeks of gestation with poor glucose control. Treatment

TABLE 2. Criteria for Determining Abnormal Result of 100-g, 3-Hour Oral GTT in Pregnancy

	Glucose Level (mg/dl)*			
	National Diabetes Data Group[10]	Carpenter and Coustan[7]	Sacks et al.[36]	O'Sullivan and Mahan[27]
Fasting	105	95	96	90
1 h	190	180	172	165
2 h	165	155	152	145
3 h	145	140	131	125

For all criteria listed, diagnosis required glucose level of at least that shown for ≥ 2 values.
* In venous plasma (National Diabetes Data Group,[10] Carpenter and Coustan,[7] Sacks et al.[36]) or venous whole blood (O'Sullivan and Mahan[27]).
From Schwartz ML, Ray WN, Lubarsky SL: The diagnosis and classification of gestational diabetes mellitus: Is it time to change our tune? Am J Obstet Gynecol 180:1560–1571, 2000, with permission.

at this time is much less effective at reducing malformations because early organogenesis has already taken place.

V. Treatment
A. Diet
Patients whose fasting glucose levels can be maintained below 100, and 2-hour postprandial values are below 120 mg/dl may be managed without insulin. Home monitoring four times a day is recommended initially with decreasing intervals as control is established. In-hospital or clinic monitoring has not shown any advantage and greatly increases the cost.[19] A typical diet is 30–35 calories/kg/day with about 20% protein and 60% carbohydrates and 20% fat (half polyunsaturated). Carbohydrates should be mainly complex, high-fiber, low glycemic index (see Chapter 3, sections A and F). A sample patient education sheet is shown in Table 3. Despite these common recommendations, a Cochrane Database review of four randomized controlled trials (RCTs) of dietary therapy in women with abnormal glucose tolerance tests concluded that there were no differences in rates of macrosomia or cesarean delivery between women managed with primary dietary therapy versus no primary dietary therapy.[43]

B. Insulin
Patients in whom diet and activity alone do not achieve desired levels of control are started on a combination of neutral protamine Hagedorn (NPH) and regular insulin once or twice per day. The percentage of gestational diabetics who require insulin varies between 23 and 66%.[7] Typically this is done when fasting blood sugar levels exceed 100–105 mg/dl or 2-hour postprandial levels exceed 120 mg/dl. The usual starting dose is 20 units of NPH and 10 units of regular insulin per day, which can be increased as needed up to 0.7 units/kg/day. Because of the relative insulin resistance, hypoglycemic reactions are rare. Nevertheless, patients and their families should be instructed in recognizing the symptoms and managing the reactions by administration of sugar-containing juices. The frequency of hypoglycemic reactions is increased with increasing "tightness" of control.[18] Thin patients with gestational diabetes may be managed with smaller doses of insulin before each meal.

TABLE 3.   Dietary Guidelines for Glucose Intolerance During Pregnancy

Avoid sugar and concentrated sweets
    No cookies, cakes, pies, soft drinks, jam, jelly, chocolate, table sugar, honey, Kool-aid, or fruit juices.
    Read labels: avoid foods containing sucrose, fructose, dextrose, honey, corn syrup, molasses, or natural sweeteners.

Eat small, frequent meals (3 meals, 3 snacks)
    Eat approximately every 3 hours.
    Include a good source of protein (meat, cheese, fish, eggs, or poultry) at every meal.
    Try to have meals at the same time every day.

Eat a very small breakfast
    Not more than one starch/bread
    No fruit or juice.
    Avoid cereals, especially sugar-coated cereals.

Choose high-fiber foods
    Whole grain breads, corn tortillas
    Hot cereals (oatmeal and oatbran—not instant)
    Dried beans
    Fresh fruits and vegetables

Lower fat intake
    Buy lean cuts of meat (no lunch meat, bacon, sausage, hot dogs).
    Bake, broil, steam, or barbecue foods (no frying)
    Use nonfat or lowfat milk.

C. Oral Hypoglycemic Agents

Oral hypoglycemic agents such as glyburide and glipizide have not been used in pregnancy because of their potential to have adverse effects on neonates such as hypoglycemia and fetal anomalies.[22] Langer et al. recently published an RCT that demonstrated that the use of glyburide was comparable to that of insulin in achieving desired glycemic control for women with type A2 gestational diabetes and was not associated with any adverse neonatal effects.[22] If further studies replicate these findings, the use of these agents offers great potential in management of this condition.

D. Effect of Glycemic Control

Farrag compared the effectiveness of three levels of control: (1) very tight, (2) tight, and (3) moderate.[13] No benefits of very tight over tight control were detected. However, tight control did show benefit compared with moderate control, where there were statistically significant decreases in the incidence of preeclampsia, urinary tract infection, cesarean birth, preterm labor, neonatal macrosomia, respiratory distress syndrome, and perinatal mortality.

E. Hypoglycemia

The conscious but symptomatic patient with hypoglycemia may be treated with sugar-containing juices. For the unconscious patient, one ampule of glucagon is administered intramuscularly or intravenously after a rapid fingerstick glucose level is checked. If the initial level is less than 50, intravenous glucose therapy is begun. If the level is greater than 50, it should be rechecked in 15 minutes.

VI. Antepartum Fetal Assessment

Although there is no evidence to support the effectiveness of antenatal fetal surveillance for women with GDM, expert opinions recommend twice-weekly antenatal testing for uncomplicated patients with insulin-requiring A2 diabetes at 32–34 weeks. This can be accomplished by a combination of BPP and NST or CST testing. Antenatal testing of patients controlled on diet alone is more controversial, but is generally suggested to begin at 38 weeks' gestation.

While macrosomia is the fetal complication most often cited as a concern in the diabetic pregnancy, ultrasound measurement of fetal weight is a poor predictor of eventual birth weight. Prediction may be improved by adding clinical information to the ultrasound, but even regular serial scanning and clinical examination do not always diagnose the macrosomic fetus in diabetic pregnancy. In many hands, clinical examination is as predictive as ultrasound measurements. As a result, ultrasound assessment of fetal weight is not sufficiently reliable to dictate mode of delivery.

VII. Delivery

A. Timing

In the absence of complications, most women may be managed expectantly until term. There is no evidence that elective induction improves perinatal mortality or morbidity.[15] A Cochrane review found only one RCT of elective delivery (either by induction or cesarean section) versus expectant management in insulin-requiring diabetic women at term. This trial suggests that induction of labor in women with GDM treated with insulin reduces the risk of macrosomia, but does not appear to modify the risk of maternal or neonatal morbidity.[5] Delayed fetal pulmonary maturation is a possibility with gestational diabetes, and induction before 38–39 weeks carries a risk of respiratory distress for the neonate. Delivery before 37 weeks should be done only for specific maternal or fetal indications.[17]

B. Optimal Route for Delivery

Controversy exists about delivery management of a fetus anticipated to have macrosomia. Two retrospective studies have looked at the cost-effectiveness of elective cesarean delivery for fetal macrosomia. In one, ultrasound diagnosis of macrosomia, followed by elective cesarean delivery for fetuses estimated to weigh > 4000 and > 4500 g was not found to be cost-effective in preventing neonatal injury (mainly brachial plexus injury) in non-diabetic patients.[32] In another study retrospectively evaluating 16,000 live births over a 10-year period, the relationship between actual neonatal birth weight and brachial plexus palsy was not significant for diabetic women with 4000-g infants, yet supportive in the 4500–5000-g category. Since 85–95% of brachial plexus injuries resolve by the first birthday, a policy of routine cesarean delivery for pregnancies complicated by GDM and suspected fetal macrosomia is not justified (see Chapter 15, section B).[5] ACOG guidelines continue to support offering elective cesarean delivery for patients with gestational diabetes and estimated fetal weights > 4500 g, although estimated fetal weights are notoriously inaccurate.[2]

C. Labor Management

Maintenance of euglycemia in order to prevent neonatal hypoglycemia is an important goal of labor management. Many women with gestational diabetes do not require insulin during labor, and those with diet-controlled GDM usually do not require monitoring. For women with insulin-requiring GDM, the usual practice is to have the patient discontinue oral intake and subcutaneous insulin at midnight before an induction, or at the onset of spontaneous labor. Bedside glucose checks are done hourly, with a target range of 70–120 mg/dl. Either subcutaneous insulin or continuous infusion may be used. If an insulin drip is required, NS is infused continuously at a constant rate of 125 ml/hour and insulin added at a drip rate based on blood sugar values obtained (Table 4).

D. Postpartum Care

1. Maternal

The immediate postpartum period is often hallmarked by a "honeymoon" phase of diabetes management, coinciding with a rapid disappearance of the physiologic alterations that impair peripheral insulin actions during pregnancy. Women who deliver vaginally usually do not require continuing intravenous fluids. Following cesarean delivery, either 5% dextrose or non-glucose-containing fluids may be continued at 125–150 ml/hour to maintain glucose levels < 200 mg/dl. Because of the rapid return of insulin sensitivity, most do not require insulin in the immediate postpartum period. Glucose levels are monitored and sliding-scale insulin administered when necessary as in the nonpregnant patient. Patients with non-insulin-dependent diabetes mellitus unrecognized before

TABLE 4.   Insulin Drip Rates Based on Blood Sugar Levels in Labor

Blood Glucose* (mg/dl)	Insulin (units/hour)
< 70	0.0
71–110	0.0 or 0.5
111–130	1.0
131–160	1.5
161–190	2.0
191–220	3.0
> 220	4.0

* Blood glucose is a capillary blood glucose checked with a reflectance meter. Cousins (California Sweet Success Program 1998).
Example protocol for a low-dose constant insulin infusion for the intrapartum period. Avoiding hypoglycemia is of paramount importance; keep maternal blood sugar between 0 and 110 mg/dl. Intravenous solution of LR or NS at 100–125 ml/hr should be used. If the blood sugar is less than 110, D5LR or D5NS can be used.

pregnancy may show an increased need for insulin on the second or third post-partum day. This may be unrecognized if the diagnosis is not suspected and the patient is discharged without further monitoring.

Breastfeeding is encouraged for diabetic mothers. Improved lipid and blood glucose measures have been noted in breastfeeding women with gestational diabetes when compared with non-breastfeeding diabetics.

2. Neonatal

Neonates should have a glucose level checked in the first 30 minutes after birth. Oral dextrose should be given for levels < 35 mg/dl. Infants with a repeat level < 45 probably require intravenous infusions. Calcium and magnesium levels may also be low and should be checked in symptomatic infants. Hyperbilirubinemia, polycythemia, and hyperviscosity are other potential neonatal problems. Finally, all infants should have a careful physical examination for cardiac, renal, gastrointestinal, or musculoskeletal anomalies. The risk of respiratory distress syndrome is not increased in infants of well-controlled diabetics at term.

VIII. Consultation and Referral

Many family physicians and midwives obtain an obstetric or perinatology consultation if the patient with gestational diabetes cannot maintain adequate glucose control with diet alone. Consultation may be helpful in any case in which the patient, family, or physician is uncomfortable or concerned. If insulin is required and consultant facilities are readily available, some clinicians prefer to transfer care of the patient for the duration of the pregnancy. If referral is less available, co-management can often be carried out by the family physician with consultation as needed by the obstetrician or perinatologist. Clinicians should monitor for complications such as hypertension, renal insufficiency, polyhydramnios, intrauterine growth restriction, suspected fetal macrosomia, preterm labor, or other signs of fetal compromise and should use their consultants in an appropriate manner to manage these conditions.

IX. Long-Term Consequences and Patient Education

A. Maternal

1. Risk of diabetes mellitus

It is estimated that 20–50% of women with gestational diabetes develop chronic diabetes later in life, and patients who had fasting hyperglycemia are very likely to have diabetes at 1 year (25%). Using a 2-hour, 75-g test, a threshold of > 140 mg/dl on fasting blood sugar, or two post-glucose measurements > 200 mg/dl are used for establishing the diagnosis of chronic diabetes. In settings where a complete 2-hour GTT cannot be done, a fasting threshold of > 126 mg/dl is considered diagnostic of diabetes. Counseling of the patient and her family regarding diet, exercise, weight control, and signs and symptoms of diabetes mellitus should continue at the postpartum visit and at yearly examinations.

2. Thyroiditis

This common postpartum problem may be overlooked by the provider, and is seen more often in women with other endocrinopathies, such as diabetes mellitus. Further discussion of this diagnosis can be found in Chapter 19, section E.

3. Birth control options

Discussion of birth control options is important in all women after childbirth. As discussed above, insulin-requiring gestational diabetics (patients with fasting hyperglycemia) are at increased risk of developing type 2 diabetes. It is important to establish euglycemia in these patients to lower the risk of birth defects in subsequent pregnancies (see Chapter 1, section A). Practitioners should make concerted efforts to provide effective and accessible contraception for these patients.

B. Pediatric

The risk of adolescent obesity has been shown to be significantly higher among macrosomic infants, although this trend did not reach statistical significance in the subgroup of infants born to diabetic mothers. Macrosomia among infants of diabetic mothers has little predictive value for obesity in late adolescence.[40] Counseling should be directed at establishing a healthy lifestyle during childhood.

X. Summary

Family physicians have an excellent opportunity to identify women with asymptomatic non-insulin-dependent diabetes mellitus during preconceptual counseling of women of childbearing age. Gestational diabetes is a common obstetric condition associated with increased perinatal morbidity and mortality. Screening pregnant patients at risk of gestational diabetes seems reasonable, although much controversy exists about who and how to screen for this diagnosis, and even if identification truly affects delivery outcomes.

Family physicians are familiar with testing, monitoring, and treatment of type 1 and type 2 diabetes mellitus in nonpregnant patients. With knowledge of modified values in the pregnant patient, family physicians are able to manage most pregnancies complicated by gestational diabetes. Consultation and referral are appropriate in selected settings and situations. There is insufficient evidence to support the need for elective induction for suspected macrosomia. Expectant management at term (using some form of antenatal fetal surveillance, usually non-stress tests) for non-insulin-requiring gestational diabetics is appropriate. The family physician should provide comprehensive postpartum care with a particular emphasis on effective contraception for women at increased risk of developing type 2 diabetes.

References

1. Acker DB, Sachs BP, Friedman EA: Risk factors for shoulder dystocia. Obstet Gynecol 66:762–768, 1985.
2. American College of Obstetricians and Gynecologists Technical Bulletin: Diabetes and pregnancy. Int J Gynecol Obstet 48:331–339, 1995.
3. American Diabetes Association: Gestational diabetes mellitus. Diabetes Care 21:S60–S62, 1998.
4. Blank A, Grave GD, Metzger BE: Effect of gestational diabetes on perinatal morbidity reassessed: Report of the International Workshop on Adverse Perinatal Outcomes of Gestational Diabetes Mellitus, Dec. 3–4, 1992. Diabetes Care 18:12–29,1995.
5. Boulvain M, Stan C, Irion O: Elective delivery in diabetic pregnant women (Cochrane Review). The Cochrane Library, Issue 4, 2000, Oxford, Update Software.
6. Canadian Task Force on the Periodic Health Examination: The Canadian Guide to Clinical Preventive Health Care. Ottawa, Canada Communication Group, 1994.
7. Carpenter MW, Coustan DR: Criteria for screening tests for gestational diabetes. Am J Obstet Gynecol 144:768–773, 1982.
8. Carr SR: Screening for gestational diabetes mellitus. Diabetes Care 21:14–18, 1998.
9. Chung CS, Myrianthopoulos NC: Factors affecting risks of congenital malformations. II. Effect of maternal diabetes. Birth Defects 11:10–14, 1975.
10. Classification and diagnosis of diabetes mellitus and other categories of glucose intolerance. National Diabetes Data Group. Diabetes 28:1039–1057, 1979.
11. Dang K, Homko C, Reece EA: Factors associated with fetal macrosomia in offspring of gestational diabetic women. J Matern Fetal Med 9:114–117, 2000.
12. Delpapa EH, Mueller-Heubach E: Pregnancy outcome following ultrasound diagnosis of macrosomia. Obstet Gynecol 78:340–343, 1991.
13. Farrag OAM: Prospective study of 3 metabolic regimens in pregnant diabetics. Aust N Z J Obstet Gynaecol 27:6–9, 1987.
14. Gabbe SG, Mestman JH, Freeman RK, et al: Management and outcome of class A diabetes mellitus. Am J Obstet Gynecol 127:465–469, 1977.
15. Gonen O, Rosen DJ, Dolfin Z, et al: Induction of labor versus expectant management in macrosomia: A randomized study. Obstet Gynecol 89:913–917, 1997.

16. Hagay Z, Reece EA: Diabetes mellitus in pregnancy and periconceptional genetic counseling. Am J Perinatol 9:87–93, 1992.
17. Hollingsworth DB: Pregnancy, Diabetes and Birth: A Management Guide. Baltimore, Williams & Wilkins, 1992.
18. Hunter DJS: Tight vs. moderate control of diabetes in pregnancy. In Chalmers I (ed): Oxford Database of Perinatal Trials. Record 4067, Version 1.3, Disk Issue 8, 1992.
19. Hunter DJS: Home vs. hospital inpatient glucose monitoring of diabetes. In Chalmers I (ed): Oxford Database of Perinatal Trails. Record 6651, Version 1.3, Disk Issue 8, 1992.
20. Hunter DJS, Keirse MJNC: Gestational diabetes. In Chalmers I (ed): Oxford Database of Perinatal Trials. Version 1.3, Disk Issue 8, 1992.
21. Johnson JW, Longmate JP, Frentzen B: Excessive maternal weight and pregnancy outcome. Am J Obstet Gynecol 167:353–370, 1992.
22. Langer O, Conway DL, Berkus MD, et al: A comparison of glyburide and insulin in women with gestational diabetes mellitus. N Engl J Med 343:1134–1138, 2000.
23. Langer O, Berkus MD, Huff RW, et al: Shoulder dystocia: Should the fetus weighing more or equal to 4000 gram be delivered by cesarean section? Am J Obstet Gynecol 165:831–837, 1991.
24. McFarland MB, Trylovich CG, Langer O: Anthropometric differences in macrosomic infants of diabetic and nondiabetic mothers. J Matern Fetal Med 7:292–295, 1998.
25. Metzger BE: Summary and Recommendations of the Third International Workshop—Conference on Gestational Diabetes Mellitus. Diabetes 40:197–201, 1991.
26. Nisswander KR, Evans AT: Endocrine disorders. In Manual of Obstetrics, 4th ed. Boston, Little, Brown, 1991.
27. O'Sullivan JB, Mahan CM: Criteria for the oral glucose tolerance test in pregnancy. Diabetes 13:278–285, 1964.
28. Ott WJ, Doyle S, Falmm S: Accurate ultrasonic estimation of weight. Am J Perinatol 2:178–182, 1985.
29. Periodic Health Examination, 1992 Update. I. Screening for gestational diabetes mellitus. Canadian Task Force on the Periodic Health Examination. Can Med Assoc J 147:435–443, 1992.
30. Pollack RN, Hauer-Pollack G, Divon MY: Macrosomia in post-dates pregnancies: Accuracy of routine ultrasonographic screening. Am J Obstet Gynecol 167:7–11, 1992.
31. Report of the Expert Committee on the Diagnosis and Classification of Diabetes Mellitus. Diabetes Care 20:1183–1197, 1997.
32. Rouse DJ, Owen J, Goldenberg RL, et al: The effectiveness and costs of elective cesarean delivery for fetal macrosomia diagnosed by ultrasound. JAMA 276:1480–1486, 1996.
33. Rouse DJ, Owen J: Prophylactic cesarean delivery for fetal macrosomia diagnosed by means of ultrasonography—A Faustian bargain? 181:332–338, 1999.
34. Rust OA, Bofill JA, Andrew ME, et al: Lowering the threshold for the diagnosis of gestational diabetes. Am J Obstet Gynecol 175:961–965, 1996.
35. Sabbagha RE, Minoque J, Tamura RK: Estimation of birth weight by use of formulas targeted to large-, appropriate-, and small-for-gestational age fetuses. Am J Obstet Gynecol 160:854–862, 1989.
36. Sacks DA, Greenspoon JS, Abu-Fadil S, et al: Toward universal criteria for gestational diabetes: The 75-gram glucose tolerance test in pregnancy. Am J Obstet Gynecol 172:607–614, 1995.
37. Santini DL, Ales KL: The impact of universal screening for gestational glucose intolerance on outcome of pregnancy. Surg Gynecol 170:427–432, 1990.
38. Schaefer UM, Songster G, Xiang A, et al: Congenital malformations in offspring of women with hyperglycemia first detected during pregnancy. Am J Obstet Gynecol 177:1165–1171, 1997.
39. Schwartz ML, Ray WN, Lubarsky SL: The diagnosis and classification of gestational diabetes mellitus: Is it time to change our tune? Am J Obstet Gynecol 180:1560–1571, 2000.
40. Seidman DS, Laor A, Stevenson DK, et al: Macrosomia does not predict overweight in late adolescence in infants of diabetic mothers. Acta Obstet Gynecol Scandi 77:58–62, 1998.
41. U.S. Preventive Services Task Force: Guide to Clinical Preventive Services, 2nd ed. Baltimore, Williams & Wilkins, 1996.
42. Vogel N, Burnand B, Vial Y, et al: Screening for gestational diabetes: Variation in guidelines. Eur J Obstet Gynecol Reprod Biol 91:29–36, 2000.
43. Walkinshaw SA: Diet Regulation for gestational diabetes (Cochrane Review). In The Cochrane Library, Issue 4, 2000 Oxford, Update Software.
44. Walkinshaw SA: Diet + insulin vs. diet alone for gestational diabetes. In Enkin MW, Keirse MJ, Renfre MT, Neilson JP (eds): Pregnancy and Childbirth Module of the Cochrane Database of Systematic Reviews: The Cochrane Collaboration. The Cochrane Pregnancy and Childbirth Database, Issue 1, Oxford, Update Software, 1995.
45. WHO Study Group on Prevention of Diabetes Mellitus: Prevention of Diabetes Mellitus: Report of a WHO Study Group. Geneva, World Health Organization. 1994.
46. Young C, Kuchl TJ, Sulak PJ, Allen SR: Gestational diabetes screening in subsequent pregnancies. Am J Obstet Gynecol 182:1024–1026, 2000.

SECTION B.
HYPERTENSION

Ellen L. Sakornbut, M.D.

Hypertension is a common cause of maternal and fetal morbidity and mortality.[1] Hypertensive diseases comprise the most common preventable cause of stillbirth near term.

I. Clinical Features
A. Incidence
Hypertension complicates 10% of all pregnancies.
B. Definition
In normal pregnancies, a reduced sensitivity to angiotensin and its associated decrease in peripheral vascular resistance and dilatation results in a physiologic decline in blood pressure at mid-trimester. Subsequently, blood pressure normally rises an average of 5 mm Hg diastolic from 24 to 30 weeks and 15 mm Hg from 30 to 40 weeks.

Blood pressure readings of 140/90 mm Hg or greater define hypertension in pregnancy. Blood pressure readings of 130/80 mm Hg or greater in the first or second trimester or absence of the physiologic decrease in pressure normally seen in the second trimester may represent chronic hypertension in pregnancy and should be observed closely.
C. Classification
Hypertension during pregnancy constitutes a heterogeneous group of disorders, with several distinct recognizable entities.[11]

    1. Chronic hypertension
This refers to blood pressure elevation that exists before pregnancy and does not regress following completion of the pregnancy. Although there are multiple causes, in most cases the underlying etiology is idiopathic. Chronic hypertension is addressed further in Chapter 7, section C.

    2. Gestational or transient hypertension
An isolated elevation of blood pressure near term is referred to as gestational or transient hypertension, also called pregnancy-induced hypertension (PIH). Up to 15–25% of patients with gestational hypertension progress to preeclampsia. This is more likely with early presentation.[25]

    3. Preeclampsia/Eclampsia
This classification is reserved for pregnancies in which hypertension is accompanied by proteinuria and edema. Eclampsia is progression of preeclampsia to include maternal seizures. Often, preeclampsia is accompanied by rapid weight gain with dependent and non-dependent edema.

        a. Mild preeclampsia. This includes patients with systolic blood pressure readings between 140 and 159 mm Hg and diastolic pressures of 90–109 mm Hg with ≤ 2+ proteinuria.

        b. Severe preeclampsia. This is defined by any of the following: blood pressure readings of 160/110 mm Hg or greater, 3 to 4+ proteinuria, epigastric pain, oliguria or HELLP syndrome (**H**emolysis, **E**levated **L**iver enzymes, **L**ow **P**latelets) (see Chapter 15, section G).

        c. Eclampsia. This refers to the development of seizure activity in patients with preeclampsia. This may present in patients who have not demonstrated significant blood pressure elevation, proteinuria, or other warning features prior to the seizure. Seizures may also occur in the postpartum period, as late as several weeks after delivery.

Preeclampsia or eclampsia may be superimposed on chronic hypertension.

D. Risk Factors for Preeclampsia
1. Nulliparity

A twofold greater risk of preeclampsia occurs in first pregnancies, and increases linearly in frequency with maternal age. Only 15% of primiparous women with preeclampsia have concomitant renal disease, contrasted with 50% of preeclamptic multiparas.[10]

2. Chronic hypertension

Similarly, there is a twofold increased risk of preeclampsia in women with underlying chronic hypertension (see Chapter 7, section C). Additionally, women with high normal blood pressures in early pregnancy and/or systolic blood pressure between 120 and 140 mm Hg at less than 20 weeks gestation,[6] appear to be at an increased risk of developing preeclampsia.[28]

3. History of preeclampsia

Women with a prior history of preeclampsia in an earlier pregnancy experience a 15% risk of recurrence in subsequent pregnancies.

4. Obesity, gestational diabetes, and insulin resistance

Obese women with metabolic features of insulin resistance (low HDL cholesterol, hyperinsulinemia, hypertriglyceridemia, hyperuricemia) have a greater chance of developing preeclampsia based on multiple recent large studies indicating increased risk with increasing body mass index and these metabolic features.[5,8,10] Another risk factor that has been associated with greater risk of cardiovascular disease is hyperhomocysteinemia, seen in 18% of patients with early-onset, severe preeclampsia according to one study.[5]

5. Thrombophilias

Patients with hypercoaguable states are at increased risk for severe, early preeclampsia. These include patients with protein C deficiency, Leiden factor V mutation, protein S deficiency, or antithrombin III deficiency (see Chapter 7, section D).[5,8]

E. Onset of Symptoms
Although preeclampsia appears to develop many weeks before clinical findings are present, recognizable features such as rapid weight gain, blood pressure elevation, and proteinuria are usually not seen until the third trimester. Early-onset preeclampsia should prompt investigation for underlying renal disease, thrombophilia, or other associated conditions. Clinical features of preeclampsia are almost never seen in the first half of pregnancy unless associated with concomitant pathology, such as molar pregnancy.

F. Fetal Outcomes
Fetal outcomes are generally good in pregnancies complicated by isolated transient hypertension. However, patients with chronic hypertension or preeclampsia have a greater risk of developing intrauterine growth restriction (IUGR) or experiencing a fetal demise. The increase in perinatal mortality is directly proportional to the mother's diastolic blood pressure. Fetal effects of antihypertensive medication are discussed in Chapter 7, section C. Newborns born to mothers with hypertension in pregnancy may experience complications of iatrogenic prematurity secondary to intervention for deterioration of the maternal or fetal condition.

G. Maternal Outcomes
Eighty-five percent of women with chronic essential hypertension preceding pregnancy do well without significant complications. Most maternal morbidity and mortality occurs in women with preeclampsia, with the most severe complications seen

in women with preeclampsia or eclampsia superimposed on chronic hypertension. Severe complications include acute renal failure, stroke, pulmonary edema, and abruption with coagulopathy.

II. Pathophysiology of Preeclampsia

A unifying mechanism in the pathophysiology of preeclampsia has yet to be solidly delineated, in part because of the heterogenous etiologies or risk factors that contribute to this condition. Numerous investigations indicate a variety of possible etiologies, including the following:

A. Defect of Trophoblastic Invasion

Some investigations suggest a defect of trophoblastic invasion of the maternal decidua[5,8] that may be at the level of the placental mitochondria.[33] Mechanisms under investigation include an imbalance or increased oxidative stress and lipid peroxidation coupled with a deficiency in antioxidant protection via the placenta.[8] This leads to increased thromboxane production and increased tumor necrosis factor-alpha (TNF) production with activated leukocytes and endothelial dysfunction.[22]

B. Reduced Smooth Muscle Sodium Pump Expression

Reduced smooth muscle sodium pump expression with resulting increase in intracellular sodium, increased pressor sensitivity, and increased direct effects on vascular tone has been postulated as a cause of preeclampsia.[17]

C. Maternal Endothelial Dysfunction

This dysfunction, resulting from a generalized intravascular inflammatory response seen in normal pregnancy, has also been considered. With this theory, the decompensation commonly seen in preeclampsia may arise from multiple varied stimuli, making it unlikely that any one predictive test or effective preventive measure will be found.[11]

D. Imbalance in Prostacyclin-Thromboxane System

Disturbances in the normal physiologic changes of pregnancy may create an imbalance in the prostacyclin-thromboxane A_2 system that results in increased sensitivity to angiotensin, increased peripheral vasoconstriction, increased blood pressure, decreased vascular volume, decreased cardiac output (variable), and decreased uteroplacental blood flow.

III. Predictive Biochemical and Biophysical Tests

No clinical test has proven useful for predicting hypertensive disease in pregnancy, including the cold pressor test, flicker infusion test, isometric exercise test, rollover test, and infusion of catecholamines, vasopressin, or angiotensin II.[31] Doppler investigation of uterine and umbilical artery waveforms performed in low-risk pregnancy between 19 and 24 weeks' gestation resulted in only limited ability to predict pregnancy-induced hypertension (59% sensitivity, 69% sensitivity) and somewhat increased ability to predict hypertension severe enough to result in premature delivery (83% sensitivity, 68% specificity).[29]

IV. Diagnosis of Preeclampsia

Hypertension and proteinuria are usually asymptomatic early in the disease process and must be detected through screening at prenatal visits. This screening underlies the common schedule of prenatal visits, with increasing frequency in the late second and third trimesters.

A. Blood Pressure Measurement

Blood pressures should be taken in the left arm, with the patient sitting, and should be recorded on at least two different occasions. Diastolic blood pressure should be recorded at the muffling of sounds (phase 4), as Korotkoff sounds may not disappear completely in pregnant patients.[31] Measurements should not be taken using the right arm if the patient is on her left side, as this results in an artificial reduction in blood pressure by 10–14 mm Hg lower than the true left atrial pressure. Other errors of blood pressure measurement are attributable to the instrument and the observer, including improper cuff size.[31] Initial blood pressure elevation may be caused by patient activity or "white coat hypertension."

Although both systolic and diastolic pressure elevation may indicate risk, some researchers advocate measuring only diastolic blood pressure, since systolic pressure is more affected by exercise or stress, and risk to the pregnancy is only increased when systolic elevations occur in conjunction with diastolic elevations. The diastolic pressure is also thought to reflect more clearly the primary circulatory problem of increased peripheral vascular resistance. Others have advocated use of the mean arterial pressure. Evidence of use of incremental increases in blood pressure is limited. A diastolic rise of 25 mm Hg, however, may help identify women who will develop preeclampsia.[20]

B. Proteinuria

A dipstick measurement of 2+ or greater on a spot urine specimen is considered significant proteinuria. This value corresponds to a level of 300 mg protein in a 24-hour specimen. False-positive dipstick reactions may occur when blood or vaginal secretions are present, or when the urine is alkaline, has a low specific gravity, or is contaminated with quaternary ammonium compounds or chlorhexidine. As such, catheterized specimens are more reliable than clean-caught specimens when a suspicion of preeclampsia is present. A 24-hour urine collection for protein should be used to confirm results of urine dipstick testing, which has a false-positive rate of 25% when a trace reaction is measured and 6% when 1+ protein is recorded by dipstick.

C. Edema

Fifty to eighty percent of women with uncomplicated pregnancies develop some degree of peripheral edema, which is generally gradual in onset. In contrast, 85% of patients with preeclampsia have edema that is typically rapid in onset and may be associated with marked weight gain over a short period of time. Facial edema is more common in preeclampsia, a finding that has been termed "leonine facies."

D. Other Clinical Symptoms and Findings

Patients with preeclampsia may present with complaints of headache, visual disturbance, chest or epigastric pain, and/or right upper quadrant pain and tenderness (which may indicate severe disease, such as HELLP syndrome). On physical examination, deep tendon reflexes may be hyperactive, and patients often have associated clonus.

E. Laboratory Evaluation

Initial laboratory studies in the evaluation of gestational hypertension and preeclampsia may vary depending on the patient's presentation. In women with mild blood pressure elevations alone, the platelet count and uric acid are poor predictors of preeclampsia.[7] However, in patients who meet criteria for preeclampsia, a CBC with platelet count, LDH, AST, ALT, uric acid, creatinine, and urinary protein determination should be obtained. Threshold values for these as predictors of preeclampsia that carries a significant risk of morbidity are: LDH > 1400 IU/L, AST > 150 IU/L, ALT > 100 IU/L, uric acid > 7.8 mg/dl, serum creatinine > 1.0 mg/dl, and 4+ urinary protein. These laboratory abnormalities result in increased morbidity when they occur in conjunction with worsening thrombocytopenia.[16]

V. Prevention

A. Low-Dose Aspirin

Prophylactic aspirin in a dose of 60–150 mg/day blocks thromboxane A_2 and its effects on vasoconstriction and platelet aggregation. Early studies demonstrated a reduction in incidence of preeclampsia with low doses of aspirin.[3,26,28,32] Although these initial studies were very promising, more recent large trials using low dose aspirin have not demonstrated a benefit in normotensive, nulliparous women,[4,21] women at high risk for preeclampsia,[9] or general obstetric populations[23] in decreasing the risk of preeclampsia. Additionally, some of these reports have shown an increase in bleeding complications (e.g., abruption) when patients were treated with low-dose aspirin.

B. Calcium Supplementation

A review in the Cochrane Library found evidence to support the use of calcium supplementation > 1 g/d for prevention of hypertensive diseases of pregnancy.[2] The largest U.S. trial (Calcium for Preeclampsia, or CPEP) did not find this effect,[15] although a systematic review of other studies suggests an overall modest reduction in the risk of hypertension, with or without proteinuria and preeclampsia, in women who take calcium supplementation. The greatest effect was noted in women at risk for hypertension and those with low calcium diets. The lack of demonstrated effect in the CPEP trial may be related to the population studied, i.e., low-risk women in five American university centers with adequate calcium in their diets. Although the evidence for routine calcium supplementation in pregnant women is questionable, no deleterious fetal or maternal effects of calcium supplementation (including nephrolithiasis) have been demonstrated.

C. Other Agents

Intake of marine n-3 fatty acids has not been found to prevent pregnancy-induced hypertension.[14] Trials using zinc and magnesium have similarly shown little to no benefit.[27]

VI. Antepartum Management (intrapartum management is reviewed in Chapter 15, section G)

A. Bed Rest

Bed rest, at home and in the hospital, has been reviewed by the Cochrane Study Group[12] relative to the following outcome measures: blood pressure > 109 mm Hg, proteinuria, preterm delivery, and perinatal mortality. When bed rest was compared to ad lib ambulation, no effect was demonstrated in reduction of the incidence of preterm delivery, low birth weight, depressed Apgar score, or admission to the neonatal intensive care unit. Recommendations for bed rest have been reported in up to 20% of all pregnancies, prescribed for a wide variety of conditions without significant evidence of effectiveness[13] or justification of its expense. Prolonged bed rest could increase the risk of deep venous thrombosis. It is, therefore, not recommended as an effective treatment, although modification of activity to eliminate high physical demand may be justified.

B. Diet

A salt-free diet has sometimes been recommended to prevent retention of salt and water. However, excessive weight gain in preeclampsia is not thought to be due to water retention, and sodium restriction potentially worsens this disease, since intravascular volume is already relatively decreased.

C. Nonemergent Pharmacologic Therapy for Preeclampsia and Gestational Hypertension

Indications for initiation of antihypertensive medication have been widely debated resulting in varying recommendations. General consensus is that blood pressure should be treated when it reaches 160/110 mm Hg.[20] The temptation to treat blood pressure elevations less than this in patients with gestational hypertension and preeclampsia may mask progression of the condition without preventing complications such as severe preeclampsia, abruption, or IUGR.

1. Diuretics

There is no evidence of improved pregnancy outcomes when diuretics are used either therapeutically or prophylactically.[10] Their use is discouraged, especially given that preeclampsia usually represents a condition with decreased intravascular volume.

2. Alpha-methyldopa

Trials of alpha-methyldopa (Aldomet), the most widely used antihypertensive agent in pregnancy, have shown a reduction in rates of severe hypertension but a nonsignificant trend toward lower rates of stillbirth and neonatal death.[10] Fewer mid-trimester pregnancy losses do occur with methyldopa therapy for chronic or early PIH. There was no significant effect on the incidence of proteinuria.

3. Beta-blockers

As with diuretics, beta-blockers are effective in reducing hypertension, and at least one randomized study showed reduction in emergency cesarean section rates for fetal distress secondary to acute hypertension.[19] Overall, insufficient data exist regarding reduction in proteinuric hypertension, perinatal mortality, or fetal growth retardation with this class of drugs.[10] With the exception of atenolol, which is pregnancy class D secondary to fetal growth restriction, beta-blockers are considered safe in pregnancy.

4. Calcium channel blockers

Nimodipine and nifedipine have both been investigated and are not associated with adverse effects to the fetus or impairment of placental circulation. The slow-release form of nifedipine should be used.

D. Emergent Pharmacologic Therapy (see Chapter 15, section G)

E. Assessment of Fetal Well-Being

1. Ultrasound

Ultrasound may help in identifying growth-restricted fetuses when lagging fundal height is discovered or fetal weight estimation by Leopold maneuver is low. IUGR and/or oligohydramnios may result from placental insufficiency.

2. Non-stress test, biophysical profile or contraction stress test

Antenatal testing should be instituted whenever the diagnosis of preeclampsia is made and used in conjunction with ultrasound diagnosis of growth restriction or oligohydramnios.

3. Doppler vascular studies

Monitoring of blood flow in the umbilical and/or uterine arteries is most useful in the severely preterm pregnancy and IUGR when conservative management is being considered. The use of Doppler sonography in the high-risk pregnancy complicated by intrauterine growth restriction to assess maternal and fetal circulation improves perinatal outcomes. Its use results in fewer inductions of labor, fewer hospital admissions, and fewer cesarean sections without demonstration of adverse effect.[18] In pregnancies complicated by hypertension, the absence of end-diastolic flow has been highly predictive of low birth weight (100%) and intrauterine fetal demise (66%).[30]

F. Timing of Delivery

1. Severe preeclampsia/eclampsia

The patient with severe preeclampsia, chronic hypertension with superimposed preeclampsia, or eclampsia warrants serious consideration of an expeditious delivery. If the patient is preterm, this decision is often made in consultation with a perinatal consultant, with consideration for maternal-fetal transfer.

2. Gestational hypertension or mild preeclampsia

Women with gestational hypertension or mild preeclampsia may be monitored, usually in the outpatient setting, for stabilization or progression of the condition.

As the patient nears term, induction of labor may be considered. If dating is well established, induction in a stable patient should be considered at 36 to 37 weeks' gestation, when fetal lung maturity is anticipated. Other indications for induction include oligohydramnios, non-reassuring fetal assessment tests (such as repeated nonreactive NSTs), intrauterine growth retardation, oligohydramnios, or abnormal Doppler testing.

3. Management of the intrapartum period and the use of magnesium sulfate
This is addressed in Chapter 15, section G.

G. Postpartum Care
Transient hypertension generally resolves without therapy in the first few weeks postpartum. However, these women are at increased risk for recurrence in future pregnancies and development of essential hypertension later in life.[11] If blood pressure values remain elevated for an extended period after delivery, the patient likely had unrecognized underlying chronic hypertension and should be evaluated and treated accordingly.

VII. Long-Term Consequences and Patient Education
The risk of developing chronic hypertension should be explained to the patient, stressing the importance of regular blood pressure monitoring. Counseling regarding diet, exercise, and weight control as means to maintain normal blood pressure and reduce overall cardiovascular risk should be emphasized.

VIII. Summary
Hypertensive disorders in pregnancy comprise a heterogeneous group of problems. Classification and risk stratification assists the clinician in determining which patients will benefit from close monitoring, pharmacologic intervention, or induction of labor.

References

1. Armstrong P: Medical treatment of pregnancy hypertension. Br J Hosp Med 36:347–353, 1986.
2. Atallah AN, Hofmeyr GJ, Duley L: Calcium supplementation during pregnancy to prevent hypertensive disorders and related adverse outcomes (Cochrane Review). In The Cochrane Library, Issue 4, 2000. Oxford, Update Software.
3. Beaufils M, Uzan S, Donsimoni R, et al: Prevention of preeclampsia by early antiplatelet therapy. Lancet 843:840–842, 1985.
4. Benigni A, Gregorini G, Frusca T, et al: Effect of low-dose aspirin on fetal and maternal generation of thromboxane by platelets in women at risk for pregnancy-induced hypertension. N Engl J Med 321:357–362, 1989.
5. Brazy JE, Grimm JK, Little VA: Neonatal manifestations of severe maternal hypertension occurring before the thirty-sixth week of pregnancy. J Pediatr 100:265–271, 1982.
6. Broughton Pipkin F, Sharif J, Lal S: Predicting high blood pressure in pregnancy: A multivariate approach. J Hypertens 16:221–229, 1998.
7. Calvert SM, Tuffnell DJ, Haley J: Poor predictive value of platelet volume, and serum urate in hypertension in pregnancy. Eur J Obstet Gynecol Reprod Biol 649:179–184, 1996.
8. Campbell S, Pearce JMF, Hackett G, et al: Qualitative assessment of uteroplacental blood flow: Early screening test for high-risk pregnancies. Obstet Gynecol 68:649–653, 1986.
9. Caritis S, Sibai B, Hauth J, et al: Low-dose aspirin to prevent preeclampsia in women at high risk: National Institute of Child Health and Human Development Network of Maternal Fetal Medicine Units. N Engl J Med 338:701–705, 1998.
10. Collins R, Wallenburg HC: Pharmacologic prevention and treatment of hypertensive disorders of pregnancy. In Chalmers I (ed): Effective Care in Pregnancy and Childbirth. Oxford, Oxford University Press, 1989, pp 512–533.
11. Cunningham FG, Lindheimer MD: Hypertension in pregnancy. N Engl J Med 326:427–432, 1992.
12. Duley L: Strict bed rest for proteinuric hypertension in pregnancy. In Enkin MW, Keirse MJNC, Renfrew MJ, Neilson JP (eds): Pregnancy and Childbirth Module. Cochrane Database of Systematic Reviews, Review No. 03373. Cochrane Updates on Disk, Oxford, Update Software, 1994.
13. Goldenberg RL, Cliver SP, Bronstein J, et al: Bed rest in pregnancy. Obstet Gynecol 84:131–136, 1994.

14. Kesmodel U, Olsen SF, Salvig JD: Marine n-3 fatty acid and calcium intake in relation to pregnancy-induced hypertension, intrauterine growth retardation, and preterm delivery: A case-control study. Acta Obstet Gynecol Scand 76:38–44, 1997.
15. Levine RJ, Hauth JC, Curet LB, et al: Trial of calcium to prevent preeclampsia. N Engl J Med 337:69–76, 1997.
16. Martin JN Jr, May WL, Magann EF, et al: Early risk assessment of severe preeclampsia: Admission battery of symptoms and laboratory tests to predict likelihood of subsequent maternal morbidity. Am J Obstet Gynecol 180:1407–1414, 1999.
17. Maxell CV, Tao QF, Seely EW, et al: Regulation of the sodium pump in pregnancy-related tissues in preeclampsia. Am J Obstet Gynecol 179:28–34, 1998.
18. Neilson JP, Alfirevic Z: Doppler ultrasound in high risk pregnancies (Cochrane Review). In The Cochrane Library, Issue 4, 2000. Oxford, Update Software.
19. Plouin PF, Breart G, Llado J, et al: A randomized comparison of early with conservative use of antihypertensive drugs in the management of pregnancy-induced hypertension. Br J Obstet Gynaecol 97:134–141, 1990.
20. Redman CW: Therapy for non-preeclamptic hypertension in pregnancy. Am J Kidney Dis 9:324–327, 1987.
21. Redman CWG, Jeffries M: Revised definition of preeclampsia. Lancet 1:809–812, 1988.
22. Roberts JM: Endothelial dysfunction in preeclampsia. Semin Reprod Endocrinol 16:5–15, 1998.
23. Rotchell YE, Cruikshank JK, Gay MP, et al: Barbados Low-Dose Aspirin Study in Pregnancy (BLASP): A randomized trial for the prevention of pre-eclampsia and its complications. Br J Obstet Gynaecol 105:286–292, 1998.
24. Rubin PC: Beta-blockers in pregnancy. N Engl J Med 305:1323–1326, 1981.
25. Saudan P, Brown MA, Buddle ML, et al: Does gestational hypertension become preeclampsia? Br J Obstet Gynaecol 105:1177–1184, 1998.
26. Schiff E, Pelleg E, Goldenberg M, et al: The use of aspirin to prevent pregnancy-induced hypertension and lower the ratio of thromboxane A_2 to prostacyclin in relatively high-risk pregnancies. N Engl J Med 321:351–356, 1989.
27. Sibai BM: Prevention of preeclampsia: A big disappointment. Am J Obstet Gynecol 179:1275–1278, 1998.
28. Sibai BM, Caritis SN, Thom E, et al: Prevention of preeclampsia with low-dose aspirin in healthy, nulliparous pregnant women. N Engl J Med 329:1213–1218, 1993.
29. Todros T, Ferrazi E, Arduini D, et al: Performance of Doppler ultrasonography as a screening test in low-risk pregnancies: Results of a multicenter study. J Ultrasound Med 14:343–348, 1995.
30. Torres PJ, Gratacos E. Alonso PL: Umbilical artery Doppler ultrasound predicts low birth weight and fetal death in hypertensive pregnancies. Acta Obstet Gynaecol Scand 74:352–355, 1995.
31. Wallenburg HCS: Detecting hypertensive disorders of pregnancy. In Chalmers I (ed): Effective Care in Pregnancy and Childbirth. Oxford, Oxford University Press, 1989, pp 382–402.
32. Wallenburg HC, Dekker GA, Makovitz JW, et al: Low-dose aspirin prevents pregnancy-induced hypertension and preeclampsia in angiotensin-sensitive primigravidae. Lancet 1:1–3, 1986.
33. Widschwendter M, Schrocksnadel H, Mortl MG: Pre-eclampsia: A disorder of placental mitochondria? Mol Med Today 4:286–291, 1998.

SECTION C.
MULTIPLE GESTATION

Ellen L. Sakornbut, M.D.

Pregnancies in which multiple gestation occur are at higher risk for many different types of complications. Many family physicians choose to refer these patients to an obstetrician or perinatalogist. Other family physicians choose to co-manage these patients with their consultants. Depending on the circumstances of the individual patient, risk status for specific complications differs. The detection of multiple gestation before the third trimester is helpful in monitoring for growth problems and prevention of preterm birth. Early diagnosis is also helpful in prognosis, especially for determination of chorionicity and amnionicity.

I. Clinical Findings
A. Presentation
Multiple gestation may present with the following:
1. Size/dates discrepancy
2. Elevated maternal serum alpha-fetoprotein level

3. Hyperemesis gravidarum
4. Auscultation of two distinctly different fetal heart rates
5. Palpation of greater than two fetal poles on Leopold maneuvers

B. Missed Presentation

A patient may not be diagnosed with multiple gestation until later in pregnancy or at term. Late onset of prenatal care and poor dating criteria increase the risk that a patient will be assigned an inaccurate and overly advanced gestational age. If preterm labor subsequently occurs, it may be assumed that the patient is at term.

C. Increased Risk of Complications

1. Low birth weight

Preterm labor, preterm spontaneous rupture of membranes, preterm birth, and low birth weight occur in up to 50% of multiple gestations. Increased rates of preterm births in monozygous multiple gestations may occur secondary to acute polyhydramnios, which has a weak association with preterm premature rupture of membranes.[17]

2. Gestational diabetes[17]
3. Pregnancy-induced hypertension[9,17]
4. Abnormal placental implantation, velamentous cord insertion, and single umbilical artery
5. Growth disturbance, including discordance
6. Manifestations of twin-twin transfusion syndrome (TTTS)
7. Malpresentation in labor
8. Uterine atony and postpartum hemorrhage
9. Congenital anomalies

This threefold increased risk occurs primarily in monozygotic twins.

10. Malformations unique to multiple gestation

These include conjoined twins and associated variations.

11. Abruption

There is a threefold increase of abruption independent of coexisting factors, such as hypertension and increasing parity.

12. Anemia

There is a 2.4 increased risk of maternal anemia.

13. Perinatal mortality

There is a five-fold increase in perinatal mortality.

14. Increased incidence of urinary tract infections
15. Increased incidence of fetal loss

This is now recognized with first-trimester ultrasound diagnosis as the disappearing twin.[7,8] Other variants of increased fetal loss include the fetus papyraceous (second trimester) and intrauterine fetal demise of one twin (late second or third trimester).

16. Increased incidence of cerebral palsy

Antenatal necrosis of cerebral white matter has been noted more frequently in association with twin-twin transfusion syndrome and death of a co-twin.[1]

D. Risk Factors for Multiple Gestation

1. Infertility therapy

There is an increased rate of dizygotic twins with gonadotrophic stimulation.

2. Family history (maternal) of dizygotic twins
3. Increasing parity and increasing maternal age

II. Types of Twins

A. Monozygous Versus Dizygous

The incidence of monozygotic twins does not vary worldwide (1 in 200–250). The incidence of dizygotic twins varies with ethnic groups.

B. Location of Placenta and Membranes[2]
1. Monochorionic
   a. Monoamnionic, monochorionic (MoMo)
   b. Diamnionic, monochorionic (DiMo)
2. Dichorionic, diamnionic (DiDi)

This type of twin gestation may be monozygotic (with early splitting of zygote) or dizygotic.

III. Complications
A. Increased Complications with Monochorionic Pregnancy
The complication rate is generally higher in monochorionic than dichorionic pregnancies. Monochorionic pregnancies carry a risk for twin-twin transfusion syndrome in up to 40% of cases,[18] may deliver at an earlier gestational age, and demonstrate higher perinatal death rates as compared to dichorionic pregnancies.

B. Twin-Twin Transfusion Syndrome[12]
1. Pathophysiology

Some degree of arterial and venous communication is found in the placental circulations of all monochorionic pregnancies. The degree of arterio-venous and arterio-arterial communication determines whether a transfusion syndrome has occurred. Characteristics of a transfusion syndrome include the following:
   a. High-to-low pressure shunting (arterial to venous). This creates a donor and a recipient twin. The degree of shunting in any given situation depends on the number of connections between the fetal circulations, the proportion of arterio-arterial, arterio-venous, and veno-venous connections, and other anatomic factors.
   b. Polyhydramnios/oligohydramnios (recipient/donor)
   c. Hypervolemia and polycythemia/anemia
   d. Growth discordance
   e. Chronic disseminated intravascular coagulation
2. Perinatal mortality

Mortality rates vary for twin A and B with degree of growth discordance. If birth weight differences are less than 10%, perinatal mortality rates are the same. As growth discordance increases to a 25% difference in birth weight, the odds ratio in perinatal death rate increases to 1.7.[17]

C. Monoamnionic, Monochorionic
Pregnancies with this type of twins are at high risk for complications. Fetal loss is common as a result of cord accidents and anomalies. Route of delivery is generally operative because of risk of cord entanglement with delivery. Fetal survival is only about 60% in the older literature but appears to be improving in more recent studies.

IV. Use of Ultrasound in Twin Gestation
Sonography has provided extremely valuable information in the diagnosis and management of multiple gestation.[3]
A. Diagnosis
A diagnosis of multiple gestation should not be made without clear visualization of two heads, two heartbeats, etc. The diagnosis of twins should not then be made until triplets are excluded. This may be more difficult in late pregnancy. Chorionicity and amnionicity should be determined as soon as possible in gestation.
1. Chorionicity

Early in pregnancy, the so-called "gestational sac" is actually a chorionic sac. Dichorionic twins will demonstrate two gestational sacs on transabdominal or transvaginal ultrasound. Ultrasound features of a dichorionic pregnancy include

the following (Fig. 1).
- a. A "thick" membrane that is easily visualized. This feature may not be reliable.
- b. Clear visualization of two distinctly separate placental masses. They may appear to be fused secondary to crowding.
- c. The "twin peak" sign. This is represented by a small triangle of chorionic tissue at the juncture of the membranes and the placenta (dichorionic).
2. Amnionicity

A twin gestation is diamnionic if a membrane can be found between the two fetuses. This is more difficult to locate in late pregnancy. In early pregnancy, the amnion has not yet fused to chorion and is seen as a wispy structure on transvaginal ultrasound surrounding the fetal pole with the yolk sac adjacent to the embryo but external to its boundaries. Dual amnionic sacs can only be visualized in this instance with transvaginal ultrasound. If a separating membrane cannot be found in late gestation, a gentle tap to the maternal abdomen may elicit a "fluid wave" across the membrane, causing sufficient displacement for visualization.

V. Management
A. Early Diagnosis of Multiple Gestation
Early diagnosis assists the practitioner in defining subsequent management strategies. Early assessment of all risk factors will aid in determining an appropriate site for care. The monoamnionic, monochorionic twin pregnancy should be referred, if possible, to a high-risk center. Multiple gestations greater than twin should be referred. Family physicians should use their best judgment regarding obstetric referral or consultation in the remaining cases. The risk associated with a first-trimester "vanishing twin" is probably not significantly increased.

B. Preterm Birth Prevention
Prophylactic hospitalization for bed rest in the third trimester has not been found to be protective against preterm labor and has been shown to be associated with poorer outcomes than outpatient management.[11,15] Some studies suggest benefit from home monitoring of uterine activity, but sufficient data from RCTs are lacking.[7] Frequent prenatal visits and cervical examinations should occur in the early third trimester. Ultrasound monitoring of cervical length and sonographically detected early changes in the internal os may be of help in predicting premature labor, as may biochemical markers such as fetal fibronectin or inflammatory cytokines. Insufficient data are available at present to recommend specific protocols for these procedures.

C. Nutrition
The prevention of anemia requires the use of iron and folate supplementation (see Chapter 7, section D). Optimal weight gain is about 44 lb (20 kg).[19]

D. Other Prenatal Surveillance
Clinicians should monitor for urinary tract infections, asymptomatic bacteriuria, and pregnancy-induced hypertension.

E. Antenatal Surveillance of Fetal Growth
Serial ultrasound scans are indicated to assess for concordant fetal growth. Fetal growth velocity appears to be diminished in twin pregnancies during the third trimester using serial measurements of fetal biparietal diameter (BPD) and abdominal circumference (AC).[20] Growth discordance of 20% or greater should alert the clinician to a potentially serious problem[4,5,16] and warrants consultation, especially in monochorionic pregnancies. "Pseudo" twin-to-twin transfusion syndrome has also been described; growth discordance appeared to have been the result of velamentous

cord insertion in half the cases seen.[13] Conventional antenatal fetal surveillance should be used if any maternal/fetal complications arise or are suspected (see Chapter 10). Doppler velocity, in particular, shows promise in predicating future compromise if intrauterine growth restriction is present.[6]

F. Management of a Second- or Third-Trimester Intrauterine Fetal Demise (IUFD)

The risk to the surviving twin appears to be significant, especially in monochorionic placentation.[6,21] One 10-year series showed 35% renal impairment in the surviving twin and almost 30% of surviving twins with abnormal brain imaging studies, 60% of which were found to have cerebral palsy.[10] Causes of IUFD in the second and third trimester include twin-twin transfusion syndrome, severe IUGR, placental insufficiency, and abruption.[14] Maternal coagulopathy, although described with IUFD, does not appear to be common in any series of surviving twin pregnancy.

References

1. Bejar R, Vigliocco G, Gramajo H, et al: Antenatal origin of neurologic damage in newborn infants. II. Multiple gestations. Am J Obstet Gynecol 162:1230–1236, 1990.
2. Benirschke K: The placenta in twin gestation. Clin Obstet Gynecol 33:18–31, 1990.
3. Benson CB, Doubilet PM: Sonography of multiple gestations. Radiol Clin North Am 28:149–161, 1990.
4. Deter RL, Stefos T, Harrist RB, et al: Detection of intrauterine growth retardation in twins using individualized growth assessment: I. Evaluation of growth outcome at birth. J Clin Ultrasound 20:573–577, 1992.
5. Deter RL, Stefos T, Harrist RB, et al: Detection of intrauterine growth retardation in twins using individualized growth assessment: II. Evaluation of third-trimester growth and prediction of growth outcome at birth. J Clin Ultrasound 20:579–585, 1992.
6. Gaziano EP, Knox GE, Bendel RP, et al: Is pulsed Doppler velocimetry useful in the management of multiple-gestation pregnancies? Am J Obstet Gynecol 164:1426–1433, 1991.
7. Keirse MHNC: Home uterine activity monitoring in twin pregnancies. In Enkin MW, Keirse MHNC, Renfrew MJ, Neilsen JP (eds): Pregnancy and Childbirth Module. Cochrane Database of Systematic Reviews, Review No. 06661. Cochrane Updates on Disk. Oxford, Update Software, 1994.
8. Landy HJ, Weiner S, Corson SL, et al: The "vanishing twin:" Ultrasonographic assessment of fetal disappearance in the first trimester. Am J Obstet Gynecol 155:14-19, 1986.
9. Levi S: Ultrasonic assessment of the high rate of multiple pregnancy in the first trimester. J Clin Ultrasound 4:3–8, 1976.
10. Lin IJ, Chen CH, Wang TM, et al: Infants in twin pregnancies with one twin demise in the uterus: A retrospective study. Chung Hua Min Kuo Hsiao Erh Koo I Hsueh Hui Tsa Chih 40:92–106, 1999.
11. Macgillivray I: Some observations on the incidence of preeclampsia. J Obstet Gynaecol Br Emp 65:536–539, 1958.
12. MacLennan AH, Green RC, O'Shea R, et al: Routine hospital admission in twin pregnancy between 26 and 30 weeks' gestation. Lancet 335:267–269, 1990.
13. Mari G, Detti L, LeviD'Ancona R, et al: "Pseudo" twin-to-twin transfusion syndrome and fetal outcome. J Perinatol 18:399–403, 1998.
14. Peterson IR, Nyholm HC: Multiple pregnancies with single intrauterine demise: Description of twenty-eight pregnancies. Acta Obstet Gynaecol Scand 78:202–206, 1999.
15. Pridjian G, Nugent CE, Barr M: Twin gestation: Influence of placentation on fetal growth. Am J Obstet Gynecol 165:1394–1401, 1991.
16. Rode ME, Jackson M: Sonographic considerations with multiple gestation. Semin Roentgenol 34:29–34, 1999.
17. Saunders MC, Dick JS, Brown IM: The effects of hospital admission for bed rest on the duration of twin pregnancy: A randomized trial. Lancet 2:793–795, 1985.
18. Snijder MJ, Wladimiroff JW: Fetal biometry and outcome in monochorionic vs. dichorionic twin pregnancies: A retrospective cross-sectional matched-control study. Ultrasound Med Biol 24:197–201, 1998.
19. Spellacy WN, Handler A, Ferre CD: A case-control study of 1253 twin pregnancies from a 1982–1987 perinatal data base. Obstet Gynecol l75:168–171, 1990.
20. Taylor GM, Own P, Mires GJ: Foetal growth velocity in twin pregnancies. Twin Res 1:9–14, 1998.
21. Van Heteren CF, Nijhuis JG, Semmekrot BA, et al: Discordant fetal growth in multiple pregnancy: Intervention should be based on chorionicity. Ned Tijdschr Geneeskd 143:1017–1021, 1999.
22. Worthington-Roberts B: Weight gain patterns in twin pregnancies with desirable outcomes. Clin Nutr 7:191–196, 1988.

SECTION D.
VAGINAL BLEEDING IN THE SECOND
AND THIRD TRIMESTER

John C. Houchins, M.D.

Vaginal bleeding late in pregnancy may represent a minor problem, such as a cervical polyp, or it may be the presenting feature of a catastrophic occurrence, such as a severe placental abruption. This section presents possible causes of vaginal bleeding, followed by a diagnostic approach and management strategies. Causes associated with preterm labor are emphasized. Chapter 15, section D contains an additional section on intra-partum management.

I. Causes of Second- and Third-Trimester Vaginal Bleeding in Pregnancy
A. Second-Trimester Miscarriage
This occurs uncommonly. Recurrent second-trimester pregnancy loss raises the diagnostic possibility of incompetent cervix (see Chapter 11, section E).
B. Onset of Labor
Often referred to as "bloody show," bleeding from cervical dilation may be heavy enough to be confused with more significant entities such as placenta previa or abruption.
C. Cervical Causes of Vaginal Bleeding
1. Cervicitis/vaginitis
These infections can be caused by numerous etiologic agents, including chlamydia, group B streptococcus, gonorrhea, trichomonas, bacterial vaginosis, candida and mycoplasma/ureaplasma.
2. Cervical polyp
3. Traumatic cervical and vaginal lacerations
4. Cervical carcinoma
D. Intrauterine Causes of Vaginal Bleeding
1. Molar pregnancy
2. Placenta previa
3. Abruptio placentae
4. Vasa previa
5. Marginal sinus rupture
6. Uterine leiomyomata
7. Coagulopathy—either pregnancy-related or preexisting

II. Diagnostic Approach
A. Patients with Minimal Bleeding
Patients with vaginal spotting or minimal bleeding can be evaluated in an expeditious manner in the office, assuming there are no other complicating factors, such as preterm labor or abdominal pain. This type of bleeding is often seen after intercourse, where the source of the bleeding is cervical.

Speculum exam should be done in an attempt to identify a source of the bleeding. There is no contraindication to a gentle speculum examination, whether or not the location of the placenta is known. This examination often provides key diagnostic information and can be performed in the office or labor room. Cervical cultures and a wet mount should be performed, if signs or symptoms indicate. If mucopurulent cervical discharge or obvious cervical inflammation is present, empiric therapy may be indicated before culture results are available. Ultrasound examination may also be necessary to identify placental location.

Patients with minimal bleeding should abstain from intercourse until the cause of bleeding is ascertained and report immediately if they experience more significant bleeding, decreased fetal movement, abdominal pain, or symptoms of labor.

B. Heavy Vaginal Bleeding

Patients experiencing significant vaginal bleeding (e.g., as much as a normal menstrual period) present an obstetric emergency and should be evaluated in labor and delivery (see Chapter 13, section D, and Chapter 16, section A). It is imperative to determine placental location in all patients with vaginal bleeding. Digital examination should never be done without knowledge of placental location, which can be determined by transvaginal or transperineal ultrasound.

III. Major Causes of Vaginal Bleeding—Clinical Features and Management Strategies

A. Placenta Previa

Placenta previa occurs when the placenta partially or completely covers the cervical os.

1. Incidence

Placenta previa is a common incidental finding on ultrasound scans obtained at an early gestational age, occurring in as many as 1 of every 20 pregnancies before 20 weeks' gestation. The incidence of placenta previa drops to 1 in 200 pregnancies after 30 weeks' gestation. This drop in frequency has been attributed to placental migration; other theories have linked this to the development of the lower uterine segment as pregnancy progresses. The concept of trophotropism has been introduced, whereby the placenta is thought to grow toward a site in the uterus with improved vascularity.[7]

2. Clinical presentation

Placenta previa occasionally presents in a previously undiagnosed patient with bleeding in labor. More often, this condition presents between 27 and 32 weeks with painless bleeding, sometimes after coitus. Patients with a large, central placenta previa tend to present earlier, and bleeding tends to recur. Placental abruption can rarely be seen in conjunction with placenta previa. One series documented the largest blood loss for patients with combined previa and abruption.[10] The incidence of placenta previa is higher for patients with a persistent transverse or breech presentation.

3. Risk factors

Risk factors for placenta previa include the following:

    a. Previous uterine scar

    b. Multiple gestation

    c. Previous abnormal placental implantation

    d. Advanced maternal age

    e. Increasing parity

4. Diagnosis

The diagnosis of true placenta previa versus a marginal or low-lying placenta often poses a diagnostic challenge. A marginal placenta previa extends to, and may partially surround, the cervical os without covering it. A low-lying placenta is close to the cervical os, but does not extend to it completely. These are often perceived to be a true previa because the chorionic surface is "rolled" over the cervical os.[7] Transvaginal ultrasound has been shown to be safe and superior to transabdominal ultrasound in diagnosing placenta previa, especially when the placenta is posterior.[15,17] This approach should be used whenever the transabdominal scan leaves the diagnosis in doubt.

5. Complications

Complications of placenta previa include:

   a. Intrauterine growth restriction

   b. Velamentous cord insertion

   c. Postpartum hemorrhage

   d. Placenta accreta, especially in multiparas with a previous uterine scar

6. Management strategies

   a. Incidental finding of low-lying placenta. When this is noted on an early ultrasound scan, a repeat scan should be obtained after 30 weeks' gestation to determine the subsequent location of the placenta. Low-lying placenta has no other particular implications for patient management.

   b. Importance of prematurity. Prematurity is the major cause of perinatal mortality and morbidity. Management is directed toward prolongation of pregnancy, if possible. In a symptomatic patient with a large central previa or a viable, but severely preterm, gestation, transfer to a perinatal center may be necessary in case of recurrent bleeding.

   c. Use of tocolysis. Although there has been some controversy about the use of tocolytic agents for late-pregnancy bleeding, they do not appear to be contraindicated, as long as the fetus is not compromised and hemorrhage is not massive. They may help to prolong the significantly preterm pregnancy. Medium-sized retrospective studies have demonstrated that tocolysis does not add any risk to the fetus, and possibly adds benefit such as increased birth weight.[2,18] However, there are RCTs that have shown a clear benefit of tocolysis. Magnesium sulfate is preferred to terbutaline, indomethacin, and nifedipine, and has been the most widely used agent for tocolysis.[10,14]

   d. Perinatal mortality. One series demonstrated a perinatal mortality of 7.6% in pregnancies with second-trimester bleeding caused by placenta previa alone, especially if pregnancy was prolonged until the third trimester.[10]

   e. Determining route of delivery. The exact relationship of the placenta to the cervical os should be determined, if necessary by transvaginal or transperineal scan.

   f. Diagnosing placenta accreta. In the presence of known placenta previa in the third trimester, it is useful to look for placenta accreta using transvaginal ultrasound with bladder filling.[7] Color Doppler imaging using a transvaginal approach has been shown to be an effective means of diagnosing placenta accreta.[8]

   g. Severe hemorrhage. Fatal or exsanguinating hemorrhage is uncommon in the absence of instrumentation or digital examination.

   h. Outpatient management. In cases when the mother and the fetus are stable and bleeding has stopped, two retrospective studies and one RCT suggest that outpatient management can be as safe as inpatient management.[6,9,19]

   i. Timing of delivery. In a stable situation, delivery should be planned once fetal lung maturity can be safely assured.

B. Placental Abruption

Placental abruption occurs when there has been a premature separation, either partial or complete, of the placenta from the uterine wall.

1. Incidence

Two percent of pregnancies are complicated by placental abruption, with approximately 0.2% severe enough to result in fetal death.

2. Clinical presentation

The presentation of this disorder is extremely variable, with hemorrhage, bloody amniotic fluid, or concealed hemorrhage being possible. A placental abruption often presents with pain in the abdomen or back, which does not diminish or go away between contractions. Clinical presentation is discussed in Chapter 15, section D.

3. Risk factors

Risk factors are additive. Hypertensive disorders are the most common risk factor, being present in 36–59% of all patients with severe abruption.[11] Uterine anomalies and leiomyomata were uncommon causes of abruption in one large series, implying less risk than previously suggested with leiomyomata.[7,11,13] Many forms of substance abuse, especially tobacco use, alcohol, and cocaine, are associated with an increased risk of placental abruption. Other conditions associated with abruption include sudden decompression of an overdistended uterus (e.g., ruptured membranes with polyhydramnios), blunt abdominal trauma (see Chapter 8, section C), grand multiparity, and history of previous abruption.

4. Diagnosis

The diagnosis of abruption is a clinical one. While ultrasound may occasionally be helpful, a negative ultrasound scan does not eliminate the diagnosis of abruption as a cause of bleeding. Greater attention should be given to features of the clinical presentation.

5. Strategies for antepartum management of abruption

    a. Second-trimester abruptions. Significant abruption in the second trimester carries a poor prognosis for the very preterm fetus. Preterm patients who are stable should be considered for transfer to a tertiary facility. A partial abruption in a preterm fetus may be managed conservatively if maternal and fetal parameters are stable.[4,10,14]

    b. Doppler flow studies. At this time, the value of Doppler testing in the management of abruption has not been demonstrated.[1,12] Antepartum assessment consists of a nonstress test and serial sonographic examination for fetal growth.[4]

    c. Tocolysis. Although previously considered controversial, tocolysis appears to be safe and helpful in delaying preterm birth and improving associated morbidity in patients with a partial abruption and a significantly preterm fetus.[4,10,14,18] Magnesium sulfate appears to be preferable to beta-sympathomimetics and nifedipine because of their hemodynamic effects. Indomethacin is contraindicated because of its antiplatelet effect.

    d. Rh-negative patients. Rh-negative women who experience any antenatal bleeding should receive Rhogam, 300 µg. If a large fetomaternal bleed is suspected, a Kleihauer-Betke test may be performed to determine the number of units of Rhogam indicated.

C. Unknown Causes of Bleeding

No etiology is found in approximately 30% of cases of second- and third-trimester bleeding. These patients remain at higher risk for premature labor and delivery and the associated morbidity and mortality. Infants of these pregnancies may also be at higher risk for minor neurodevelopmental abnormalities compared to gestational and birth weight-matched controls.[3,16]

References

1. Ajayi RA, Soothill PW, Campbell S, et al: Antenatal testing to predict outcome in pregnancies with unexplained antepartum hemorrhage. Br J Obstet Gynaecol 99:122–125, 1992.
2. Besinger RE, Moniak CW, Paskiewicz LS, et al: The effect of tocolytic use in the management of symptomatic placenta previa. Am J Obstet Gynecol 172:1770–1775, 1995.
3. Chan CCW, To WWK: Antepartum hemorrhage of unknown origin—what is its clinical significance? Acta Obstet Gynaecol Scand 78:186–190, 1999.
4. Combs CA, Nyberg DA, Mack LA, et al: Expectant management after sonographic diagnosis of placental abruptio. Am J Perinatol 9:170–174, 1992.

5. Davis JL, Ray-Mazumder S, Hobel CJ, et al: Uterine leiomyomas in pregnancy: A prospective study. Obstet Gynecol 75:41–44, 1990.
6. Droste S, Keil K: Expectant management of placenta previa: Cost-benefit analysis of outpatient treatment. Am J Obstet Gynecol 170:1254–1257, 1994.
7. Finberg HJ, Benirschke K: Recent observations on the ultrasound diagnosis of placenta previa and placenta accreta with correlation to the principles of placental pathophysiology. Proceedings of the American Institute of Ultrasound in Medicine Annual Meeting, 1992.
8. Lerner JP, Deane S, Timor-Tretsch IE: Characterization of placenta accreta using transvaginal sonography and color Doppler imaging. Ultrasound Obstet Gynecol 5:198–201, 1995.
9. Mouer JR: Placenta previa: Antepartum conservative management, inpatient versus outpatient. Am J Obstet Gynecol 170:1683–1685, 1994.
10. Nielson EC, Varner MW, Scott JR: The outcome of pregnancies complicated by bleeding in the second trimester. Surg Gynecol Obstet 173:371–374, 1991.
11. Pritchard JA, Cunningham G, Pritchard SA, et al: On reducing the frequency of severe abruptio placentae. Am J Obstet Gynecol 165:1345–1351, 1991.
12. Rafla NM: The use of Doppler umbilical artery waveforms in placental abruptio: A report of two cases. Eur J Obstet Gynaecol 38:167–168, 1990.
13. Rice, Kay HH, Mahony BS: The clinical significance of uterine leiomyomas in pregnancy. Am J Obstet Gynecol 160:1212–1216, 1989.
14. Saller DN, Nagey DA, Pupkin MJ, et al: Tocolysis in the management of third-trimester bleeding. J Perinatol 10:125–128, 1990.
15. Sherman SJ, Carlson DE, Platt ID, et al: Transvaginal ultrasound: Does it help in the diagnosis of placenta previa? Ultrasound Obstet Gynecol 2:256–260, 1992.
16. Spinillo A, Fazzi E, Stronati M, et al: Early morbidity and neurodevelopmental outcome in low-birth-weight infants born after third trimester bleeding. Am J Perinatol 11:85–90, 1994.
17. Timor-Tritsch IE, Yunis R: Confirming the safety of transvaginal sonography in patients suspected of placenta previa. Obstet Gynecol 81:742–744, 1993.
18. Towers CV, Pircon RA, Heppard M: Is tocolysis safe in the management of third-trimester bleeding? Am J Obstet Gynecol 180:1572–1578, 1999.
19. Wing DA, Paul RH, Millar LK: Management of the symptomatic placenta previa: A randomized, controlled trial of inpatient versus outpatient expectant management. Am J Obstet Gynecol 175:806–811, 1996.

SECTION E.
PREVIOUS UTERINE SCAR

Ellen L. Sakornbut, M.D.

I. Patient Education
Patient education regarding vaginal birth after cesarean section (VBAC) should begin before hospital discharge at the time of the first cesarean section. This counseling should continue at the first postpartum follow-up visit, since 56% of VBAC patients have already made their decision regarding mode of delivery before the first prenatal visit for a subsequent pregnancy. Fear of a repeated long and difficult labor; convenience of scheduling; and opinions of partner, family, or friends were rated as important as medical estimates of the relative risks and benefits of VBAC by patients. However, physician attitudes are still an important influence on decision making. Women should be provided with objective information on the medical risks and benefits of both methods of delivery, including the higher rate of uterine rupture with VBAC and the higher rates of infection and bleeding with elective repeat cesarean section (ERCS).[10] Patient preference may take into account other factors, such as desire for tubal ligation.

II. Evidence on Trial of Labor (TOL) after VBAC
A. ACOG Guidelines for VBAC
ACOG published guidelines for consideration of VBAC in 1999. They contain the following circumstances in which VBAC is considered appropriate and well-supported by the literature.

   1. One or two previous lower uterine segment transverse cesarean sections
   2. Clinically adequate pelvis
   3. No other uterine scars or previous uterine rupture
   4. A physician readily available throughout labor for emergency cesarean section
   5. Availability of anesthesia and surgery personnel for emergency cesarean section

B. Contraindications for VBAC

ACOG also listed circumstances in which VBAC was contraindicated. These circumstances include.

   1. Prior classic or T-shaped incision, other transfundal surgery
   2. Contracted pelvis
   3. Medical/obstetric complication that precludes vaginal delivery
   4. Inability to perform immediate cesarean section

C. Uncertain Support for VBAC

ACOG considers some circumstances potentially appropriate for TOL consideration, but notes that less evidence is available to substantiate their use. These are:

   1. Previous low vertical incision
   2. More than two previous cesarean sections
   3. Induction of labor by oxytocin and prostaglandin gel requires close monitoring.

D. General Studies about Efficacy and Safety

Success rates of VBAC in most studies range between 65 and 85% of patients attempting a trial of labor. In a 10-year study with over 160,000 deliveries, 80% of women with one previous cesarean delivery underwent a trial of labor with an 83% success rate. Uterine rupture rates range from 1 to 2%. Over half (54%) of women with two previous cesarean deliveries had a 75% success rate with VBAC. However, uterine rupture was three times more common in women with two or more previous cesarean deliveries.[6]

In one study following a protocol for active management of labor, 82% of women undertook TOL with an 88% success rate. Older women, women of higher parity, and women with preterm births were more likely to have cesarean delivery. Women requiring oxytocin use in labor, epidural anesthesia, or those treated for chorioamnionitis were more likely to fail trial of labor. Uterine rupture was less than 1%.[12]

Epidemiologic studies show lower success rates in women undergoing a trial of labor.[2] A population-based study in Washington state showed 64% of pregnancies attempting VBAC, with 62% successful for an overall VBAC rate of 40%. The highest success rates were in women without prior labor problems. A preliminary study of VBAC attempt rates and success rates found both to be lower in rural settings than in urban settings. The author concluded this disparity was probably due to a lack of local resources (in-house surgical, anesthesia, NICU) and physician factors.[11] Factors reported to be predictive of successful VBAC include the following.[13]

   1. Prior malpresentation, odds ratio 1.9
   2. Prior fetal distress
   3. Prior placental indication
   4. Previous vaginal delivery before cesarean section, odds ratio 1.8
   5. Prior pregnancy-induced HTN, odds ratio 2.3
   6. Bishop score > 4 , odds ratio 6.0
   7. Cesarean section for herpes infection
   8. Previous cephalopelvic disproportion (CPD), odds ratio 0.8 (64% of women who underwent trial of labor were successful in delivering vaginally)

Information is less clear about the likelihood of successful trial of labor when timing of the previous cesarean delivery is considered. For cesarean section performed during the second stage of labor (arrest disorder), success rates of VBAC range from 13% to 80%.[3,4] VBAC attempts in women with a previous vertical lower uterine segment incision have had reported success rates up to 82%, with approximately a 1% rate of uterine rupture.[5,8] A few studies suggest that vaginal birth can also be accomplished safely in twin gestations if they would otherwise be considered for vaginal delivery.[7,9]

III. Careful Dating

Careful dating is important, as with all pregnancies, to avoid postterm pregnancy and macrosomic infants if VBAC is going to be considered. Well-documented dates in pregnancies that have been followed since the first trimester may eliminate the need for amniocentesis to determine fetal lung maturity if ERCS is chosen.

IV. Records

Prior to considering a trial of labor in a patient with a previous uterine scar, it is imperative that operative reports from the previous surgery be obtained. These should accompany the prenatal records from the current pregnancy to the hospital.

V. Antenatal Consultation

For maternity care providers who do not perform cesarean sections, antenatal consultation with a provider who performs operative deliveries (an obstetrician, surgeon, or family physician trained to do cesarean sections) is recommended. The timing of this consultation varies by local practice, making it important to know the consultant's preferences for notification and discussion of the patient in whom VBAC is being considered. It is equally important to notify the consultant at the time the patient is admitted to the hospital in labor. It is essential that the clinician set up a system in which a cesarean section can be performed in an expeditious manner. ACOG's most recent technical bulletin regarding the management of VBAC recommended that the ability to perform a cesarean section be "immediately" available, but the timing from the decision to perform a cesarean section to delivery of the infant was not defined.[1]

VI. Facilities

The same facilities required for all laboring patients are satisfactory for patients attempting a VBAC. Personnel for surgery, anesthesia, neonatal resuscitation, laboratory, and blood bank must be available so that cesarean section can be started in an expeditious manner as described above. Family physicians should take an active role in helping to design a quick response system in their local setting.

VII. Informed Consent

Informed consent should be obtained from all patients, including discussion of the standard risks associated with a major operative procedure if ERCS is chosen, the risks of uterine rupture with TOL, and the increased risks of infection in women with failed TOL (see Chapter 13, section H for a discussion of intrapartum management of VBAC candidates).

References

1. American College of Obstetricians and Gynecologists Technical Bulletin: Vaginal birth after previous cesarean section. ACOG, July, 1999.
2. Holt VL, Mueller BA: Attempt and success rates for vaginal birth after cesarean section in relation to complications of the previous pregnancy. Paediatr Perinat Epidemiol 11(Suppl 1):63–72, 1997.
3. Hoskins IA, Gomez JL: Correlation between maximum cervical dilatation at cesarean delivery for failure of the second stage of labor. Obstet Gynecol 89:591–593, 1997.
4. Jongen VH, Halfwerk MG, Brouwer WK: Vaginal delivery after previous cesarean delivery for failure of the second stage of labor. Br J Obstet Gynaecol 105:1079–1081, 1998.
5. Martin JN, Perry KG Jr, Roberts WE, et al: The case for a trial of labor in the patient with a prior lower uterine segment vertical cesarean incision. Am J Obstet Gynecol 177:144–148, 1997.

6. Miller DA, Diaz FG, Paul RH: Vaginal birth after cesarean section: a ten year experience. Obstet Gynecol 84:255–258, 1994.
7. Miller DA, Mullin P, Hou D, et al: Vaginal birth after cesarean section in twin gestation. Am J Obstet Gynecol 175:194–199, 1996.
8. Naef RW 3rd, Ray MA, Chauhan SP, et al: Trial of labor after cesarean delivery with a lower-segment, vertical incision: Is it safe? Am J Obstet Gynecol 172:1666–1673, discussion 1673–1674, 1995.
9. Odeh M, Tarazova L, Wolfson M, et al: Evidence that women with a history of cesarean section can deliver twins safely. Acta Obstet Gynaecol Scand 76:663–666, 1997.
10. Roberts RG, Bell HS, Wall EM, et al: Trial of labor or repeated cesarean section. The woman's choice. Arch Fam Med 6:120–125, 1997.
11. Sieck CC: Vaginal birth cesarean section: A comparison of rural and metropolitan rates in Oklahoma. J Okla State Med Assoc 90:444–449, 1997.
12. Videla FL, Satin AJ, Barth WH Jr, et al: Trial of labor: A disciplined approach to labor management resulting in a high rate of vaginal delivery. Am J Perinatol 12:181–184, 1995.
13. Weinstein D, Benushushan A, Tanos V, et al: Predictive score for vaginal birth after cesarean section. Am J Obstet Gynecol 174:192–198, 1996.

SECTION F.
SMALL-FOR-DATES PREGNANCY

Ellen L. Sakornbut, M.D.

I. Pregnancy Dating by Clinical Examination

Fetuses that are discovered to be small for dates are typically first suspected during prenatal visits when the uterine size is routinely measured and compared to established pregnancy dating parameters.

A. Prior to 20 Weeks' Gestation

With ample clinical experience, first-trimester uterine size as determined by bimanual examination can be accurately correlated with dates; however, this is not a period in which concern for a small-for-dates fetus is of clinical relevance. Size-date discrepancy in early pregnancy usually represents abnormal pregnancy (missed abortion, molar pregnancy, etc.), uterine abnormality (such as fibroids), or wrong dates. Size-date correlation may become more difficult between 10 and 20 weeks' gestation, particularly in the presence of clinical factors such as uterine retroversion or maternal obesity.

B. Between 20 and 32 Weeks' Gestation

Assessing the small-for-dates pregnancy becomes easier after 20 weeks' gestation, when fundal height measurements typically correlate well (within 2 cm) with gestational age. Generally speaking, the fundus should be at the umbilicus at 20 weeks' gestation, and rise by 1 cm per week. Reliability of the size-date correlation should remain consistent until 32 weeks' gestation, after which time fundal height may less well predict fetal size depending on descent into the pelvis, fetal lie, and abdominal laxity. The acquisition of physical examination skills in assessment of uterine and fetal size requires experience and repeated correlation with outcome. Accuracy in suggesting a deviation from normal is dependent on both patient and clinician factors.

II. Etiology of a Small-for-Dates Presentation

A. Inaccurate Pregnancy Dating

Many women are unsure of the exact dates of their last menstrual period (LMP), particularly if they have recently discontinued hormonal contraceptive methods. Even the more certain LMP may be unreliable because of menstrual cycle lengths that are either shorter or longer than the traditional 28 days, or when the last known bleeding is associated with implantation of the pregnancy.

II. Improper Measurement of Fundal Height

Fundal height is measured from the symphysis pubis to the top of the uterine fundus. Errors in measurement can be made by extending the tape only to the top of the fetus and not all the way to the most superior aspect of the fundus. A limited amount of normal variation can be seen with measurements of different providers, such that continuity of providers is important in assessing for size-date discrepancies.

III. Transverse Lie

A fetus in a transverse lie causes the fundal height measurement to be artificially low compared to the actual size of the fetus. Determination of the fetal lie is an important component of the clinical evaluation of small-for-dates pregnancies.

IV. Pregnancy Complications

The pregnancy complicated by intrauterine growth restriction (IUGR) or oligohydramnios will initially present as a size-date discrepancy in which the fundal height lags behind the established gestational age. While small discrepancies in size and dates during the 20–32-week period are usually not significant, a fundal height measurement that lags 3–4 cm may be a matter of concern.

V. Constitutionally Small Fetus

Not all small-for-dates pregnancies result from a pregnancy complication. A small fetus may be normal for some parents. This is usually a diagnosis of exclusion after a thorough evaluation for intrauterine growth restriction and oligohydramnios. Parental height and ethnic background may be contributory.

VI. Intrauterine Growth Restriction

The incidence of IUGR is about 5% in the general pregnant population, but can rise to as much as 10% in high-risk populations.

A. Asymmetric Intrauterine Growth Restriction (AIUGR)

The majority (70%) of growth restriction in fetuses is asymmetric, in which growth of the head and long bones is spared relative to that of abdomen and viscera. This pattern reflects compromised fetal nutrition, with decreased subcutaneous fat, brown fat, and liver glycogen stores.

1. Risk factors

Risk factors are listed in Table 5 along with possible pathophysiology of these conditions.

2. Fetal complications of AIUGR

These include a greater likelihood of encountering fetal intolerance of labor, higher rates of meconium aspiration syndrome, and increased incidence of stillbirth related to chronic uteroplacental insufficiency.

3. Maternal complications

Pregnancies in which AIUGR occurs have a higher prevalence of several maternal complications, including preeclampsia and antiphospholipid antibody syndromes.

4. Neonatal complications

After delivery, neonates that had AIUGR are at increased risk for hypoglycemia, hypothermia, polycythemia with hyperbilirubinemia, and possibly hyperviscosity syndrome. In addition, they may initially be poor feeders. Although it has been theorized that premature newborns who underwent the stress of intrauterine growth restriction would have less neonatal pulmonary complications, recent studies indicate a poorer prognosis for growth-restricted than for AGA counterparts.[6,23]

TABLE 5. Conditions Associated with Intrauterine Growth Restriction

Chronic Medical Conditions	Obstetric Complications
Chronic hypertension and chronic renal disease	Pregnancy-induced hypertension (preeclampsia)
Diabetes mellitus, class C, D, or R	Multiple gestation
Systemic lupus erythematosus	Placental abnormalities—partial abruption,
Sickle cell anemia and other severe anemias	placenta previa, circumvallate placenta, and
Cyanotic congenital heart disease	velamentous cord insertion
Other maternal cardiac diseases with poor	Intrauterine infection (TORCH infections,
cardiac output	listeria)
Therapeutic medications, including phenytoin	Previous history of IUGR
(Dilantin), trimethadione, warfarin (Coumadin)	Fetal abnormalities
Tobacco use	Chromosomal abnormalities—trisomies, Turner's
Alcohol and other substance abuse (opiates,	syndrome, cri-du-chat
cocaine)	Congenital malformations
Thrombophilias (APA, Factor V Leiden, protein C	
and S)	
Malnutrition	
Chronic lead poisoning	
Low socioeconomic status, especially with poor	
social support	

5. Long-term sequelae

AIUGR has been postulated to result in long-term subtle neurologic manifestations, such as learning disabilities and attention deficit disorder. Confounding factors, such as maternal smoking, make it difficult to substantiate these concerns. A cohort study that assessed the relative significance of small-for-gestational age versus parental factors found that childhood cognitive development was strongly associated with parental factors, such as child-rearing style and maternal smoking, and only marginally associated with intrauterine growth restriction.[20]

Evidence continues to accumulate linking AIUGR with an increased risk for essential hypertension, non-insulin-dependent diabetes mellitus, ischemic heart disease, and other manifestations of insulin resistance.[1] Prospective cohort study of term singleton children from the Avon longitudinal study found those gaining greater than 0.67 SD in weight between ages 0 and 2 (defined as catch-up growth) had lower weight, length, and ponderal index at birth. Their mothers were more likely to smoke. At age 5 these children were heavier, taller, and fatter, with greater central fat distribution.[17] Mechanisms that influence this early catch-up growth are postulated to alter adult metabolism. Insulin resistance has been demonstrated both in children[3] and in young adults[14] who were growth-restricted in utero as compared to their counterparts who had normal intrauterine growth.

B. Symmetric Intrauterine Growth Restriction (SIUGR)

Thirty percent of all patients with IUGR have fetuses with symmetrically disturbed growth velocity in the head, abdomen, and long bones. This usually reflects an early and continuing insult to the fetus, such as first-trimester intrauterine infections or chromosomal anomalies.

Neonatal and long-term complications vary according to the etiology of the growth restriction, whether genetic, infectious, or otherwise.

C. Diagnosis of IUGR

1. Clinical Diagnosis

A diagnosis of growth restriction can be suspected on the basis of lagging fundal height, palpation of a fetus that seems small-for-dates, or abnormal measurements on ultrasound. The diagnosis of growth restriction almost always relies upon previous accurate establishment of the gestational age. It has been proposed that accuracy of fundal height measurements may be improved by using customized fundal height charts adjusted to a woman's height, weight, parity, and ethnic group,[5] but the results of this study have not been duplicated.

2. Use of growth charts

Growth charts for all biometric measurements of the fetus exist with established percentiles for each gestational age. If a fetus is assigned an average uterine age of 18 weeks, this merely implies that the fetal measurements, on average, are at the 50th percentile for 18 weeks. Growth charts should be used that are compatible with the ethnic composition of the population measured. Once a fetus has been assigned a gestational age by thorough and accurate means of clinical and/or ultrasound dating, growth percentiles for a given gestational age can be assigned on later ultrasound exams.

3. Other markers of IUGR

Growth restriction has been defined as less than the 10th percentile for gestational age (some authors use less than the 5th percentile). A more specific definition of AIUGR is a fetal ponderal index (the weight of the fetus divided by the length) that is less than the 10th percentile.[21] This defines the "thin" fetus, as described previously, but may be difficult to prove by clinical or ultrasound means because the length and weight of the fetus can only be estimated in utero. Multiple body ratios have been developed to define normal proportions of fetal measurements; the most pertinent in growth assessment are the femur length to abdominal circumference ratio[10,11] and the head circumference to abdominal circumference ratio.[2] Others advocate the use of the abdominal circumference alone as most reflective of fetal nutritional status.[18,22] Single ultrasound examinations are rarely helpful because the most meaningful information is obtained by plotting serial fetal measurements with an abnormal growth velocity (see Table 6 for a comparison of sonographic methods).

4. Diagnosis of SIUGR

SIUGR is diagnosed using serial ultrasound scans demonstrating abnormal progression of all fetal growth parameters. Rarely, it may be diagnosed by a single ultrasound scan that can be compared with unequivocal information about the gestational age of the fetus.

5. Screening for IUGR

Routine use of third-trimester screening for IUGR shows low sensitivity and has not been demonstrated to be of benefit. A prospective European study of all admissions to a tertiary facility in one year examined outcomes of 2,378 births that were routinely screened for growth restriction. They found an increased risk of preterm delivery and NICU admissions among neonates from pregnancies that were diagnosed as growth-restricted, primarily due to iatrogenic prematurity. This study found the sensitivity in ultrasound detection of IUGR to be only

TABLE 6. Sonographic Detection of Intrauterine Growth Restriction

Method	Sensitivity	Specificity	Positive Predictive Value	Gestational Age–Dependent
HC/AC[2]	0.70	NA	NA	Yes
AC Percentile[18,22]	0.72	0.69	0.19	Yes
EFW Percentile[21]	0.25	0.97	0.47	Yes
FL/AC[10,11]	0.64	0.90	0.25	No
FPI[21]	0.77	0.82	0.35	No

HC/AC, Head circumference to abdominal circumference ratio; AC, abdominal circumference; EFW, estimated fetal weight; FL/AC, femur length to abdominal circumference ratio; FPI, fetal ponderal index.

32%.[13] In contrast, while medical interventions for growth restriction were associated with newborn iatrogenic complications, newborns whose restricted growth was undetected prior to delivery were not more likely to have low Apgar scores or low cord pH.

Because the risk of asymmetric IUGR is higher in women with hypertension in pregnancy, ultrasound examination of the fetus is of benefit in assessment of chronic hypertension in pregnancy (suggested at 32–34 weeks)[19] and pre-eclampsia (as part of the work-up when the diagnosis is established). Other patients who should be screened include pregnancies with poor fundal height progression between 20 and 32 weeks (fundal height lagging behind gestational age by greater than 3 cm), women who are drug users, heavy smokers, those with known or suspected vascular disease, and those with known thrombophilic disorders.

Doppler flow velocimetry of the uterine arteries has not been found reliably predictive for intrauterine growth restriction.[4] Additionally, changes in fetal circulation detected by Doppler are preceded by slowing of growth velocity, especially growth velocity of the abdominal circumference.[12] Thus, Doppler flow velocimetry is not recommended as a screening modality.

D. Management of IUGR

In the presence of otherwise reassuring fetal assessment, or in cases in which the diagnosis is not well established, conservative management is justified with modification of risk factors where possible. In general, treatment of hypertension with antihypertensives in preeclampsia has not been found to prevent growth restriction.

1. Evidence for treatment

A series of Cochrane reviews found insufficient evidence to support modalities such as bed rest,[7] nutritional supplements,[9] and calcium channel blockers for suspected impaired fetal growth, although one trial of pregnant smokers found significant increases in birth weight of women given a calcium channel blocker (flunarizine).[8]

2. IUGR and antenatal surveillance

Further antenatal testing may include Doppler velocimetry, amniotic fluid assessment, non-stress testing, and biophysical profile. A Cochrane Systematic Review of randomized trials utilizing Doppler flow velocimetry of the umbilical artery identified eleven trials in high-risk women. These trials demonstrated a reduction in the risk of perinatal death that narrowly misses statistical significance (OR 0.47, CI 0.47–1.07, ARR 0.4%). The use of Doppler was associated with fewer admissions to hospital, fewer inductions of labor, and fewer cesarean sections without adverse effect.[16]

3. Further evaluation

Genetic amniocentesis and/or TORCH titers may be performed if an anatomic survey indicates major anomalies, a large (hydropic) placenta, and/or other findings indicative of intrauterine infections, although no data exist regarding the change in outcome. Routine screening of IUGR infants with postnatal workups for TORCH infections produces minimal yields.[15]

VII. Summary of Management of Small-for-Dates Pregnancy

A. Establishment of Accurate Dating

Establishing an accurate gestational age and estimated date of delivery should be done by using multiple parameters (LMP, initial uterine size, fetal heart tone, initial ultrasound, serial growth, quickening, fundal height at umbilicus, etc.), with a careful review of these criteria at 20 weeks when possible. Follow-up ultrasound scans should never be used to "redate" a pregnancy when a reliable, early ultrasound scan is available. Dating parameters become less certain as the pregnancy progresses.

B. Use of Ultrasound

Ultrasound evaluation should be obtained in selected patients at high risk. If a patient is to be screened, this should be performed between 32 and 34 weeks' gestation or as part of an overall assessment of a significant pregnancy complication, such as preeclampsia. Ultrasound examinations for growth must include a measurement of the abdomen, head, and femur, with attention to normal body ratios and using previously recorded measurements for comparison. A careful anatomic survey should be performed, as well as an assessment for fluid volume.

C. Fetal Surveillance and the Timing of Delivery

Since intrauterine growth restriction may occur in conjunction with significant maternal complications, the timing of maternal delivery may be determined by deterioration of maternal condition. Oligohydramnios is considered to be a serious finding, signifying uteroplacental insufficiency in the absence of severe urinary obstruction or bilateral renal agenesis (see section H). The use of Doppler flow velocimetry of the umbilical artery has been found to result in reduced perinatal mortality and decrease interventions. In the premature fetus, the risks of continuation of the pregnancy must be balanced against the risks of prematurity, and perinatal consultation or referral is recommended.

D. Late-Onset Prenatal Care

If a patient presents late in pregnancy without any reliable method of establishing dates, sonographic evaluation may provide limited information suspicious for growth restriction, such as severe discrepancy in abdominal versus head and long bone growth. A normal anatomic survey and symmetric growth in the absence of known risk factors likely indicate a fetus that is within 2 to 3 weeks of sonographically measured uterine age. This pregnancy can be managed expectantly. Recognition of significant risk factors, such as preeclampsia, should prompt the physician to further investigate the well-being of the pregnancy.

References

1. Barker DJ: In utero programming of cardiovascular disease. Theriogenology 53:555–574, 2000.
2. Campbell S, Thomas A: Ultrasound measurement of the fetal head to abdomen circumference ratio in the assessment of growth retardation. Br J Obstet Gynaecol 84:165-174, 1977.
3. Chiarelli F, diRicco L, Mohn A, et al: Insulin resistance in short children with intrauterine growth retardation. Acta Paediatr Suppl 88:62–65, 1999.
4. Chien PF, Arnott N, Gordon A, et al: How useful is uterine artery Doppler flow velocimetry in the prediction of preeclampsia, intrauterine growth retardation, and perinatal death? An overview. Br J Obstet Gynaecol 107:196–208, 2000.
5. Francis A: Controlled trial of fundal height measurement plotted on customised antenatal growth charts. Br J Obstet Gynaecol 106:309–317, 1999.
6. Gortner L, Wauer RR, Stock GJ, et al: Neonatal outcome in small-for-gestational-age infants: Do they really do better? J Perinat Med 27:484–489, 1999.
7. Gulmezoglu AM, Hofmeyr GJ: Bed rest in hospital for suspected impaired fetal growth (Cochrane Review). In The Cochrane Library, Issue 4, 2000. Oxford, Update Software.
8. Gulmezoglu AM, Hofmeyr GJ: Calcium channel blockers for potential impaired growth (Cochrane Review). In The Cochrane Library, Issue 4, 2000. Oxford, Update Software.
9. Gulmezoglu AM, Hofmeyr GJ: Maternal nutrient supplementation for suspected impaired fetal growth. Cochrane Database Syst Rev 2000;(2):CD000148.
10. Hadlock FP, Deter RL, Harrist RB, et al: A date-independent predictor of intrauterine growth retardation: Femur-length/abdominal circumference ratio. Am J Roentgenol 141:979–984,1983.
11. Hadlock FP, Deter RL, Harrist RB: Sonographic detection of abnormal fetal growth patterns. Clin Obstet Gynecol 27:342–351, 1984.
12. Harrington K, Thompson MO, Carpenter RG, et al: Doppler fetal circulation in pregnancies complicated by pre-eclampsia or delivery of a small for gestational age baby: Longitudinal analysis. Br J Obstet Gynaecol 106:453–466, 1999.

13. Jahn A, Razum O, Berle P: Routine screening for intaruterine growth retardation in Germany: Low sensitivity and questionable benefit for diagnosed cases. Acta Obstet Gynaecol Scand 77:643–648, 1998.
14. Jaquet D, Gaborian A, Czernichow P, et al: Insulin resistance early in adulthood in subjects born with intrauterine growth retardation. J Clin Endocrinol Metab 85:1401–1406, 2000.
15. Khan NA, Kazzi SN: Yield and costs of screening growth-retarded infants for TORCH infections. Am J Perinatol 17:131–135, 2000.
16. Nielson JP, Alfirevic Z: Doppler ultrasound in high risk pregnancies (Cochrane Review).In The Cochrane Library, Issue 4, 2000. Oxford, Update Software.
17. Ong KK, Ahmed ML, Emmett PM, et al: Association between catch-up growth and obesity in childhood: Prospective cohort study. BMJ 320:967–971, 2000.
18. Seeds JW: Impaired fetal growth: Ultrasonic evaluation and clinical management. Obstet Gynecol 64:577–584, 1984.
19. Skovron ML, Berkowitz GS, Lapinski RH, et al: Evaluation of early third-trimester ultrasound screening for intrauterine growth retardation. J Ultrasound Med 10:153–159, 1991.
20. Sommerfelt K, Andersson HW, Sonnander K, et al: Cognitive development of term small for gestational age children at five years of age. Arch Dis Child 83:25–30, 2000.
21. Vintzileos AM, Lodeiro JG, Feinstein SJ, et al: Value of fetal ponderal index in predicting intrauterine growth retardation. Obstet Gynecol 67:585–588, 1986.
22. Warsof, SL, Cooper DJ, Little D, Campbell S: Routine ultrasound screening for antenatal detection of intrauterine growth retardation. Obstet Gynecol 67:33–39, 1986.
23. Witlin AG, Saade GR, Mattar F, et al: Predictors of neonatal outcome in women with severe preeclampsia or eclampsia between 24 and 32 weeks' gestation. Am J Obstet Gynecol 182:607–611, 2000.

SECTION G.
LARGE-FOR-DATES PREGNANCY

Elizabeth G. Baxley, M.D.

I. Clinical Presentation
A. Obesity
In obese women who are pregnant, the measured fundal height may appear to be increased in all trimesters of pregnancy. Macrosomia, however, is also more common in the obese patient. When a patient with risk factors for macrosomia is discovered to measure large-for-dates late in pregnancy, fetal macrosomia should be suspected.
B. Short Stature
Women whose height is short also may appear to be larger than their dates suggest, although the fundal height measurements typically correlate properly between 20 and 32 weeks.
C. Uterine Enlargement
Fundal height measurements that exceed menstrual or ultrasound dates may signify an increase in uterine size. Diagnoses to be considered include polyhydramnios, multiple gestation, fetal macrosomia, or growth of uterine leiomyomata (see below).

II. Etiologies of Large-for-Dates Pregnancy
A. Inaccurate Dates
The most common cause of fundal height measurements exceeding menstrual dates is improper dating of the pregnancy. In these cases, the designated last menstrual period (LMP) may actually represent bleeding that took place after the onset of pregnancy, such as implantation bleeding of the placenta. The patient who presents late for prenatal care poses a significant diagnostic problem when fetal size exceeds that expected with menstrual dating, since reliability of ultrasound dating lessens with advancing gestational age.
B. Inaccurate Measurement
Fundal height measurements carry a measure of subjectivity, such that variation of several centimeters may be recorded by different examiners on the same patient at

the same gestational age. This variation is enhanced in the patient with obesity or excessive maternal weight gain.

C. Fetal Macrosomia

When fetal growth exceeds the range of normal rates, macrosomia causes the uterine size to be large for dates. This occurs predominantly in the third trimester. A history of previous large infants, large parental size, or gestational diabetes may predict a subsequent large fetus. It is difficult to predict macrosomia at, or close to, term. It is important to determine whether diabetes is present (see Chapter 6, section A). The uterus may be enlarged in diabetes as a result of polyhydramnios, fetal macrosomia, or both. There is greater fetal soft tissue mass proportionate to head size.[1]

Birth weight estimation by ultrasound, and thus prediction of shoulder dystocia risk, is no more accurate than 10–15%.[2–4,6] Prediction of fetal macrosomia may be more accurate when patients have well-established dates and an estimated fetal weight exceeds the 90th percentile early in the third trimester. Prediction of macrosomic status antenatally has been demonstrated in one series to result in increased rates of elective cesarean section.[2] Induction before 40 weeks based on the diagnosis of macrosomia, and recommendations for elective cesarean section based on an arbitrary weight cut-off in nondiabetic pregnancies do not appear to be justified.[1,2,4] One decision analysis model determined that 3695 elective cesarean deliveries would be needed to prevent one permanent brachial plexus injury among nondiabetic patients with an estimated fetal weight > 4500 grams.[5]

D. Polyhydramnios

The increase in uterine size may represent an increase in amniotic fluid rather than fetal size. This is more common in the late second and third trimester (see section I).

E. Multiple Gestation

Any number of fetuses greater than one causes the fundal height to measure large for dates. Multiple gestation is often discovered by ultrasound obtained because of concern over a large fundal height measurement (see section C).

F. Uterine Leiomyomata

Women with preexisting leiomyomata may experience growth of these benign tumors during pregnancy. Even when fibroid growth does not occur, their mere presence may cause the uterus to measure larger than would be expected by the fetus, amniotic fluid, and placenta alone.

G. Molar Pregnancy

In the first trimester, an enlarged uterus may signify a molar pregnancy, particularly if fetal heart tones are not heard by Doppler when anticipated.

III. Summary

Patients with large-for-dates pregnancy should have sonographic evaluation because of potential diagnosis of complications such as multiple gestation and polyhydramnios. The large-for-gestational-age fetus may be seen in both diabetic and normal pregnancies. Diagnosis of macrosomia in late pregnancy is a poor predictor of actual birth weight and of pregnancy outcome, including the need for operative delivery of the occurrence of birth trauma.

References

1. Acker DB, Sachs BP, Friedman EA: Risk factors for shoulder dystocia. Obstet Gynecol 66:762–768, 1985.
2. Delpapa EH, Mueller-Heubach E: Pregnancy outcome following ultrasound diagnosis of macrosomia. Obstet Gynecol 78:340–343, 1991.
3. Ott WJ, Doyle S, Falmm S: Accurate ultrasonic estimation of weight. Am J Perinatol 2:178–182, 1985.
4. Pollack RN, Hauer-Pollack G, Divon MY: Macrosomia in post-dates pregnancies: Accuracy of routine ultrasonographic screening. Am J Obstet Gynecol 167:7–11, 1992.

5. Rouse DJ. Owen J, Goldenberg RL, et al: The effectiveness and costs of elective cesarean delivery for fetal macrosomia diagnosed by ultrasound. JAMA 276:1480–1486, 1996.
6. Sabbagha RE, Minoque J, Tamura RK: Estimation of birth weight by use of formulas targeted to large-, appropriate-, and small-for-gestational age fetuses. Am J Obstet Gynecol 160:854–862, 1989.

SECTION H.
OLIGOHYDRAMNIOS

Janis E. Byrd, M.D.

I. Physiology

The primary contributors to amniotic fluid volume (AFV) in late gestation are fetal urine and lung secretion, while fetal swallowing and intramembranous absorption are responsible for fluid clearance.[1]

II. Clinical Significance

The clinical significance of oligohydramnios is highly dependent upon gestational age at diagnosis, the presence or absence of underlying fetal anomalies or maternal disease, associated premature rupture of membranes (PROM) or intrauterine growth restriction (IUGR), and cut-off values used for diagnosis. Pathologic conditions commonly associated with oligohydramnios include maternal hypertension, postmaturity, multiple gestation, and placental abruption. Genetic factors also contribute to the incidence of oligohydramnios. Over all gestational ages the aneuploidy rate is 4.4%, although this rate is quite variable depending upon the population being studied.

Fetal renal anomalies or, less commonly, anomalies of the central nervous system, cardiovascular, and skeletal systems are present in about half of second-trimester pregnancies with oligohydramnios.[13] Survival rates of only 10% have been reported when severe oligohydramnios is present in conjunction with fetal anomalies. Pregnancies diagnosed with severe oligohydramnios in the third trimester have a much lower rate of anomalies (22.1%) and a survival rate of 85.3%.

In the absence of IUGR, PROM, or anomalies, one study of patients with oligohydramnios diagnosed between 17 and 37 weeks found a higher incidence of preterm delivery but no increased risk of intrauterine death or birth asphyxia over controls.[4] Another study of isolated oligohydramnios (no fetal or maternal complications) in women undergoing induction at 37–41 weeks[6,7] found no difference in neonatal outcomes. However, there were significantly more cesarean deliveries (15.8% vs. 6.6%, p < 0.01, OR 2.7),[2] which were attributable to non-reassuring fetal heart rate tracings. Oligohydramnios does not alter fetal lung maturity studies but in polyhydramnios the results are low.[12]

III. Diagnosis

Although the diagnosis may be suspected clinically by fundal height measurements that lag behind calculated weeks of gestation, it is usually made or confirmed by semi-quantitative sonographic analysis.[6,8] A single vertical pocket < 2 cm, or a sum of the largest pockets in each uterine quadrant of < 5 cm (AFI) are the most commonly used parameters for making a diagnosis of oligohydramnios. Higher positive predictive values are obtained at AFI values of 3 or 4 cm (85%) as compared to 50% at AFI value of 5 cm.[9]

Once the diagnosis of oligohydramnios has been confirmed, ultrasound assessment should include a careful search for fetal anomalies and placental pathology. Genetic amniocentesis is recommended for detection of aneuploidy when severe oligohydramnios is discovered in the second trimester or fetal anomalies are seen on ultrasound.

IV. Management

A. Second Trimester

Specific fetal therapies are now available for some conditions, e.g., bladder-amniotic fluid shunt for posterior urethral valves. Transabdominal amnioinfusion is most useful to improve sonographic diagnosis of the underlying cause of the oligohydramnios and may offer some improvement in outcome for neonates without lethal anomalies.[5,7] Patients with lethal fetal anomalies can be counseled accordingly.

B. Third Trimester

1. Antepartum testing

Wing[14] has addressed the important clinical question of how frequently to obtain AFI measurements in women with oligohydramnios. Testing intervals of 4 versus 7 days were compared. Patients with AFI > 8 had a 2.3% chance of subsequently having an AFI < 5 in 4 days and a 2.2% chance in 7 days. Patients with AFI of 5–8 had a 16.2% chance of AFI < 5 in 4 days and 16.3% in 7 days. At > 41 weeks' gestation, if the initial AFI was > 8, the chance of the AFI being < 5 in 4 days was 7.4%. If the initial AFI was 5–8, however, the chance of oligohydramnios increased to 23.3% in 4 days. Patients who are < 41 weeks' gestation with an initial AFI of 5–8, and patients who are > 41 weeks' gestation, are best followed with twice-weekly AFI assessment. For women < 41 weeks' gestation undergoing antepartum testing with initial AFI > 8, weekly testing is probably adequate.

2 Prophylactic intrapartum amnioinfusion

Five RCTs have failed to show improved maternal or neonatal outcome with prophylactic intrapartum amnioinfusion for oligohydramnios only (known oligohydramnios with a reassuring fetal heart rate tracing).[7] There are considerable data, however, to support amnioinfusion when meconium or variable decelerations are noted.[11] The procedure can be safely performed in women with a prior cesarean delivery.[10]

3. Maternal hydration

An RCT comparing various methods of maternal hydration (isotonic IV fluids, hypotonic IV fluids, or oral water @ 2 L/2 hr) found that either oral water or hypotonic IV fluids increased AFI by about 30% in women with oligohydramnios. Maternal osmotic change, rather than volume expansion, appears to be the major influence on AFV. Whether maternal hydration is an appropriate therapy depends on the underlying condition(s).[7] There are no data to show improved outcomes, although hydration could delay induction and/or prevent meconium complications.

V. Summary

The causes of oligohydramnios are varied, with associated clinical significance ranging from lethal fetal anomalies to isolated benign oligohydramnios in otherwise normal term pregnancies requiring no intervention. Diagnosis is based on ultrasound measurements of the AFI of < 5 cm, with 5–8 cm being considered low-normal or borderline and requiring close follow-up. Assessment for fetal anomalies and maternal disease are key to diagnosis of the underlying cause and consideration of possible interventions. Weekly assessment of AFI is sufficient unless the patient is > 41 weeks' gestation or has an initial AFI < 8. Fetal lung maturity tests are not affected by oligohydramnios.

References

1. Brace RA: Physiology of amniotic fluid volume regulation. Clin Obstet Gynecol 40:280–289, 1997.
2. Conway Dl, Adkins WB, Schroeder B, et al: Isolated oligohydramnios in the term pregnancy: Is it a clinical entity? J Matern Fet Med 7:197–200, 1998.
3. Doi S, Osada H, Seki K, et al: Effect of maternal hydration on oligohydramnios: A comparison of three volume expansion methods. Obstet Gynecol 92:525–529, 1998.

4. Garmel SH, Chelmow D, Sha SJ, et al: Oligohydramnios and the appropriately grown fetus. Am J Perinatol 14:359–363, 1997.
5. Gramellini D, Piantelli G, Delle Chiaie L, et al: Amnioinfusion in the management of oligohydramnios. J Perinatal Med 26:293–301, 1998.
6. Hill L: Oligohydramnios: Sonographic diagnosis and clinical implications. Clin Obstet Gynecol 40:314–327, 1997.
7. Kilpatrick SJ: Therapeutic interventions for oligohydramnios: Amnioinfusion and maternal hydration. Clin Obstet Gynecol 40:328–336, 1997.
8. Moore TR: Clinical assessment of amniotic fluid. Clin Obstet Gynecol 40:303–313, 1997.
9. O'Reilly-Green CP, Divon MY: Predictive value of amniotic fluid index for oligohydramnios in patients with prolonged pregnancies. J Matern Fet Med 5:218–226, 1996.
10. Ouzounian JG, Miller DA, Paul RH: Amnioinfusion in women with previous cesarean births: A preliminary report. Am J Obstet Gynecol 174:783–786, 1996.
11. Ouzounian JG, Paul RH: Clinical role of amnioinfusion. Baillieres Clin Obstet Gynaecol 10:259–272, 1996.
12. Piazze JJ, Maranghi L, Cosmi EV, et al: The effect of polyhydramnios and oligohydramnios on fetal lung maturity indexes. Am J Perinatol 15:249–252, 1998.
13. Shipp TD, Bromlley B, Pauker S, et al: Outcome of singleton pregnancies with severe oligohydramnios in the second and third trimesters. Ultrasound Obstet Gynecol 7:108–113, 1996.
14. Wing DA, Fishman A, Gonzalez C, et al: How frequently should the amniotic fluid index be performed during the course of antepartum testing? Am J Obstet Gynecol 174:33–36, 1996.

SECTION I.
POLYHYDRAMNIOS

Janis E. Byrd, M.D.

I. Epidemiology

Approximately two-thirds of women with polyhydramnios during pregnancy have an idiopathic cause of increased amniotic fluid volume (AFV) and 40% of these show spontaneous resolution. However, polyhydramnios is associated with overall higher rates of maternal and fetal complications, primarily maternal diabetes mellitus and fetal gastrointestinal tract abnormalities. Other less common anomalies involve the central nervous system, cardiovascular or urinary tract. If fetal hydrops is associated with this diagnosis the cause may be either immune or nonimmune. In 95% of cases polyhydramnios is classified as mild to moderate in severity. The risk of fetal abnormalities increases from 17% with mild hydramnios to 86% with severe hydramnios.

II. Definition

In singleton pregnancies, an amniotic fluid index (AFI, see section H) of > 24 cm is defined as polyhydramnios, and is two standard deviations above normal for pregnancies at 26–39 weeks' gestation.[3] An AFI of 20–24 cm is considered borderline elevated. Mild, moderate, and severe categories are based on the largest vertical pocket of 8–11 cm, 12–15 cm, and ≥ 16 cm, respectively. For normal values in twin gestations the reader is referred to Chau et al.[1]

III. Evaluation

Fetal evaluation begins with an anomaly scan targeting the systems mentioned above as well as a search for a "stuck twin" or fetal hydrops. Genetic amniocentesis may be indicated. If hydrops is noted, a maternal antibody screen should determine whether it is of immune or nonimmune origin. If nonimmune, further maternal testing should include a search for intrauterine infections, including syphilis, parvovirus, cytomegalovirus, and varicella (see Chapter 8, section A). Maternal glucose tolerance screening is indicated in most cases of hydramnios as anomalies can coexist and do not rule out diabetes mellitus as a contributing cause.

IV. Management

Patients with idiopathic polyhydramnios are usually followed at 3–4-week intervals with serial ultrasound examinations for AFI and fetal growth. Most patients with non-idiopathic polyhydramnios require referral for definitive evaluation and treatment of the underlying cause. Fetal transfusion is available for immune hydrops fetalis and chronic fetomaternal hemorrhage. Supraventricular fetal cardiac arrhythmias may be successfully treated with various antiarrhythmic agents, and some therapies may have limited success in twin-twin transfusion syndrome.[2]

Preterm labor or maternal respiratory compromise often complicate polyhydramnios, and can be treated with abdominal decompression or indomethacin administered rectally or orally in a dose of 25 mg every 6 hours. Amniotic fluid volume is monitored twice weekly for oligohydramnios and the maintenance dose adjusted to twice daily or less. Six percent of fetuses in one review of 56 series developed renal complications, usually transient but occasionally permanent or even lethal.[2] Sulindac may prove to be a good agent, but is still experimental. Other potential fetal complications of prostaglandin inhibitor therapy include constriction of the ductus arteriosus (the risk of which increases with advancing gestational age), and perforation of the ileum. Maternal problems are primarily limited to the well-known gastrointestinal side effects of these agents. The complications of polyhydramnios are often jointly managed by family physicians and their obstetrical or perinatal consultants.

If polyhydramnios persists at the time of labor, consideration should be given to needling the membranes or abdominal decompression to prevent cord prolapse or placental abruption, which can occur with rapid changes in uterine pressure that sometimes accompany spontaneous or artificial rupture of the membranes. This can be done by using the pudendal block trumpet and needle. The potential risk of an umbilical cord prolapse should be weighed and steps to respond to this emergency identified.

V. Summary

Most polyhydramnios is idiopathic, mild and will resolve spontaneously. Once fetal anomalies, fetal hydrops, multiple gestation and maternal diabetes mellitus have been excluded, the patient may be followed with ultrasound every 3–4 weeks. Treatment should be instituted only if maternal symptoms develop, as fetal side effects of treatment may be severe. This treatment is usually done in conjunction with an obstetrical or perinatal consultant. Consideration can be given to slow decompression of amniotic fluid at the time of labor although the potential risk of umbilical cord prolapse should be weighed. Most causes of non-idiopathic hydramnios will require referral for definitive evaluation and treatment of the underlying cause.

References

1. Chau AC, Kjos SL, Kovacs BW: Ultrasonographic measurement of amniotic fluid volume in normal di-amniotic twin pregnancies. Am J Obstet Gynecol 174:1003–1007, 1996.
2. Moise KJ Jr: Polydramnios. Clin Obstet Gynecol 40:266–279, 1997.
3. Moore TR, Cayle JE: The amniotic fluid index in normal human pregnancy. Am J Obstet Gynecol 162:1168–1173, 1990.

SECTION J.
POSSIBLE INDICATORS OF FETAL ABNORMALITIES

Louise Acheson, M.D.

Most pregnancies that progress beyond the first trimester result in the birth of a normal infant. Of fetal abnormalities encountered, those associated with disturbed fetal growth are the most common. Intrauterine growth retardation and macrosomia were discussed in sections F and G in this chapter. Other indirect indicators of potential fetal abnormality, polyhydramnios and oligohydramnios, were also covered in this chapter (sections H and I). While discussion of congenital anomalies as individual entities is beyond the scope of this text, the focus of this section is to provide an overall approach to the possibly abnormal fetus and review some commonly encountered situations when specific fetal abnormalities should be considered. Assessment of the potentially abnormal fetus requires that the family physician be skilled in taking a genetic history (see Chapter 1), appropriately use screening tests for birth defects (see Chapter 4, section E) and pursue further testing when indicated.

I. Abnormal Maternal Serum Alpha-Fetoprotein, Estriol, and Human Chorionic Gonadotropin
A. Overview
Evaluation of a pregnancy with an abnormal maternal serum alpha-fetoprotein (MSAFP) or triple marker screen includes detailed ultrasound examination in order to determine accuracy of pregnancy dating and to assess fetal anatomy. Inaccurate dating is the most common cause of abnormal results on either MSAFP or triple screen testing. If dates are confirmed and values remain abnormal after recalculation, amniocentesis may be offered for chromosome analysis and measurement of amniotic fluid AFP and acetylcholinesterase levels.[2] If MSAFP is elevated but no fetal anomaly is detected, further tests of fetal growth and well-being may be indicated later in the pregnancy.

Many patients with uncomplicated pregnancies have levels of MSAFP that fall outside the normal ranges set by diagnostic laboratories. When these tests are offered for screening, it may start a cascade effect in which diagnostic evaluations are performed on many patients in order to make a definitive diagnosis of an abnormality in one fetus (Table 7).[2,8,21,25] Because of this, pretest counseling regarding benefits and limitations of serum marker testing should precede any decision to screen. Prospective parents vary in the value they place on such information; some desire

TABLE 7.   Hypothetical Results of Screening 10,000 Pregnant Women* with Maternal Serum Triple Markers

Condition	Trisomy 21 (Down Syndrome)	Trisomy 18	Neural Tube Defects
Number with initial screen indicating increased risk	587	23	500–1000
Still abnormal after dating sonography and repeat MSAFP (if MSAFP elevated)	380	23	300–600
Number of affected fetuses## Detected	87	3	4 spina bifida + 5–10 anencephaly
Undetected	57**	2**	1 closed spina bifida
Number of diagnostic evaluations (amniocentesis or detailed sonography) offered per case detected	23–87	8	20–67 (90% detected by ultrasound, 10% by amniocentesis)

* Representative of U.S. population
\# Example based on notification of elevated risk if it is greater than 1 in 190 [Ross]
\## Calculated based on proportion of U.S. *live births* affected by the condition
** Additional cases would be detected by performing chromosome analysis on all pregnancies at advanced maternal age[2,8,21,25]

screening and accept the potential for further testing, whereas others decline screening. In one study, when parents were offered amniocentesis because of triple screen findings that indicated increased risk of Down syndrome, 21–31% declined.[8]

B. Low Maternal Serum Alpha-Fetoprotein and the Detection of Chromosomal Abnormalities

Low MSAFP is associated with trisomy 21 and trisomy 18, but it is an imperfect screening test because of its low sensitivity and specificity, especially in women with advanced maternal age. For example, universal screening of women under 35 with MSAFP and screening combined with genetic amniocentesis for women over 35 would result in the detection of only 45% of fetuses with trisomy 21 and would require amniocentesis for 10–12% of the general population of pregnant women.[17]

1. Multiple marker screening

Approximately 75% of all infants with trisomy 21 are born to mothers younger than 35 years of age. Yet, the risk of trisomy 21 increases to nearly 1 in 270 pregnancies in women 35 years of age. Triple marker screening combines maternal age with the measurement of MSAFP, maternal serum estriol (low levels associated with trisomy 21 and 18), and hCG (high in trisomy 21, low in trisomy 18).[2] The use of triple marker screening in women younger than 35 results in an estimated 58% detection rate (sensitivity) for trisomy 21, specificity of 96.3%, and a positive predictive value of 1.9% (i.e., 98% of positive tests are false-positives).[8] The sensitivity for trisomy 18 is 60% and specificity is 99%.[21] Elevated maternal serum inhibin A in the second trimester and low pregnancy-associated plasma protein A in the first trimester have also been associated with Down syndrome.[31]

   a. Use of the triple screen, with or without ultrasound, improves the specificity of screening for chromosome defects in women under age 35.
   b. In patients 35 years and older, triple marker screening would result in a 75% reduction in amniocenteses performed, with a 15% reduction in detection of trisomy 21 (85% rather than 100% detection rate).[25] Although ACOG does not recommend substitution of maternal serum screening and sonography for prenatal diagnosis in women over 35, some women may choose this option.[2]
   c. The interpretation of multiple marker screening is highly dependent on accurate pregnancy dating; a 2-week difference in gestational age may make a tenfold difference in risk. Because the most common reason for an "abnormal" result is inaccurate dating, sonography should be performed as the first step in assessing any "abnormal" triple marker screen. A repeat serum test is not indicated.[2]
   d. In cases where sonography and/or triple marker screening with accurate dating indicate a significant probability of trisomy 21 or 18, amniocentesis for chromosome analysis should be offered.

2. Sonographic features of trisomy 21 and trisomy 18

Down syndrome has been associated with sonographic findings of a thickened nuchal skin-fold (6 mm or more) and a shortened femur (actual to expected femur length ratio of 0.91 or less). In a high-risk population of patients undergoing genetic amniocentesis who received ultrasound screening at a tertiary care facility, Down syndrome was detected using these sonographic features with a sensitivity of 75% and a specificity of 98%.[4] However, this degree of accuracy has not been demonstrated in ordinary practice. Patients noted to have these findings on routine ultrasound scans should be considered for amniocentesis.[2] Sonographic evaluation is more accurate in identifying fetuses with trisomy 18, because of the multiple anatomic abnormalities usually present.[5] Fetal chromosome analysis is indicated for definitive diagnosis.

C. High Maternal Serum Alpha-Fetoprotein

Elevated levels of maternal serum alpha-fetoprotein most frequently reflect inaccurate dating or undiagnosed multiple gestation. Fetal demise is also a reason for an elevated MSAFP. In the absence of these, the most well known etiology of an elevated MSAFP is an open neural tube defect or other congenital anomalies. After definitive testing, some abnormally high levels of MSAFP remain unexplained. An MSAFP level of 2.5 to 2.99 MoM prior to 19 weeks' gestation warrants a repeat MSAFP test in addition to sonography.[25]

1. Neural tube defects

Neural tube defects occur in 1 to 2 per 1000 pregnancies in the United States; the incidence appears to be decreasing. This disorder appears to display polygenic inheritance, but 90–95% occur in families without known history of neural tube defects.[1,2]

   a. Anencephaly

   This condition is incompatible with prolonged postnatal survival. It should be detected on any second-trimester sonogram and may be detected on some first-trimester scans. MSAFP levels tend to be higher than with other neural tube defects.

   b. Open spina bifida, meningocele, and myelomeningocele

   These may all be detected on ultrasound, with one large, prospective case series reporting sensitivity rates of 90%.[23] In referral facilities among patients being evaluated for elevated MSAFP, detection rates > 95% have been reported,[2] but such results may not be realistic for community practice.

   All second- and third-trimester sonographic examinations should include views of the spine,[3] although fetal position or maternal body habitus may sometimes prevent adequate examination, causing small defects to be missed. Targeted scans in women with elevated MSAFP levels should include, if possible, evaluation of the integrity of each vertebral element. Other findings that assist in the detection of small neural tube defects include the presence of a "lemon sign" of frontal bone deformation and the "banana sign," which represents an Arnold Chiari malformation of the posterior fossa.[22] Closed neural tube defects, which represent 15% of spina bifida cases, are not associated with elevated MSAFP levels.[25]

2. Ventral defects

Gastroschisis, omphalocele, and exstrophy of the urinary bladder can be discovered as the result of finding an elevated MSAFP. These anomalies are detectable in most second-trimester ultrasound examinations. Patients with an omphalocele should be offered genetic amniocentesis because of a significant risk for coexisting chromosomal abnormalities.[2]

3. Other defects

Other defects with elevated MSAFP include Finnish nephrosis, Turner syndrome with cystic hygroma, fetal bowel obstruction, and sacral teratoma.[25]

4. Ultrasound screening for aneuploidy

The association of aneuploidy with major structural fetal defects has been known for some time. More recently, studies performed in high-risk populations referred for genetic amniocentesis because of advanced maternal age or abnormal triple screen testing have revealed a number of sonographic findings associated with trisomy 21, such as a thickened nuchal skin-fold ≥ 6 mm (second trimester). Table 8 summarizes sonographic findings, both major and minor, that have been associated with aneuploidy.

   Two separate large U.S. studies involving a total of approximately 2200 patients referred for genetic amniocentesis utilized sonographic scoring criteria to

TABLE 8.   Ultrasound Findings of Aneuploidy[7,11,15,18,19,20]

Finding	Trisomy	Likelihood Ratio (LR)
Cardiac defects	21, 18, 13	25
Duodenal atresia	21	25
Cystic hygroma	21, 18, 13	25
Omphalocele	21	25
Hydrops/hydrothorax	21	25
Nuchal skin fold thickness ≥ 6 mm	21, 18	18.6
Echogenic bowel	21	5.5
Echogenic intracardiac focus	21	2.0
Renal pyelectasis	21	1.6
Choroid plexus cyst	18	7
Short humerus, femur	21	2.5
Mild cerebral ventricular dilatation	21, 18, 13	
Other CNS anomalies	18, 13	

predict trisomy 21. Using structural and nonstructural findings as listed in Table 8, the detection of trisomy 21 by ultrasound was 62–68%.[7,20] When combined with amniocentesis for all pregnancies with maternal age of 40 or greater, the accuracy of these protocols increased to 74–75% detection rate with amniocentesis performed in 26% of normals. Additionally, reserving amniocentesis for women with a positive ultrasound or maternal age of 40 would reduce the percent of women needing amniocentesis in the 35–39-year age group from 100% to 12.5%.[7] Another large European study found ultrasound markers that were independent predictors of trisomy 21 were cardiac abnormalities, other structural abnormalities, and a nuchal skin-fold thickness ≥ 6 mm.[29] Because of the overlap in sonographic markers for trisomy 21, these authors recommend using only markers that have been shown to be independent predictors of trisomy 21.

Less promising markers for aneuploidy include choroid plexus cysts that may be predictive of trisomy 18[11] but not trisomy 21.[6] A widened fetal iliac angle (≥ 90°) has been associated with trisomy 21 but does not appear to be useful as a single screening test due to a high false-positive rate.[26] Although multiple studies have found an increased incidence of shortened femur and humerus length in fetuses with trisomy 21,[19] its predictive ability has been inconsistent when performed in second-trimester scans.[30] Ultrasound findings associated with trisomies 18 and 13 are present even more frequently than with trisomy 21, and CNS defects and intrauterine growth restriction are more common.[15,18]

A number of European studies have focused on the use of first-trimester ultrasound screening for aneuploidy, several involving low-risk populations presenting for routine dating ultrasound at 10–14 weeks. In these studies, measurement of a fetal nuchial translucency (NT) ≥ 3 mm than the 95th percentile for gestational age has been associated with detection of 40–80% of aneuploidy.[12,27] Preliminary studies combining first-trimester ultrasound with serum screening for human chorionic gonadotropin and pregnancy-associated plasma protein A suggest increased effectiveness.[14,28] Overall rates of screen-positive patients in NT protocols are approximately 5%. Benefits of earlier screening include the possibility of first-trimester termination, but risks include a higher rate of procedure-associated loss with chorionic villus sampling.

At the present time in the United States, the value of ultrasound in assessment of the fetus with genetic risk appears to be twofold. First, all pregnancies diagnosed with major structural defects associated with aneuploidy, such as endocardial cushion defect (AV canal) or omphalocele, should be offered genetic amniocentesis. Genetic diagnosis of the fetus with trisomy at any gestational age may enhance the ability of the medical team and the parents to make decisions regarding management. Second, the use of an ultrasound risk assessment combined with age-adjusted risk may substantially reduce the number of genetic amniocenteses performed on women under 40 years of age. The initiation of first-trimester screening appears to be investigational at this time, and its incorporation into U.S. care systems would involve additional changes in pregnancy care in order to be used effectively.

5. Abnormal ultrasound screening

If any abnormalities are noted on sonographic examination, or if the patient desires, amniocentesis should be offered. Patients in whom normal fetal spine and CNS anatomy can be visualized may decide to forgo invasive testing of amniotic fluid, but must be counseled that sonography may miss some neural tube defects.[2] When a defect is detected, options available to the family should be discussed in a nondirective manner and genetic counseling provided about treatment, prognosis, and recurrence risk.[2]

6. Delivery of a fetus with spina bifida

One retrospective study suggests that the neurologic outcome is better for infants with open neural tube defects if they are delivered by cesarean section without labor.[16] Although the benefit has not been proven by prospective trials, cesarean delivery should be considered in cases of open spina bifida.[2]

7. Isolated elevated MSAFP

Elevated MSAFP with a normal anatomic survey and amniocentesis delineates a population at risk. Twenty to 38% of all women with unexplained MSAFP elevations have been shown to still be at risk for the following poor pregnancy outcomes, even without evidence of fetal anomalies, and whether or not they have had amniocentesis:[13]

a. Two- to fourfold increase in rates of low birth weight both from preterm delivery and IUGR
b. Tenfold increase in placental abruption
c. Tenfold increase in perinatal mortality
d. Two- to eightfold increase in stillbirth
e. Increased risk (up to twofold) of preeclampsia in some studies
f. Two- to threefold increase in rates of vaginal bleeding and higher rates of fetal-maternal hemorrhage. It is hypothesized that some abnormality is present in the placenta, causing a transplacental alpha-fetoprotein leak into the maternal serum. However, amniotic fluid alpha-fetoprotein levels are normal in these patients. Well-defined protocols and experimental evidence of efficacy are not available to guide the management of patients with unexplained MSAFP elevations. Possible management schemes include the following:[2,13]

    i. Kleihauer-Betke test should be performed initially if the patient is Rh-negative because of the small risk that fetal-maternal hemorrhage and isoimmunization have occurred.
    ii. Patients with a history of pregnancy loss or vascular thromboses should have tests for acquired and inherited thrombophilia, possibly including antiphospholipid antibodies and Factor V Leiden.
    iii. Follow-up ultrasound scan between 28 and 32 weeks should be considered because of the increased risk of IUGR.
    iv. Third-trimester antenatal testing or fetal movement counting may be considered.

II. Other Evidence of Fetal Abnormality

Several additional findings should prompt consideration that the possibility of an anatomically abnormal fetus exists, even in the face of no apparent anomalies by ultrasound examination.[3] These include the following:

A. Polyhydramnios
B. Oligohydramnios
C. Single Umbilical Artery

This deviation from the normal 3-vessel cord has been associated with other structural anomalies in 15–40% of fetuses in which it has been detected. However, this information is largely derived from tertiary referral facilities and may be skewed.

D. Fetal Choroid Plexus Cysts

These occur in about 2% of fetuses and are associated with chromosomal abnormalities in up to 10% of cases. If the cysts are large (> 5 mm in diameter) the incidence of abnormalities increases to 24% of affected fetuses.[24] Most (75–90%) choroid plexus cysts are found in normal fetuses and typically disappear in serial ultrasound examinations by the third trimester.

III. Women at Increased Risk for Fetal Anomaly

A. Teratogenic Exposures

A common concern expressed by both patient and physician is whether or not a medication or other exposure, especially early in pregnancy, has been teratogenic to the fetus. These concerns range in severity from minor exposures with minimal risk, such as taking an over-the-counter "cold" medication, to serious exposure during a crucial stage of gestation to medications of known teratogenicity, such as lithium.[1] Information about teratogenicity can be obtained through the National Library of Medicine's TOXLINE database. Exposure to radiologic procedures, although anxiety-provoking, is rarely significant, even if multiple films are obtained (e.g., upper gastrointestinal series).

B. Evaluation Options

The physician is often faced with diagnostic decisions regarding the use of high-resolution ultrasound, maternal-fetal medicine consultation, or amniocentesis to evaluate these concerns.

1. Minor exposure

The physician and patient can usually be reassured in the case of a minor exposure by a routine sonographic examination that includes an anatomic survey.[3] This is not necessary in all cases of minor exposure (e.g, over-the-counter use of decongestants) and a decision whether to pursue further testing should be made by the physician and patient reviewing the evidence on any specific exposure.

2. Missed anomalies

A number of structural defects that may be missed by either routine or high-resolution ultrasound are of less consequence to the management of a pregnancy (e.g., diagnosis of isolated cleft palate or a small muscular ventricular septal defect). When anomalies are diagnosed, referral for genetic counseling is appropriate.

3. Indication for genetic evaluation

Any patient in whom the medical history or a routine evaluation raises suspicion for abnormality should be referred for consultation.

C. Role of Genetic Evaluation

Genetics consultation is often helpful in order to determine the etiology and risk of recurrence when there is a history of a congenital or chromosomal abnormality in a current or prior pregnancy or in the family.[1]

D. Increased Fetal Surveillance

Patients who may require more intensive fetal evaluation include women with insulin-dependent diabetes, those with a family history of neural tube defects, and those with exposures to medications and agents that are known teratogens.[1] Couples whose previous pregnancies have resulted in a child with a congenital anomaly or perinatal death may also be at risk for recurrence. Even when the risk for recurrence is low, patients may benefit from a consultative ultrasound examination to decrease anxiety.

IV. Discovery of a Fetal Abnormality

A. Counseling Patients and Their Families

Women and their family members often respond with shock and disbelief when faced with a diagnosis of an abnormality that has poor or fatal prognosis. Even minor or treatable conditions may cause great anxiety, especially when the prognosis is uncertain. Reactions by the parents and other family members often encompass the stages of grieving (denial, anger, bargaining, depression, and acceptance), and may be further complicated by diagnostic and prognostic uncertainty. The threat of serious illness or death of one's child is generally viewed as one of the most stressful events in life. The caregiver must be prepared to assist the family in dealing with the loss and grieving (see Chapter 12).

B. Maternal Response

The revelation of a fetal abnormality significantly challenges the well-being and self-esteem of the pregnant woman, because she and/or others may secretly or openly blame the mother for the abnormality. The physician and other members of the health care team must communicate to the family that many fetal abnormalities represent random occurrences. Even in pregnancies in which an abnormality can be linked to a specific exposure, blaming the mother is problematic and should be viewed by the physician as an opportunity to help the family deal with the grief. Caregivers must be cautioned about their own tendency to be judgmental, because causality is often difficult to determine.

C. Resources

Patient self-help groups (e.g., local groups for parents who have experienced perinatal losses, national support organizations like SHARE and RESOLVE, support groups for particular genetic disorders), clergy, social workers, and maternal-child nurse educators may provide valuable assistance to the family by helping them to understand and address their feelings. The same resources can also help the parents and physician by providing valuable information about caring for children with special needs.[9,10]

References

1. Acheson LS, Root S, Tyler CV Jr: Clinical Genetics: Monograph. Edition number 240, Home Study Self-Assessment Program. Kansas City, MO, American Academy of Family Physicians, 1999, pp 24–31.
2. American College of Obstetricians and Gynecologists: Maternal Serum Screening. ACOG Educational Bulletin Number 228, September 1996.
3. Antepartum Guidelines for the Routine Ultrasound Exam. American Institute of Ultrasound in Medicine, 1988.
4. Benacerraf BR, Gelman R, Frigoletto FD: Sonographic identification of second trimester fetuses with Down's syndrome. N Engl J Med 317:1371–1376, 1987.
5. Benacerraf BR, Neuberg D, Bromley B, et al: Sonographic scoring index for prenatal detection of chromosomal abnormalities. J Ultrasound Med 11:449–458, 1992.
6. Bromley B, Lieberman R, Benacerraf BR: Choroid plexus cysts: Not associated with Down's syndrome. Ultrasound Obstet Gynecol 8:232–235, 1996.
7. Bromley B, Shipp T, Benacerraf BR: Genetic scoring index: Accuracy and clinical utility. J Ultrasound Med 18:523–528, 1999.

8. Dick PT: Periodic Health Examination, 1996 Update: 1. Prenatal screening for and diagnosis of Down syndrome. Canadian Task Force on the Periodic Health Examination. CMAJ 154:465–479, 1996.
9. Directory of National Genetic Voluntary Organizations (http://medhlp.netusa.net/agsg/agsgsup.htm): Lists support groups and other resources for persons with genetic disorders and their families.
10. Family Village (http://www.familyvillage.wisc.edu): This site links to medical information, resources, and support organizations for families of children with mental retardation and other disabilities.
11. Ghidini A, Strobelt N, Locatelli A, et al: Isolated fetal choroid plexus cysts: Role of ultrasonography in establishment of the risk of trisomy 18. Am J Obstet Gynecol 182:972–977, 2000.
12. Jackson M, Rose NC: Diagnosis and management of fetal nuchal lucency. Semin Roentgenol 88:333–338, 1998.
13. Katz VL, Chescher NC, Cefalo RC: Unexplained elevations of maternal serum alpha-fetoprotein. Obstet Gynecol Surv 45:719–726, 1990.
14. Krantz DA, Hallahan TW, Orlandi F, et al: First-trimester Down's syndrome screening using dried blood biochemistry and nuchal translucency. Obstet Gynecol 96:207–213, 2000.
15. Lehman CD, Nyberg DA, Winter TC, et al: Trisomy 13 syndrome: Prenatal U.S. findings in a review of 33 cases. Radiology 194:217–222, 1995.
16. Luthy DA, Wardinsky T, Shurtleff DB, et al: Cesarean section before the onset of labor and subsequent motor function in infants with meningomyelocele diagnosed antenatally. N Engl J Med 324:662–666, 1992.
17. New England Regional Genetics Group: Study of Down syndrome screening: Combining maternal serum alpha-fetoprotein measurements and age to screen for pregnant women under age 35. Am J Obstet Gynecol 160:575–579, 1989.
18. Nyberg DA, Kramer D, Resta RG, et al: Prenatal sonographic findings of trisomy 18: Review of 47 cases. J Ultrasound Med 12:103–113, 1993.
19. Nyberg DA, Resta RG, Luthy DA, et al: Humerus and femur length shortening in the detection of Down's syndrome. Am J Obstet Gynecol 168:534–538, 1993.
20. Nyberg DA, Luthy DA, Resta RG, et al: Age-adjusted ultrasound risk assessment for fetal Down's syndrome during the second trimester: Description of the method and analysis of 142 cases. Ultrasound Obstet Gynecol 12:8–14, 1998.
21. Palomaki GE, Haddow JE, Knight GJ, et al: Risk-based prenatal screening for trisomy 18 using alpha-fetoprotein, unconjugated estriol, and human chorionic gonadotropin. Prenat Diagn 15:713–723, 1995.
22. Penso C, Redline RW, Benacerraf BR: A sonographic sign which reliably predicts which fetuses with hydrocephalus have an associated neural tube defect. J Ultrasound Med 6:307–311, 1987.
23. Platt LD, Feuchtbaum L, Filly R, et al: The California Maternal Serum Alpha-fetoprotein Screening Program: The role of ultrasonography in the detection of spina bifida. Am J Obstet Gynecol 166:1328–1329, 1992.
24. Porto M, Murata Y, Warneke LA, et al: Fetal choroid plexus cysts: An independent factor for chromosomal anomalies. J Clin Ultrasound 21:103–108, 1993.
25. Ross HL, Elias S: Maternal serum screening for fetal genetic disorders. Obstet Gynecol Clin North Am 24:33–47, 1997.
26. Shipp TD, Bromley B, Lieberman E, et al: The second-trimester fetal iliac angle as a sign of Down's syndrome. Ultrasound Obstet Gynecol 12:15–18, 1998.
27. Snijders RJ, Noble P, Sebire N, et al: UK multicentre project on assessment of risk of trisomy 21 by maternal age and fetal nuchal-translucency thickness at 10–14 weeks' gestation. Fetal Medicine Foundation First Trimester Screening Group. Lancet 352:343–346, 1998.
28. Spencer K, Spencer CE, Power M, et al: One-stop clinic for assessment of risk for fetal abnormalities: A report of the first year of prospective screening for chromosomal anomalies in the first trimester. Br J Obstet Gynaecol 107:1272–1275, 2000.
29. Vergani P, Locatelli A, Piccoli MG, et al: Best second-trimester sonographic markers for the detection of trisomy 21. J Ultrasound Med 18:469–473, 1999.
30. Vergani P, Locatelli A, Piccoli MG, et al: Critical reappraisal of the utility of fetal femur length in the prediction of trisomy 21. Prenat Diagn 20:210–214, 2000.
31. Wald NJ, Watt HC, Hackshaw AK: Integrated screening for Down's syndrome based on tests performed during the first and second trimesters. N Engl J Med 341:461–467, 1999.

CHAPTER 7

Chronic Medical Conditions in Pregnancy

Women of childbearing age should receive preconception counseling for any increased risks they may face for chronic medical conditions. These increased risks may adversely affect pregnancy outcome (see Chapter 1). Some women benefit from preconception interventions or changes in medication to enhance fetal outcome. A number of medical diagnoses impart significant risks to the pregnant woman; a few conditions are extremely dangerous.

This chapter covers a number of chronic medical conditions seen in primary care. Each section focuses on preconception and early antenatal risk assessment, antenatal management guidelines, complications, and intrapartum management. Many pregnant patients with increased medical risk benefit from high-risk obstetric or medical subspecialty consultation. Even when the patient is receiving obstetric management from high-risk consultants, it may be necessary for the family physician to manage the patient's medical care.

SECTION A.
PULMONARY CONDITIONS

Ellen L. Sakornbut, M.D.

I. Asthma
A. Preconception Counseling and Management
The treatment goal is optimal asthma control. The vast majority of patients with asthma can expect a positive pregnancy outcome. Women with severe, steroid-dependent asthma may experience an increase in pregnancy-induced hypertension.[2]
B. Epidemiology
1. Asthma in pregnancy
Asthma complicates 4–6% of pregnancies. The severity of asthma worsens in about 20–35% of pregnant women, remains stable in 40–50%, and improves in 20–30%.[2,5,13,15] In a large, control-matched study, 40% of women were successfully managed on the same medication regimen as before pregnancy, 18% needed less medication, and 42% required more medication.[20] Acute exacerbations occur with increasing frequency in the early third trimester.
2. Asthma-related complications
Although earlier literature suggests increased pregnancy complications with asthma, current management strategies for asthma control during pregnancy should result in satisfactory outcomes. Studies from the early 1990s reported increased risk for antepartum and postpartum hemorrhage,[1] preterm birth, low-birth-weight babies, pregnancy-induced hypertension, cesarean section, and placenta previa.[7] However, a later study found no association except an increased use of cesarean delivery for non-cephalic presentation.[9]

TABLE 1.   Management of Asthma in Pregnancy

Asthma severity	Medication	Comments
Mild, rare symptoms	Beta-agonist inhalers as rescue medication	Avoidance of irritants, allergens
Exercise-induced only	Beta-agonist inhalers, nedocromil, or cromolyn	Peak-flow meter to evaluate non-exercise-induced symptoms
Mild asthma, including any patient with previous ED visit	Inhaled corticosteroids , beta-agonist rescue	Peak-flow meter self-monitoring; may add cromolyn
Severe asthma	Inhaled corticosteroids, night-time long-acting beta-agonist therapy; also consider nedocromil, cromolyn	Also consider theophylline, toxicity concerns; daily home peak-flow monitoring
Severe, refractory	Oral corticosteroids in lowest doses or alternate-day doses preferred; leukotriene receptor antagonists or 5-lipo-oxygenase inhibitors if good pre-pregnancy response	Stress-dose corticosteroids in labor if chronic systemic steroids; consultation; breast-feeding contraindicated if using zafirlukast

C. Antenatal Management (Table 1)

1. Medications considered safe in pregnancy

These include beta-agonists (including albuterol, metaproterenol, and terbutaline), nedocromil, theophylline, cromolyn, and inhaled steroids. Theophylline clearance is increased during pregnancy[11] (see Chapter 2, section G).

3. Inhaled steroids

These should be used prophylactically in any pregnant woman with asthma exacerbations that occur on a regular basis. This is done to reduce the incidence of acute asthma attacks. Even patients with rare exacerbations should be considered for inhaled steroids if these attacks have been severe enough to warrant an emergency room visit. This therapy may be successful in reducing acute exacerbations by as much as four times.[19]

4. Systemic steroids

These should be used at the lowest possible dose. Although there is a theoretical risk of effects on the fetal adrenal gland, this occurrence has been extremely rare in pregnancies in which steroids have been used throughout gestation. This is probably due to the fact that prednisone is not converted to its active form, prednisolone, by the placenta or fetus.

   a. Effects on fetal growth. There is some suggestion of effects on fetal growth with long-term use.[13]

   b. Risk of cleft palate. There is a possible low risk of cleft palate with first-trimester use.[14]

   c. Steroid-dependent asthmatics. These patients need stress-dose coverage during labor and delivery.

5. Leukotriene receptor antagonists

Although these agents are categorized as FDA class B, little information is available from large clinical trials. Animal studies have shown tumorigenicity with zafirlukast but not with montelukast. At this time, the use of leukotriene receptor antagonists should be restricted to severe asthmatics with a demonstrated positive response to these medications prior to pregnancy.[17] Zileuton should probably not be used in pregnancy, since little information is available.

6. Medications to avoid

These include $F_{2\alpha}$ prostaglandins (Hemabate) and beta-blockers that may cause bronchospasm. Bronchospasm has also been encountered with the use of misoprostol and dinoprostone.

7. Clinical management
   a. Influenza vaccination. This should be provided although first-trimester use is discouraged.
   b. Self-monitoring. The patient should self-monitor on a daily basis with the use of a peak-flow meter.
   c. Exercise-induced asthma. This common condition may be treated with albuterol inhalation 30 minutes prior to exercise, cromolyn, or nedocromil as chronic therapy.
   d. Difficult to manage asthmatics. If a patient has regular, daily or near-daily symptoms requiring the use of a rescue beta-agonist therapy, she should be started on an inhaled steroid with the hope that use of rescue medication will be reduced. For patients with moderate or severe asthma, control of nocturnal symptoms may improve with long-acting beta-sympathomimetics, such as bitolterol or salmeterol. Other medications that may be used to control severe asthma include cromolyn sodium or nedocromil in combination with inhaled corticosteroids and beta-agonists or the addition of theophylline.
8. Acute exacerbations
Usual protocols followed in the nonpregnant state should be used. Hypoxia should be treated aggressively. Steroids, beta-agonists, and theophylline can be used. The normal pCO_2 in pregnancy is 32 torr owing to the effects of progesterone (hyperventilation) and decrease in residual volume. This should be considered in any assessment of arterial blood gases.

II. Other Pulmonary Disease
A. Cystic Fibrosis
Women with cystic fibrosis are subfertile, while men are generally infertile. Decreased fertility may result from changes in the mucosal surfaces producing thick cervical mucus. Increased rates of prematurity and perinatal mortality and maternal morbidity and mortality have been observed.[12] Cystic fibrosis is an autosomal recessive disease with a risk of transmission of 2.5%. Prognosis for the mother appears to be poorer in patients with more severe disease before pregnancy and better in patients without significant pancreatic insufficiency[6,10] and when the FEV_1 is > 80% of predicted.[8]

B. Sarcoidosis
Most patients either improve or experience no change in their condition with pregnancy.[1] There are no effects on fertility. Use of steroids is based on pulmonary manifestations and individual patient response.

C. Tuberculosis
Skin testing and shielded chest films are valid means of screening and assessment for selected patients in pregnancy. High-risk patients include those with a positive HIV test and some immigrants. The course of the disease and prognosis are not altered by pregnancy. Diagnosis and treatment are important, however, because of the effects on maternal health and the risk to the infant of tuberculous meningitis.
1. Isoniazid
Isoniazid does not appear to be teratogenic. It is recommended that prophylaxis (treatment of inactive disease) be withheld until after pregnancy, unless there is a strong risk of recent infection.[3] Supplemental pyridoxine should be given.[4]
2. Ethambutol
Ethambutol appears to be safe in pregnancy.[18]
3. Rifampin
There is a possible association of rifampin use with limb reduction defects, so it should be used with caution in pregnancy.[18] It is clearly indicated if miliary, meningeal, or extensive pulmonary tuberculosis is present.

4. Streptomycin/ethionamide

Streptomycin has been associated with fetal ototoxicity. Ethionamide is believed to be teratogenic.[21]

References

1. Agha FP, Vade A, Amendola MA, et al: Effects of pregnancy on sarcoidosis. Surg Gynecol Obstet 155:817–822, 1982.
2. Alexander S, Dodds L, Armson BA: Perinatal outcomes in women with asthma during pregnancy. Obstet Gynecol 92:435–440, 1998.
3. American Thoracic Society: Treatment of tuberculosis and other mycobacterial diseases. Am Rev Respir Dis 127:790–796, 1983.
4. Atkins JN: Maternal plasma concentration of pyridoxal phosphate during pregnancy: Adequacy of vitamin B6 supplementation during isoniazid therapy. Am Rev Respir Dis 126:714–716, 1982.
5. Burdon JG and Goss G: Asthma and pregnancy. Aust N Z J Med 24:3–4, 1994.
6. Corkey CWB, Newth CJL, Corey M, et al: Pregnancy in cystic fibrosis: A better prognosis in patients with pancreatic function? Am J Obstet Gynecol 140:737–742, 1981.
7. Demissie K, Breckenridge MB, Rhoads GG: Infant and maternal outcomes in the pregnancies of asthmatic women. Am J Respir Crit Care Med 158:1091–1095, 1998.
8. Jackelson D, Robinson M, Parsons S, et al: Cystic fibrosis and pregnancy. Aust N Z J Obstet Gynecol 38:180–184, 1998.
9. Minerbi-Codish I, Fraser D, Avnum L, et al: Influence of asthma in pregnancy on labor and the newborn. Respiration 65:130–135, 1998.
10. Palmer J, Dillon-Baker C, Teklin JS, et al: Pregnancy in patients with cystic fibrosis. Ann Intern Med 99:596–600, 1983.
11. Patterson R, Greenberger PA, Frederickson MC: Asthma and pregnancy: Responsibility of physicians and patients. Ann Allergy 65:469–472, 1990.
12. Phillipson G: Cystic fibrosis and reproduction. Reprod Fertil Dev 10:113–119, 1998.
13. Reinisch JM, Simon NG, Karow WG, et al: Prenatal exposure to prednisone in humans and animals retards intrauterine growth. Science 202:436–438, 1978.
14. Schatz M, Patterson R, Zeitz S, et al: Corticosteroid therapy for the pregnant asthmatic patient. JAMA 233:804–807, 1975.
15. Schatz M, Harden K, Forsythe A, et al: The course of asthma in pregnancy, post-partum, and with successive pregnancies: A prospective analysis. J Allergy Clin Immunol 81:509–517, 1998.
16. Sims C, Chamberlain G, DeSwiet M: Lung function test in bronchial asthma before, during and after pregnancy. Br J Obstet Gynaecol 83:434–437, 1976.
17. Smith LJ: A risk-benefit assessment of antileukotrienes in asthma. Drug Saf 19:205–218, 1998.
18. Snider DE, Layde PM, Johnson MW, et al: Treatment of tuberculosis during pregnancy. Am Rev Respir Dis 122:65, 1980.
19. Stenius-Aarniala B, Hedman J, Teramo KA: Acute asthma in pregnancy. Thorax 51:411–414, 1996.
20. Stenius-Aarniala B, Piirila P, Teramo KA: Asthma and pregnancy: A prospective study of 198 pregnancies. Thorax 43:12–18, 1998.
21. Warkany J: Antituberculous drugs. Teratology 20:133–137, 1979.

SECTION B.
CARDIOVASCULAR CONDITIONS

Ellen L. Sakornbut, M.D.

I. Structural Heart Disease
A. General Approach

Some patients with heart conditions can be safely managed in pregnancy by the family physician. Other patients should receive consultation or referral for pregnancy management. Nonetheless, the family physician may encounter these referred patients in emergency situations, particularly in rural areas. Additionally, patients with heart disease should receive preconception counseling.[9] The number of women with heart disease in pregnancy is approximately 1%; this number may increase as improved therapy of pediatric heart disease allows for greater survival to adulthood.

TABLE 2.   Cardiac Conditions Associated with High Maternal/Fetal Mortality

Condition	Maternal effects	Fetal effects
Mitral stenosis, severe, valve < 1.0 cm	Up to 25% maternal mortality if pulmonary hypertension present	
Aortic stenosis, severe	Cardiac, cerebral ischemia	Decreased uterine blood flow; 30% fetal loss
Eisenmenger's syndrome	30–40% maternal mortality	30% fetal loss if mother survives
Marfan's syndrome, with dilated aortic root > 4 cm or valvular lesions	30–50% maternal mortality secondary to aortic dissection	
Primary pulmonary hypertension	Up to 50% maternal mortality	40% perinatal mortality if mother survives

B. Fetal Outcomes

Patients with New York Heart Association (NYHA) classification I or II (no symptoms or symptoms only with heavy activity) experience only slightly increased perinatal mortality rates. The perinatal mortality rates with class III or IV are 12% and 31%, respectively. More than 40% of patients with rheumatic heart disease develop pulmonary edema for the first time during pregnancy.[6] Table 2 summarizes cardiac conditions associated with high maternal and fetal mortalities.

C. Changes in Pregnancy

Cardiovascular changes in pregnancy (Table 3) that affect the patient with structural heart disease include the following:

1. Increased intravascular volume

A 50% increase in intravascular volume by the early to middle third trimester may lead to congestive heart failure or increased ischemia in patients with valvular heart disease or myocardial dysfunction. It may result in formation or dissection of an aneurysm in patients at risk, such as those with Marfan's syndrome.

2. Decreased systemic vascular resistance

This may worsen a right-to-left shunt.

3. Pregnancy-associated hypercoagulability

This increases the risk of arterial thromboembolic disease, especially for patients with atrial fibrillation and artificial valves.

4. Peripartum physiologic changes

Marked shifts in cardiac output and intravascular volume occur in the peripartum period. Cardiac output increases during the first stage of labor. Preload may be increased by the release of pressure on the inferior vena cava and a physiologic transfusion from the contracted uterus, or it may be decreased with postpartum hemorrhage. Decreases in preload adversely affect patients with pulmonary hypertension or fixed cardiac output. Tachycardia may be poorly tolerated in patients with valvular obstructive lesions.

TABLE 3.   Cardiovascular Changes in Pregnancy

Blood volume	40–50% increase
Heart rate	10–20% (15 bpm) increase
Cardiac output	30–50% increase (4.5–6.8 L/min)
Systemic vascular resistance	Decreased
Mean arterial blood pressure	Decreased

D. Labor Management in Patients with Significant Structural Heart Disease

1. Subacute bacterial endocarditis prophylaxis

Many patients with structural heart disease require subacute bacterial endocarditis (SBE) prophylaxis for delivery.

2. Labor management

Labor management for patients with significant structural heart disease includes careful monitoring of fluid status, often with the use of central catheter monitoring to assess right and left heart pressures. Epidural anesthesia is used in most patients to prevent fluctuations in cardiac output. Lateral recumbent positioning and oxygen administration are used if there are any concerns about fetal well-being. Clinical setting and resources for management should be appropriate to the risk status of these patients. Nevertheless, family physicians in small hospitals may encounter these patients for emergency care, even if referral had been arranged.

3. Preterm labor

Preterm labor should be treated with magnesium sulfate and avoidance of beta-sympathomimetic agents.

4. Ergot alkaloids

Ergot alkaloids, such as methergine, should be avoided for patients at risk for pulmonary congestion.[6]

5. Oxytocin

A bolus injection of oxytocin may cause transient but significant hypotension.[4]

E. Specific Diagnoses[1,7,8]

1. Mitral stenosis

Mitral stenosis may be relatively asymptomatic until pregnancy-associated hemodynamic changes (increased cardiac output and heart rate) cause an increase in the diastolic pressure gradient across the mitral valve. This results in increased left atrial and pulmonary capillary wedge pressure, leading to pulmonary edema. Severe mitral stenosis, with a valve cross-section of < 1.0 cm,[8] carries a poor prognosis in pregnancy.

    a. Tachycardia. Tachycardia or atrial fibrillation results in decreased filling of the left ventricle with resultant pulmonary edema, although left ventricular function is normal. Atrial fibrillation increases the risk of embolic phenomena and cerebrovascular accident.

    b. Treatment. Digitalization should be used in atrial fibrillation to prevent a rapid ventricular rate. Beta-blockade may be used with tachycardia that is not due to atrial fibrillation. High dosage of beta-blockers may be necessary because of high circulating levels of catecholamines. Salt restriction, bed rest, and diuretics may be necessary.

    c. Antibiotic prophylaxis. Rheumatic fever prophylaxis with daily oral penicillin V or monthly benzathine penicillin is indicated as well as SBE prophylaxis.

    d. Labor management. In addition to the general measures described, patients should not bear down. Epidural anesthesia is commonly used; assisted delivery is often used.

    e. Pulmonary edema. There is increased risk of postpartum pulmonary edema with mobilization of extravascular fluid.

2. Aortic stenosis

Aortic stenosis carries high maternal mortality rates if the stenosis is severe, with high fetal loss rates (about 30%), especially if surgical correction is necessary during pregnancy.

    a. Angina and syncope. These are worrisome symptoms associated with transient inadequacy of cardiac output.

    b. Intrapartum management. This includes avoidance of acute increase in afterload or decrease in preload. Regional anesthesia may cause hypotension and a decrease in cardiac output.

3. Atrial septal defect (ASD)

ASD (specifically secundum ASD) is the most common congenital lesion that may escape diagnosis in childhood. Most patients with ASD tolerate pregnancy well. A few patients develop congestive heart failure.

    a. Arterial embolus. A right to left embolus is possible with Valsalva maneuver with potentially devastating results.

    b. Eisenmenger's syndrome. If Eisenmenger's syndrome (pulmonary hypertension with a right-to-left intracardiac shunt) is present, maternal mortality is > 40%.[10]

4. Ventricular septal defect

Ventricular septal defects are usually detected early in childhood. Surgical correction should take place before pregnancy. Patients with a small ventricular septal defect or previous surgery tolerate pregnancy well. SBE prophylaxis is indicated.

    a. Pulmonary hypertension. A large left-to-right shunt puts the patient at risk for development of pulmonary hypertension and Eisenmenger's syndrome with the high maternal mortality rates as above.

    b. Congestive heart failure. There is an increased risk of congestive heart failure.

5. Marfan's syndrome

Marfan's syndrome carries a significant risk of aortic dissection, with higher risk in symptomatic patients with mitral prolapse, aortic insufficiency, or aortic root dilatation. SBE prophylaxis is indicated. Offspring of a patient with Marfan's syndrome carry a 50% risk of inheriting the autosomal dominant gene for this syndrome.

    a. Risk of dissection. This is as high as 60% in patients with an aortic root > 4 cm; pregnancy should not be undertaken.

    b. Management during pregnancy. Patients at high risk who choose to undertake or continue pregnancy are treated with bed rest and beta-blockade.

    c. Diagnosis. Transesophageal echocardiography and magnetic resonance imaging may be used to diagnose aortic dissection.

    d. Surgical correction. Patients with progressive aortic root dilation during pregnancy should have surgical correction when or before the aortic root reaches 5.5 cm.[2] SBE prophylaxis is indicated.

6. Mitral valve prolapse

Mitral valve prolapse is common in young women, most of whom are asymptomatic.

    a. Antenatal treatment. No antenatal treatment is indicated if symptoms are minor.

    b. Symptomatic arrhythmias. These arrhythmias are treated with activity restriction and beta-blockers if needed.

    c. SBE prophylaxis. This is indicated for patients who have a murmur consistent with mitral regurgitation (holosystolic, heard best at the fourth left intercostal space and radiating to the apex and axilla). Echocardiography may occasionally be helpful in defining the cause of a murmur that seems to be different than the common flow murmur heard in many pregnant women. However, clinicians should be aware that modern color-flow Doppler techniques demonstrate clinically insignificant regurgitant flow across normal heart valves in significant numbers of patients who have no disease state and are not at risk for endocarditis.

7. Idiopathic hypertrophic subaortic stenosis (IHSS)

IHSS carries a good prognosis for most patients in pregnancy because of the increased blood volume.

    a. Syncope. This may occur with vasovagal attacks or blood loss.

    b. Drug treatment. Beta-blockade is indicated for symptoms of dyspnea and angina.

    c. Avoidance of regional anesthesia. Epidural anesthesia with systemic vasodilatation and postpartum hemorrhage should be avoided.

    d. SBE prophylaxis is indicated.

8. Dilated cardiomyopathy

    a. Peripartum cardiomyopathy. This condition is defined as occurring in the peripartum period in a patient without a prior history of heart disease, thus excluding other cardiologic diagnoses.

    b. Incidence. The incidence of peripartum cardiomyopathy is from 1 in 1300 to 1 in 4000 pregnancies; occurrence is more common in older patients, multiparas, African-Americans, and patients with multiple gestations. The cause is unclear, but possible linkages include pregnancy-induced hypertension, viral myocarditis, autoimmune disorders such as lupus and antiphospholipid antibody syndrome, and beri-beri. Transvenous myocardial biopsy may be helpful. Multiple causes may indicate a number of medical illnesses manifesting in a similar fashion.

    c. Natural history. The onset of this disorder is from the 7th month of pregnancy to 6 months postpartum, most commonly in the 2nd month postpartum. One series showed an 18% mortality rate, with 11% of patients receiving transplants, the majority continuing with cardiac impairment, and only 7% regression of cardiomyopathy.[12]

    d. Prognosis. The prognosis is poor for future pregnancies, with congestive heart failure occurring in 60–80% of patients and maternal mortality rates up to 60%. Prognosis is better if cardiac function normalizes within 6 months. Other types of dilated cardiomyopathies carry a poor prognosis for mother and fetus.

9. Coarctation of the aorta

Coarctation of the aorta may go undiagnosed until pregnancy and may be associated with bicuspid aortic valve, ASD, or congenital cerebral aneurysm. There is increased risk of aortic dissection, stroke, congestive heart failure, or endocarditis. Fetal growth is normal.

    a. Activity is limited with increased bed rest.

    b. SBE prophylaxis is indicated.

    c. Labor management includes avoidance of bearing down and systolic blood pressure elevation.

10. Cyanotic congenital heart disease

Cyanotic congenital heart disease carries an increased risk of congenital heart disease in the fetus, as do other congenital heart lesions.

    a. Poor prognostic indicators include polycythemia with a hematocrit > 60 and oxygen saturation < 80%.

    b. IUGR is increased.

    c. SBE prophylaxis is indicated.

    d. Patients with surgical correction tend to do better, but some have residual valvular defects or postoperative effects that may affect status.

11. Other valvular heart disease

Other valvular defects, such as aortic insufficiency and mitral insufficiency, are generally tolerated better in pregnancy than stenotic lesions. Acquired valvular disease may include women with valvular insufficiency who have taken appetite-suppressant medication. These patients need SBE prophylaxis.

12. Prosthetic valves

Patients with mechanical valves receiving warfarin (Coumadin) for anticoagulation should be switched to heparin before conception. Patients with heterograft prostheses (e.g., porcine) have a much lower risk of embolic phenomena and need not be anticoagulated if asymptomatic. All patients with prosthetic valves require SBE prophylaxis. The subcutaneous dosage of heparin for anticoagulation is 150–250 units/kg every 12 hours.

13. Pulmonary hypertension

Pulmonary hypertension generally carries a poor prognosis with maternal mortality rates of 30% and 56% in primary and secondary pulmonary hypertension, respectively.[11] Neonatal survival in this study ranged from 87–89%. A recent small series demonstrated improved pregnancy performance in patients treated with right pulmonary artery catheterization, intravenous prostacyclin, and oral nifedipine. Women in this small study who normalized right ventricular function were able to successfully complete pregnancies.[3]

II. Arrhythmias
A. Prevention
Use of medications depends on indications as in the nonpregnant state. Elimination of stimulants and avoidance of fatigue may be helpful.
B. Medications and Other Therapies[5,6]
1. Adenosine

Adenosine is safe in pregnancy and is the drug of choice for acute termination of maternal supraventricular tachycardia.

2. Verapamil

Verapamil may be used to treat maternal supraventricular tachycardia and is not teratogenic.

3. Digoxin

Digoxin is not teratogenic and appears to be without fetal toxicity. An increased dose may be needed in pregnancy.

4. Quinidine

Quinidine appears to be non-teratogenic; plasma levels are the same in mother and fetus.

5. Lidocaine

Lidocaine is generally safe in pregnancy; fetal levels are half of maternal levels. Uterine artery constriction has been noted at high levels but not at therapeutic levels. Fetal accumulation may be greater in the presence of fetal acidosis.

6. Procainamide

Procainamide has not been shown to be teratogenic. It should be used as the first-line treatment in undiagnosed wide-complex tachycardia.

7. Flecainide

Flecainide has been shown to be effective in treating fetal supraventricular tachycardia complicated by hydrops.

8. Amiodarone

Amiodarone has been associated with congenital abnormalities; it should be used only after the first trimester for arrhythmias refractory to other medications.

9. Cardioversion

Cardioversion is safe in pregnancy when indicated.

III. Subacute Bacterial Endocarditis Prophylaxis

A. Protocol for SBE Prophylaxis

Aqueous penicillin, 2 million units, or ampicillin 1 g, intravenously or intramuscularly, 30 minutes to 1 hour before procedure; repeat every 8–12 hours for two doses *or* Vancomycin 1 g intravenously for penicillin-allergic patient

plus

Gentamicin 1.5 mg/kg intramuscularly or intravenously; repeat every 8 hours for two doses *or*

Streptomycin 1 g intramuscularly; repeat every 12 hours for two doses

B. Cardiac Conditions Requiring SBE Prophylaxis[1,7,8]

1. Prosthetic valves
2. Valvular disease such as mitral or aortic stenosis
3. Ventricular septal defect (not ASD)
4. Patent ductus arteriosus
5. Idiopathic hypertrophic subaortic stenosis
6. Mitral valve prolapse with murmur suggestive of valvular regurgitation
7. Marfan's syndrome
8. Coarctation of the aorta

References

1. Cardiac Disease in Pregnancy. ACOG Technical Bulletin, No. 168, 1992.
2. Elkayam U, Ostrzega E, Shotan A, et al: Cardiovascular problems in pregnant women with the Marfan's syndrome. Ann Intern Med 123:117–122, 1995.
3. Easterling TR, Ralph DD, Schmucker BC: Pulmonary hypertension in pregnancy: Treatment with pulmonary vasodilators. Obstet Gynecol 93:494–498,1999.
4. Hendricks CH, Brenner WE: Cardiovascular effects of oxytocic drugs used postpartum. Am J Obstet Gynecol 108:751–760, 1970.
5. Joglar JA, Page RL: Treatment of cardiac arrhythmias during pregnancy: Safety considerations. Drug Saf 20:85–94,1999.
6. Lavin JP, Shaub TF: Cardiac drugs during pregnancy. In Rayburn WF, Zuspan FP (eds): Drug Therapy in Obstetrics and Gynecology, 3rd ed. St Louis, Mosby, 1992.
7. McAnulty JH, Metcalfe J, Ueland K: Cardiovascular disease. In Burrow GN, Ferris TF (eds): Medical Complications During Pregnancy, 3rd ed. Philadelphia, W.B. Saunders, 1988.
8. Oakley CM: Cardiovascular disease in pregnancy. Can J Cardiol 6:3B–9B, 1990.
9. Villablanca AC: Heart disease during pregnancy: Which cardiovascular changes reflect disease? Postgrad Med 105:149–156, 1998.
10. Vongpatanasin W, Brickner ME, Hillis LD, et al: The Eisenmenger syndrome in adults. Ann Intern Med 128:745–755, 1998.
11. Weiss BM, Zemp L, Seifert B, et al: Outcome of pulmonary vascular disease in pregnancy: A systematic overview from 1978 through 1996. J Am Coll Cardiol 31:1650–1657, 1998.
12. Witlin AG, Mabie WC, Sibai BM: Peripartum cardiomyopathy: An ominous diagnosis. Am J Obstet Gynecol 176:182–188, 1997.

SECTION C.
CHRONIC HYPERTENSION

Ellen L. Sakornbut, M.D.

Pre-existing hypertension is a common condition affecting women of childbearing age. In some populations, hypertensive conditions are significant contributors to a higher rate of preterm birth.[12] Pregnancy-induced hypertension (PIH) and preeclampsia/eclampsia are addressed in Chapter 6, section B. This section discusses chronic hypertension and the patient who is suspected to be a chronic hypertensive, although pre-pregnancy blood pressure is unknown.

I. Preconception Evaluation

There is a direct correlation between severity of blood pressure and pregnancy complications.

A. Patients with Mild Chronic Hypertension

Patients with mild chronic hypertension (diastolic blood pressure < 100 mm Hg) and normal renal function do not have significantly increased risks for preeclampsia or severe exacerbations of blood pressure during pregnancy.[8]

B. Patients with Moderate Hypertension

Patients with diastolic blood pressure 100–105 mm Hg experience an increased rate of complications.

C. Patients with Severe Hypertension

Patients with diastolic blood pressure consistently > 105 mm Hg or requiring high-dose or multiple antihypertensives for control experience a 20–30% chance of superimposed preeclampsia, increased risk of abruption, and cardiac failure.

D. Renal Insufficiency

A creatinine value > 3.0 or blood urea nitrogen (BUN) value > 30 indicates a much greater risk of maternal or fetal complications.

E. Hypertension Work-up

A preconception or early pregnancy work up of the hypertensive patient may include EKG or echocardiogram, particularly if the patient has been hypertensive for many years or if there are any signs of hypertensive end organ damage. Urinalysis, BUN, and creatinine values are obtained to assess renal function.[8] Other laboratory evaluations in the preconception and early antenatal period depend on the severity of hypertension and the likelihood of secondary causes of hypertension. Some rare causes of hypertension, such as pheochromocytoma, may be exacerbated by pregnancy. Secondary hypertension from renal causes carries a worse prognosis in pregnancy.

F. Medication

If medication is needed to control the diastolic blood pressure > 100 mm Hg before conception, alpha-methyldopa, diuretics, hydralazine, beta-blockers, and calcium channel blockers in therapeutic doses all appear to be without teratogenic effects (see Chapter 6, section B).[15] Although some beta-blockers, such as atenolol, appear to carry a risk for fetal growth restriction if used throughout pregnancy, this is not a teratogenic effect and does not preclude the patient continuing her hypertensive medication prior to conception or during the first trimester (see below). Angiotensin-converting enzyme inhibitors have been associated with limb defects and increased rates of abortion. Reserpine is also associated with fetal defects. Patients desiring pregnancy should be switched from these agents before conception.

II. Antenatal Management

A. Trial Discontinuance of Medication

Many patients with mild hypertension become normotensive by the end of the first trimester. This is of some prognostic value. Patients who remain normotensive with a trial discontinuance of medication should be managed with increased rest and close monitoring of blood pressure, fetal growth, and observation for signs of superimposed preeclampsia.

B. Self Blood Pressure Determination

Patients should be taught self blood pressure determination. They may be better able to modify their own activities based on response of blood pressure.[13]

C. Institution of Antihypertensive Medication

Recommendations vary regarding the diastolic pressure at which antihypertensive medication should be initiated (85–100 mm Hg). Evidence from RCTs demonstrates

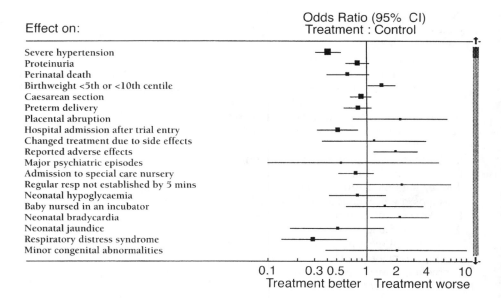

Effect on:

Odds Ratio (95% CI)
Treatment : Control

Severe hypertension
Proteinuria
Perinatal death
Birthweight <5th or <10th centile
Caesarean section
Preterm delivery
Placental abruption
Hospital admission after trial entry
Changed treatment due to side effects
Reported adverse effects
Major psychiatric episodes
Admission to special care nursery
Regular resp not established by 5 mins
Neonatal hypoglycaemia
Baby nursed in an incubator
Neonatal bradycardia
Neonatal jaundice
Respiratory distress syndrome
Minor congenital abnormalities

0.1   0.3 0.5   1   2   4   10

Treatment better   Treatment worse

FIGURE 1. Treatment of mild-to-moderate hypertension: antihypertensive therapy for pregnancy hypertension (23 trials reviewed). (From Collins R, Duley L: Any hypertensive therapy for pregnancy hypertension. In Enkin MW, Keirse MHNC, Renfrew MJ, Neilson JP (eds): Cochrane Database of Systematic Reviews: Review No. 04426. Cochrane Updates on Disk. Oxford, Update Software, 1994, with permission.)

the ability of antihypertensive agents to lower maternal blood pressure.[2] Evidence-based guidelines recommend institution of hypertensive medication for pre-existing hypertension at gestational ages less than 28 weeks with a blood pressure of 140/90 and after 28 weeks for blood pressures of 150/95.[10] Lowering of blood pressure does not prevent such complications as IUGR, preterm delivery, and placental abruption. There is a trend that does not reach statistical significance for treatment with antihypertensive medication to lower the incidence of proteinuria and perinatal mortality (Fig. 1). The following classes of antihypertensive medications are presented with respect to their use in pregnancy.

1. Alpha-methyldopa

Alpha-methyldopa has the longest track record of efficacy and safety in pregnancy. Side effects that may necessitate discontinuance include sedation, fatigue, and Coombs'-positive hemolytic anemia.

2. Beta-blockers

Beta-blockers have been extensively studied in pregnancy, but most studies were small or performed in heterogeneous populations of patients with pregnancy-induced hypertension and chronic hypertension. Propranolol and atenolol (class D) have been associated with intrauterine growth restriction.[5,6,8] Oxprenolol, pindolol, metoprolol, and acebutolol have not. These studies are difficult to interpret because of methodologic differences. Besides possible effects on fetal growth, fetal bradycardia may be encountered with normal reactivity. Neonatal effects observed include hypoglycemia and respiratory depression. For these reasons, beta-blockers should probably be considered as second-line drugs, with alpha-methyldopa as a first-line agent.[6,8] Labetalol is an agent that may have a salutary effect on renal function.[3]

3. Diuretics

Because diminished extravascular volume has been implicated in some of the hemodynamic changes of preeclampsia, many authors have argued against use of diuretics as antihypertensives in pregnancy. Diuretics cause multiple metabolic abnormalities and have no place as first-line therapy but may have an ancillary role in some patients, usually those with cardiac disease. They should not be used if there is concern about reduced uteroplacental flow.

4. Vasodilators

Vasodilators, such as hydralazine, have been used effectively for acute management of hypertension in the intrapartum setting. Their long-term use is limited because of reflex tachycardia and tachyphylaxis. In combination with labetalol, these agents have been used effectively for severe hypertension. Prazosin has been used but much less extensively.

5. Calcium channel blockers

Calcium channel blockers have not been used as extensively as other agents for treatment of hypertension but have been used in treatment of preterm labor. Nifedipine, nicardipine, and verapamil have been studied with respect to effects on uterine blood flow. No reduction in uterine blood flow has been noted by Doppler examination in patients with pregnancy-induced hypertension and chronic hypertension.[1] A prospective, multi-site study of calcium-channel blockers in human pregnancy found no increased risk of teratogenicity and lower birth weights of infants in the study group attributable to maternal disease.[7] When used in conjunction with magnesium sulfate, calcium channel blockers may cause significant hypotension and neuromuscular blockade as a result of interference with contraction-excitation coupling.[14]

6. Angiotensin-converting enzyme inhibitors

Besides previously mentioned fetal limb defects, reduction of uterine blood flow has been noted in animal models, and fatal neonatal renal failure has been reported.[11] There is consensus that these agents should not be used in pregnancy.

D. Fetal Growth

Establishment of accurate ultrasound dating before 20 weeks' gestation can be carried out as a baseline measurement. This may be followed by repeat scans at the end of the second trimester and between 32 and 34 weeks if inadequate fetal growth is suspected (see Chapter 6, section F, regarding asymmetric growth restriction).[13]

E. Fetal Well-Being Assessment

Antenatal assessment of fetal well-being is begun at 34–36 weeks' gestation (see Chapter 10, section B).[13]

F. Serum Uric Acid Determinations and Monitoring of Renal Function

Serum uric acid determinations and monitoring of renal function may be helpful in detecting the onset of superimposed preeclampsia when performed in the early third trimester.[8]

G. Low-Dose Aspirin

At this time, there is insufficient evidence to support the use of low-dose aspirin for preeclampsia prevention (see Chapter 6, section B).

H. Intrapartum Management (see Chapter 15, section G).

References

1. Carbonne B, Jannet D, Touboul C, et al: Nicardipine treatment of hypertension during pregnancy. Obstet Gynecol 81:908–914, 1993.
2. Collins R, Duley L: Any hypertensive therapy for pregnancy hypertension. In Enkin MW, Keirse MHNC, Renfrew MJ, Neilson JP (eds): Pregnancy and Childbirth Module. Cochrane Database of Systematic Reviews, Review No. 04426. Cochrane Updates on Disk. Oxford, Update Software, 1994.

3. el-Qarmalawi AM, Morsy AH, al-Fadly A, et al: Labetalol vs. methyldopa in treatment of pregnancy-induced hypertension. Int J Gynaecol Obstet 49:125–130, 1995.
4. Imperiale TF, Petrullis AS: A meta-analysis of low-dose aspirin for the prevention of pregnancy-induced hypertensive disease. JAMA 266:260–264, 1991.
5. Lip GY, Beevers M, Churchill D: Effect of atenolol on birth weight. Am J Cardiol 79:1436–1438, 1997.
6. Lowe SA, Rubin PC: The pharmacologic management of hypertension in pregnancy. J Hypertens 10:201–207, 1992.
7. Magee LA, Schick B, Donnefeld AE, et al: The safety of calcium channel blockers in human pregnancy: A prospective, multicenter cohort. Am J Obstet Gynecol 174:823–828, 1996.
8. National High Blood Pressure Education Program Working Group: Report on high blood pressure in pregnancy. Am J Obstet Gynecol 163:1691–1712, 1990.
9. Oakley CM: Cardiovascular disease in pregnancy. Can J Cardiol 6:3B–9B, 1990.
10. Rey E, LeLorier J, Burgess E, et al: Report of the Canadian Hypertension Society Consensus Conference: Pharmacologic treatment of hypertensive disorders in pregnancy. CMAJ 157:1245–1254, 1997.
11. Rosa FW, Bosco LA, Graham CF, et al: Neonatal anuria with maternal angiotensin-converting enzyme inhibitor. Obstet Gynecol 74:371–374, 1989.
12. Samidi AR, Mayberry RM: Maternal hypertension and spontaneous preterm birth among black women. Obstet Gynecol 91:899–904, 1998.
13. Sibai BM: Diagnosis and management of chronic hypertension in pregnancy. Obstet Gynecol 78:451–461, 1991.
14. Snyder SN, Cardwell MS: Neuromuscular blockade with magnesium sulfate and nifedipine. Am J Obstet Gynecol 161:35–36, 1989.
15. Zuspan FP, Zuspan KJ: Antihypertensive therapy during pregnancy. In Rayburn WF, Zuspan FP (eds): Drug Therapy in Obstetrics and Gynecology, 3rd ed. St Louis, Mosby, 1992.

SECTION D.
THROMBOEMBOLIC DISEASE AND CHRONIC ANTICOAGULATION

Donald Marquardt, M.D., Ph.D.

I. Preconception
A. Chronically Anticoagulated Women
Women who receive chronic anticoagulation must be switched from warfarin (Coumadin) prior to conception due to its multiple teratogenic effects.

    1. Embryopathy
First-trimester fetal exposure to warfarin may result in nasal hypoplasia and skeletal abnormalities.

    2. CNS abnormalities
Multiple central nervous system abnormalities, including optic atrophy, may result during any trimester.

B. Anticoagulant of Choice
Subcutaneous heparin is the current drug of choice for anticoagulation in preconception and pregnancy, although benefits should be weighed against risks. It is administered every 12 hours in a dose (usually 150–250 units/kg from a 25,000 units/ml solution) that maintains the mid-interval activated partial thromboplastin time (PTT) at 1.5 to 2 times baseline. Injection sites on the inner and outer thighs and lower abdomen should be rotated and must be compressed for 5 minutes postinjection to minimize local bruising.

C. Low-Molecular-Weight Heparanoids
The newer low-molecular-weight heparin-like compounds are not currently approved for use in either treatment or prophylaxis of deep venous thrombosis (DVT) during pregnancy. Since they do not cross the placenta and, in nonpregnant situations, appear to have benefits in ease of usage and (no necessary) monitoring, there is interest and

some experimental use. However, the inability to monitor or reverse its action and the prolonged duration of action make it more difficult to discontinue expediently, thus increasing the risks of many pre- and intrapartum situations/procedures.

D. History of Thrombophilic Disease

Careful evaluation of a woman's personal and family history of thromboembolic disease, and possible screening for inherited thrombophilic diseases should be considered. This is particularly important in women with previous untoward obstetric outcomes such as severe preeclampsia, abruptio placentae, fetal growth retardation, or stillbirth.[5]

II. Antenatal Management

A. Women with Previous Thromboembolic Events

Depending whether the previous thromboembolic event was associated with pregnancy, women should be treated in either of two ways.

1. Events associated with pregnancy

Women with previous events associated with pregnancy should receive "minidose heparin," antepartum, intrapartum, and continued until 6 weeks postpartum. Minidose heparin is usually empirically given as 5000 units subcutaneously every 12 hours and, once verified that the current dose is not generating full therapeutic anticoagulation, does not require monitoring as needed for therapeutic use of heparin described above.

2. Events not associated with pregnancy

Women with previous events not associated with pregnancy and considered at low risk for recurrent disease, may receive intrapartum and 1 week postpartum minidose heparin. High-risk patients, such as those with active DVT, should receive treatment as for thromboembolic events associated with pregnancy.

B. Diagnosis of DVT

The diagnosis of DVT during pregnancy is generally similar to the diagnosis in the nonpregnant patient except for the confounding factor that pregnant women may experience unilateral or bilateral leg swelling from iliac vein compression that may mimic DVT, especially after 20 weeks.[1,4,9]

1. Venous Doppler

Doppler ultrasound, by looking at flow, augmentation, and effects of compression, is sensitive as a diagnostic tool in proximal vein thrombosis but less sensitive in calf thrombosis (treatment of which, in the absence of thigh disease, is controversial). False-positive results can also occur in late pregnancy with compression of the iliac veins by the gravid uterus. The sensitivity and specificity are 96% and 99% prior to 20 weeks.[7]

2. Magnetic resonance imaging (MRI)

MRI venography has demonstrated the ability to diagnose pelvic extension of thrombus as well as isolated pelvic thrombosis, generally distinguishing between thrombus and pelvic vein compression by the gravid uterus.[8] In the diagnosis of extremity thrombosis, MRI has a sensitivity of 90% and a specificity of 100%.[2] With no ionizing radiation, the electromagnetic fields of MRI have not shown any risk to the fetus.

3. Venography

Limited venography for calf vessel disease can be performed (with lead shielding of the fetus) visualizing the deep calf veins, popliteal vein, and distal three quarters of the superficial femoral vein. Full visualization of the pelvic system by conventional venography requires simultaneous injection of both feet. Venography should be restricted to those patients with abnormal or inconclusive noninvasive testing, or in whom it is crucial to determine patency of the calf vessels. Risks include systemic reactions, contrast extravasation/tissue necrosis, induction of venous thrombosis, and the risk of radiation in the third trimester (plain films and attendant fetal irradiation are estimated to increase the risk of childhood cancer by 2.4 times[3]).

4. Radioisotope studies

Due to radiation exposure, radioisotopes should be avoided during pregnancy or breastfeeding if possible. However, with pulmonary embolism among the major causes of maternal death, ventilation-perfusion scintigraphy (V/Q scan) may be necessary if less invasive testing cannot establish the diagnosis before embarking on a potentially dangerous course of therapy.

C. Antepartum Therapy

1. DVT occurring in the antepartum period

This should include short-term IV heparin as well as prolonged prophylaxis against recurrent disease for the duration of that pregnancy and through the first 6 weeks postpartum. See section I.B. above for dosage regimen.

2. Presumptive treatment

If the above procedures are unavailable or inconclusive, presumptive treatment based on clinical findings may be a viable option.

D. Intrapartum and Emergency Management of DVT

The management of intrapartum and emergent DVT is discussed in Chapter 15, section H.

E. Intravenous Heparin during Labor

Intravenous heparin should be stopped at the onset of labor and can be restarted within 2 hours post-delivery unless factors, such as surgery, lacerations, or thrombocytopenia lead to excessive blood loss. The IV heparin is continued for several days while the patient is switched to subcutaneous heparin or oral anticoagulants. Anticoagulation should be continued at least 1 month postpartum because heightened risk of venous thrombosis in this period.

F. Reversal of Effects of Heparin

Intended therapeutic or unintended supratherapeutic effects of heparin may be reversed in an emergency by protamine sulfate (pregnancy category C) at a dose of 1 mg to neutralize approximately 100 units of heparin, administered IV in doses of less than 50 mg over a 10 minute course. More rapid injection increases risk of dyspnea, flushing, bradycardia, and hypotension; hypersensitivity reactions are more common in patients allergic to fish (especially the family Salmonidae from which protamine is isolated).

G. Breastfeeding and Anticoagulants

Breastfeeding is not a contraindication to either the use of heparin or warfarin.[6]

References

1. Berquist A, Berquist D, Hallbrook T: Deep vein thrombosis during pregnancy: A prospective study. Acta Obstet Gynaecol Scand 62:443–448, 1983.
2. Erdman WA, Jayson HT: Deep venous thrombosis of extremities: Role of MR imaging in the diagnosis. Radiology 174:425–431, 1990.
3. Harvey EB, Boice JD, Honeyman M, et al: Prenatal x-ray exposure and childhood cancer in twins. N Engl J Med 312:541–545, 1985.
4. Kierkegaard A: Incidence and diagnosis of deep vein thrombosis associated with pregnancy. Acta Obstet Gynaecol Scand 62:239–243, 1983.
5. Kupperminic M, Eldor A, Steinman N: Increased frequency of genetic thrombophilia in women with complications of pregnancy. N Engl J Med 340:9–13, 1999.
6. McKenna R, Cole ER, Vasan V: Is warfarin sodium contraindicated in the lactating mother? J Pediatr 103:325–327, 1983.
7. Polak JF, Wilkinson DL: Ultrasonic diagnosis of symptomatic deep venous thrombosis in pregnancy. Am J Obstet Gynecol 165:625–629, 1991.

8. Spritzer C, Evans A, Kay H: Magnetic resonance imaging of deep venous thrombosis in pregnant women with lower extremity edema. Obstet Gynecol 85:603–607, 1995.
9. Villasanta U: Thromboembolic disease in pregnancy. Am J Obstet Gynecol 93:142–160, 1965.

SECTION E.
HEMATOLOGIC CONDITIONS

Donald Marquardt, M.D., Ph.D.

I. Anemia
Anemia during pregnancy is defined by the Centers for Disease Control and Prevention as a hemoglobin < 11 g/dl, in first and third trimesters, or < 10.5 g/dl in the second trimester.

A. Iron Deficiency Anemia
The most common cause of anemia in pregnancy is iron deficiency, but controversy exists as to whether or not it represents a significant problem warranting routine iron therapy (see Chapters 3 and 4, section A). Cochrane Reviews indicate improved hematologic indices in pregnant women routinely receiving iron, but "no detectable effect on any substantive measures of either maternal or fetal outcome" with routine iron supplementation.[8]

1. Severe anemia
Anemia with < 6 g/dl of hemoglobin is considered severe and can be associated with high-output congestive heart failure during pregnancy as well as increased intrapartum complications with excessive blood loss. Severe anemia must be treated.

2. Effect on infants
Infants born to severely iron-deficient women are not usually anemic, but do have lower iron stores and may be more likely to develop iron deficiency during infancy.

3. Effect on premature birth
Previously derived associations of anemia and premature birth are probably spurious, caused by a normal rise in hemoglobin between 28 and 40 weeks.[3]

4. Empiric treatment
Most patients with iron deficiency anemia can be empirically treated based on a typical presentation with anemia, hypochromia, and microcytosis. If there is a doubt as to the diagnosis or failure to respond, serum ferritin levels are more accurate than either serum iron (which falls during pregnancy) or total iron-binding capacity (which rises during pregnancy).

5. Therapy
Oral iron preparations, in full therapeutic doses, are most commonly employed if anemia is shown to exist. Generous fiber and fluid recommendations, as well as careful timing of doses, may minimize the gastric distress and constipation frequently associated with oral iron replacement. The usual elemental iron therapeutic daily dose is approximately 200 mg (2–3 mg elemental iron/kg) and may be provided by several common preparations:

   a. Ferrous sulfate, 300 mg (containing 60 mg elemental iron) taken 3–4 times daily.
   b. Ferrous gluconate, 320 mg (containing 39 mg elemental iron) taken 4–5 times daily.
   c. Ferrous fumarate, 200 mg (containing 66 mg elemental iron) taken 3–4 times daily. Absorption is from the proximal gut, so enteric-coated preparations may be better tolerated but are definitely less effective. Similarly,

absorption is decreased by 50–60% in the non-fasting state, so the most effective dosing would be while fasting. Different iron formulations and gradually increasing the doses may assist women who poorly tolerate their initial iron preparation.

  d. Parenteral iron. Although bypassing the gut may improve compliance, parenteral iron does not increase the patient's hematologic response and has specific risks. Given intramuscularly, it is painful, can stain the skin, and has the risk of potential malignant degeneration at the site. Intravascular dosing avoids local reaction, but not infrequently results in headache, lymphadenopathy, fever, arthralgias, and urticaria, not to mention the risk of fatal anaphylactic reaction. Providers using parenteral iron should familiarize themselves with the drug's complete profile and have specific indications therefor.

B. Megaloblastic Anemia

Several deficiencies/processes may cause a megaloblastic anemia.

  1. Vitamin B_{12} deficiency

Primary inability to absorb vitamin B_{12} is extremely rare in pregnancy. B_{12} deficiency is more likely related to ethanol abuse, gastric or ileal resection, or inflammatory bowel disease. Patients with a severe deficiency are usually sterile.

  2. Folate deficiency

Folic acid deficiency is the most common cause of megaloblastic anemia in pregnancy. This deficiency is usually due to increasing folate requirements from 0.1 mg/day baseline to 0.4 mg/day in pregnancy. Note that folate absorption is decreased for patients on many drugs, notably phenytoin. The Cochrane Review clearly demonstrates that hemoglobin and folate levels are improved in pregnant women routinely supplemented with folate, but insufficient evidence exists to show either benefit or harm to the mother or fetus in studies to date.[7] Folate supplementation recommendations for pregnancy differ from recommendations prior to pregnancy. Relative folate deficiency prior to conception is linked to congenital malformations, especially neural tube defects. For pre-conception prevention, the World Health Organization recommends 0.5 mg/day supplemental folate, and therapeutic doses at 1 mg/day or more depending on special needs, such as poor absorption or high turnover of cells (sickle cell disease).

  3. Iron deficiency and folate deficiency

With its characteristic microcytosis, iron deficiency coexisting with folate deficiency may mask the macrocytosis. Serum folate falls naturally during pregnancy. Red cell folate is more reflective of tissue levels, but abnormal and normal values can overlap.

C. Hemoglobinopathies

Abnormal hemoglobin biosynthesis is responsible for a diverse group of inherited diseases. Several of the more common/morbid include:

  1. Sickle hemoglobin[9,10]

Hbg-S can present as either the homozygous [Hbg-S—Hbg-S] disease, the heterozygous (Hbg-S—Hbg-A) trait, or in combination with other altered hemoglobins (the most concerning being Hbg-S—Hbg-C and Hbg-S—Hbg-Ǝ-thalasemia). Sickle cell disease occurs in 0.2% of the African-American population, with sickle cell trait occurring in 6–13%. Patients with sickle cell anemia demonstrate reduced fertility, a 20% spontaneous abortion rate, a 1% stillborn rate, and a maternal mortality rate of approximately 2%. Maternal risks include congestive heart failure, pulmonary infarction, preeclampsia/eclampsia, and infection. Risks to the surviving fetus include placental infarction, growth retardation, and prematurity. Overall fetal survival is only 70%.

    a. Sickle cell trait. Patients with the trait may demonstrate a renal concentrating defect and hematuria owing to sickling in the renal medulla. They have an increased risk of bacteriuria and urinary tract infections, but overall prognosis in pregnancy is good. These patients should receive genetic counseling.

    b. Sickle cell disease.[9] Patients with the homozygous disease usually benefit from referral, due to increased risk to both mother and fetus. Treatment for crises is exchange transfusion, and prophylactic transfusions are advocated by some, but each transfusion increase risks of red cell alloantibodies as well as blood-borne diseases.[4,5]

2. Alpha-thalassemias and beta-thalassemias5

Both thalassemias present in multiple genotypes and phenotypes with very different prognoses.

    a. Alpha-thalassemia. There are four forms, presenting with three different outcomes.

        i. Bart hemoglobin. All four alpha chains are missing [–,–], which results in hydrops fetalis and fetal or neonatal death.

        ii. Hemoglobin H. Three alpha chains are missing [–,-alpha], usually presenting with hemoglobin levels that are 7–10 g/dl. The prognosis for pregnancy outcome is usually good.

        iii. Alpha-thalassemia minor and carrier state. Both alpha-thalassemia minor [-α,-α] and the (silent) alpha-thalassemia carrier state [-α, $\alpha\alpha$] bear no clinical significance for pregnancy outcome. Depending on the father's hemoglobin genotype, genetic counseling may be in order.

    b. Beta-thalassemia. Since there are over 100 different mutations of variable morbidity, these present a wide spectrum of diseases. Recognizing that there are many forms with intermediate morbidity, the beta-thalassemias are broadly grouped into two forms.

        i. Beta-thalassemia major. This homozygous form is rarely seen in pregnancy because patients tend to die in childhood of severe anemia and failure to thrive; survivors have reduced fertility.

        ii. Beta-thalassemia minor. In the heterozygous form of the disease, there is rarely any effect on pregnancy outcome unless heterozygous with another hemoglobinopathy, e.g., Hbg-S. It may manifest as a hypochromic, microcytic anemia, usually with a hemoglobin in the range of 9–10 mg/dl, but frequently may be distinguished from iron deficiency anemia by a relatively normal red cell count (approximately 5×10^6 RBC/ml vs. reduced red cell count in iron deficiency of 3×10^6 RBC/ml). Ferritin levels may assist in the diagnosis; however beta-thalassemia patients may also be iron-deficient. Hemoglobin electrophoresis is definitive. Beta-thalassemia patients should not receive iron unless proved iron-deficient because of the risk of iron overload.

II. Bleeding Disorders[5]
A. Thrombocytopenia

A myriad of problems in pregnancy may present with an abnormally low platelet count.[1]

1. Underproduction

Folate deficiency may lead to underproduction of platelets, but it is rare as an isolated abnormality.

2. Severe preeclampsia[4]

Consumptive thrombocytopenia may be seen in 15% of preeclamptic patients and higher in eclampsia. Platelet-released thromboxane A may contribute to vasospastic changes. The bleeding time may be disproportionately prolonged because of an acquired platelet function defect, and 25% have abnormal bleeding times with platelet counts between 50,000 and 100,000/mm^3.

3. Septicemia

Thrombocytopenia, possibly resulting from an immune mechanism, may be found in septicemia (not always associated with disseminated intravascular coagulation).

4. Drug-induced thrombocytopenia

This may occur with quinine, quinidine, heparin, and many antibiotics.

5. Idiopathic thrombocytopenic purpura

Idiopathic thrombocytopenic purpura (ITP) is seen most frequently in women of reproductive age.[5]

   a. Maternal risk. The possibility of increased bleeding exists at delivery, usually with platelet counts < 20,000 to 30,000/mm^3. Most patients do not reach these levels.
   b. Fetal risks. There is a 5% incidence of intrauterine demise and 10% of surviving fetuses have serious defects in hemostasis. Fifty percent have abnormal platelet counts, the nadir of which is usually 1 week post-delivery with recovery about 2 weeks later.
   c. Prognosis. Thrombocytopenia in early pregnancy is worse, since platelet counts usually drop during pregnancy.
   d. Management.[4] Based on platelet count and bleeding complications, treatment may be initiated with corticosteroids. Generally, these patients benefit from tertiary center referral.
   e. Intracranial hemorrhage. The risk of fetal thrombocytopenia and intracranial hemorrhage is not predictable by monitoring maternal platelet count. One management strategy is to obtain a fetal scalp platelet count in early labor, proceding with vaginal delivery only if the platelet count is > 50,000/mm^3.
   f. Mild thrombocytopenia. If maternal platelet count remains in the range of 100,000 to 150,000/mm^3 in the peripartum period, postpartum care is handled in a routine fashion except for obtaining a platelet count on the newborn.

B. Common Coagulopathies[5]

Abnormalities in the blood clotting factors VIII and IX have variable clinical courses.

1. Hemophilias A and B

Defined as deficiencies of factor VIII and factor IX, respectively, the hemophilias are X-linked disorders and do not affect heterozygous women. It is rare to see a woman (homozygous) with hemophilia in pregnancy; she would benefit from tertiary care referral. The primary physician is more likely to see the potentially devastating effects on male offspring (100% from homozygous women, 50% from heterozygotes). Genetic counseling in affected families is best accomplished during a preconceptual evaluation (see Chapter 1, section A).

2. von Willebrand's disease

As a heterogenous mix of factor VIII-platelet complex deficiencies, it is characterized by a prolonged bleeding time, is not X-linked and usually autosomal dominant, and thus more commonly affects women. Affected patients have easy bruising, frequent nose/mucosal bleeds, and have excessive bleeding with trauma/surgery. Bleeding times are frequently prolonged, PTT increased, and specific factor VIII assays abnormal. Unless severe, there is little risk of significant bleeding. If severe bleeding occurs, fresh frozen plasma is the preferred treatment (cryoprecipitate is less commonly used because of the pooled blood product risk).

C. Thrombophilic Disorders

Both hereditary and acquired processes promoting pathologic coagulation are increasingly associated with severe ante-, intra-, and postpartum consequences for both maternal and fetal units. The number of identified defects is increasing yearly in the literature. Several occur in the general population several times more frequently than the better known coagulopathies. Some of these diseases and apparent complications are listed below, some with known/defined gene mutations.[4]

1. Disorders associated with known gene mutations
   a. Factor V Leiden. A mutation of adenine to guanine at nucleotide 506 in factor V gene, this mutation renders factor Va resistant to proteolysis by active protein C and doubles the risk of recurrent thrombophlebitis.[9] Factor V Leiden is seemingly responsible for trebling the risk of women to experience severe preeclampsia, abruptio placentae, and stillbirth.[6] This mutation may also be responsible for an increased risk of thromboembolic disease in the neonate.[10]
   b. Two other single gene mutations. Cytosine to thymine at nucleotide 677 in methylenetetrahydrofolate reductase gene, which leads to an increase in plasma homocysteine, and guanine to adenine at nucleotide 20210 in prothrombin gene, which leads to increased concentrations of prothrombin, have been implicated in obstetric complications. The former appears to treble the risks of the group of severe complications. The latter is significantly more common in women experiencing abruptio placentae and fetal growth retardation without apparently affecting the risk of preeclampsia.[4] Studies into the clinical manifestations of individuals heterozygous with more than one mutation clearly delineate an even greater risk of recurrent DVT.[11]
2. Disorders unrelated or less clearly related to genetic mutations
   a. Protein deficiencies in the coagulation cascade. Protein C deficiency, antithrombin III deficiency, and protein S deficiency are other inherited disorders that appear to increase the risk of severe obstetrical complications.[4]
   b. Antiphospholipid antibodies. These specific antibodies, including lupus anticoagulant and anticardiolipin, are associated with arterial and venous thromboses increasing fetal death rates and perhaps other complications.
3. Diseases worsened by thrombophilic disorders
   a. Negative history of thromboembolic disease. One or more of the above mentioned three thrombophilic mutations was present in 52% of women with severe complications of pregnancy and only 17% of matched controls. These numbers approached 65% of women with severe pregnancy complications compared to 18% of matched controls when the other thrombophilic conditions were included.[4] These mutations predispose the maternal-fetal unit to multiple pregnancy complications by microvascular thrombosis, from preeclampsia to incremental infarction of the placenta and resultant growth retardation, abruptio, and stillbirth.
   b. Deep venous thrombosis. The relative risk of DVT is approximately 9.0 (95% CI 4.7–17.4) or 10.8 (95% CI 2.9–40.3) for Factor V Leiden and the G20210 prothrombin mutation, respectively, in individuals heterozygous for both Factor V Leiden and the G20210. A prothrombin mutation has a relative risk calculated at 69 and 152 (confidence intervals not calculable) for pregnant women with initial or recurrent thromboembolic disease, respectively.[12]
   c. Neonatal complications. The complications are more rare in the neonate, but these same genetic abnormalities may increase the risk of thrombotic complications to the newborn.[10]

4. Screening for thrombophilia

Gene mutations may be screened by blood tests available through reference laboratories as either single tests (if family history suggests a specific disease) or screening panels. Screening should be done prior to or early in pregnancy to prepare for possible complications, especially when there is a family history of thromboembolic disease or maternal history of previous severe obstetric complications. Although prophylaxis of these increased risks of complications is speculative, prior knowledge and consideration, with effective patient education of potential problems, may be conducive to proactive management and may decrease morbidity. Clearly further studies are needed to determine what, if any, obstetric implications exist for other mixed heterozygous states. More information on the natural history of these diseases will provide for more rational and effective screening and treatment strategies.

References

1. DeStefano V, Martinelli I, Mannucci PM: The risk of recurrent deep venous thrombosis among heterozygous carriers of both Factor V Leiden and the G20210A prothrombin mutation. N Engl J Med 341:801–806,1999.
2. Gerhardt A, Scharf RE: Prothrombin and Factor V mutations in women with a history of thrombosis during pregnancy and the puerperium. N Engl J Med 342:374–380, 2000.
3. Klebanoff MA, Shiono PH, Berendes HW, et al: Facts and artifacts about anemia and preterm delivery. JAMA 262:511–515, 1989.
4. Kupperminc M, Eldor A, Steinman N: Increased frequency of genetic thrombophilia in women with complications of pregnancy. N Engl J Med 340:9–13, 1999.
5. Larus RK: Maternal hematologic disorders. In Creasy RK, Resnik R (eds): Maternal Fetal Medicine: Principles and Practice, 3rd ed. Philadelphia, W.B. Saunders, 1994, pp 923–925.
6. Lieberman E, Ryan KJ, Monson RR, et al: Association of maternal hematocrit with premature labor. Obstet Gynecol 159:107–114, 1988.
7. Mahomed K: Iron and folate supplementation in pregnancy (Cochrane Review). In The Cochrane Library, Issue 4, 2000, Oxford, Update Software.
8. Mahomed K: Folate supplementation in pregnancy (Cochrane Review). In The Cochrane Library, Issue 4, 2000, Oxford, Update Software.
9. Miller JM, Horger EO, Key TC, et al: Management of sickle hemoglobinopathies in pregnant patients. Am J Obstet Gynecol 141:237–241, 1981.
10. Morrison JC, Blake PG, Reed CD: Therapy for the pregnant patient with sickle hemoglobinopathies: A national focus. Am J Obstet Gynecol 144:268–269, 1982.
11. Newman R, Spear G, Kirshbaum N: Postmortem DNA diagnosis of Factor V Leiden in a neonate with systemic thrombosis and probable antithrombin deficiency. Obstet Gynecol 92:702–705, 1998.
12. Simioni P, Prandoni P, Lensing A: The risk of recurrent venous thromboembolism in patients with an Arg^{506} →Gln mutation in the gene for Factor V (Factor V Leiden). N Engl J Med 336:399–403, 1997.

SECTION F.
GASTROINTESTINAL CONDITIONS

Ellen L. Sakornbut, M.D.

I. Inflammatory Bowel Disease
A. Ulcerative Colitis

1. Impact on perinatal outcomes

There are no increases in abortion, stillbirth, or fetal abnormalities in quiescent disease. Fertility remains normal.

2. The risk of exacerbation

This is cited as between 20–35% and 50% (the yearly risk in nonpregnant patients) and relapse rate decreases in both ulcerative colitis and Crohn's disease postpartum.[1] The risk is decreased if the disease is quiescent at conception. The most serious prognosis occurs with new onset of disease occurring during pregnancy.[4]

3. Genetic link
There is increased risk of familial transmission.
4. Pharmacologic treatment[3]
   a. Sulfasalazine. This drug is safe during pregnancy. Discontinuing briefly when the patient is close to delivery may be advisable because of binding to fetal albumin with resultant hyperbilirubinemia. It should be started immediately postpartum to avoid relapse and is safe for breastfeeding.
   b. Mesalazine. The dose should be limited to 2 g/d.
   c. Prednisone. This drug is discussed previously in other sections of this chapter. Prednisone is relatively safe for use in pregnancy.

B. Crohn's Disease
1. Impact on perinatal outcomes
Reduced fertility is noted, but no increases in abortion, fetal abnormality, or stillbirths occur when disease is quiescent. If Crohn's disease is active at conception, the spontaneous abortion rate is increased.[5] Onset of Crohn's disease during pregnancy is associated with increased fetal risk. Most patients experience improvement during pregnancy.
2. Crohn's-associated complications
Patients with a previous ileostomy may deliver vaginally. A history of previous surgery for Crohn's disease is associated with a higher spontaneous abortion rate.[2]
3. Treatment
Sulfasalazine and steroids, as discussed previously, are safe medications.
4. Genetic link
There is an increased risk of familial transmission.

II. Peptic Ulcer Disease
Peptic ulcer disease is not increased in pregnancy. Most patients with dyspepsia have gastroesophageal reflux (see Chapter 3, section E). Medications that can be safely used include sucralfate, antacids, H_2-blockers and proton pump inhibitors.

References
1. Castiglione F, Pignata S, Morace F, et al: Effect of pregnancy on the clinical course of a cohort of women with inflammatory bowel disease. Ital J Gastroenterol 28:199–204, 1996.
2. Hudson M, Flett G, Sinclair TS, et al: Fertility and pregnancy in inflammatory bowel disease. Int J Obstet Gynecol 58:229–237, 1997.
3. Modigliani R: Drug therapy for ulcerative colitis in pregnancy. Eur J Gastroenterol Hepatol 9:854–857, 1997.
4. Nielsen OH, Andreasson B, Bondesen S, et al: Pregnancy in ulcerative colitis. Scand J Gastroenterol 18:735–742, 1983.
5. Nielsen OH, Andreasson B, Bondesen S, et al: Pregnancy in Crohn's disease. Scand J Gastroenterol 19:724–732, 1984.

SECTION G.
NEUROLOGIC CONDITIONS

Ellen L. Sakornbut, M.D.

I. Seizure Disorders
A. Clinical Background
Seizure disorders occur in 0.3–0.6% of pregnancies. Approximately 1 million women of childbearing age in the United States have epilepsy. The cause of seizures, whether epileptic or of other etiologies, may be of prognostic importance in pregnancy.

1. Genetic links

Epilepsy is transmitted genetically. The risk of congenital defects is increased 2.4-fold, independent of medication.

2. Arteriovenous malformations

There is an increased risk of arteriovenous malformation hemorrhage or enlargement during pregnancy.

3. Post-traumatic seizures

If the seizure disorder is post-traumatic in origin, the risk for malformation is increased only because of teratogenic effects of medication.

4. Tuberous sclerosis

If the patient has tuberous sclerosis, genetic counseling is indicated.

B. Preconception Assessment and Planning

Antiepileptic medication may decrease ovulatory function and fertility. However, enzyme-inducing antiepileptic drugs may decrease the effectiveness of oral contraceptives. A higher-dose oral contraceptive or another method may be indicated in these patients. Newer antiepileptic medications such as felbamate, gabapentin, lamotrigine, tiagabine, and vigabatrin do not interfere with hormonal contraception.[14] Women desiring pregnancy should be supplemented with folic acid and treated, if at all possible, with monotherapy to reduce the risk of major congenital anomalies.

Preconception assessment includes consideration of the frequency of seizures and number of medications needed for control with a reduction in number of medications or trial off medications in selected patients.[2] While biologic evidence exists for a number of recommendations about medications and other preventive measures, there is limited RCT evidence to guide decisions in many situations.[31]

C. Effects of Pregnancy on Seizures

Recent studies show that about 20% of patients with epilepsy have worsening of seizures during pregnancy.[22,27] Patients with rare seizures are less likely to deteriorate; patients with seizures occurring at least monthly almost always experience increased seizures. These effects are usually temporary and revert after delivery.

1. Physiologic changes of pregnancy

These changes, such as increased minute ventilation, hyponatremia, hypocalcemia, and expanded extracellular volume, may precipitate seizures. Fatigue and emotional stress may make patients more prone to seizures.

2. Anticonvulsant levels

These levels may fluctuate as a result of changes in extravascular fluid, nausea and vomiting, metabolism, or with noncompliance because of patient anxiety about the medication.

D. New-Onset Seizures

Patients who have new-onset seizures during pregnancy (and who are determined not to be eclamptic) or who have seizures which only occur in pregnancy, should be worked up for vascular malformations, such as a cavernous angioma[3] and intracranial hemorrhage.[6] Diagnostic testing should include computed tomography or magnetic resonance imaging if CT is negative.

E. Effects of Seizures on Pregnancy

1. Fetal loss

Spontaneous abortion appears to be increased.[25]

2. Increased incidence of fetal anomalies

Large population-based studies and drug surveillance studies have found that major congenital anomalies are increased about 3 times that of the general population,[10,18] although some studies show more facial dysmorphism and minor abnormalities.[9,16] The risk of major anomalies is substantially increased with combinations of medications.[24]

3. Increased perinatal mortality

Perinatal mortality is two times that of the general population in some studies,[13] mainly because of increased congenital malformations and neonatal hemorrhages.

4. Maternal folate absorption

Anticonvulsants may decrease maternal folate absorption.

5. Impact of seizures on fetal health

Fetal acidosis, hypoxia, and fetal heart rate abnormalities may accompany seizures. Seizures, especially status epilepticus, may result in fetal death, presumably as a result of altered uteroplacental circulation and hypoxia.

F. Medications

1. Phenytoin

Phenytoin is indicated in generalized tonic-clonic seizures.

  a. Dosage. The dosage of phenytoin generally increases in pregnancy.[5] Levels should be checked throughout pregnancy.

  b. Fetal and maternal levels are identical. Neonatal depression or withdrawal does not occur.

  c. Teratogenesis occurs in 7–10% of fetuses. Phenytoin embryopathy features include:[5]

    i. fetal growth restriction and postnatal growth problems

    ii. mild motor and development delays

    iii. facial dysmorphism with hypertelorism

    iv. frontal bossing

    v. a long upper lip and midfacial hypoplasia

    vi. nail hypoplasia

    vii. hirsutism

    viii. other major congenital anomalies such as congenital heart disease, microcephaly, diaphragmatic hernias, cleft lip/palate, or abnormal genitalia in 50% of infants with fetal hydantoin syndrome.

    There is an increased incidence of this syndrome with combination medications because of competition for metabolism.

  d. Cognitive function. A well-controlled prospective comparison of phenytoin and carbemazepine monotherapy in patients with generalized seizures demonstrated a significant effect on cognitive function in children with intrauterine exposure to phenytoin,[13] but mild mental retardation has been found as well in children exposed to carbamazepine monotherapy in utero.[19]

  e. Coagulopathy. Fifty percent of exposed fetuses develop coagulopathy, and 50% of these experience bleeding complications, many during the first 24 hours (pleural, pericardial, intracranial, peritoneal, retroperitoneal). This coagulopathy is due to a deficiency of vitamin K–dependent clotting factors II, VII, IX, and X secondary to altered absorption of vitamin K.

    i. Neonatal treatment is 1 mg vitamin K intramuscularly

    ii. Antenatal vitamin K during the last months of pregnancy is recommended.[15] Alternate regimens include 10 mg orally daily or 2.5 to 5 mg intravenously or subcutaneously while in labor.

    iii. Cord blood should be sent for clotting studies; if highly abnormal, the neonate should receive fresh frozen plasma and additional vitamin K because delayed treatment may be fatal.

  f. Interference with folate metabolism. Folate acts as cofactor in metabolism, which is increased by microsomal enzyme induction. Phenytoin also interferes with folate absorption. Patients need supplemental folate given as 4 mg every day in the periconceptional period and during pregnancy.

The exact dose of folic acid is not well established by outcome studies at this time.

g. Calcium metabolism and absorption are altered. Neonatal hypocalcemia and tetany may result. Patients should receive supplemental vitamin D (1000 mg/day) during pregnancy.

h. Breastfeeding. Breast milk contains 25–35% of maternal levels of phenytoin. Breastfeeding is not contraindicated.

2. Phenobarbital

Phenobarbital is indicated in generalized tonic-clonic seizures.

a. Increased dosage in pregnancy. Phenobarbital dosing usually increases during pregnancy to maintain therapeutic levels.

b. Fetal levels are similar to maternal levels. Phenobarbital is metabolized slowly by the fetus and may cause neonatal depression and withdrawal 10–20% of the time.

c. Teratogenicity. Controversial evidence exists regarding teratogenicity, but it appears to be much lower than phenytoin. For this reason, phenobarbital has been recommended as the drug of choice during pregnancy for grand mal seizures.[5] Unfortunately, this may not always be the best choice for an individual patient because control may not be optimal with phenobarbital.

d. Coagulopathy. Coagulopathy in neonates has been noted. For this reason, many clinicians administer vitamin K during the third trimester to avoid bleeding complications.

e. Breastfeeding. Breast milk levels are 10–30% of maternal levels. Neonatal depression may decrease the neonate's adaptation to breastfeeding by about 48 hours. Breastfeeding is not contraindicated unless the newborn continues to show signs of depression.

3. Primidone

Primidone is indicated in generalized tonic-clonic seizures.

a. Primidone is metabolized to phenobarbital.

b. Primidone embryopathy (suspected) results in craniofacial and cardiac anomalies.

c. Very little medication crosses into breast milk.

4. Carbamazepine

Carbamazepine is indicated in complex, partial motor, and generalized tonic-clonic seizures.

a. Serum levels. These levels may decrease during pregnancy.

b. Metabolism. Carbamazepine is eliminated from the mother and neonate at the same rate without incidence of neonatal depression.

c. Teratogenicity. The incidence of this is probably less than that for phenytoin and includes:
   i. craniofacial defects
   ii. fingernail hypoplasia
   iii. developmental delays[11,13]

Neurodevelopmental effects appear to be less in one study.[11] Because carbamazepine is often effective in the control of generalized seizures, it may be a reasonable alternative when phenobarbital is not effective in generalized seizures.

d. Breastfeeding. Breast milk levels are 40% of maternal serum levels. There are no contraindications to breastfeeding.

5. Ethosuximide

Ethosuximide is indicated for the treatment of petit mal seizures.

   a. Teratogenicity. Ethosuximide crosses the placenta rapidly but is much less teratogenic than trimethadione, with malformations occurring in about 6% of exposed fetuses.
   b. Natural history. Petit mal epilepsy usually resolves in adolescence, so patients may be able to discontinue medication.
   c. Metabolism. Levels are almost the same in breast milk as in maternal serum, but no harmful effects are found in exposed fetuses.
6. Valproic acid
Valproic acid is indicated in generalized tonic-clonic seizures and is also used in some patients with partial complex seizures.
   a. Teratogenicity. Neural tube defects (especially spina bifida) occur in 2.5%; MSAFP and targeted ultrasound examinations are indicated. Valproate enhances teratogenicity of other anticonvulsants. It should be used as monotherapy if possible.[5] Recent information suggests that valproate teratogenicity is dose-related; doses greater than 1000 mg/day are associated with greater risk of major congenital malformations than pregnancies exposed to lower daily doses.[24] Other malformations seen include cardiac, oral clefts, hypospadias, and limb reduction defects.[4]
   b. Metabolism. Fetal levels are the same or higher than maternal levels.
   c. Breastfeeding. Breast milk levels are 2% of maternal serum levels and there are no contraindications to breastfeeding.
7. Trimethadione
Trimethadione is indicated for control of petit mal seizures.
   a. Teratogenicity. This drug is most teratogenic of all anticonvulsants—83% major fetal malformations and a high rate of spontaneous abortions are noted.[10] Use of this agent during pregnancy should be avoided because of the associated anomalies that include multiple facial anomalies, congenital heart defects, microcephaly, mental retardation, developmental delays, multiple gastrointestinal and genitourinary defects.
   b. Avoid use. Patients with petit mal epilepsy should be switched to ethosuximide or clonazepam, preferably before conception.
8. Diazepam
Diazepam is indicated only for control of status epilepticus.
   a. Teratogenicity. There is a probable increase in oral clefts with first-trimester use.
   b. Metabolism. Fetal levels and levels of active metabolites exceed maternal levels; newborn metabolism is slow.
   c. Intrapartum use. If administered during labor, the neonate may have low Apgar scores with apneic spells, hypotonia, poor suckling, and hypothermia. The use of diazepam during labor can result in decreased beat-to-beat variability. Diazepam manifests extremely slow metabolism and elimination in the newborn.
   d. Breastfeeding. Diazepam may cause lethargy and poor feeding; it is best avoided in breastfeeding.
9. Newer antiepileptic medications
None of the newer antiepileptic agents are studied well. Very little in the way of adverse events has been reported, but cardiac and neural tube defects have been reported in pregnancies with zonisamide polypharmacy.[12] Lamotrigine passes extensively across the placenta; levels in breast milk are approximately 25% of maternal serum.[28] Vigabatrin is transferred slowly across the placenta and is poorly excreted in human milk.[29]

G. Management Summary

1. Preconception care (see Chapter 1, section A)
   a. Patients with poor seizure control. These patients may want to avoid pregnancy and should be counseled about probable diminished control during pregnancy.
   b. Recent-onset seizures. Patients who had new-onset seizures in pregnancy (not eclampsia) or seizures that only occurred during pregnancy should undergo work-up for possible causes of seizures other than epilepsy, such as an arteriovenous malformation.
   c. Idiopathic epilepsy. Patients with idiopathic epilepsy should be advised that the risk of their children developing epilepsy is 2–3%, five times that of the general population. They should be advised that the risk of malformations is slightly higher than that of the general population independent of medications.
   d. Candidates for drug withdrawal. If patients have been seizure-free for several years and have a normal EEG, they should be slowly withdrawn from medications before conception. If they need to remain on medications, an attempt should be made to control seizures on a single agent of the lowest teratogenic potential. Patients should not be given trimethadione.

2. Antepartum care
   a. Initial management. If the patient is first seen in early pregnancy and is in good control, she should not be withdrawn from those medications because there is a high risk of status epilepticus.
   b. Monitoring drug levels. Serum anticonvulsant levels should be monitored monthly with adjustments to maintain therapeutic levels.
   c. Prevention of related complications. Prophylactic folic acid (4.0 mg/day starting before conception) and vitamin K (5 to 10 mg/day during the last 2 months of pregnancy) is advisable with phenytoin, phenobarbital, and primidone.

3. Intrapartum and postpartum care
   a. Parenteral anticonvulsants. These may be administered during labor if there are concerns about the patient receiving medication because of vomiting or delayed gastric emptying. This is probably not necessary in early labor, when oral medication is suitable.
   b. Prevention of neonatal coagulopathy. Clotting studies are performed on cord blood with maternal use of phenytoin, phenobarbital or primidone; neonatal vitamin K (1 mg) is administered. Infants with abnormal studies may need additional measures.
   c. Breastfeeding. Infants should be monitored for lethargy, poor feeding, and signs of withdrawal, depending on maternal medication used.

II. Migraine Headache

Patients with catamenial migraine (related to menses) generally improve with pregnancy. The frequency of migraine headache, regardless of type, is decreased in 55–90% of women, generally in the second and third trimester.[20]

A. Treatment

Most patients can be treated with analgesics and antiemetic medication. Prophylaxis with beta-blockers should be considered only in patients with frequent, severe migraine, using metoprolol and pindolol.

B. Medications to Avoid

Ergots (dihydroergotamine and ergotamine tartrate) and the "triptans" (sumatriptan, zolmitriptan, naratriptan) are contraindicated according to most experts. However, a controlled clinical trial of sumatriptan showed no adverse pregnancy outcome compared to disease-matched and non-teratogen controls.[26] This study does not address effects later in pregnancy.

III. Multiple Sclerosis

A. Relapse Rates
Relapse rates are not increased with pregnancy and may be decreased. The disease appears to have no specific effects on the course of pregnancy. In addition, pregnancy does not appear to contribute to the progression of multiple sclerosis.[7,23] There may be an increased risk of multiple sclerosis in the nulliparous woman and a decreased risk of progressive course in women who become pregnant after multiple sclerosis onset.[21]

B. Urinary Tract Infection
Patients with urinary retention caused by a neurogenic bladder are at increased risk for urinary tract infection. Besides more frequent urine cultures, patients may need to practice intermittent self-catheterization.

C. Postpartum
Although findings in studies vary, the six months following delivery appear to be associated with an increase in the rate of relapse.[8] Half of the relapses that occur in the pregnancy year are in the first 3 months postpartum. There is no contraindication to breastfeeding. Patients should be careful to get extra rest because fatigue influences symptoms.

IV. Myasthenia Gravis
Myasthenia gravis may complicate the course of pregnancy in multiple ways. Because of the complexity of management and risks to the neonate, these patients should be delivered in a tertiary setting. The following information is provided for assistance in emergency management and patient counseling.[1]

A. Increase in Preterm Labor
The risk of premature labor is increased as a result of anticholinesterase medication. Beta-sympathomimetic drugs and betamethasone have been associated with a respiratory crisis.

B. Myasthenic Crisis
This crisis presents as severe weakness and respiratory insufficiency, and may be precipitated by labor. It must be distinguished from cholinergic crisis, which is usually associated with nausea, tearing, cramping, and diarrhea. Edrophonium improves myasthenic crisis but not a cholinergic crisis.

C. Contraindicated Medications
Magnesium sulfate should not be used because high levels inhibit the release of acetylcholine, causing collapse and apnea. Numerous anesthetics can also cause untoward effects.

D. Neonatal Myasthenia
This occurs in 4–20% of neonates due to transplacental passage of acetylcholine receptor antibodies. This syndrome is more severe in the premature infant.

E. Postpartum Exacerbations
These exacerbations are common in the first 6 weeks. Patients may breastfeed while taking anticholinesterase medications.

V. Paraplegia and Quadriplegia

A. Urinary Tract Infections
Urinary tract infections are common complications and more so in women who have a pre-pregnancy history of such.[30]

1. Bladder evacuation

This may be managed by the Credé maneuver, self-catheterization, or self-voiding. Urinary retention should be avoided.

2. Urine cultures

Urine cultures should be done on an intermittent basis dependent on patient history.

3. Acidification of the urine

This may be accomplished with vitamin C, 500 mg four times a day, and may be helpful to prevent recurrent infection.[17]

B. Preterm Labor

Preterm labor is increased (19% in one series).[30] Patients should be followed closely in the third trimester for signs and symptoms of preterm labor.[17]

C. Labor Management

All patients have sacral anesthesia. If the lesion is above T11, labor is painless. If the lesion is above T5–T6, it is above the level of splanchnic outflow. Autonomic hyperreflexia may occur during labor, because of bladder distention before labor occurs, or with cesarean section. Signs and symptoms of this massive sympathetic outflow include hypertension, severe vasoconstriction, secondary bradycardia, sweating, pounding headache, and flushing.[17] Normal blood pressures in Westgren et al[30] series of spinal cord injury patients were low. Regional anesthesia (epidural) is indicated to prevent or treat autonomic hyperreflexia.[30] If the patient has autonomic hyperreflexia caused by a distended bladder, it should be emptied. The cesarean section rate is increased for patients with spinal cord injury.[30]

References

1. Aminoff M: Neurologic disorders. In Creasy RK, Resnik, R (eds): Maternal Fetal Medicine: Principles and Practice, 3rd ed. Philadelphia, W. B. Saunders, 1994, pp 1094–1095.
2. Ann Pharmacother 32:794–801, 1996.
3. Awada A, Watson T, Obeid T: Cavernous angioma presenting as pregnancy-related seizures. Epilepsia 38:844–846, 1997.
4. Bradai R, Robert E: [Prenatal ultrasonographic diagnosis in epileptic mother on valproic acid: Retrospective study of 161 cases in central eastern France register of congenital malformations.] J Gynecol Obstet Biol Reprod (Paris) 27:413–419, 1998.
5. Buehler BA, Stempel LE: Anticonvulsant therapy during pregnancy. In Rayburn WF, Zuspan FP (eds): Drug Therapy in Obstetrics and Gynecology, 3rd ed. St Louis, Mosby, 1992.
6. Cheng AY, Kwan A: Perioperative management in intra-partum seizure. Anaesth Intensive Care 25:535–538, 1997.
7. Damek DM, Shuster EA: Pregnancy and multiple sclerosis. Mayo Clin Proc 72:977–989, 1997.
8. Flachenecker P, Hartung P: Multiple sclerosis and pregnancy: Overview and status of the European multicenter PRIMS study. Nervenarzt 66:97–104, 1995.
9. Garza-Morales S, Ibarra-Puig JM, Poblano-Luna A, et al: [Epilepsy and pregnancy: Prospective study of 100 cases]. Ginecol Obstet Mex 64:449–454, 1996.
10. Jick SS, Terris BZ: Anticonvulsants and congenital malformations. Pharmacotherapy 17:561–564, 1997.
11. Jones KL, Lacro RV, Johnson BA, et al: Pattern of malformations in children of women treated with carbemazepine during pregnancy. N Engl J Med 320:1661–1666, 1989.
12. Kondo T, Kaneko S, Amano Y, et al: Preliminary report on teratogenic effects of zonisamide in the offspring of treated women with epilepsy. Epilepsia 31:1242–1244, 1996.
13. Lindhout D, Hoppener RJ, Meinhard H: Teratogenicity of antiepileptic drug combinations with special emphasis on epoxidation of carbemazepine. Epilepsia 25:77–83, 1984.
14. Morrell MJ: The new antiepileptic drugs and women: Efficacy, reproductive health, pregnancy, and fetal outcome. Epilepsia 37 (Suppl 6)S34–S44, 1996.
15. Mountain KR, Hirsch J, Gallus AS: Neonatal coagulation defect due to anticonvulsant drug treatment in pregnancy. Lancet 1:265–268, 1970.
16. Nulman I, Schonik D, Chitayat D, et al: Am J Med Genet 68:18–24, 1997.
17. Obstetric management of patients with spinal cord injury. ACOG Committee Opinion. Number 121, 1993.
18. Olafussib E, Hallgrimsson JT, Hauser WA, et al: Pregnancies of women with epilepsy: A population-based study in Iceland. Epilepsia 39:887–892, 1998.
19. Ornoy A, Cohen E: Outcome of children born to mothers treated with carbamazepine during pregnancy. Arch Dis Child 75:517–520, 1996.

20. Pfaffenrath V, Rehm M: Migraine in pregnancy: What are the safest treatment options? Drug Saf 19:383–388, 1998.
21. Runmarker B, Andersen O: Pregnancy is associated with a lower risk of onset and a better prognosis in multiple sclerosis. Brain 118:253–261, 1995.
22. Sabers A, Rogvi-Hansen B, Dam M, et al: Pregnancy and epilepsy: a retrospective study of 151 pregnancies. Acta Neurol Scand 97:164–170, 1998.
23. Sadovnick AD, Eisen K, Hashimoto SA, et al: Pregnancy and multiple sclerosis: A prospective study. Arch Neurol 51:1120–1124, 1994.
24. Samren EB, van Duijin CM, Koch S, et al: Maternal use of antiepileptic drugs and the risk of major congenital malformations: A joint European prospective study of human teratogenesis associated with maternal epilepsy. Epilepsia 38:981–990, 1997.
25. Schupf N, Ottman R: Reproduction among individuals with idiopathic/cryptogenic epilepsy: Risk factors for spontaneous abortion. Epilepsia 38:824–829, 1997.
26. Shuhaiber S, Pastiszak A, Schick B, et al: Pregnancy outcome following first trimester exposure to sumatriptan. Neurology 51:581–583, 1998.
27. Taganelli P, Regesta G: Epilepsy, pregnancy, and major birth anomalies: an Italian prospective, controlled study. Neurology 42(Suppl 5):89–93, 1992.
28. Tomson T, Ohman, I, Vitols S: Lamotrigine in pregnancy and lactation: A case report. Epilepsia 38:1039–1041, 1997.
29. Tran A, O'Mahoney T, Rey E, et al: Vigabatrin: Placental transfer in vivo and excretion into breast milk of the enantiomers. Br J Clin Pharmacol 45:409–411, 1998.
30. Westgren N, Hultling C, Levi R, et al: Pregnancy and delivery in women with a traumatic spinal cord injury in Sweden, 1980–91. Obstet Gynecol 81:926–930, 1993.
31. Zahn CA, Morrell MJ, Collins SD, et al: Management issues for women with epilepsy: A review of the literature. Neurology 51:949–956, 1998.

SECTION H.
RENAL DISEASE

Ellen L. Sakornbut, M.D.

I. Effects of Chronic Renal Failure on Pregnancy Outcome
A. Mild Renal Insufficiency
A creatinine level of 0.85 mg/dl and BUN of 15 mg/dl, which are normal values in nonpregnant patients, may suggest mild renal insufficiency during pregnancy.

1. Pregnancy outcomes

Patients with chronic renal disease but normal or mildly decreased function usually have good pregnancy outcomes. Stable patients with mild glomerular disease also usually have successful outcomes if they are normotensive.[2] Less favorable outcomes may be seen in patients with certain diagnoses, including lupus nephropathy, certain glomerulopathies, and reflux nephropathy.

2. Proteinuria

In patients with chronic renal insufficiency, proteinuria increases in 50% of pregnancies and may lead to nephrotic syndrome with edema.

B. Moderate and Severe Renal Insufficiency
Most experts agree that pregnancy should be avoided in patients with a baseline creatinine level > 2.0 mg/dl. The incidence of maternal and fetal complications, including preeclampsia, IUGR, and abruption, is significantly increased in patients with a creatinine of 3.0 mg/dl or more. Most patients with severe renal insufficiency are infertile.

1. Dialysis

Recent literature has published rates of 50–70% successful pregnancies in women who were able to become pregnant while undergoing long-term dialysis or who were started on dialysis after diagnosis of pregnancy. Fertility is markedly reduced, however. Maternal protocols included increase in erythropoietin dosage to maintain a hemoglobin of 10 or 11 and an increase in dialysis frequency and volumes. Fetal outcomes included prematurity and low birth weight in 100% of pregnancies, with other complications including hypertension, disorders of amniotic fluid volume (both oligohydramnios and polyhydramnios), and second- and third-trimester losses.[1,4]

2. Transplant recipients

Kidney recipients have been successfully treated with prednisone, azathioprine, cyclosporine, and tacrolimus without adverse effects to the fetus except an increase in small-for-gestational age fetuses and prematurity. Transplant recipients are also at risk for intrauterine infections with cytomegalovirus, toxplasmosis, and herpes simplex.[3]

II. Specific Diagnoses and Need for Specialized Management

A. Chronic Pyelonephritis (see Chapter 8, section A)

Outcomes are better if renal function is well preserved and blood pressure normal. Prognosis is better in this tubulointerstitial disease than in glomerular diseases.

1. Increased incidence of urinary tract infections

Urinary tract infections are more frequent during pregnancy.

2. Role of antibiotic suppression

Patients may benefit from antibiotic suppressive therapy.

B. Nephrolithiasis

Genitourinary infections occur more frequently than in the nonpregnant state.

C. Nephrotic Syndrome

Pregnancy prognosis depends on cause and presence or absence of hypertension and renal function compromise. If renal function is normal, and the patient is not hypertensive, outcomes are generally good.

1. Albumin levels in pregnancy

These levels are normally 1 gram lower in pregnancy.

2. Diuretics are contraindicated

With nephrotic syndrome, the patient may become significantly edematous; diuretics should not be used because intravascular volume is decreased.

D. Glomerulonephritis

Outcomes are generally poorer if renal function is decreased or if hypertension is present. The incidence of preeclampsia is increased.

E. Diabetic Nephropathy

The incidence of preeclampsia is increased. Prognosis is worse with concomitant hypertension (see section I on diabetes mellitus).

F. Lupus-Related Renal Disease

Prognosis is poorer with high rates of preeclampsia. About 7% of patients develop end-stage renal disease, and a higher number have progression of disease in pregnancy (see section J).

G. Permanent Urinary Diversion

Patients usually do well, but they may develop acute pyelonephritis or outflow obstruction in late pregnancy.

H. Polycystic Kidney Disease

There is a slight increase in preeclampsia, but patients generally do well. Genetic counseling is indicated because adult polycystic kidney disease is autosomal dominant.

I. Single Kidney

Renal function should be monitored serially. Most patients experience no difficulties.

J. Pelvic Kidney

This type of kidney may be more prone to infection. Some types of urinary tract anomalies may interfere with fetal descent.

References

1. Bagon JA, Vernaeve H, De Muylder X, et al: Pregnancy and dialysis. Am J Kidney Dis 31:756–765, 1998.
2. Hidaka M, Ohi H, Ohsawa I, et al: [Three cases of pregnancy with successful outcomes in spite of severe histological findings.] Nippon Jinzo Gaddai Shi 41:454–459, 1999.
3. Hou S: Pregnancy in chronic renal insufficiency and end-stage renal disease. Am J Kidney Dis 33:235–245, 1999.
4. Romaoo JE Jr, Luders C, Kahhale S, et al: Pregnancy in women on chronic dialysis: A single center experience with 17 cases. Nephron 78:416–422, 1998.

SECTION I.
ENDOCRINE CONDITIONS

David Turok, M.D., and Ted Schultz, M.D.

I. Diabetes Mellitus

The ability to improve perinatal outcomes for patients with gestational diabetes is uncertain (see Chapter 6, section A). However, there is vast potential to improve these outcomes for patients with preexisting diabetes. Because pregnancy risks are high in this group, every office visit with diabetic women of childbearing age should include a clear plan for contraception or preconceptional planning (see Chapter 1, section A).

A. Type 1 Diabetes

Prior to the discovery of insulin in 1922, the maternal mortality rate in diabetic pregnancies was > 50%. These patients have increased risk of miscarriage, fetal malformations, pre-eclampsia, birth trauma, and progression of maternal retinopathy. Tight glycemic control from the preconception period through delivery has normalized the majority of the above risks in this patient group. Thus, preconception care is crucial for the well-being of these patients and their potential offspring. It is best to develop a plan of care for type 1 diabetics prior to conception that involves all available resources, including nutrition/diabetes counselors, endocrinology, ophthalmology, and perinatology/obstetrics back-up or referral if available.

B. Type 2 Diabetes

Non–insulin-dependent or type 2 diabetic patients are commonly encountered in family practice and comprise 90% of all diabetics. This condition is increasingly common for patients over the age of 30. In addition, the family physician may provide care for women whose family histories or ethnic backgrounds put them at increased risk. Screening for diabetes in early pregnancy for patients at high risk enhances the likelihood of diagnosing previously undetected non–insulin-dependent diabetes. Because there are no available trials on pregnancy outcomes of type 2 diabetics, management recommendations for IDDM mothers seem appropriate for this group. Data to support the recommendations come from studies of type 1 diabetics and collections of type 1, type 2, and gestational diabetics.

C. Definition/Classification Systems

The American Diabetes Association (ADA) and the World Health Organization (WHO) revised diagnostic criteria for diabetes mellitus in 1997 to a random venous plasma glucose (PG) > 200 mg/dl in the presence of symptoms (polyuria, polydipsia, ketoacidosis) or a fasting PG of > 126 mg/dl on 2 different days. The older WHO definition of a 2-hour oral glucose tolerance test of > 200 mg/dl following a 75-g glucose load is no longer recommended for routine clinical use.[4]

    1. The White classification system of diabetes in pregnancy
    This system established the following classes:[24]
        a. Class A1 and A2: gestational diabetes (see Chapter 6, section A)
        b. Class B: onset of disease after age 20, no vascular complications

    c. Class C: onset between ages 10 and 19 or duration 10 to 19 years, no vascular complications

    d. Class D: onset of disease before age 10 or greater than 20 years' duration and those with benign retinopathy including microaneurysms, exudates, or venous dilatation.

    e. Class F: patients with renal disease who have impaired creatinine clearance or proteinuria of at least 400 mg/24 hours, measured in the first trimester

    f. Class R: patients with proliferative retinopathy

    g. Class T: patients who have undergone renal transplant

    h. Class H: patients with diabetes and coronary artery disease

2. Alternative classification system

    a. Class I: pregnancy-induced glucose intolerance; treatment is with nutritional adjustment alone

    b. Class II: abnormal glucose tolerance requiring insulin for management, no vascular involvement

    c. Class III: abnormal glucose tolerance requiring insulin, with vascular involvement

    d. Class IV: atherosclerotic ischemic heart disease

D. Risk Assessment/Preconception Care

1. General considerations

The chances of a successful pregnancy outcome are influenced by patient involvement and compliance, the presence or absence of vascular complications, and contributions from several members of the health care team. Class A diabetics usually have good pregnancy outcomes. Class B and C patients require intensive supervision, education, and good control to maximize their chances for successful pregnancies. Patients in classes D, F, and R are at significant risk for both maternal and fetal complications and should be referred for specialist care. Class H patients are at high maternal risk and should not become pregnant.

2. Preconception diabetic control

Women should be counseled on the importance of achieving tight control of their diabetes before they become pregnant to reduce the risk of congenital anomalies related to hyperglycemia during the period of organogenesis.[14,17] Tight control is defined as maintaining euglycemia as measured by normal glycohemoglobin levels. Effective family planning is critical. Preconception and early pregnancy control of diabetes has been shown to reduce the incidence of anomalies to that of the general population.[6]

3. Congenital anomalies

Congenital anomalies are the leading cause of perinatal mortality in diabetes.[2,3] The relative risk of congenital anomalies ranges from 2.0 to 7.9 compared to the rate in the nondiabetic population.[2,3,8,17] The most common anomalies are cardiac defects, neural tube defects (especially anencephaly), and hemivertebrae.[15,24] MSAFP levels may be up to 60% lower in diabetics than in non-diabetic women with pregnancies of the same gestational age. Therefore, thresholds for detection of neural tube defects must be set lower if the patient is diabetic.

4. Risk of preterm labor

The incidence of preterm deliveries is increased because of conditions such as IUGR, polyhydramnios, and preeclampsia.

5. Risk of abnormal fetal growth

Macrosomia is found in all classes of diabetics. There are data to support a relative risk of 5.2 for shoulder dystocia in diabetics, an effect which is compounded by increasing neonatal weight. Despite the increased risk of shoulder dystocia, the rate of birth trauma in 118 diabetics was not significantly different than 354 normal controls (3.4% vs. 2.5%).[16]

6. Intrauterine growth restriction (IUGR)

IUGR is common for patients with microvascular disease, especially those with diabetic nephropathy.

E. Maternal Considerations

1. Nephropathy

In mothers with nephropathy, generally good fetal outcomes occur in the absence of abnormal creatinine clearance or hypertension. It has been recommended that pregnancy be restricted to patients with a creatinine level < 2.0 mg/dl and diastolic blood pressure < 90 mm Hg.[7] Some women experience irreversible worsening of renal function with pregnancy.

2. Retinopathy

No clear trend in progression of retinopathy is associated with pregnancy. Laser photocoagulation has been used extensively during pregnancy.

3. Pregnancy-induced hypertension (PIH)

PIH occurs in 25% of diabetics.

F. Antepartum Care Guidelines

1. Tests

Early in pregnancy, the patient should undergo a dilated retinal examination and studies of renal function, including BUN, creatinine, 24-hour urine for creatinine clearance, and protein. Evaluation of glycemic control during the periconception and organogenesis periods can be made with home glucose monitoring and following glycohemoglobin levels. If an early glycohemoglobin is > 8.5%, the patient should undergo fetal echocardiography in the second or third trimester because of the increased risk of cardiac defects.[23] Septal defects, either ventricular or atrial, may nonetheless be missed with this procedure, but this should not significantly affect management.

2. Dating

Accurate dating of pregnancy should be accomplished by clinical measures and ultrasonography. Screening for anomalies should be performed in the second trimester, with follow-up of fetal growth in the early third trimester. Macrosomia may be an indicator of poor control but can be found even in patients who have been well controlled.[14] Polyhydramnios may indicate poor control or a fetal anomaly.

3. Diet

There is no single "diabetic" or "ADA" diet, as there is no one proven strategy. A regular diet is crucial to maintain good glycemic control and should be based on formal nutritional assessment. A successful diet should be culturally appropriate and account for obesity, desired weight gain during pregnancy (13-18 kg for BMI < 19.8, 12–16 kg for BMI 20–29, ~7 kg for BMI > 29), gestational age, exercise, coexisting renal disease and lipid goals. A starting point is a diet consisting of the 30–kcal/kg of ideal body weight divided into three meals and three snacks per day. The diet composition should be high fiber with limited foods that cause a glycemic response (e.g., simple sugars) and calorie distribution as follows:

    a. 50–60% carbohydrates

    b. 10–20% protein

    c. 20–30% fat, less than 10% saturated fat, the rest monounsaturated.

G. Insulin Therapy—Goals and Management

1. Baseline hemoglobin A1c

This test is helpful in identifying patients who are under good control (HgbA1c < 7.0) and those who need stricter control. It is not necessary to repeat this during the pregnancy but can be useful to demonstrate long-term progress to patients. Home glucose monitoring is an essential step in assessing the adequacy of current treatment and modifying it to meet goals.

2. Tight glycemic control

This is the major strategy to prevent maternal, fetal, and neonatal complications. The ACOG recommends "normalization" of blood glucose with fasting values < 90 mg/dl (5.0 mmol/L), 2-hour postprandial values < 120 mg/dl (6.6 mmol/L), and < 105 mg/dl (5.8 mmol/L) before a meal. While there is broad agreement that euglycemia is beneficial, the ACOG Technical Bulletin cites no specific papers for these values. Blood sugar control in this range was associated with the fewest neonatal complications and maternal hypoglycemia in 60 pregnant diabetics divided into three levels of control.[5] Tight control is advocated rather than very tight control (all blood glucose levels < 5.6 mmol/L = 100 mg/dl) because very tight control has not been shown to result in improved outcomes but is associated with high incidence of hypoglycemia, especially in the first trimester.[5] The increased attention to 2-hour postprandial blood sugars is based on The Diabetes in Early Pregnancy Study, which showed that the incidence of macrosomia was 20% when these values were < 120 and 30% when they were greater.[10]

   a. Maintaining euglycemia. Blood sugars should be checked often enough to maintain euglycemia and recorded in a log book. There is no definitive answer of exactly how often this should be from the literature. A common practice is to check five times daily: a.m. fasting, 2 hour postprandial, and bedtime. A large prospective study with over 1000 gestational diabetics in each arm showed that the group that monitored 7 values a day (the above schedule plus 2 preprandial checks) had fewer cesarean deliveries and NICU admissions than a group that monitored 4 times daily.[12] There are no similar data for type 1 and 2 diabetics during pregnancy.

   b. Insulin administration. Just as with glucose monitoring, there is no one best method for use of insulin in pregnancy. Insulin administration now occurs via several practices.

      i. The standard approach is to divide total daily insulin use into regular and NPH. Two-thirds of the daily dose is given in the morning, 30 minutes prior to breakfast. Of this 2/3 is NPH and 1/3 is standard regular. Half of the remaining 1/3 is given as regular prior to dinner and the other half as NPH at bedtime. A recent study has shown improved glycemic control with four times daily vs. two times daily insulin in pregnancy. This study had both gestational and type 1 and 2 diabetics.[19] Because of the shorter half-life of insulin during pregnancy, it is convention to change the evening NPH dose to bedtime. This is done to avoid nocturnal hypoglycemia when the NPH effect would be peaking at 2–3:00 a.m.

      ii. Using a night-time dose of Ultralente and quick-acting Humalog or lispro before meals is becoming increasingly popular in the management of type 1 diabetes. Use of this very-short-acting insulin allows patients to inject it immediately before meals and avoid the postprandial hypoglycemia that occurs when regular insulin is still working but the meal has already been absorbed. Humalog is pregnancy category B and is now being used in pregnancy.[9]

      iii. Another option is the insulin pump that is an excellent option in a patient who cannot attain adequate glycemic control with other methods. Continuous subcutaneous insulin infusion uses Humalog insulin at an adjustable basal rate and gives boluses at mealtimes. There are several reports of successful use of the pump in pregnancy dating back to 1981.[21]

    iv. There is preliminary evidence that the sulfonyl ureas may be used safely and effectively in pregnancy. Further studies are needed before clinicians consider their use in pregnancy.[12A]

  c. Hypoglycemic reactions. Early in pregnancy, most patients require less insulin; hypoglycemic reactions are encountered more frequently. Hypoglycemia occurring after fetal beta cell hyperplasia has occurred may present a severe stress to the fetus and is thought to be a cause of unexplained stillbirth.[17]

  d. Insulin requirements. These increase with rising levels of human placental lactogen at 14–16 weeks. Numerous metabolic changes occur, which result in fetal organ hypertrophy and hyperplasia as well as increased maternal triglyceride levels.[14]

  e. Diabetic ketoacidosis. This may be precipitated by infection or other stressors. Its incidence has decreased since the advent of home glucose monitoring. It represents a major hazard to the fetus and the mother.

3. Other management issues

  a. Infection. Urine cultures should be performed at least every trimester. The patient should be taught to report immediately any signs of viral or bacterial infection.

  b. Preeclampsia. Patients with associated hypertension, renal compromise, or other high risks for pregnancy-induced hypertension should have uric acid, creatinine levels, urine protein and creatinine clearance monitored. Low-dose daily aspirin therapy and calcium supplementation, which showed promise in early clinical trials, have not proven to prevent preeclampsia in large multicenter randomized trials.[1,13]

4. Assessment of fetal well-being

  a. Third-trimester ultrasound. This should be obtained to document fetal growth and rule out IUGR.

  b. Antepartum testing. This should begin at 32 weeks for type A diabetics and at 36 weeks for non-insulin-requiring diabetics. This may consist of biweekly nonstress tests or weekly biophysical profiles or modified BPPs. Doppler flow studies have been demonstrated to improve perinatal outcomes in the presence of IUGR (see Chapter 10, section B)

H. Intrapartum Management

1. Timing of delivery

The timing of delivery is somewhat controversial. The well-controlled diabetic without other complications can be allowed to continue pregnancy until 38–40 weeks. If complications such as preeclampsia or IUGR are present, management should follow guidelines for those conditions.

2. Intrapartum control of glucose

This is managed with insulin infusion and hourly glucose monitoring.[18]

3. Preterm delivery/complications of prematurity

If delivery before 37 weeks is contemplated, ascertaining fetal lung maturity is desirable because of delayed fetal lung maturity that may accompany this condition. Fetal lung maturity may be delayed due to poor diabetic control. A lecithin-sphingomyelin ratio of 2.0 with phosphatidylglycerol > 2 to 5% and optical density at 650 nm > 0.150 should be predictable of fetal lung maturity.[11] Other causes of respiratory distress syndrome encountered in infants of diabetic mothers include transient tachypnea of the newborn, hypertrophic cardiomyopathy, and pneumonia.

I. Postpartum Issues

1. Neonatal conditions

Infants of diabetic mothers need to be observed for hypoglycemia and are at increased risk for other neonatal complications, including hypocalcemia, hypomagnesemia, polycythemia, hyperbilirubinemia, renal vein thrombosis, and the above mentioned respiratory issues (see Chapter 18).

2. Breastfeeding

Breastfeeding should be strongly encouraged as it has shown to significantly decrease the future likelihood of type 2 diabetes in infants who were exclusively breastfed versus those exclusively bottlefed (odds ratio 0.41).[20]

3. Maternal glucose control and follow-up care

It is likely that insulin requirements will decrease after delivery and that many of these diabetic women may return to using oral agents to achieve desirable glycemic control. Effective family planning should be instituted and the cycle of preconception care should be re-started.

J. Summary

Diabetes mellitus presents many preconceptional and perinatal management challenges to the family physician. This section outlines how to manage diabetic women in pregnancy, often in consultation with high-risk obstetrical or perinatologist consultation.

References

1. Caritis S, Sidai B, Hauth J, et al: Low-dose aspirin to prevent pre-eclampsia in women at high risk. N Engl J Med 338:701, 1998.
2. Chung CS, Myrianthopoulos NC: Factors affecting risks of congenital malformations. II. Effect of maternal diabetes. Birth Defects 11:1–38, 1975.
3. Cousins L: Congenital anomalies among infants of diabetic mothers: Am J Obstet Gynecol 147:333–338, 1983.
4. Expert Committee on the Diagnosis and Classification of Diabetes Mellitus. Diabetes Care 20:1183–1197, 1997.
5. Farrag OM: Prospective study of 3 metabolic regimens in pregnant diabetics. Aust N Z J Obstet Gynaecol 27:6–9, 1987.
6. Fuhrman K, Reiher H, Semmler K, et al: The effect of intensified conventional insulin therapy before and during pregnancy on malformation rate in offspring of diabetic mothers. Exp Clin Endocrinol 83:173–177, 1984.
7. Gabbe SG: Management of diabetes mellitus in pregnancy. Am J Obstet Gynecol 153:824–828, 1985.
8. Grix A: Malformations in infants of diabetic mothers. Am J Med Genet 13:131–137, 1982.
9. Jovanovic L, Ilic S, Petett DJ, et al: Metabolic immunologic effects of insulin lispro in gestational diabetes. Diabetes Care 22:1422–1427, 1999.
10. Jovanovic-Peterson L, Peterson CM, Red DG, et al: Maternal postprandial glucose levels and infant birth weight: The diabetes in early pregnancy study. Am J Obstet Gynecol 164:103–111, 1991.
11. Kjos SL, Walther FJ, Montoro M, et al: Prevalence and etiology of respiratory distress in infants of diabetic mothers: Predictive value of fetal lung maturation tests. Am J Obstet Gynecol 163:898–903, 1990.
12. Langer O, Rodriquez DA, Xenakis EMJ, et al: Intensified versus conventional management of gestational diabetes. Am J Obstet Gynecol 171:1036–1047, 1994.
12A. Langer O, Conway D, Berkus M, et al: A comparison of glyburide and insulin in women with gestational diabetes mellitus. N Engl J Med 343:1134–1138, 2000.
13. Levine RJ, Hauth JC, Curet LB, et al: Trial of calcium to prevent preeclampsia. N Engl J Med 337:69–76, 1997.
14. Miller E, Hare JW, Cloherty JP, et al: Elevated maternal hemoglobin A1c in early pregnancy and major congenital anomalies in infants of diabetic mothers. N Engl J Med 304:1331–1334, 1981.
15. Milunsky A, Alpert A, Kitzmiller JL, et al: Prenatal diagnosis of neural tube defects. VIII. The importance of serum alpha-fetoprotein screening in diabetic pregnant women. Am J Obstet Gynecol 142:1030–1032, 1982.
16. Mimouni F, Miodovnik M, Rosenn B, et al: Birth trauma in insulin-dependent diabetic pregnancies. Am J Perinatol 9:205–208, 1992.
17. Molsted-Peterson L, Tygstrup I, Pedersen J: Congenital malformations in newborn infants of diabetic women. Lancet 1:1124–1126, 1964.

18. Moore TR: Diabetes in pregnancy. In Creasy RK, Resnik R (eds): Maternal Fetal Medicine. Philadelphia, W.B. Saunders, 1999, p 989.
19. Nachum Z, Ber-Shlono I, Weives E, et al: Twice daily leisure four times daily insulin dose regimens in pregnancy: Randomized control trial. Br Med J 319:1223–1227, 1999.
20. Perez-Brazo F, Carrusco E, Gutierrez-Lopez MD, et al: Genetic predisposition and environmental factors leading to the development of insulin dependent diabetes mellitus in Chilean children. J Md Med 74:105–109, 1996.
21. Potter JM, Reckless JPD, Cullen DR: The effect of continuous subcutaneous insulin infusion and conventional insulin regimens on 24-hour variations of blood glucose and intermediary metabolism in the third trimester of diabetic pregnancy. Diabetologia 21: 534–539, 1981.
22. Reece EA, Lockwood CJ, Tuck ST, et al: Pregnancy outcome and severe diabetic retinopathy. Sixth Annual Meeting, The Society of Perinatal Obstetricians, 1986, A40.
23. Shields LE, Gan EA, Murphy HF, et al: The prognostic value of hemoglobin A1c in predicting fetal heart disease in diabetic pregnancies. Obstet Gynecol 81:954–957, 1993.
24. White P: Diabetes in Childhood and Adolescence. Philadelphia, Lea & Febiger, 1932, pp 224–225.

II. Thyroid Disease

This section describes normal changes in thyroid function during pregnancy and common thyroid disorders in pregnancy.

A. Normal Changes in Thyroid Function with Pregnancy

Normal thyroid values in pregnancy are summarized in Table 4.

    1. Increase in thyroxine-binding globulin (TBG)

Elevation in estrogen levels during pregnancy causes an increase in TBG.

    2. First-trimester changes

During the first trimester as serum levels of hCG peak, and free T_4 levels increase initially causing depressed TSH levels. This is due to hCG having a mild thyroid stimulating activity.[1,10,15] After the first trimester free T_4 and TSH levels return to normal.

    3. Free T_4 and T_3 during pregnancy

These range from nonpregnant levels to as much as 25% lower.[2,12]

    4. Increased glomerular filtration rate (GFR)

The increase of GFR has a significant effect on the excretion of iodide.[10] In areas of iodide deficiency this has dramatic implications.

B. Fetal Thyroid Function

Fetal thyroid hormone production does not start until the end of the first trimester. Normal fetal development is dependent on normal maternal thyroid function.

C. Epidemiology

The incidence of hyperthryoidism in pregnancy is 2 per 1000 and hypothyroidism is 1 per 2000.

D. Preconception Care and Risk Assessment

Patients usually require a euthyroid state in order to conceive. Infertility is common in clinically hypothyroid patients with anovulatory cycles. Treatment of hypothyroidism reverses this problem. Careful attention and evaluation is warranted if a

TABLE 4.   Changes in Thyroid Function with Pregnancy

Test	Changes	Normal values
Thyroxine-binding globulin	Increased	30–50 mg/L
T_3RU	Decreased	25–35
T_4 (total)	Increased	9–16 mg/dl
TSH	Unchanged except decreased first trimester	0.3–6 (varies with laboratory)
Free T_4	Unchanged except increased first trimester	2.5–3.5 ng/100 ml
Serum T_3	Unchanged	150–250 ng/100 ml

medical history includes thyroid problems, medications, prior or current use of iodine- or lithium-containing products, or head and or neck radiation. Physical exam findings of thyroid enlargement or neck scars require further work-up.

E. General Screening for Maternal Hypothyroidism

Universal screening for hypothyroidism in pregnancy has been advocated by some.[13] Haddow et al. in 1999 reported that 7–9-year-old children of women with hypothyroidism during pregnancy had lower IQ scores than control children.[13] These interpretations are controversial because of methodologic and testing differences. Universal screening for thyroid disease with thyroid function tests during pregnancy is not recommended, but should be based on symptoms and history of thyroid disease.[26]

F. Hyperthyroidism in Pregnancy

1. Clinical diagnosis of hyperthyroidism

This is difficult since many of the signs of hyperthyroidism can also be found in normal pregnancy. Anxiety, increased appetite, fatigue, heat intolerance, tremor, emotional instability, and thyroid enlargement are common to both conditions. Signs of hyperthyroidism that are uncommon in normal pregnancy include unanticipated weight loss and sinus tachycardia.

2. Laboratory diagnosis of hyperthyroidism

A decrease in serum TSH and an increase in free T_4 are seen. However, these findings are common in the first trimester because beta HCG has a TSH-like effect on maternal thyroid function. Abnormalities can be detected first in free T_4 levels when compared to TSH. Since mild to moderate hyperthyroidism is generally tolerated, borderline tests may be repeated in 3–4 weeks. An elevated thyroid-stimulating immunoglobulin (TSI) performed at 28–30 weeks can help predict fetal hyperthyroidism.[19]

3. Differential diagnosis

The most common cause of hyperthyroidism during pregnancy is Graves' disease. It accounts for 90–95% of all cases. Graves' disease is caused by hyperstimulation of the thyroid follicle cell by TSI antibodies. Graves' disease has the distinguishing features of nontender goiter and ophthalmopathy. An elevated serum TSI assists in making the diagnosis. During pregnancy the natural history of Graves' disease is one of aggravation in the first trimester, spontaneous improvement during the second half of pregnancy, and worsening in the postpartum period.

    a. Previously diagnosed Graves' disease, now off medication. Patients previously diagnosed with Graves' disease but not taking any antithyroid medication require early and frequent thyroid function monitoring due to the risk of recurrence during pregnancy.

    b. Previously diagnosed and treated patients with Graves' disease. Patients who are taking antithyroid medication require close thyroid function monitoring, and the decision to continue medication should rest on thyroid function evaluation.[9]

4. Other causes of hyperthyroidism

Other causes of hyperthyroidism in pregnancy include gestational trophoblastic disease (i.e., hydatidiform mole and choriocarcinoma) and hyperemesis gravidarum. Both of these diseases must be ruled out in hyperthyroidism.

5. Treatment

    a. Preconception concerns. Because hyperthyroidism may complicate pregnancy, every effort should be made to provide definitive treatment before pregnancy.[4,14] and to ensure effective contraception for the patient until her medical condition is stabilized. Improved outcomes with preconceptive treatment vs. during pregnancy have been documented.[5]

b. Radioactive iodine (inadvertent). Fetuses who are inadvertently exposed to ^{131}I are at high risk for the athyreotic state with all the problems of congenital hypothyroidism because the fetus concentrates iodine starting in the 12th week of pregnancy. Recommendations include consideration of therapeutic abortion.

c. Antithyroid drugs. Antithyroid drugs appear to be the treatment of choice for sustained hyperthyroidism needing treatment during pregnancy. More transient conditions, such as viral thyroiditis, rarely need treatment; symptomatic patients may benefit from short-term administration of blockers in this circumstance. Propylthiouracil (PTU) is the drug of choice because methimazole has been associated with aplasia cutis (a reversible scalp defect) and crosses the placenta more readily than PTU. If antithyroid medication must be discontinued because of serious reactions to the drug (agranulocytosis), beta-blockade may be used with consideration of partial thyroidectomy.

 i. PTU should be administered in larger doses initially to shorten the duration of hyperthyroidism with tapering of doses as the patient's condition permits. One third of patients improve sufficiently so that PTU may be discontinued in the third trimester.[14] Because the fetus is more sensitive to the effects of PTU than the mother, the dosage should be adjusted to maintain the patient in the mildly hyperthyroid range. This minimizes the risks of hypothyroidism to the fetus.[14] Patient noncompliance and failure to maintain adequate supervision of PTU therapy pose a significant hazard to the fetus.

 ii. Beta-blockers may be used on a short-term basis for control of symptoms. A goal of therapy is maternal heart rate less than 90 bpm. Long-term administration of beta-blockers in pregnancy has been associated with growth restriction and poor fetal outcome, but most of these studies are difficult to interpret because of methodologic problems and the confounding influence of the disease state treated.[22] Beta-blockers do not offer any advantage for long-term treatment of hyperthyroidism and do not prevent fetal hyperthyroidism, whereas PTU does treat the fetal thyroid gland.

d. Surgical intervention. In cases of severe complications due to thyrotoxicosis when medical management has failed, a thyroidectomy or subtotal thyroidectomy must be considered.

e. Treatment of thyroid storm or congestive heart failure. One gram of potassium iodide and 1 gram of PTU can be given orally or via nasogastric tube, with careful attention to exacerbating factors, such as infection and anemia. Beta-blockade can be used to treat the hemodynamic state. Caution has been urged regarding the use of beta-blockade in congestive heart failure, but most cases of congestive heart failure should be amenable to this therapy because failure from hyperthyroidism is generally high-output congestive heart failure. Potassium iodide (Lugol's solution) should not be used for more than 1 to 2 weeks.

6. Fetal and neonatal concerns

a. Fetal effects. When a pregnancy is complicated by thyrotoxicosis and the accompanying medications, the fetus is at risk for hyperthyroidism or hypothyroidism. Fetal hyperthyroidism may be characterized by fetal tachycardia (> 160 beats/min), IUGR, and craniosynostosis.[3] The fetal thyroid can be stimulated by TSIs starting between 20–24 weeks.[5,14] A difficult diagnostic situation occurs when the maternal thyroid function is normal but fetal thyrotoxicosis exists if previous treatment for Graves' disease included radioactive iodine or thyroidectomy.[5] If fetal hypothyroidism or hyperthyroidism is detected, these patients should be managed in a tertiary setting. Fetal hyperthyroidism has been treated with maternal administration of PTU.

b. Neonatal effects. When maternal hyperthyroidism is controlled by thionamides, neonatal hyperthyroidism may not be present at birth. Falling maternal immunoglobulins and decreasing thionamide levels can to symptoms such as mild irritability, tachycardia, poor feeding, goiter, heart failure, jaundice, exophthalmos, and thrombocytopenia.[5] Cord blood and fetal serum (day of life 1–2) should be used for diagnostic thyroid evaluation (free T_4/TSH).

G. Hypothyroidism in Pregnancy

1. Maternal Effects

   a. Diagnosis. As with hyperthyroidism, the diagnosis of hypothyroidism is complicated by pregnancy being a hypermetabolic state. Classic symptoms include modest weight gain, fatigue, cold intolerance, dry skin, and constipation. The thyroid gland may be enlarged or undetectable. Making the diagnosis is imperative due to its complications. Spontaneous abortion and stillbirth rates are doubled if hypothyroidism is untreated. Institution of treatment prevents the increase in stillbirth and abortion but not an increased rate of congenital anomalies.[23] Preeclampsia, anemia, placental abruption, and heart failure have an increased frequency.[7] Maternal hypothyroidism may be a predisposing factor to aneuploidy and Down syndrome in young women.[11]

   b. Laboratory diagnosis of primary hypothyroidism. This is made when TSH is elevated and free T_4 is decreased. In subclinical hypothyroidism TSH is elevated with a normal free T_4.

   c. Differential diagnosis

      i. Hashimoto's thyroiditis. The most common cause of hypothyroidism in pregnancy is Hashimoto's thyroiditis. Autoantibodies to thyroglobulin and antimicrosomal antibodies can be measured. This is pertinent because these autoantibodies can cross the placenta and cause hypothyroidism in the neonate.[18] Hashimoto's thyroiditis is common in insulin-dependent diabetics, occurring in 20% of class D and F diabetics.[23]

      ii. Other causes of hypothyroidism in pregnancy include Hashimoto's disease, post-thyroid ablation, iodine defiency, primary atrophic hypothyroidism, and infiltrative disease.[10] Drugs associated with hypothyroidism include carbamazepine, phenytoin, lithium, iodides, and thionamides. There is a causal association between lithium and iodides with hypothyroidism. An unusual cause of maternal and fetal hypothyroidism in the U.S. is iodine deficiency with subsequent goiter. This is a common cause of goiter in many endemic areas in the world.

2. Treatment

   a. Pre-existing hypothyroidism. This condition may require up to a 50% increase in dosage during pregnancy, thus close monitoring of levels is important.[17,24] If there is a previous diagnosis of hypothyroidism that is in doubt, and the patient is on replacement therapy, medication should be continued. A therapeutic trial off thyroid replacement medication should not be attempted during pregnancy.

   b. Increased risk for anomalies. Patients who were hypothyroid in early pregnancy should have ultrasound evaluation for congenital anomalies.[21]

    c. Initiation of therapy in a newly diagnosed patient. This may be started at an average daily dose of 0.10–0.15 mg/day of L-thyroxine. Increases can be made every 4 wks. TSH levels need to be monitored at least every 6 weeks since increased levels of thyroid are needed in the later stages of pregnancy.

3. Fetal and neonatal concerns

    a. Fetal hypothyroidism is associated with craniosynostosis, cardiomegaly, and prematurity. Fetal hypothyroidism may be accompanied by goiter sufficient to prevent vaginal delivery and polyhydramnios (probably owing to inadequate fetal swallowing). Fetal hypothyroidism may be the result of inadvertent ^{131}I administration before the diagnosis of pregnancy or due to maternal PTU therapy, because PTU crosses the placenta. It may also occur with prolonged exposure to iodide, which readily crosses the placenta after 10–12 weeks' gestation. Fetal hypothyroidism is a theoretical risk for any pregnancy occurring within 12 months of ^{131}I administration, although this has not been observed clinically.[4] Fetal hypothyroidism has been documented with percutaneous umbilical vein sampling and treated with intramniotic instillation of L-thyroxine.

    b. Neonatal hypothyroidism. This may present with prolonged gestation, macrosomia, feeding and respiratory difficulties, constipation, abdominal distention, vomiting, and prolonged jaundice. Other features are a large posterior fontanelle (delayed bony maturation); coarse, dry skin; hypothermia; and umbilical hernia. Although routine neonatal screening occurs in most states, diagnosis should not await the results of this routine screen in an infant with suspicious findings or in situations of known increased risk (in which cord blood studies may be sent immediately). T_4 values < 4 µg/100 ml and TSH > 80 µU/100 ml are diagnostic. T_4 values of 4–7 µg/100 ml and TSH values of 20–80 µU/100 ml are borderline and require further evaluation. Bone-age films, especially delayed ossification of the distal or proximal femoral epiphysis, are helpful.

H. Evaluation of Goiter and Thyroid Masses During Pregnancy

Slight enlargement of the thyroid is common in pregnancy. The enlarged gland should be soft and homogeneous in texture and nontender to palpation. Patients with a thyroid mass should have an ultrasound scan of the thyroid as well as thyroid function tests. Radionucleotide scanning should not be performed. Fine-needle aspiration of a single nodule is safe during pregnancy. Thyroid cancer is rare in pregnancy.

References

1. Amir SM, Osanthonondh R, Berkowitz RW, et al: Human chorionic gonadotropin and thyroid function in patients with hydatiform mole. Am J Obstet Gynecol 150:723–728, 1984.
2. Ball R, Freedman DB, Holmes JC, et al: Low-normal concentrations of free thyroxine in serum in late pregnancy: Physiological fact, not detected artifact. Clin Chem 35:1891–1896, 1989.
3. Becks GP, Burrow G: Thyroid disease and pregnancy. Med Clin North Am 75:121–150, 1991.
4. Cefalo RC: Thyroid disorders. In Cefalo RC, Moos MK (eds): Preconceptional Health Promotion: A Practical Guide. Rockville, MD, Aspen Publishers, 1988, pp 112–115.
5. Creasy RK, Resnik R: Maternal-Fetal Medicine, 4th ed. Philadelphia, W.B. Saunders, 1999.
6. Crump WJ, Aten LA: Hyperemesis, hyperthyroidism, or both? J Fam Pract 35:450–456, 1992.
7. Davis LF, Leveno KJ, Cunningham FG: Hypothyroidism complicating pregnancy. Obstet Gynecol 72:108–112, 1988.
8. Davis LE, Lucas MJ, Hankins GDV, et al: Thyrotoxicosis complicating pregnancy. Am J Obstet Gynecol 160:63–70, 1989.
9. Deutchman M: Thyroid disease during and after pregnancy. Utah Family Practice Refresher Course, March 29, 2000.
10. Fantz CR, Fantz CR, Dagogo-Jack S, Ladenson JH, Gronowski AM: Thyroid function during pregnancy. Clin Chem 45:2250–2258, 1999.

11. Fialkow PJ, Glinoer D, de Nayer P, Bourdoux P, et al: Autoimmunity and chromosomal aberrations. Am J Hum Genet 18:93–108, 1966.
12. Glinoer D, et al: Regulation of maternal thyroid during pregnancy. J Clin Endocrinol Metab 71:276–287, 1990.
13. Haddow JE, Palomaki GE, Allan WC, et al., Maternal thyroid deficiency during pregnancy and subsequent neuropsychological development of the child. N Engl J Med 341:549–555, 1999.
14. Hamburger JL: Diagnosis and management of grave's disease in pregnancy. Thyroid 2:219–225,1992.
15. Kimura M, Amino N, Tamaki H, et al: Physiologic thyroid activation in normal early pregnancy is induced by circulating hCG. Obstet Gynecol 75:775–778, 1990.
16. Lazarus JH: Hyperthyroidism. Lancet 349:339–343, 1997.
17. Mandel SJ, Larsen PR, Seely EW, et al: Increased need for thyroxine during pregnancy in women with primary hypothyroidism. N Engl J Med 323:91–96, 1990.
18. Matsuura N, Konishi J, Fujieda K, et al: TSH-receptor antibodies in mothers with Graves' disease and outcome in their offspring. Lancet 1:14–17, 1988.
19. Mitsuda N, Tamaki H, Amino N, et al: Risk factors for developmental disorders in infants born to women with Graves' disease. Obstet Gynecol 80:359–364, 1992.
20. Mori M, Amino N, Tamaki H, et al: Morning sickness and thyroid function in normal pregnancy. Obstet Gynecol 72:355–359, 1988.
21. Potter JD: Hypothyroidism and reproductive failure. Surg Gynecol Obstet 150:251–255, 1980.
22. Rubin PC: Beta-blockers in pregnancy. N Engl J Med 305:1323–1326, 1981.
23. Soler NG, Nicholson H: Diabetes and thyroid disease during pregnancy. Obstet Gynecol 54:318–321, 1979.
24. Tamaki H, Amino N, Takeoka K, et al: Thyroxine requirement during pregnancy for replacement therapy of hypothyroidism. Obstet Gynecol 76:230–233, 1990.
25. Thyroid Disease in Pregnancy. ACOG Technical Bulletin, Number 181, 1993.
26. U.S. Preventive Task Force Guidelines: Metabolic, nutritional, and environmental disorders. In Guide to Clinical Preventive Services, 2nd ed, 1996, pp 209–218.

SECTION J.
AUTOIMMUNE CONDITIONS

Multiple conditions are noted in pregnancy in which autoantibodies affect pregnancy outcome by transplacental passage or effects on the placenta or maternal physiology. In general, autoimmune conditions that necessitate corticosteroid therapy are best treated with prednisone or hydrocortisone because these substances are oxidized to relatively inactive forms by the placenta, decreasing the effect on the fetus. Fetal adrenal suppression is an extremely rare event in patients treated with steroids. Consideration of maternal steroid therapy should be based on maternal indications and also may be influenced by the desirable effect on the fetus of stabilizing the maternal condition. Patients who are on long-term steroid therapy require stress doses of corticosteroids for infection, the intrapartum period, and operations.

I. Rheumatoid Arthritis
A. Natural History in Pregnancy
The clinical course of rheumatoid arthritis is generally improved during pregnancy, with more than 70% experiencing improvement.[6] This appears to be related to maternal T cell function in some maternal HLA types. Other than rare cases of vasculitis, there do not appear to be any increased risks to the fetus for patients with rheumatoid arthritis.
B. Use of Medications
Drugs commonly used in disease-modifying therapy (gold, methotrexate, and penicillamine) are not recommended in pregnancy. The following medications may be used and in some cases require special precautions.
    1. Corticosteroids
    Corticosteroids may be used and require close monitoring for complications such as steroid-induced hyperglycemia.

2. Antimalarials

These agents may be used to treat either rheumatoid arthritis or systemic lupus, erythematosus with hydroxychloroquine exhibiting less toxicity than chloroquine.

3. Nonsteroidal anti-inflammatory agents

Non-steroidal anti-inflammatory medications should be stopped at least 8 weeks prior to anticipated delivery to prevent problems in the fetus such as persistent fetal circulation, premature constriction of the ductus, and impaired renal function as well as bleeding risks in the mother.[7]

4. Other agents

Sulfasalazine may also be continued, as well as cyclosporine in women with severe rheumatoid arthritis.[18,19]

C. Intrapartum Management

A few patients with hip contractures may experience some need for modification of delivery practices. A lateral Sims' position may be more comfortable.

II. Systemic Lupus Erythematosus (SLE) and Antiphospholipid Syndrome

These conditions are discussed together because there is some overlap in patients with SLE and patients with lupus anticoagulant and anticardiolipin antibody.

A. Effect of Pregnancy on SLE

The natural history of lupus in pregnancy is variable. Patients with quiescent disease often do well. Conflicting information exists about the tendency for lupus to flare during pregnancy. Recent studies have found no increase in lupus flares and no long-term impact on the disease except in certain situations.[13,17] Other studies have found increased flares, whether or not the patient was taking steroids, but these flares were not more severe than outside of pregnancy.[22] Specific situations that increase maternal risk include:

1. Lupus nephritis

This condition has been associated with a significant risk of deterioration in renal function. In several case series, approximately 7% of patients progressed to end-stage renal disease.[1,2] Creatinine values > 1.5 mg/dl are indicators of greater risk for deterioration. Preeclampsia is extremely common in patients with nephropathy, occurring in 72% of patients in one series.[17] The incidence of preeclampsia was 22% in patients without nephropathy.

2. First episode of lupus in pregnancy

The initial presentation of lupus during pregnancy is often predictive of a severe course. Indeed, if the disease is active at the time of conception, there is more chance of exacerbation during pregnancy. Termination of pregnancy does not seem to alter the course of the disease.

3. Treatment

Medications that may be continued through pregnancy include systemic steroids (prednisone and prednisolone) and hydroxychloroquine.[21]

B. Effect of SLE on Pregnancy

1. Increased perinatal morbidity/mortality

This includes an increased incidence of spontaneous abortions (especially in active, uncontrolled disease), premature labor and delivery, small-for-gestation fetuses, and intrauterine fetal demise.

2. Increased severity of lupus

The same patient characteristics that are predictive of the course of lupus in pregnancy are predictive of fetal outcome.

3. Neonatal lupus

This may occur as a complication for patients who have anti-SSA (Ro) and anti-SSB/La antibodies. The neonate may demonstrate typical skin lesions, hemolytic anemia, and thrombocytopenia. The most serious manifestation of neonatal lupus is congenital complete heart block, caused by fibrosis and inflammation of the cardiac conduction system. The dermatologic and hematologic manifestations of neonatal lupus resolve within 6 months, suggesting mediation by maternal antibodies. Many infants affected by complete heart block require permanent cardiac pacing. If complete heart block affects the fetus sufficiently, fetal hydrops and demise may result.

4. Antiphospholipid antibody (APA) syndrome

Another risk factor for poor fetal outcome is the APA syndrome. The APA syndrome is the most highly predictive factor in fetal mortality and morbidity.

C. Antiphospholipid Antibody Syndrome

Ten to thirty percent of patients with SLE are at increased risk for fetal loss, preeclampsia, and IUGR as a result of APA syndrome.

1. Antiphospholipid antibodies

These include lupus anticoagulant and anticardiolipin (ACL) antibody. Other autoantibodies that have been identified include anti-prothrombin (aPT), which appears to be a marker for risk of thrombosis,[1] anti-endothelial cell antibodies (AECA), and von Willebrand factor antigen.[8]

2. Asymptomatic patients with APA

There are women with APA who do not experience fetal loss.[9] The incidence of antiphosholipid antibodies in normal obstetric patients appears to be approximately 5%. ACL antibodies are found in 20% of women with recurrent pregnancy loss, 37% of women with lupus, and 24% of women requiring in vitro fertilization.[11]

3. Symptomatic patients with APA syndrome

These women may demonstrate ACL antibodies (IgG) or lupus anticoagulant. They may also demonstrate thrombocytopenia, hemolytic anemia, arterial or venous thromboses, and placental infarction. Lupus anticoagulant and ACL antibody are also found in women who have no other evidence of SLE and are thus classified as APA syndrome, without lupus.

4. Antiphospholipid antibodies in other illnesses

APA are known to be present in other rheumatic illnesses, and infectious illnesses such as syphilis and HIV infection. Patients with infection-related antibodies have predominantly IgM antibodies and do not demonstrate the syndrome of fetal loss. IgM anticardiolipin antibodies alone do not support the diagnosis of APA syndrome;[4] patients with APA syndrome should demonstrate IgG antibodies.

5. Pathophysiology

Mechanisms that have been proposed include decreased prostacycline production by endothelial cells, increased thromboxane production by platelets, and decreased protein C activation. The antiphospholipid antigen appears to be a complex formed between beta-2 glycoprotein 1 and phospholipids.[17]

6. Lupus anticoagulant

This antibody appears to be more predictive of thrombotic complications. IgG APA measured by enzyme-linked immunosorbent assay (otherwise referred to as ACL antibody) in high titers is more predictive of pregnancies at risk for fetal death. Titers > 40 GPL units are significant. Low titers of 5–40 GPL are nonspecific and of little clinical significance.[23]

D. Management of Lupus in Pregnancy

1. Screening for APA syndrome

Current recommendations include screening of patients with two or more pregnancy losses for APA syndrome.[23] The frequency of moderate-to-high-titer IgG antiphospholipid antibodies in this subset of patients is about 10%. Pregnancy losses should be defined as fetal (not early pregnancy). In a study of recurrent pregnancy loss in a tertiary center, fetal death (one or more) was 76% specific for the presence of APA IgG. Early first-trimester losses were only associated with APA in 6% of cases.[20]

2. Management of APA syndrome

Both low-dose aspirin and prednisone or prednisolone and low-dose aspirin and heparin have been investigated as a means of improving pregnancy outcome in APA syndrome.[7,16] This area remains somewhat controversial, since a large study has found that prednisone and aspirin did not increase the rate of live birth but increased the rate of prematurity, hypertension, and diabetes.[12] Another small study using only low dose aspirin (LDA) showed an improved perinatal survival rate of 95% in the APA syndrome with 14% prematurity.[3]

3. Management of the patient with SLE: preconception and early pregnancy

    a. Laboratory evaluation. This includes urinalysis, BUN, creatinine, and 24-hour urine for creatinine clearance and protein, complete blood count, erythrocyte sedimentation rate, antinuclear antibody titers, anti-SSA and anti-SSB, lupus anticoagulant test, and ACL antibody.

    b. Patients with complications. Women with lupus complications who strongly desire pregnancy may benefit from preconception consultation with a perinatologist. High-risk referral is appropriate for most of these patients.

    c. Referral. All patients with antiSSA/Ro or antiSSB/La or APA should be referred.

III. Other Connective Tissue Disorders

A. Sjögren's Syndrome

This syndrome has been studied in a relatively small series demonstrating increased fetal loss with a relative risk of 2.7 (95% CI 1.1–6.5; $p = 0.023$). This risk is similar to that with SLE, but fetal growth restriction and prematurity were seen less frequently than in pregnancies with lupus.[10]

B. Scleroderma

Limited information is available about scleroderma. It appears that the extent of cardiac, renal, and pulmonary disease is more important than duration of disease.[2]

References

1. Bertolaccini ML, Atsumi K, Khamashta MA, Amengual O, Hughes GR: Autoantibodies to human pro-thrombin and clinical manifestations in 207 patients with systemic lupus erythematosus. J Rheumatol 25:1104–1108, 1998.
2. Bobrie G, Liote F, Houillier P, et al: Pregnancy in lupus nephritis and related disorders. Am J Kidney Dis 9:339–343, 1987.
3. Botet F, Romera G, Montagut P, et al: Neonatal outcome in women treated for antiphospholipid syndrome during pregnancy. J Perinat Med 25:192–196, 1997.
4. Branch DW: Antiphospholipid antibodies and reproductive outcome: The current status of affairs. J Reprod Immunol 38:75–87, 1998.
5. Burkett G: Lupus nephropathy and pregnancy. Clin Obstet Gynecol 28:310–323, 1985.
6. Buyon JP: The effects of pregnancy on autoimmune diseases. J Leukoc Biol 63:281–287,1998.
7. Cowchock FS, Reece EA, Balaban D, et al: Repeated fetal losses associated with antiphospholipid antibodies: A collaborative randomized trial comparing prednisone to low-dose heparin treatment. Am J Obstet Gynecol 166:1318–1323, 1992.
8. Direskenili H, Buchanan NM, Khamashta MA, et al: Markers of vascular damage in lupus pregnancy. Clin Exp Rheumatol 15:535–539, 1997.
9. Harris EN, Spinnato JA: Should anticardiolipin tests be performed in otherwise healthy pregnant women? Am J Obstet Gynecol 165:1272–1277, 1991.
10. Julkunen H, Kaaja R, Kurki P, Pauusuo T, Friman C: Fetal outcome in women with primary Sjögren's syndrome. A retrospective case-control study. Clin Exp Rheumatol 13:65–71, 1995.

11. Kutteh WH: Antiphospholipid antibodies and reproduction. J Reprod Immunol 35:151–171, 1997.
12. Laskin CA, Bombardier C, Hannah ME, et al: Prednisone and aspirin in women with autoantibodies and unexplained recurrent fetal loss. N Engl J Med 337:148–153, 1997.
13. Lockshin MD: Antiphospholipid antibody syndrome. JAMA 268:1451–1453, 1992.
14. Lockshin MD, Qamar T, Druzin ML: Hazards of lupus pregnancy. J Rheumatol 14:214–217, 1987.
15. Lockshin MD, Sammaritano LR: Antiphospholipid antibodies and fetal loss. N Engl J Med 326:951–952, 1992.
16. Lubbe WF, Palmer SJ, Butler WS, Liggins GC: Fetal survival after prednisone suppression of maternal lupus-anticoagulant. Lancet 1:1361–1363, 1983.
17. Mintz R, Niz J, Gutierrez G, et al: Prospective study of pregnancy in systemic lupus erythematosus: Results of a multidisciplinary approach. J Rheumatol 13:732–739, 1986.
18. Oetesen M: Optimisation of antirheumatic drug treatment in pregnancy. Clin Pharmacokinet 27:486–502, 1994.
19. Oetesen M, Ramsey-Goldman R: Treatment of inflammatory rheumatic disorders in pregnancy: What are the safest treatment options? Drug Saf 19:389–410, 1998.
20. Ohiro BT, Silver RM, Scott JR, et al: Antiphospholipid antibodies and fetal death. Obstet Gynecol 87:489–493, 1996.
21. Parke A, West B: Hydroxychloroquine in pregnant patients with systemic lupus erythematosus. J Rheumatol 23:1715–1718, 1996.
22. Ruiz-Irastorza G, Lima F, Alves J, et al: Increased rate of lupus flares during pregnancy and the puerperium: A prospective study of 78 pregnancies. Br J Rheumatol 35:133–138, 1996.
23. Stuart RA, Kornman LH, McHugh NJ: A prospective study of pregnancy outcome in women screened at a routine antenatal clinic for anticardiolipin antibodies. Br J Obstet Gynaecol 100:599–600, 1993.

CHAPTER 8

Commonly Encountered Medical Problems in Pregnancy

This chapter provides the practitioner with relevant information about the medical care of pregnant patients. Problems covered include frequently encountered infections, abdominal pain, trauma, cervical dysplasia, and dermatologic conditions. Chronic medical conditions are covered in Chapter 7.

The general format of each section includes clinical information such as prevalence and presentation of the condition, how the presentation and clinical course may be affected by pregnancy, how the condition may affect pregnancy outcome, and specific management guidelines appropriate to pregnancy. Commonly used medications are discussed.

These chapters on common and chronic conditions are not intended to provide in-depth information on complex illnesses. The family physician may provide care for such a patient during her pregnancy, but this often occurs with consultation or referral for high-risk services.

SECTION A.
INFECTIONS IN PREGNANCY

Stephen D. Ratcliffe, M.D., M.S.P.H.

Infectious illnesses are commonly encountered in pregnancy. Many are self-limited and can be addressed solely from the perspective of patient comfort and safe use of medication in pregnancy. Some have substantial impact on the course and outcome of pregnancy. Others pose a significant danger to the neonate. Several conditions are associated with increased complications in pregnancy.

I. General Guidelines for the Use of Antibiotics in Pregnancy
A. Safe Use in Pregnancy (see Chapter 2, section E)
Antibiotics that are classified as category A or B in pregnancy include penicillins, cephalosporins, clindamycin, erythromycin (except estolate because of increased hepatotoxicity in pregnancy), nitrofurantoin, nystatin, azithromycin, and spectinomycin.
B. Use with Caution in Pregnancy
Antibiotics that are classified as category C include acyclovir, vancomycin, and miconazole. Class C antibiotics that should be used only with specific precautions include metronidazole, aminoglycosides, sulfonamides, chloramphenicol, and trimethoprim.
    1. Chloramphenicol
    Chloramphenicol is classified as category C but its use may result in "gray baby syndrome" if used close to term, so it should be avoided except in situations of specific need.

2. Sulfonamides

Sulfonamides theoretically increase the risk of kernicterus in the neonate because of competitive binding of albumin sites. Their use should be avoided in late pregnancy, if possible.

3. Gentamycin

Gentamycin and other aminoglycosides may cause ototoxicity in the fetus. Their use should include the monitoring of levels.

4. Trimethoprim

Trimethoprim is a folate antagonist. There are concerns about its teratogenicity; it should not be used in the first trimester. In the second and third trimesters, concern for its antagonistic effects on folate should be balanced with other clinical considerations.

5. Metronidazole

Metronidazole should not be used in the first trimester although a recent meta-analysis did not find an association between its use in this period and an increased risk of birth defects.[3] It has a class B designation.

C. Unsafe for Use in Pregnancy

Antibiotics classified as category C that should be completely avoided during pregnancy except in severe circumstances in which other medications are not efficacious.

1. Quinolones

Quinolones, category C, have been found to cause cartilage degeneration in animal studies; no information is available about human fetal effects. Quinolones should not be used if class A or B antibiotics can be used as effective treatment.

2. Tetracycline and derivatives

Tetracycline and derivatives are associated with staining of the teeth in the fetus and in young children. Their use should be avoided in pregnancy, but inadvertent first-trimester use is not known to be teratogenic. Severe hepatic toxicity has been reported with use during pregnancy.

3. Newer macrolides

Azithromycin is a category B drug and can be used safely. Clarithromycin has been associated with increased embryonic loss and malformations in animal studies. It is classified as category C and should not be used if at all possible.

II. Chlamydia

A. Epidemiology

1. Incidence/Prevalence

Chlamydia trachomatis is the most common bacterial sexually transmitted disease. An estimated 4 million cases occur each year in the United States. Clinicians can expect to find chlamydial infection in 2–25% of their patients.[17]

2. At-risk groups

Chlamydial infections are encountered in all age and socioeconomic groups, although teenage and college-age women are at increased risk, particularly if they have been engaged in unsafe sexual practices and have had multiple sexual partners.[12]

B. Natural History

1. Signs and symptoms

Chlamydia infections may demonstrate no specific signs or symptoms. They also may present with mucopurulent cervicitis, excessive friability of the cervix at the time of pelvic examination, or spotting.

2. Pelvic inflammatory disease

Approximately 25% of untreated chlamydial infections develop into pelvic inflammatory disease (PID) with a number of life-long sequelae including ectopic pregnancy and infertility.

3. PID and pregnancy

Upper genital tract infection (pelvic inflammatory disease) is an unusual complication during pregnancy. This may pose a confusing and concerning clinical picture because of consideration of ectopic pregnancy. Demonstration of an intrauterine gestation is essential in a first-trimester patient with pelvic pain (see Chapter 5, section A).

4. Differential diagnosis

The differential diagnosis of chlamydia cervicitis includes trichomonal, gonorrheal, ureaplasma, and mycoplasma infections.

C. Effects on Perinatal Outcome

1. Prenatal

Chlamydia infections are associated with increased rates of preterm labor and premature rupture of membranes, particularly if infection is recent or invasive as evidenced by IgM antibodies.

2. Neonatal

Chlamydia conjunctivitis occurs in about 20% of neonates whose mothers are infected with chlamydia despite the prophylactic use of topical silver nitrate and antibiotic ointment. Pneumonia occurs in 11–18% of these infants.

3. Late-onset endometritis

More than 50% of patients presenting with late-onset endometritis following vaginal delivery have positive cultures for chlamydia.[7] Chlamydia does not have an association with early-onset endometritis.[16]

4. Treatment of chlamydia in pregnancy

Successful treatment of patients with chlamydia infection has been shown to decrease rates of preterm labor and preterm premature rupture of the membranes in one study. In this study, the comparison groups were women who were not successfully treated and a control group that was at risk for chlamydia infection but had negative antepartum cultures.[13] This favorable outcome was not demonstrated in the Vaginal Infections and Prematurity Study (VIPS) group.[10] Antepartum treatment of infected pregnant women has been shown to decrease rates of infection in offspring from 70% to 50%.[5]

D. Diagnosis

1. Symptomatic infection

Identification of cervicitis occurs via mucopurulent discharge, excessive friability, or complaints of spotting (including post-coital). Wet preparation demonstrates increased leukocytes.

2. Routine screening

Routine screening in populations at increased risk is recommended. The CDC defines this group to include women less than 20 years old, with other STDs, with a new partner or more than one in the preceding 3 months, and women who do not use a barrier method of contraception. The CDC also recommends repeat screening for these at-risk groups early in the third trimester.[4]

3. Preterm labor

Chlamydia testing of any patient who presents with preterm labor or preterm premature rupture of membranes should be considered because of the high rates of transmitted infection to the fetus, although there are no randomized controlled trial (RCT) data to support this intervention.

4. Testing techniques

Acceptable testing techniques include rapid monoclonal fluorescent-antibody staining, enzyme-linked immunoassay, culture, direct gene probe, and DNA amplification assays (polymerase chain reaction, ligase chain reaction).[17] The first three testing techniques have a sensitivity of about 75%, which means about one in four cases of chlamydia will be missed (25% false-negative rate); the direct gene probe technology has a sensitivity of approximately 90%. The ligase chain reaction technology can be used using urine specimens and achieve a sensitivity of 96% and a specificity of 99%.[6] The superior sensitivity and specificity of the DNA amplification tests result in a higher positive and negative predictive value for at-risk populations. Practitioners should check the availability and costs of the newer technologies to determine what is most cost-effective in their practices.

E. Treatment

1. Erythromycin

Erythromycin base 500 mg four times a day for 7 days or 250 mg base four times a day for 14 days has been the standard treatment of choice. An alternative is erythromycin ethylsuccinate 800 mg four times a day for 7 days or 400 mg four times a day for 14 days. Erythromycin estolate should not be used in pregnancy.

2. Amoxicillin

An emerging alternative is amoxicillin, 500 mg three times a day for 7 days. Meta-analyses confirm equivalent test of cure rates and compliance with this regimen is superior to that of erythromycin.[2,15] This regimen has also been deemed most cost-effective.[8]

3. Clindamycin

Clindamycin, 450 mg four times a day for 2 weeks, is also an acceptable regimen but is much more costly than those listed above.

4. Azithromycin

Azithromycin, 1 g as a single dose or 500 mg in two doses is as effective as a 7-day course of doxycycline in nonpregnant women.[9] Azithromycin is a class B agent. In a recent RCT, a 1-g dose of azithromycin was as efficacious as a 7-day course of erythromycin with fewer gastrointestinal side effects.[1]

5. Tetracycline

Tetracycline derivatives, quinolones, and clarithromycin are not indicated in pregnancy.

6. Test-of-cure/treatment of partners

Test-of-cure culture or other testing technique should be performed after completion of therapy. Treatment of the patient's sexual partner is essential.

7. Repeat screening for high-risk patients

Patients judged to be at high risk of contracting chlamydia, such as adolescents, should undergo repeat chlamydial testing in the third trimester because recurrent infection is common.[11]

F. Prevention

There is strong evidence that population-based screening for asymptomatic chlamydia infections results in a decreased prevalence of this infection and its complications.[14] The CDC recommends screening women who are 24 or younger. Women older than 24 who have recently begun a new sexual relationship are also candidates for screening in the asymptomatic state.

References

1. Adair C, Gunter M, Stovall T, et al: Chlamydia in pregnancy: A randomized trial of azithromycin and erythromycin. Obstet Gynecol 91:165–168,1998.
2. Brocklehurst P, Rooney G: The treatment of genital chlamydia infection in pregnancy. (Cochrane Review). In The Cochrane Library, Issue 4, 2000. Oxford, Update Software.
3. Cano-Paton T, Carvajal A, Martin de Diego I, et al: Is metronidazole teratogenic? A meta-analysis. Br J Clin Pharmacol 44:179–182, 1997.
4. Centers for Disease Control: Recommendations for the prevention and management of *Chlamydia trachomatis* infections. MMWR 42:1–39, 1993.

5. Cohen I, Veille JC, Calkins BM: Improved pregnancy outcome following successful treatment of chlamydial infections. JAMA 263:3160–3163, 1990.
6. Gaydos C, Howell M, Quinn T, et al: Use of ligase chain reaction with urine versus cervical culture for detection of *Chlamydia trachomatis* in an asymptomatic military population of pregnant and non-pregnant females attending papanicolaou smear clinics. J Clin Microbiol 36:1300-1304, 1998.
7. Hoyme VB, Kiviat N, Eschenbach DA: The microbiology and treatment of late post-partum endometritis. Obstet Gynecol 68:226–230, 1986.
8. Hueston W, Lenhart J: A decision analysis to guide antibiotic selection for *Chlamydia* infection during pregnancy. Arch Fam Med 6:551–555, 1997.
9. Martin D, Mroczkowski T, Dalu Z, et al: A controlled trial of a single dose of azithromycin for the treatment of chlamydial urethritis and cervicitis. N Engl J Med 327:921–925, 1992.
10. Martin D: Vaginal Infections and Prematurity Study Group: Erythromycin treatment of *Chlamydia trachomatis* infections during pregnancy. Abstract No. 683. 30th Interscience Conference on Antimicrobial Agents and Chemotherapy. Atlanta, GA, October 1990.
11. Miller J: Recurrent chlamydial colonization during pregnancy. Am J Perinatol 15:307–309, 1998.
12. Oh M, Richey C, Pate M, et al: High prevalence of *Chlamydia trachomatis* infections in adolescent females not having pelvic examinations: Utility of PCR-based urine screening in urban adolescent clinic setting. J Adolesc Health 21:80–86, 1997.
13. Ryan G, Abdella T, McNeeley S, et al: *Chlamydia trachomatis* infection in pregnancy and effect of treatment on outcome. Am J Obstet Gynecol 162:34–39, 1990.
14. Scholes D, Stergachis A, Heidrich F, et al: Prevention of pelvic inflammatory disease by screening for cervical chlamydial infection. N Engl J Med 334:1842–1846, 1994.
15. Turrentine MA, Newton ER: Amoxicillin or erythromycin for the treatment of antenatal chlamydial infection: A meta-analysis. Obstet Gynecol 86:1021–1025, 1995.
16. Watts DH, Eschenbach DA, Kenny GE: Early post-partum endometritis: The role of bacteria, genital mycoplasmas, and *Chlamydia trachomatis*. Obstet Gynecol 73:52–57, 1989.
17. Wendel P, Wendel G: Sexually transmitted diseases in pregnancy. Semins in Perinatol 17:443–451, 1993.

III. Gonorrhea

A. Epidemiology[2]

The prevalence is estimated to be 1–7.5% and is greater in inner-city and low socioeconomic status populations. Over the past 25 years, the overall incidence of gonorrhea has declined.

B. Natural History[1–3]

The endocervical canal and urethra are usually infected with these bacteria. Symptoms include dysuria, vaginal discharge, and abnormal vaginal bleeding. Signs include mucopurulent endocervical discharge and/or cervical friability and erythema.

C. Diagnosis

Recovery rate of cultures is higher if appropriate technique is observed (endocervical canal thoroughly swabbed, careful use of transport media or direct plating on Thayer-Martin culture media, increased pick-up with urethral and anal culture). The sensitivity of culture is between 80% and 90%.[2] Gram stain of cervical discharge is unacceptable for diagnosis owing to normal vaginal commensal organisms (sensitivity 50–70%, specificity 97%). There is insufficient evidence to support the use of wet mount to predict which patients are at increased risk of gonorrhea.[4,8] DNA probe technology and polymerase chain reaction techniques are now readily available in many practice settings. These tests are rapidly replacing culture techniques.

D. Effects on Perinatal Outcome[1,2,6]

1. Effects on the mother and fetus
   a. Pelvic inflammatory disease (rare, in first trimester)
   b. Septic abortion
   c. Preterm premature rupture of membranes
   d. Preterm labor
   e. Chorioamnionitis
   f. Puerperal sepsis

2. Effects on the neonate

About one third of exposed neonates (including infants born by cesarean section after rupture of membranes) develop infection.[2,7]

    a. Gonococcal ophthalmia neonatorum.[7] This results in acute purulent conjunctivitis in the first week of life; untreated infants may develop corneal ulceration, panophthalmitis, and loss of the eye. Before topical silver nitrate or erythromycin prophylaxis, this was a major cause of blindness.

    b. Other neonatal infections include:

       i. Gonococcemia
       ii. Septic arthritis
       iii. Pharyngitis
       iv. Proctitis
       v. Vaginitis
       vi. Scalp abscesses
       vii. Meningitis

E. Management Guidelines[2,5]

1. Beta-lactamase resistance

This is common in the United States at this time; recommended first-line therapy is ceftriaxone 250 mg intramuscularly once.

2. Cephalosporin allergy

If cephalosporin allergy is present, give spectinomycin 2 g intramuscularly.

3. Other precautions

The patient's partner should be treated. A test-of-cure culture and a third-trimester culture should be performed because of risk of treatment failures and recurrent infection.

References

1. Ament LA, Whalen E: Sexually transmitted diseases in pregnancy: Diagnosis, impact, and intervention. JOGNN 25:657–666, 1996.
2. American College of Obstetricians and Gynecologists Technical Bulletin: Gonorrhea and chlamydial infections. Number 190, March 1994.
3. Blanchard AC, Pastorek JG, Weeks T: Pelvic inflammatory disease during pregnancy. South Med J 80:1363–1365, 1987.
4. Bohmer JT, Schemmer G, Harrison F, et al: Cervical wet mount as a negative predictor for gonococci- and *Chlamydia trachomatis*-induced cervicitis in a gravid population. Am J Obstet Gynecol 181:283–287, 1999.
5. Brocklhurst P: Treatment of gonorrhea in pregnancy (Cochrane Review), In The Cochrane Library, Issue 4, 2000. Oxford, Update Software.
6. Edwards LE, Barrada MI, Hamann AA, et al: Gonorrhea in pregnancy. Am J Obstet Gynecol 132:637–641, 1978.
7. Fletcher JL, Gordon RC: Perinatal transmission of bacterial sexually transmitted diseases. Part I: Syphilis and gonorrhea. J Fam Pract 30:448–456, 1990.
8. Majeroni BA, Schank JN, Horwitz M, et al: Use of wet mount to predict *Chlamydia trachomatis* and *Neisseria gonorrhoeae* cervicitis in primary care. Fam Med 28:580–583, 1996.
9. Rothenberg R: Ophthalmia neonatorum due to *Neisseria gonorrhoeae*: Prevention and treatment. Sex Transm Dis 6:187–191, 1979.

IV. Syphilis

A. Epidemiology

1. Incidence/Prevalence

Syphilis is a life-threatening, chronic infection caused by the *Treponema pallidum* spirochete. It is acquired via sexual or congenital transmission. An increase in congenital syphilis occurred in the late 1980s, especially in populations in which drug abuse is common and among patients with late entry into prenatal care.[10] This occurred, in part, because of a revised case definition by the Centers for Disease Control and Prevention (CDC) that considers infants of mothers who have not received any or appropriate treatment during pregnancy to have presumed congenital infection.[11]

B. Natural History

1. Primary syphilis

This is the initial phase of infection and is usually accompanied by the presence of a painless chancre and regional lymphadenopathy. The chancre can persist up to 8 weeks if the infection is untreated. The lymphadenopathy persists well after this.

2. Secondary syphilis

This phase of the infection begins about 6 weeks after the appearance of the chancre and is marked by the following signs and symptoms.[13]

    a. Macular papular rash (90%)

    b. Silver-gray mucosal patches (30%)

    c. White-gray intertriginous patches (condylomata lata) (20%)

    d. Constitutional symptoms, such as fever, headache, malaise, arthralgia, myalgia (70%)

3. Latent syphilis

The signs and symptoms of secondary syphilis resolve in 3–12 weeks without treatment. About 25% of patients will have relapsing symptoms during the first 12-month period, called early latent syphilis. During this initial asymptomatic period, patients are still highly infectious. Late latent syphilis begins after a period of 12 months. Relapses are uncommon and overall infectivity is less.

4. Late/Tertiary syphilis

About 25% of patients who do not receive treatment develop late or tertiary syphilis. Manifestations include:

    a. Gummata. These are locally destructive granulomatous lesions that occur in body tissues including muscle, bone and skin.

    b. Cardiovascular disease. This results in a vasculitis of the aorta that leads to the formation of an aneurysm, most commonly in the ascending portion.

    c. Neurosyphilis. Meningovascular disease results in stroke-like syndromes or in seizure disorders. Parenchymal involvement also can result in stroke-like symptoms or in tabes dorsalis.

C. Effects on Perinatal Outcome[11,13]

Pregnancy does not appear to affect the natural history of syphilis. Syphilis, however, exerts many deleterious effects on pregnancy.

1. Increased perinatal morbidity/mortality

Forty to fifty percent of women who do not receive treatment for syphilis during pregnancy experience the following complications. These risks are also increased when syphilis occurs in its earlier stages (primary, secondary, early latent).

    a. Spontaneous abortion. This can occur throughout pregnancy.

    b. Stillbirth. This is a major cause of stillborn infants in the third world where the diagnosis of syphilis is often missed in pregnancy.[12]

    c. Prematurity

2. Congenital syphilis[13]

Vertical transmission is more common in primary syphilis (70–100%), secondary syphilis, and early latent syphilis with bacteremic relapse (30%).[5] The revised CDC definitions of confirmed and presumed congenital syphilis are found in Table 1. There are two phases of congenital syphilis:

    a. Early congenital syphilis. In neonates with early congenital syphilis, clinical presentation includes hepatosplenomegaly, abdominal distention, nephrotic syndrome, petechiae, hemolytic anemia, thrombocytopenia,

TABLE 1.   Congenital Syphilis Case Definition

Case Type	Description
Confirmed	Infant in whom *T. pallidum* is identified by darkfield microscopy, fluorescent anti-body, or other specific stains in specimens from lesions, placenta, umbilical cord, or autopsy material
Presumed	An infant whose mother had untreated or inadequately treated syphilis at delivery, regardless of findings for the infant Any infant or child with a reactive treponemal test for syphilis and one of the following: Evidence of CS upon physical examination Evidence of CS on long bone radiograph Reactive CSF on a VDRL test Elevated CSF cell count or protein (without other cause) Non-treponemal serologic titers 4-fold higher than the mother's (drawn at birth) Reactive test for FTA-ABS-19S-IgM antibody

From Centers for Disease Control and Prevention: Guidelines for the prevention and control of congenital syphilis. MMWR 37:1–13, 1988.
Inadequate treatment consists of any non-penicillin therapy or penicillin given less than 30 days before delivery.

osteochondritis, periostitis, CNS involvement, and mucocutaneous manifestations. Full discussion of congenital infection and its management is beyond the scope of this chapter.

b. Late congenital syphilis. This is a clinical syndrome that presents after 2 years of age and is a result of an inflammatory response to the initial or persistence of infection. Malformations/abnormalities include abnormal teeth (Hutchinson's teeth), healed chorioretinitis, eighth nerve deafness, cranial nerve palsies, mental retardation, and bony abnormalities such as frontal bossing and saddle-nose deformities.

D. Diagnosis

1. Maternal infection[7]

a. Direct detection. Fluid can be expressed from cutaneous lesions or aspirated from lymph nodes and examined using a darkfield microscope to directly visualize spirochetes. High spirochete loads and an experienced examiner are required. When these conditions are met, the sensitivity is about 80%.

b. Non-treponemal tests. The VDRL or RPR are the screening tests of choice. The sensitivity is only 78–86% for primary infections, increases to 100% for secondary, remains high at 95–98% for latent infections, and drops to 72–73% for tertiary syphilis. The specificity remains at 97–99% for all stages of the infection yielding a false-positive rate of 1–3%. False-positive tests may occur in the setting of other infections, malignancies, autoimmune disorders, aging, and illicit parenteral drug use.[13]

c. Treponemal tests. The two available tests are the fluorescent treponemal antibody absorption (FTA) and the microhemagglutination (MHA). These tests have sensitivities and specificities comparable to the non-treponemal methods and are used to confirm the diagnoses of a positive VDRL or RPR. If the non-treponemal test is positive and the treponemal test is nonreactive without clinical evidence of disease, both tests should be repeated within 4 weeks. If the FTA or MHA remain negative, it can be assumed that the non-treponemal test was a false-positive result.

2. Prenatal diagnosis of fetal syphilis[11]

The diagnosis of fetal syphilis can be made when the mother is seropositive for infection and the ultrasound identifies hydrops fetalis characterized by skin

thickening, intra-abdominal and pleural effusions, hepatomegaly, and polyhydramnios. Cordocentesis and amniocentesis may be used to confirm the diagnosis.
3. Diagnosis of congenital syphilis (see Table 1)

E. Treatment

If clinical or serologic evidence of infection is present, the patient should be treated per CDC guidelines.
1. Primary, secondary and early latent disease[13]
Administer benzathine penicillin 2.4 million units intramuscularly once. Some authors recommend two injections spaced by 1 week. For latent disease with unknown duration or greater than 1 year, treatment should be weekly for 3 weeks. RPR or VDRL titers should be monitored on a monthly basis to document response to therapy. A four-fold drop in the titer should occur after 3–6 months, and an eightfold drop by 6–12 months.[11] The treponemal antibody level (FTA or MHA) will remain positive despite treatment. Treatment failures are rare among women with primary or tertiary syphilis.[1,4] Failure rates of 5-6% in secondary and 2% in early latent syphilis have been reported.
2. Penicillin-allergic patients
The approximate 5–10% of women who are penicillin-allergic can be identified with skin testing and safely undergo oral penicillin desensitization.[15]
3. Jarisch-Herxheimer reaction[6]
The Jarisch-Herxheimer reaction is common in the earlier stages of syphilis (60–100%), characterized by maternal fever, tachycardia, hypotension, myalgias, and headache. Pregnant patients may experience, in addition, uterine contractions, decreased fetal movement, fetal tachycardia, and decreased variability noted by fetal monitoring. Transient late decelerations have also been noted with monitoring of contractions. This reaction should be treated with hydration, rest, and acetaminophen for fever. Patients with reduced fetal movement and contractions should receive fetal heart rate monitoring until signs and symptoms resolve. Klein et al. have recommended obtaining a baseline fetal ultrasound prior to initiating syphilitic therapy and providing more intensive monitoring and follow-up for women with abnormal studies.[6]
4. Congenital syphilis
Treatment regimens are available through the CDC and are beyond the scope of this book.[3]

F. Prevention

Clinicians can largely prevent congenital syphilis by screening all pregnancies for the maternal syphilis and tracking all confirmed cases with serial serologies to confirm successful treatment. Clinicians working with at-risk populations (inner-city populations with suspected use or access to illicit drugs, especially cocaine) should screen for maternal syphilis at the onset of care, at 28 weeks' gestation, and again at birth.[3] There is good evidence that models of clinician-community partnerships with WIC, Medicaid, AFDC, and family-planning clinics improve the detection and treatment of maternal syphilis.[14]

References

1. Alexander J, Sheffield J, Sanchez P, et al: Efficacy of treatment for syphilis in pregnancy. Obstet Gynecol 93:5–8, 1999.
2. Centers for Disease Control and Prevention: Guidelines for the prevention and control of congenital syphilis. MMWR 37:1–13, 1988.
3. Centers for Disease Control and Prevention: 1998 guidelines for treatment of sexually transmitted diseases. MMWR 47:288–299, 1998.
4. Conover C, Rend C, Miller G, et al: Congenital syphilis after treatment of maternal syphilis with a penicillin regimen exceeding CDC guidelines. Infect Dis Obstet Gynecol 6:134–137, 1998.

5. Fletcher JL, Gordon RC: Perinatal transmission of bacterial sexually transmitted diseases. Part I: Syphilis and gonorrhea. J Fam Pract 30:448–456, 1990.
6. Klein VR, Cox SM, Mitchell MD, et al: The Jarisch-Herxheimer reaction complicating syphilotherapy in pregnancy. Obstet Gynecol 375–380, 1990.
7. Larsen S, Steiner B, Rudolph A: Laboratory diagnosis and interpretation of tests for syphilis. Clin Microbiol Rev 8:1–21, 1995.
8. McFarlin B, Bottoms S: Maternal syphilis: The next pregnancy. Am J Perinatol 13:513–518, 1996.
9. Mobley J, McKeown R, Jackson K, et al: Risk factors for congenital syphilis in infants of women with syphilis in South Carolina. Am J Public Health 88:597-602, 1998.
10. Rolfs RT, Nakashima AK: Epidemiology of primary and secondary syphilis in the United States, 1981 through 1989. JAMA 264:1432–1437, 1990.
11. Sanchez P, Wendel G: Syphilis in pregnancy. Clin Perinatol 24:71–90, 1997.
12. Schultz K, Cates W, O'Mara P: Pregnancy loss, infant death, suffering: Legacy of syphilis and gonorrhea in Africa. Genitourin Med 63:320–327, 1987.
13. Sheffield J, Wendel G: Syphilis in pregnancy. Clin Obstet Gynecol 42:97–106, 1999.
14. Swain G, Kowalewski S, Schubot D: Reducing the incidence of congenital syphilis in Milwaukee: A public private partnership (letter). Am J Public Health 88:1101–1102, 1998.
15. Wendel GD, Stark BJ, Jamison RB, et al: Penicillin allergy and desensitization in serious infections during pregnancy. N Engl J Med 322:270–271, 1985.

V. Group B Streptococcus
A. Epidemiology
1. Prevalence

About 30% of women are colonized with group B streptococcus (GBS) at some time during pregnancy with two thirds of them being colonized at the time of delivery.[13] Of the women who are culture-positive at the time of labor, neonatal colonization of the mucous membranes occurs in 50–70%. Of these colonized infants, 1–3% will develop symptomatic infection.[8,17] The overall number of infants who develop early-onset group B streptococcus (EOGBS) is about 1.8 per 1000. The GBS "attack" rate varies greatly depending on the presence or absence of concurrent risk factors. There are approximately 8,000 neonatal GBS infections in the U.S. each year. Eighty to eighty five percent of these infections occur in the first 7 days of life, are thought to occur from vertical transmission at or before birth and are termed EOGBS. The remaining are called late-onset GBS infections and occur from 7 days to 3 months of age.

2. Risk factors for colonization with GBS
   a. Age < 21
   b. Low socioeconomic status
   c. Sexual activity
   d. Low parity
   e. Swabbing multiple sites for GBS culture (proximal vagina, perineum, anorectum)
   f. Hispanic and African-American ethnicity[9]

B. Natural History
1. Timing of colonization[13]

Women who are GBS-positive during pregnancy have the following natural history: one third remain culture positive throughout the pregnancy; one third are intermittently positive; and one third are positive only once.

2. Risk factors that affect vertical transmission of GBS:
   a. Women who are chronically colonized with heavy GBS growth
   b. Women with GBS bacteriuria[17]
   c. Prematurity (less than 37 weeks' gestation)
   d. Rupture of membranes greater than 18 hours
   e. Intrapartum fever
   f. Having a sibling with previous invasive GBS

3. Early-onset GBS

The case fatality rate for EOGBS infections has dropped from about 50% in the 1970s to 10% in the 1990s.[19] Nevertheless, these are otherwise healthy infants who continue to experience significant morbidity and mortality from vertical transmission of GBS at or before birth.

4. Late-onset GBS

These infections can also be devastating to the older neonate and may be acquired by vertical or horizontal spread. Intrapartum interventions described in this section are not effective in preventing the late-onset type.

C. Effects on Perinatal Outcome

1. Association with preterm labor (PTL) and preterm premature rupture of membranes (PPROM)

Heavy, persistent growth of GBS as well as GBS bacteriuria are associated with an increased risk of PTL and PPROM.[17] RCTs have not been able to demonstrate a reduction in PTL or PPROM with the treatment of this infection in pregnancy.[11]

2. Asymptomatic bacteriuria (ASB)

15% of ASB in pregnancy is caused by GBS. This condition is associated with increased risk of PTL, PPROM, chorioamnionitis, and increased EOGBS.

3. Increased risk of chorioamnionitis and endometritis

Women who are chronic carriers of GBS are at increased risk of having these intra- and postpartum complications.

4. Other puerperal infections

Women colonized with GBS are at increased risk of pelvic cellulitis and septic thrombophlebitis.[23]

5. Early-onset GBS neonatal infection

6. Late-onset GBS neonatal infection

D. Diagnosis

1. Culture

Culture remains the gold standard. However, clinicians should use selective broth medium and obtain cultures from the anterior vagina, perineum, and anorectal area to assure accurate detection of the GBS. Failure to use this culture medium and the multiple culture sites results in a false-negative rate or sensitivity of about 50%.[13]

2. Rapid streptococcal tests

It is desirable to have a rapid turn-around test that a clinician could use in the intrapartum setting. The sensitivity of the currently available tests is not sufficient to detect GBS in patients who are not heavily colonized. In 1997 the FDA issued a warning not to use these rapid strep tests but to rely instead on cultures using the selective broth medium.[22] There is preliminary evidence that the rapid detection of GBS in the intrapartum setting can be done using polymerase chain reaction (PCR) testing with a sensitivity of 97% and specificity of 98.8%.[4] If this technology is confirmed and adopted on a widespread basis, it will lead to a screening and treatment paradigm that is very different to that recommended in this section.

E. Management: Prevention of Early-Onset GBS Infection

The focus on management has shifted over the past decade to the intrapartum setting. There are four RCTs that show that the vertical transmission of GBS from an infected mother to the newborn can be effectively prevented with the use of intrapartum antibiotics.[5,20,21] Infant colonization is decreased (OR 0.10, CI 0.07–0.14, NNT = 2.3) and neonatal GBS infection is decreased (OR 0.17, CI 0.07–0.39, NNT = 20). On the basis of the studies, neonatal mortality is not improved (OR 0.12, CI 0.10–2.00). This is likely due to insufficient numbers in the studies. Further RCTs in this area will most likely not occur because of the risk posed to infants in the control group.

1. Antibiotic selection
    a. Aqueous penicillin G (5 million units every 6 hours until delivery) is the treatment of choice because of its narrow antimicrobial spectrum, thus having less of a chance of inducing antibiotic-resistant bacteria.[19]
    b. Ampicillin (2 g bolus intravenously followed by 1 g every 4 hours until delivery)
    c. Clindamycin for penicillin-allergic mother (300 mg intravenously every 6 hours). There are no prospective trials that measure the effectiveness of clindamycin in the treatment of GBS. Pearlman et al. recently found that 15% of genitourinary GBS isolates are resistant to clindamycin.[14]
    d. Erythromycin (500 intravenously every 6 hours) is a less desirable alternative because of unpredictable levels of antibiotic crossing the placenta. Pearlman et al. also found a 16% of GBS isolates were resistant to erythromycin.[14]
    e. Broad-spectrum coverage. Regimens such as ampicillin and gentamicin should be used if clinically apparent chorioamnionitis is present (see Chapter 15, section C).
2. Timing of antibiotic use in labor
Two or more doses of intravenous antibiotics or having an interval of 4 or more hours between antibiotic dosing and delivery are effective in reducing infant colonization rates to less than 3%.[15]
3. Current CDC treatment strategies
Until 1996 there was considerable controversy as to the best approach to prevent EOGBS. The American Academy of Pediatrics (AAP) recommended screening cultures at 26–28 weeks' gestation and the intrapartum treatment of positive cultures when one of the following obstetrical risk factors (fever, rupture of membranes > 18 hours, history of sibling with invasive GBS, gestational age < 37 weeks, GBS bacteriuria in current pregnancy) were present.[1] The American College of Obstetricians and Gynecologists (ACOG) recommended that no prenatal cultures be performed but that a risk factor-guided intrapartum treatment regimen should be followed.

In 1996, the CDC issued consensus guidelines that were endorsed by the AAP and ACOG.[3,6] They provide clinicians with two treatment strategies:
    a. Culture- and risk factor-based approach. Clinicians obtain GBS cultures from the lower genital tract of all of their patients between 35 and 37 weeks' gestation and offer chemoprophylaxis for culture-positive women when they are in labor. If culture results are not available, patients receive intrapartum chemoprophylaxis if one or more of the following risk factors are present: gestation less than 37 weeks, duration of membrane rupture greater than 18 hours, maternal temperature greater than 100.4°F, and a previous infant with GBS infection. It is estimated that this approach would result in intrapartum antibiotic use for about 27% of women and should prevent 90% of EOGBS cases.[18]
    b. Risk factor-alone approach. This approach would offer antibiotic chemoprophylaxis to those women who have one or more of the above-mentioned risk factors. It is estimated that this approach would result in intrapartum antibiotic use for about 18% of women and should prevent 69% of EOGBS cases.[18]

F. Impact of CDC Screening Recommendations
    1. Hospitals with GBS policies
By 1997, 46% of hospitals had a written GBS policy compared to 14% in 1994. Both teaching and non-teaching hospitals followed this trend.[7]

2. Decreasing incidence of EOGBS

The CDC's Active Bacterial Core Surveillance, reflecting data collected in California, Georgia, Tennessee, and Maryland, documented a 50% decrease in EOGBS to a rate of 0.8 per 1000 births.[7] The policy of intrapartum chemoprophylaxis had no impact on the incidence of late-onset GBS.

3. Association between prenatal screening and decrease in maternal morbidity

Locksmith et al. analyzed the impact of using one of three GBS treatment strategies over a 7-year period involving more than 20,000 deliveries.[12] Two of the three strategies were the ones recommended by the CDC in 1996. They were unable to detect an improvement in neonatal outcome under the universal screening protocol. The group that underwent universal screening had a 30% decrease in chorioamnionitis (RR 0.7, CI 0.6–0.8, NNT = culture 23 patients and treat 4 patients in labor) and endometritis (RR 0.7, CI 0.6–0.8, NNT = culture 31 patients and treat 5.3 patients in labor).

4. Number of women screened and treated to prevent one case of EOGBS

One thousand and seven women needed to be cultured resulting in 142 women receiving intrapartum antibiotics to prevent one case of EOGBS.[12]

G. Primary Prevention: Development of a GBS Vaccine

Extensive research has been undertaken to develop conjugated vaccines against the major serotypes of GBS. One of these vaccines produced a fourfold or greater rise in antibody production in more than 90% of women of child-bearing age.[10] The primary prevention of EOGBS is a promising strategy for the future.

References

1. American Academy of Pediatrics, Committee on Infectious Diseases 1991–1992: Recommendations for Prevention of Early-Onset Neonatal GBS Infection, 1992.
2. American Academy of Pediatrics: Revised guidelines for prevention of early-onset group B streptococcal (GBS) infection. American Academy of Pediatrics Committee on Infectious Disease and Committee on Fetus and Newborn. Pediatrics 99:489–496, 1997.
3. American College of Obstetricians and Gynecologists Committee Opinion: Prevention of early-onset group B streptococcal disease in newborns. No.173, June 1996.
4. Bergeron MG, Danbing K, Menard C, et al: Rapid detection of group B streptococci in pregnant women at delivery. N Engl J Med 343:175–179, 2000.
5. Boyer KM, Gotoff SP: Prevention of early onset neonatal group B streptococcal disease with selective intrapartum chemoprophylaxis. N Engl J Med 314:1665–1669, 1986.
6. CDC: Prevention of perinatal group B streptococcal disease: A public health perspective. MMWR 45(RR-7), 1996.
7. CDC: Adoption of hospital policies for prevention of perinatal group B streptococcal disease; United States, 1997. MMWR 47(32), 1998.
8. Ferrieri P, Cleary P, Seeds A: Epidemiology of group B streptoccocal carriage in pregnant women and newborn infants. J Med Microbiol 10:103–114, 1976.
9. Goldenberg R, Klebanoff M, Nugent, et al: Bacterial colonization of the vagina during pregnancy in four ethnic groups. Am J Obstet Gynecol 174:1618–1621, 1996.
10. Kasper D, Paoletti L, Wessels M, et al: Immune response to type III group B streptococcal polysaccharide-tetanus toxoid conjugate vaccine. J Clin Invest 98:2308–2314, 1996.
11. Klebanoff M, Regan J, Rau A, et al: Outcome of the Vaginal Infections and Prematurity Study: Results of a clinical trial of erythromycin among pregnant women colonized with group B streptococci. Am J Obstet Gynecol 172:1540–1545, 1995.
12. Locksmith G, Clark P, Duff P: Maternal and neonatal infection rates with three different protocols for prevention of group B streptococcal disease. Am J Obstet Gynecol 180:416–422, 1999.
13. McKenna D, Iams J: Group B streptococcal infections. Semin Perinatol 22:267–276, 1998.
14. Pearlman M, Pierson C, Faix R: Frequent resistance of clinical group B streptococci isolates to clindamycin and erythromycin. Obstet Gynecol 92:258–261, 1998.
15. Pylipow M, Gaddis M, Kinney J: Selective intrapartum prophylaxis for group B streptococcus colonization: Management and outcome of newborns. Pediatrics 93:631–635, 1994.
16. Regan JA, Klebanoff MA, Nugent RP: The epidemiology of group B streptococcal colonization in pregnancy. Obstet Gynecol 77:604–610, 1991.

17. Regan J, Klebanoff M, Nugent R, et al: Colonization with group B streptococci in pregnancy and adverse outcome. VIP Study Group. Am J Obstet Gynecol 174:1354–1360, 1996.
18. Rouse D, Goldenberg R, Cliver S, et al: Strategies for the prevention of early-onset neonatal group B streptococcal sepsis: A decision analysis. Obstet Gynecol 83:483–494, 1994.
19. Schuchat A: Group B streptococcus. Lancet 353:51–56, 1999.
20. Smaill F: Intrapartum antibiotics for group B streptococcal colonisation (Cochrane Review). In The Cochrane Library, Issue 4, 2000, Oxford, Update Software.
21. Tuppurainen N, Hallman M: Prevention of neonatal group B streptococcal disease: Intrapartum detection and chemoprophylaxis of heavily colonized parturients. Obstet Gynecol 73:583–587, 1989.
22. United States Food and Drug Administration. FDA safety alert: Risks of devices for direct detection of group B streptococcal antigen. Rockville, MD, Department of Health and Human Services, 1997.
23. Yancey M, Duff P, Clark P, et al: Peripartum infection associated with vaginal group B streptococcal colonization. Obstet Gynecol 84:816–819, 1994.

VI. Bacterial Vaginosis

A. Epidemiology

Bacterial vaginosis (BV) is the most common vaginal infection. It affects between 15% and 20% of women. It is a clinical syndrome where the vaginal flora has changed from one of being 95% lactobacilli to a mixed one where there are increased concentrations of *Gardnerella vaginalis*, *Mobiluncus*, *Bacteroides*, and *Mycoplasma* species.[9]

B. Natural History

Women who are symptomatic with BV present with a malodorous, homogeneous vaginal discharge. Vulvar pain, irritation, and itching are usually not present with BV infections. About 50% of BV infections are asymptomatic.

C. Effect on Perinatal Outcome

Prospective studies show an independent association between BV and increased rates of preterm premature rupture of membranes, preterm labor, chorioamnionitis, and post-cesarean endometritis.[3,5,7,9] Several RCTs show that screening and treatment of BV in pregnancy for women who have either had previous premature deliveries or whose pre-pregnancy body mass index is less than 19.8 results in an approximate 70% decrease in subsequent low-birth-weight outcomes.[6,13] This improvement in birth outcomes has not been demonstrated in otherwise low-risk women.[2,11]

D. Diagnosis/Management

The Amsel criteria developed in 1983 is the method most commonly used.[1] They include the following factors.

1. Thin, homogeneous discharge
2. pH greater than 4.5
3. Positive whiff test (fishy odor) after placing a few drops of potassium hydroxide with the vaginal specimen
4. Presence of 25% or greater of clue cells, which are epithelial cells heavily coated with bacilli that cause a stippled appearance.

The presence of three or more of these factors indicates a diagnosis of BV.

Other techniques that have been used include Gram stain, DNA probe technology, and a swab test that identifies diamines. The latter test has a sensitivity of 97% and a specificity of 83% and may prove to be efficient and practical for office use.[14]

Treatment in pregnancy should be initiated if the patient is symptomatic.[4] As noted above, the detection and treatment in *asymptomatic* women should be relegated to those women with previous premature outcomes or those with low prepregnancy weights.

E. Management

1. Metronidazole

Metronidazole (second and third trimester) 500 mg orally twice a day for 7 days or 250 mg three times a day for 7 days.

2. Metronidazole vaginal gel
One applicator, twice a day for 5 days.
3. Clindamycin vaginal cream (2%)
One applicator (5 g) at bedtime for 7 days or clindamycin orally 300 mg twice a day for 7 days. This treatment is the preferred one for symptomatic infections in the first trimester to avoid the use of metronidazole. Systemic clindamycin would appear to be more effective than topical in terms of prolonging gestational age and increasing birth weight.[8,12]

References

1. Amsel R, Totten P, Spiegel C, et al.: Nonspecific vaginitis: Diagnostic and microbial and epidemiological associations. Am J Med 74:14–22, 1983.
2. Carey J, Klebanoff A, Hauth J, et al: Metronidzole to prevent preterm delivery in pregnant women with asymptomatic bacterial vaginosis. N Engl J Med 342:534–540, 2000.
3. Eschenbach D: Bacterial vaginosis and anaerobes in obstetric-gynecologic infection. Clin Infect Disease 16:S282–S287, 1993.
4. Ferris D: Management of bacterial vaginosis during pregnancy. Am Fam Physician 57:1215–1228, 1998.
5. Gibbs R: Chorioamnionitis and bacterial vaginosis. Am J Obstet Gynecol 169:460–462, 1993.
6. Hauth J, Godenberg R, Andrews W, et al: Reduced incidence of preterm delivery with metronidazole and erythromycin in women with bacterial vaginosis. N Engl J Med 333:1732–1736, 1995.
7. Hillier S, Nugent R, Eschenbach D, et al: Association between bacterial vaginosis and preterm delivery of a low-birth-weight infant. N Engl J Med 333:1737–1742, 1995.
8. Joesoef M, Hillier S, Wiknjosastro G, et al: Intravaginal clindamycin treatment for bacterial vaginosis: Effects on preterm delivery and low birth weight. Am J Obstet Gynecol 173:1527–1531, 1995.
9. Kimberlin D, Andrews W: Bacterial vaginosis: Association with adverse pregnancy outcome. Semin Perinatol 22:242–250, 1998.
10. Martius J, Eschenbach DA: The role of bacterial vaginosis as a cause of amniotic fluid infection, chorioamnionitis, and prematurity—a review. Arch Gynecol Obstet 247:1–13, 1990.
11. McDonald H, O'Loughlin J, Vigneswaran R, et al: Impact of metronidazole therapy on preterm birth in women with bacterial vaginosis flora (*Gardnerella vaginalis*): A randomised, placebo-controlled trial. Br J Obstet Gynaecol 104:1394–1397, 1997.
12. McGregor J, French J, Seo K: Adjunctive clindamycin therapy for preterm labor: Results of a double-blind, placebo-controlled trial. Am J Obstet Gynecol 165:867–875, 1991.
13. Morales W, Schorr S, Albritton J: Effect of metronidazole in patients with preterm birth in preceding pregnancy and bacterial vaginosis: A placebo-controlled, double-blind study. Am J Obstet Gynecol 171:345–349, 1994.
14. O'Dowd T, West R, Winterburn P, et al: Evaluation of a rapid diagnostic test for bacterial vaginosis. Br J Obstet Gynaecol 103:366–370, 1996.
15. Watts D, Krohn M, Hillier S, et al: Bacterial vaginosis as a risk factor for post-cesarean endometritis. Obstet Gynecol 75:52–56, 1990.

VII. Candida Vulvovaginitis
A. Epidemiology
Candida vulvovaginitis is one of the most common vaginal infections causing 15–30% of all infections. There is evidence that the incidence of this condition is increasing in the United States and England.[3] There are approximately 13 millions cases reported in the United States per year.[5]

1. Microbiology
The great majority of infections are caused by *Candida albicans*. Non-albicans species such as *C. tropicalis* and *C. glabrata* are becoming increasingly common and can be a source of antifungal resistance.
2. Conditions that are associated with candidal infections[3]
    a. Diabetes mellitus
    b. Cushing's or Addison's disease
    c. Hypo- or hyperthyroidism
    d. Malignancies
    e. HIV

   f. Pregnancy
   g. Vaginal trauma
 3. Other predisposing risk factors[3]
   a. Antibiotic therapy
   b. Hormone therapy
   c. Corticosteroids
   d. Radio- or chemotherapy
   e. Immunosuppressive therapy
   f. Multiple sexual partners

B. Natural History
Candida vaginitis may be asymptomatic or symptomatic; it is characterized by heavy, white, curd-like vaginal discharge, often with severe vaginal or vulvar pruritus and inflammation.

C. Effect on Perinatal Outcome
Infection in pregnancy may be more difficult to eradicate; recurrence is common. Otherwise, there are no other untoward effects on perinatal outcome.

D. Diagnosis
 1. Physical examination
Marked vulvar erythema and swelling may be seen in women with symptomatic infections. A thick, white, "curd-like" discharge is often present.
 2. Microscopic diagnosis
This infection can be detected as budding yeast or hyphae on KOH preparation. It may be seen on Pap smear or on urinalysis if there is a contaminated specimen.

E. Management
Multiple regimens and a generally longer course of any medication used are more likely to effect remission of symptoms during pregnancy. Note that oral therapy is contraindicated during pregnancy.[5]
 1. Clotrimazole (over the counter, class B)
1% cream, 5 grams for 7 to 14 days or vaginal tablets 100 mg for 7 days, 200 mg for 3 days or 500 mg for a single dose
 2. Miconazole (over the counter, class C)
2% cream, 5 grams for 7 to 14 days or 100 mg vaginal tablet 200 mg for 3 days or 500 mg vaginal tablet for one dose
 3. Nystatin (prescription, class B)
100,000 U vaginal tablet for 14 days
 4. Butoconazole (prescription, class C)
2% cream, 5 grams for 3 days
 5. Terconazole (prescription, class C)
0.4% cream, 5 grams for 7 days or 0.8% cream 5 grams for 3 days
 6. Ticonazole (prescription, class C)
6.5% ointment, 5 grams single dose
 7. Nystatin cream (prescription, class B)
14-day treatment, not as effective
 8. Boric acid capsules
600-mg gelatin capsules per dose for two doses.
 9. Gentian violet
One application a week for 2 weeks (effective but messy).

References

1. American College of Obstetricians and Gynecologists Technical Bulletin: Vaginitis. Number 226, July 1996.
2. Association of Reproductive Health Professionals Clinical Proceedings: Risk/benefit of antifungal therapy for vulvovaginal candidiasis, April 1–8, 1995.

3. Cullins V, Ford M, Harper E, et al: Vulvovaginitis: A practice protocol for the managed care clinician. In National Association of Managed Care Physicians Roundtable Highlights, January, 1996.
4. Horowitz B, Kent H, Marinoff S, et al: Vaginitis: The total picture. In International Society for the Study of Vulvar Disease, January 1995.
5. Tobin M: Vulvovaginal candidiasis: Topical vs. oral therapy. Am Fam Physician 51:1715–1720, 1995.

VIII. *Trichomonas vaginalis*

A. Epidemiology

The prevalence of *Trichomonas vaginalis*, a unicellular flagellated protozoan, in the prospective VIP study was 12.6% (n = 13,816).[3] In this study, the prevalence among African-American women was 22.8% compared to 6.6% among Hispanic and 6.1% among white women. Other factors that were associated with an increased risk of trichomonas infection include being unmarried, lower income, lower educational attainment, and smoking. Trichomonas infection is also associated with an increased risk of concurrent gonorrhea, chlamydia, group B streptococcus, and bacterial vaginosis.[5]

B. Natural History[1]

Infection often presents with copious frothy, greenish to clear, watery vaginal discharge; vaginal pruritus; dyspareunia; or dysuria. Spotting may be a common presentation because of cervical inflammation. Physical examination may reveal vaginal erythema, often accompanied by cervicitis, sometimes described as a strawberry cervix.

C. Effect on Perinatal Outcome

Trichomonas vaginalis infection in pregnancy is associated with a 40% increase in premature, low-birth-weight infants.[3,7] Women with this infection are also more likely to have preterm premature rupture of fetal membranes, postpartum endometritis, stillborns and neonatal deaths than are women without trichomonas infection. Neonatal infections are an uncommon occurrence but have been reported.[4] An RCT is currently underway in the National Institute of Child Health and Human Development's Maternal-Fetal Medicine Units Network that should determine if treatment of trichomonas in pregnancy results in an improvement in perinatal outcomes.

D. Diagnosis

Most office settings use a microscopic vaginal wet prep to diagnose symptomatic infections. Motile flagellated organisms are diagnostic of infection. However, the VIP study demonstrated that trichomonas infections are common in the absence of the classical symptoms and thus are often underdiagnosed.[5] Using culture as the standard diagnostic test, the sensitivity of the wet prep was 55.8%, specificity 98.5%, positive predictive value 78.4%, and negative predictive value 95.7%. Clinicians serving at-risk populations should consider the routine use of cultures for the detection of trichomonas infections in pregnancy.

E. Management

1. Delay treatment in first-trimester[1]

Treatment with topical clotrimazole should alleviate symptoms.

2. Treatment with metronidazole

Evidence supports that metronidazole is not teratogenic in humans although many clinicians delay the use of metronidazole past the period of organogenesis.[2] Metronidazole (category C), 2 g for one dose or 250 mg three times a day for 7 days is the drug of choice. Topical metronidazole does not effectively eradicate *Trichomonas vaginalis* from the Bartholin or Skene's glands. Sexual partners should receive contemporaneous treatment. Given the increased risk of adverse outcome, it is prudent to apply a test of cure to assure eradication of this organism.

References

1. Ament L, Whalen E: Sexually transmitted diseases in pregnancy: Diagnosis, impact, and intervention. JOGNN 25:657–666, 1996.
2. Burtin P, Taddio A, Ariburnu O, et al: Safety of metronidazole in pregnancy: A meta-analysis. Am J Obstet Gynecol 172:525–529, 1995.
3. Cotch M, Pastorek J, Nugent R, et al: *Trichomonas vaginalis* associated with low birth weight and preterm delivery. Sex Transmit Dis 24:353–560, 1997.
4. Danesh I, Stephen J, Gorbach J: Neonatal *Trichomonas vaginalis* infection. J Emerg Med 13:51–54, 1995.
5. Pastorek J, Cotch M, Martin D, et al: Clinical and microbiological correlates of vaginal trichomoniasis during pregnancy. Clin Infect Dis 23:1075–1080, 1996.
6. Saurina G, McCormack W: Trichomoniasis in pregnancy. Sex Transmit Dis 24:361–362, 1997.
7. Sutton M, Sternberg M, Nsuami M, et al: Trichomoniasis in pregnant human immunodeficiency virus-uninfected Congolese women: Prevalence risk factors, and association with low birth weight. Am J Obstet Gynecol 181:656–662, 1999.

IX. Herpes Simplex, Type II (Genital)

A. Epidemiology

The third National Health and Nutrition Examination Surveys (NHANES III) showed that the age-adjusted prevalence of herpes simplex virus type 2 (HSV-2) among women is 25.6%, a 30% increase compared to the last survey done in 1980.[6] The groups identified as having the highest seroprevalence include African-American, Mexican-American, and women living in poverty, having numerous sexual partners, and using illicit drugs. Since 1980, there has been a fivefold increase in the seroprevalence of HSV-2 among white adolescents and a twofold increase among white women in their twenties.

B. Natural History

1. Primary genital HSV infection

A large prospective study of HSV-seronegative women demonstrated that approximately 2% of these women acquire this infection during pregnancy. Thirty percent are acquired in the first and second trimesters and 40% in the third trimester.[5] It is this latter group that is at increased risk of vertical transmission of the virus to the newborn because of insufficient time to mount an IgG response to help protect the newborn. HSV-2 virus accounts for 80% of genital infections and HSV-1 causes the remaining 20%. The primary genital HSV infection is characterized by multiple vesicular lesions and may have systemic symptoms of fever and regional lymphadenopathy. Antibodies to HSV-1 and HSV-2 are absent. This initial infection can be asymptomatic. The initial infection lasts from 2–3 weeks. HSV-2 ascends along proximal nerve fibers to establish a latent infection in the lumbosacral sensory ganglia.[1]

2. Non-primary first-episode genital HSV

This occurs with a first-time genital infection to HSV-1 when antibodies to HSV-2 were already present or with a first time genital infection with HSV-2 when antibodies to HSV-1 were already present. Nonprimary first-episode infections have fewer systemic symptoms and a briefer duration of viral shedding.[2]

3. Recurrent infection

Recurrent infections are usually accompanied by single or few lesions, often with some prodromal itching, hyperesthesia or dysesthesia in the affected area, and last from 5–7 days. Reactivation of HSV-2 may be completely asymptomatic such that about 1% of infected persons are shedding the virus at a given time.[1]

C. Effects on Perinatal Outcome

1. Spontaneous miscarriage

The medical literature provides conflicting evidence as to whether HSV-2 is associated with an increased risk of spontaneous miscarriage.[4]

2. Increased risk of preterm labor and delivery

Primary infections in the second half of pregnancy have been associated with an increased risk of premature labor and delivery as well as an increased risk of vertical transmission.[4]

3. Vertical transmission to the newborn

About 70–85% of infections occur in infants in which there is no history of maternal peripartum genital herpes infection. Transmission rates vary depending on whether viral shedding takes place with or without symptoms or during an initial or recurrent infection. Mortality or neurologic impairment occurs in 40% of infected neonates. As noted above, the highest risk of infection appears to be in late third trimester primary herpes infections when women have not yet seroconverted.[5] The rate of transmission is much lower in recurrent infections, estimated to be about 1 in 100.[4,5]

D. Diagnosis

1. Culture

Culture of unroofed lesions remains the gold standard although this test has a limited sensitivity because the herpes virus stops shedding before the lesion resolves; hence, the culture may have a false-negative result about 25% of the time. The yield of positive cultures on recurrent lesions is only 50%. The clinician should keep this mind when interpreting the culture results. This test does have a 100% specificity, i.e., no false-positive results.

2. DNA polymerase chain reaction (PCR) testing

This is the emerging diagnostic test of choice because of its very high sensitivity (95%) that can detect the presence of the virus as long as the ulcer is present. This modality also has a specificity of 90%. The higher cost of this test is limiting its use in primary care practices at this time.

3. Serologic testing

Commercial tests can differentiate between HSV-1 and HSV-2 IgG antibodies in selected settings. Clinicians should check to see if their reference lab can perform this test. This testing is primarily helpful for the clinician to diagnose a case of primary herpes when the culture or PCR is positive and the serology for HSV IgG is negative.[14]

E. Management during Pregnancy to Prevent Neonatal Herpes

1. Primary genital HSV

    a. Prenatal care. The initial prenatal assessment should include a careful history for genital lesions, specifically "blisters," ulcers, painful lesions, lesions associated with genital dysesthesias, and prodromal symptoms. Women with no known history of HSV whose partners have a history of recurrent herpes should be counseled to use condoms throughout pregnancy and to report if they have symptoms suggestive of HSV.

    b. Primary HSV. Special attention must be given to women who may have contracted primary HSV during pregnancy, particularly if this has occurred well into the late third trimester. Women at this stage of pregnancy with positive cultures or PCR testing and negative serologies are at very high risk of vertical transmission of HSV to their newborn and should be comanaged with a perinatologist if possible.[16]

2. Recurrent genital HSV

    a. Routine third-trimester cultures. These cultures are not indicated because of an inability to predict viral shedding at the time of delivery. Multiple RCTs have demonstrated that this practice has not been shown to decrease viral transmission rates.[1]

    b. Labor room assessment. This should include inquiries regarding recent lesions, even if the patient has no prior history. All patients with lesions or symptoms should be examined for herpes. Lesions that are distant from the vulva, vagina, and cervix are not a contraindication to vaginal delivery.[2] They should be covered with a dressing to prevent direct contact with the newborn.

    c. Indication for cesarean section. Cesarean intervention has been recommended for active herpes lesions or prodromal symptoms such as vulvar pain or burning. There appears to be no arbitrary time after rupture of the membranes when performing a cesarean section is not beneficial in preventing vertical transmission of the virus.[10] Current controversy exists as to the cost-effectiveness of performing cesarean section for patients with recurrent, active lesions because the neonatal transmission rate is low.[12]

    d. Acyclovir prophylaxis to prevent recurrent lesions. Several RCTs have investigated the use of acyclovir, 400 mg po twice daily from 36 to 40 weeks to prevent the recurrence of symptomatic herpes.[8,14] This approach has been associated with decreased cesarean section rates without any increase in neonatal herpes infections. Acyclovir, a class C agent, appears to be safe in pregnancy. Thus, this approach may have merits in preventing cesarean section in patients with frequent recurrences of lesions.[15]

References

1. Arvin A, Hensleigh P, Prober C, et al: Failure of antepartum maternal cultures to predict the infant's risk of exposure to herpes simplex virus at delivery. N Engl J Med 35:796–800, 1986.
2. Baker D: Management of herpes in pregnancy. ACOG Practice Bulletin Number 8, October, 1999.
3. Boursnell M, Entwisle C, Blakeley D: A genetically inactivated herpes simplex virus type 2 vaccine provides effective protection against primary and recurrent HSV-2 disease. J Infect Dis 175:16–25, 1997.
4. Brown Z, Benedetti J, Ashley R, et al: Neonatal herpes simplex virus infection in relation to asymptomatic maternal infection at the time of labor. N Engl J Med 324:1247–1252, 1991.
5. Brown Z, Selke S, Zeh J, et al: The acquisition of herpes simplex virus during pregnancy. N Engl J Med 337:509–515, 1997.
6. Fleming D, McQuillan G, Johnson R, et al: Herpes simplex virus type 2 in the United States, 1976–1994. N Engl J Med 337:1105–1111, 1997.
7. Gibbs R, Amstey M, Lezotte D: Role of cesarean delivery in preventing neonatal herpes virus infection. JAMA 270:94–95, 1993.
8. Haddad J, Langer B, Astruc D, et al.: Oral acyclovir and recurrent genital herpes during late pregnancy. Obstet Gynecol 82:102–104, 1993.
9. Hensleigh P, Andrews W, Brown Z, et al: Genital herpes during pregnancy: Inability to distinguish primary and recurrent infections clinically. Obstet Gynecol 89:891–895, 1997.
10. Nahmias A, Josey W, Naib Z, et al: Perinatal risk associated with maternal genital herpes simplex virus infection. Am J Obstet Gynecol 110:825–837, 1971.
11. Randolph A, Washington E, Prober C: Cesarean delivery for women presenting with genital herpes lesions: Efficacy, risks, and costs. JAMA 270:77–82, 1993.
12. Randolph A, Hartshorn R, Washington A: Acyclovir prophylaxis in late pregnancy to prevent neonatal herpes: A cost-effectiveness analysis. Obstet Gynecol 88:603–610, 1996.
13. Riley L: Herpes simplex virus. Semin Perinatol 22:284–292, 1998.
14. Scott L, Sanchez P, Jackson G: Acyclovir suppression to prevent cesarean delivery after first-episode genital herpes. Obstet Gynecol 87:69–73, 1996.
15. Scott L, Alexander J: Cost-effectiveness of acyclovir suppression to prevent recurrent genital herpes in term pregnancy. Am J Perinatol 15:57–62, 1998.
16. Smith J, Cowan F, Munday P, et al: The management of herpes simplex virus infection in pregnancy. Br J Obstet Gynaecol 105:255–260, 1998.

X. Human Papillomavirus

This segment provides an overview of the highly prevalent sexually transmissible disease caused by the human papillomavirus (HPV).

A. Epidemiology[7]

1. Prevalence

Between the mid-1960s and the 1980s, there has been an estimated sevenfold increase in the prevalence of HPV infections. Koutsky has estimated the prevalence of HPV among men and women 15–49 years of age to be as follows.[7]

   a. Genital warts: 1%
   b. Subclinical HPV detected by colposcopy or cytology: 4%
   c. Subclinical HPV detected by DNA amplification: 10%
   d. Prior infection with antibodies to HPV: 60%
   e. No prior infection: 25%

2. Associated risk factors

   a. Age. Women less than 25 have a consistently higher prevalence even after adjusting for other risk factors. This is most likely due to the development of progressive immunity to HPV as a function of age.
   b. Sexual activity. This risk factor is related to the number of partners, frequency of intercourse, and presence of genital warts on sex partners.
   c. Oral contraceptive (OC) use. The use of OCs does not increase the prevalence of HPV but may increase the progression of the disease process.[10]
   d. Pregnancy. There is a higher HPV viral load during pregnancy. There are conflicting results as to whether pregnancy is associated with an increased prevalence of HPV infections.[5,9]
   e. Immune status. Patients who are immunocompromised appear to have more infections as well as higher viral loads.[7]

B. Natural History

1. Relationship of HPV to intraepithelial neoplasia

HPV is a DNA virus that infects epithelial cells and induces proliferative changes.[2] This virus is known to cause many genitourinary epithelial cancers.[7]

2. Relationship of HPV type to grade of cervical intraepithelial neoplasia (CIN)

There are more than 80 subtypes of HPV. HPV subtypes 16 and 18 are strongly associated with high-grade CIN and invasive cervical cancer. Subtypes 6 and 11 are seldom found in invasive cancers and instead are found in the exophytic lesions known as condylomata on the external surfaces of the vagina, vulva, and anus.

C. Effects on Perinatal Outcome

1. Maternal effects

Rapid growth of condyloma is possible during pregnancy accompanied with discomfort and with the risk of tearing, bleeding, and poor perineal healing with delivery.

2. Fetal/neonatal effects

Perinatal transmission to the neonate is uncommon. A recent prospective study that used DNA polymerase testing followed the offspring of 112 infected women for 36 months after birth.[13] It found that, at the most, the perinatal transmission rate was 2.8%.

D. Diagnosis

1. Physical exam

There are four types of external genital warts.[6]

   a. Condylomata acuminata. These have the shape of small cauliflowers.
   b. Smooth dome-shaped papules. These are flesh colored and about 1–4 millimeters in width.
   c. Keratotic genital warts. These tend to resemble a typical wart or seborrheic keratosis.

d. Flat-topped papules. These are flat to slightly raised.
Clinicians need to perform a careful examination of the external genitalia, perineum, and anus to detect the presence of these lesions.

2. Papanicolaou smear findings

Abnormal cytology found on the Pap smear is a common way to detect HPV infections. The Bethesda system classifies cytologic features of HPV as low-grade squamous intraepithelial lesions or mild dysplasia (CIN 1). This is known as koilocytosis that occurs with nuclear enlargement and a perinuclear halo.

3. HPV subtyping

DNA hybridization techniques can be used to determine which HPV subtypes are found in infected tissues. Polymerase chain reaction (PCR) is the most sensitive technique.[3] Clinical applications of this technology are still in the investigative stage.

E. Management of Condylomata in Pregnancy

Management of dysplasia in pregnancy in discussed in section F. Treatment of condylomata aims for removal of lesions but not for cure of viral infection.

1. Cryosurgery with liquid nitrogen
2. Electrodesiccation/curettage, scissor excision
3. Trichloroacetic acid (TCA)

Apply repeated applications of 80–85% TCA to affected areas every 7–10 days. TCA can be safely used during pregnancy. Avoid placing this caustic medicine on "unaffected" areas. In the event of intense pain, the acid can be neutralized with soap and sodium bicarbonate.

4. Laser

Laser therapy has been used in pregnancy.

5. Podophyllin

Podophyllin is an antimitotic agent that causes local tissue destruction. It is potentially fetotoxic and is *contraindicated* for use during pregnancy.

6. Interferon alfa-2b

This medicine is also contraindicated in pregnancy.

7. Imiquimod cream

Imiquimod is an inducer of interferon alpha and other cytokines. The safety of this agent in pregnancy has not been established.

8. Cesarean section

Cesarean section may be necessary if lesions are extremely large and preclude safe vaginal delivery but not because of transmission of infection.

References

1. Ahdoot D, Van Nostrand K, Nguyen J, et al: The effect of route of delivery on regression of abnormal cervical cytologic findings in the postpartum period. Am J Obstet Gynecol 178:1116–1120, 1998.
2. Alania R, Munger K: Human papillomaviruses and associated malignancies. J Clin Oncol 16:330–337, 1998.
3. American College of Obstetricians and Gynecologists Technical Bulletin: Genital Human Papillomavirus Infections. No. 193, 1994.
4. Apgar B, Zoschnick L: Triage of the abnormal Papanicolaou smear in pregnancy. Prim Care 25:483–501, 1998.
5. De Roda Husman A, Walboomers J, Hopman E, et al: HPV prevalence in cytomorphologically normal cervical scrapes of pregnant women as determined by PCR: The age-related pattern. J Med Virol 46:97–102, 1995.
6. Evans R, Wiley D, Cole H: External genital warts: Diagnosis and treatment. American Medical Association, 1–34, 1997.
7. Koutsky L: Epidemiology of genital human papillomavirus infection. Am J Med. 102:3–8, 1997.
8. Lungu O, Xiao W, Felix J, et al: Relationship of human papillomavirus type to grade of cervical intraepithelial neoplasia. JAMA 267:2493–2496, 1992.

9. Morrison E, Gammon M, Goldberg G, et al: Pregnancy and cervical infection with human papillomaviruses. Internat Fed Gynecol Obstet 54:125–130, 1996.
10. Negrini B, Schiffman M, Kurman R, et al: Oral contraceptive use, human papillomavirus infection, and risk of early cytological abnormalities of the cervix. Cancer Res 50:4670–4675, 1990.
11. Pakarian F, Kaye J, Cason J, et al: Cancer-associated human papillomaviruses: Perinatal transmission and persistence. Brit J Obstet Gynaecol 101:514–517, 1994.
12. Stillson T, Knight A, Elswick R: The effectiveness and safety of two cervical cytologic techniques during pregnancy. J Fam Pract 45:159–163, 1997.
13. Watts D, Koutsky L, Homes K, et al: Low risk of perinatal transmission of human papillomavirus: Results from a prospective cohort study. Am J Obstet Gynecol 178:365–373, 1998.

XI. Hepatitis B

Hepatitis B is caused by a highly infectious DNA virus.

A. Epidemiology

Hepatitis B accounts for about 35% of all viral hepatitis infections. The incidence of acute hepatitis B in pregnancy is 1 to 2 per thousand and the prevalence of chronic hepatitis B is 5 to 15 per thousand. Certain groups have an increased prevalence of this infection.[8]

1. Southeast Asians
2. Pacific Islanders
3. Alaskan Native Americans
4. Drug addicts
5. Transfusion recipients
6. Dialysis patients
7. Patients in chronic residential facilities
8. Recipients of tattoos

B. Natural History[6,8]

1. Natural history of hepatitis B

After an acute case of hepatitis B, 85–90% of patients resolve physical and laboratory findings, eradicate the viremia and acquire life-long immunity. The remaining patients become chronically infected. Of these patients 15–30% develop chronic liver disorders including chronic active or persistent hepatitis, cirrhosis, and hepatocellular carcinoma. These patients will always test positive for the hepatitis B surface antigen (HBsAg), which is the antigen marker of the active virus. Chronically infected patients who carry the hepatitis B e antigen (HBeAg) have an increased risk of developing the hepatic complications noted above. All chronically infected patients pose a risk to any individual who could come into direct contact with their body fluids (blood, urine, semen).

2. Perinatal transmission of acute hepatitis B

First-trimester infection results in transmission to the newborn about 10% of the time, whereas acute infection in the third-trimester results in about 75% transmission if immunoprophylactic intervention is not carried out.

3. Perinatal transmission of chronic hepatitis B

In the absence of chemoprophylaxis with the use of vaccinations or hepatitis B gammaglobulin, perinatal transmission to the newborn occurs in the following forms.

   a. HBsAg carrier only. There is a 12% vertical transmission rate.
   b. HBeAg carrier state. The hepatitis B e antigen is a marker of extreme infectivity. Women who carry the e antigen will pass the hepatitis B virus to 80–90% of their infants. Eighty five percent of these infants become chronic carriers and have the possibility of developing chronic liver disease.[15]
   c. Transplacental transmission. Congenital infection occurs in about 10% of cases.

C. Effect on Perinatal Outcome[3,7]

Acute hepatitis B results in an increased risk of perinatal transmission (as noted above) and increased risk of preterm labor. In 1–3% of patients acute hepatitis B can result in liver failure with life-threatening effects on mothers and their fetuses. Likewise, women with chronic hepatitis B infections who have significant hepatic insufficiency will encounter increased risks of adverse perinatal outcomes and should be managed in a high-risk fashion with available obstetric or perinatal consultation.

D. Diagnosis

The initial diagnostic test of choice is the HBsAg. This antigen measures the presence of the hepatitis B virus. The sensitivity and specificity of this test are estimated to be 98–99%.[13] If the HbsAg is positive, it may be important to distinguish between acute and chronic hepatitis B infection. This is done by checking the hepatitis B core antibody (anti-HBc). The presence of anti-HBc IgM confirms that the infection is acute; the presence of anti-HBc IgG confirms a chronic infection. If the HBsAg is negative, the patient is either susceptible to the infection or is immune. Immune patients have detectable levels of hepatitis B surface antigen antibodies (anti-HBs) and also have anti-HBc IgG.

E. Management

1. Prenatal management
   a. Acute hepatitis B. Clinicians should assess for evidence of severe liver toxicity by assessing liver function tests and coagulation studies. Acute hepatitis in the third trimester is associated with an increased risk of vertical transmission of the virus. Patients should receive immunoprophylaxis with hepatitis B immunoglobulin (HBIG), 0.06 ml/kg intramuscularly.
   b. Chronic hepatitis B. Clinicians should check basic liver function tests to rule out significant liver dysfunction. Otherwise, attention is focused on the administration of passive and active chemoprophylaxis of the neonate to minimize congenital infection.

2. Intrapartum management

There is no evidence to support cesarean intervention to lower the risk of congenital infection. It is prudent to avoid unnecessary invasive procedures such as placement of fetal scalp electrode or performance of fetal scalp sampling.

3. Newborn management[1]

Infants should undergo bathing soon after birth to remove maternal blood.[1] Hepatitis B immune globulin (0.5 ml) should be administered immediately after birth for infants when the mother is HBsAg-positive and the hepatitis B vaccination series should be started within 2 hours of birth. These infants must be closely tracked to ensure compliance with hepatitis vaccination, 0.5 ml of the recombinant DNA product at birth, 1 month, and 6 months.

If the maternal hepatitis B status is unknown, the neonate should only receive the vaccine. Administration of HBIG can be deferred up to 7 days until results of maternal testing are known.

4. Breastfeeding for mothers who have chronic hepatitis B infection[11]

Breast milk contains very low concentrations of the hepatitis B virus. Active and passive chemoprophylaxis should provide effective protection against congenital infection, thus allowing breastfeeding to occur. Breastfeeding should be withheld if the mother carries the HBeAg because of the marked increase in the infectivity of the virus.

F. Prevention

The prevention of congenital hepatitis B with the use of HBIG and HBV vaccines has been a major public health success. Additional strategies to prevent the horizontal and vertical transmission of this virus are presented.

1. Universal screening for hepatitis B in pregnancy

Maternal screening in pregnancy for HBV that is directed only at women with apparent risk factors miss up to 50% of women who are HBV-positive. Arevalo demonstrated that it was cost-effective to perform universal HBV screening in pregnancy if the prevalence of this infection exceeded 6%.[4] Although most practices do not have prevalence rates that approach 6%, universal screening for HBV has been adopted in most practices in the U.S. This has occurred in part because of the 1991 CDC guideline that recommended universal screening in pregnancy as a major strategy to eliminate hepatitis B.[5] Despite the recommendation for universal screening, a recent study in North Carolina indicated that only 92% of women underwent screening for HBV and that 86% received the first dose of HBV vaccine.[14]

2. Vaccination of "at-risk" patients during pregnancy

Ten percent of the general population has received the HBV vaccine. The safety of this vaccine in pregnancy has been demonstrated.[12] ACOG has recommended the HBV vaccine series in pregnancy for HBsAg-negative patients who are judged to be at increased risk of contracting HBV infection in the pregnancy or at a subsequent time in the future.[2] The risk factors cited include:

    a. Presence of sexually transmitted infections

    b. Personal or significant other's use of illicit drugs

    c. Multiple sexual partners

    d. Working in a health care or public safety field

    e. Household contact with HBV carrier

    f. Working with patients who live in chronic residential units or who undergo dialysis

3. Efficacy of the HBV vaccine during pregnancy

Although the HBV vaccine can be safely administered in pregnancy, preliminary data indicate that certain subgroups of women were less likely to acquire serologic immunity.[9] Women with marked obesity (BMI > 34) were 16 times less likely to achieve immunity after two HBV vaccines compared to nonobese women. Other groups who were less likely to acquire protective immunity included smokers (OR 7.5, CI 2.0–27.7) and women 25 and older (OR 3.9, CI 1.1–14.4).

References

1. American Academy of Pediatrics: Hepatitis B and hepatitis C. In Peter G (ed): 1997 Red Book: Report of the Committee on Infectious Diseases, 24th ed. Elk Grove Village, IL, American Academy of Pediatricians, 1997.
2. American College of Obstetricians and Gynecologists Committee Opinion: Guidelines for hepatitis B virus screening and vaccination during pregnancy. Int J Gynaecol Obstet 40:172–174, 1993.
3. American College of Obstetricians and Gynecologists Educational Bulletin: Viral Hepatitis in Pregnancy. July 1998, 248.
4. Arevalo JA, Washington AE: Cost-effectiveness of prenatal screening and immunization for hepatitis B virus. JAMA 259:365–369, 1988.
5. Centers for Disease Control. Hepatitis B virus: A comprehensive strategy for eliminating transmission in the United States through universal childhood vaccination: Recommendations of the Immunization Practices Advisory Committee (ACIP). MMWR 40:1–25, 1991.
6. Culpepper L: Preventing hepatitis B: Focus on women and their families. J Am Board Fam Pract 6:483–491, 1993.
7. Dinsmoor M: Hepatitis in the obstetric patient. Infect Dis Clin North Am 11:77–91, 1997.
8. Duff P: Hepatitis in pregnancy. Semin Perinatol 22:277–283, 1998.
9. Ingardia C, Kelley L, Steinfeld, J, et al: Hepatitis B vaccination in pregnancy: Factors influencing efficacy. Obstet Gynecol 93:983–986, 1999.
10. Jordan R and Law M: An appraisal of the efficacy and cost-effectiveness of antenatal screening for hepatitis B. J Med Screening 4:117–127, 1997.

11. Kane MS, et al: Prenatal screening for hepatitis B antigen (reply). JAMA 261:1728–1732, 1989.
12. Levy M, Koren G: Hepatitis B vaccine in pregnancy: Maternal and fetal safety. Am J Perinatol 8:227–232, 1991.
13. McCready J, Morens D, Fields H, et al: Evaluation of enzyme immunoassay (EIA) as a screening method for hepatitis B markers in an open population. Epidemiol Infect 107:673–684, 1991.
14. Pierce R, Smith S, Rowe-West B, et al; Hepatitis B maternal screening infant vaccination, and infant prophylaxis practices in North Carolina. Arch Pediatr Adolesc Med 153:619–623, 1999.
15. Sinatra FR, Shah P, Weissman JY, et al: Perinatal transmitted acute icteric hepatitis B in infants born to hepatitis B surface antigen-positive and anti-hepatitis Be-positive carrier mothers. Pediatrics 70:557–559, 1982.
16. Smith N, et al: Surveillance and prevention of hepatitis B transmission. Am J Public Health 89:11–13, 1999.

XII. Human Immunodeficiency Virus (HIV)

This is summary of a rapidly evolving body of knowledge. For a more in-depth discussion of this topic, the reader is referred the Public Health Service web site, www.HIVATIS.org, for recommendations for the management of HIV infections in pregnancy that are updated on a regular basis.

A. Epidemiology[1]

There are approximately 6000 HIV-infected women who deliver babies in the United States each year with 0.17% of all pregnant women being infected. Twenty per cent of all new cases of HIV disease occur in women, compared with a 5% incidence in the mid-1980s.

B. Natural History

1. Acquisition of HIV disease
   a. Sexual contact. The vast majority of women contract HIV infection from their sexual partners. Factors that are associated with an increased risk of heterosexual transmission include high viral loads (HIV RNA loads of 50,000 or more), presence of genital discharge or dysuria, advanced HIV disease, and lack of circumcision.[13]
   b. Blood products. HIV is transmitted by direct contact with infected blood products, i.e., sharing contaminated needles, receiving infected blood products, or inadvertent needle stick injuries.
   c. Congenital acquisition. In the U.S., about 25% of newborn infants acquire HIV disease from their infected mothers before, during, and after labor if antiretroviral treatment if not used. In Africa, vertical transmission rates are as high as 40%.

2. HIV and maternal fertility
   Chu et al. analyzed surveillance data on 3915 HIV-positive women in more than 90 private and public clinics in 9 U.S. cities between January of 1990 and August of 1994.[5] Maternal fertility was reduced among women with advanced HIV disease. It remained high among women who are younger (age 15–19 47%, age 20–24 30%). African-American women had higher pregnancy rates compared to other ethnic groups. Twelve per cent of this population had more than one pregnancy.

3. Vertical transmission
   a. Intrauterine. Twenty five to forty percent of congenital transmission of HIV occurs during pregnancy. There is a higher rate of transplacental transmission if the mother contracts HIV during pregnancy. Her immune system is unable to mount an immediate immune response. RNA loads of 20,000 or more copies/ml are needed to cause a fetal infection.[10,21]
   b. Intrapartum. Fifty to eighty percent of HIV transmission occurs during labor and delivery. Factors associated with an increased risk of transmission include chorioamnionitis, rupture of membranes greater than 4 hours,

preterm delivery, advanced maternal disease, vitamin A deficiency, invasive procedures (fetal scalp electrode, artificial rupture of membranes), and illicit drug use in pregnancy.[13,24]

c. Postpartum. Breastfeeding may account for a transmission rate up to 14% of all congenital infection. In developed countries, breastfeeding should be avoided. In developing and underdeveloped countries, this is a more complex issue because the lack of affordable formula and clean water increase the risk of enteric infection and infant malnutrition. Other factors associated with an increased risk of HIV transmission in breast milk include breast infection, vitamin A deficiency, and bleeding due to nipple trauma.[16]

4. Reducing HIV transmission: Impact of AIDS Clinical Trial 076

The AIDS Clinical Trial 076 demonstrated that the use of zidovudine after the first trimester, during labor, and for the first 6 weeks of life was associated with an approximate 70% reduction in vertical transmission of the HIV virus.[6] There has been rapid dissemination of this evidence and introduction into clinical practice. Clinical outcomes have confirmed the effectiveness of the use of zidovudine.[7]

C. Effects of HIV on Perinatal Outcome

1. Maternal outcome

Alger et al. in a prospective study, compared 101 seropositive women with 98 control women in an urban, indigent American setting who were matched for similar risk factors and demographic characteristics to measure the effect of HIV on pregnancy outcomes.[2] The only differences between the two groups were a higher incidence of condylomata, elevated temperatures upon admission to labor and delivery, and use of intrapartum antibiotics among seropositive women. Temmerman et al. also in a prospective study, compared 406 HIV seropositive and 407 seronegative pregnant women (matched for age and parity) in Nairobi, Kenya to measure the effect of HIV disease on pregnancy outcome.[22] The following maternal outcomes were increased among women with HIV infection:

a. Genital ulcers
b. Genital warts
c. Positive syphilis serology
d. Low-birth-weight infants
e. Prematurity

Temmerman et al. did not match for maternal risk factors or for demographic characteristics as did Alger. On the basis on these studies, clinicians should primarily focus on their patients' risk factors and adjust their prenatal care accordingly.

2. Fetal/neonatal outcome

Alger's prospective study that matched HIV-positive women with seronegative women with similar risk factors did not find different fetal or neonatal outcomes.[2] Any fetus or neonate who acquires HIV infection has a profound lifelong disease.

D. Management Guidelines

1. Preconception

Family physicians should conduct screening of high-risk patients, using informed consent, as in the nonpregnant patient. Some authors recommend offering this test to all patients as a means of decreasing stigma attached to the test and increasing the number of patients detected. Patients who are routinely offered the test need not admit socially unsanctioned behaviors. CDC recommends offering to all pregnant women because treatment in pregnancy is effective in preventing HIV transmission. Preconception counseling for patients with HIV disease about the risks of pregnancy complications and vertical transmission has enormous potential benefit.

2. Prenatal care for women with HIV disease

    a. Prenatal care. Patients with HIV should be screened for a wide variety of sexually transmitted diseases as well as tuberculosis and have baseline cytomegalovirus and toxoplasmosis titers performed. HIV-1 RNA levels should be obtained approximately once each trimester. These levels correlate with the risk of vertical transmission of the virus.[18]

    b. Medication usage. Zidovudine therapy should be employed in an effort to prevent congenital transmission. It can be safely used in pregnancy.[17] Culnane et al. have studied the long-term effects of zidovudine in pregnancy among a cohort of 234 uninfected children born to 230 HIV-infected women who were followed up to 5.6 years after birth and found no apparent adverse treatment effects.[8] It does not completely prevent perinatal transmission. CDC guidelines recommend that zidovudine therapy used only for the purpose of reducing the risk of perinatal infection should not be started until the 14th week of gestation.[9] The treatment protocol used in this study is shown in Table 2. The Public Health Service recommends that combination drug regimens that maximally suppress viral replication be offered to HIV-infected women.[18] Clinicians must work closely with their local or regional HIV infectious disease consultant to develop specific treatment regimens to be offered to their patients. Clinicians are strongly encouraged to report cases of prenatal exposure to antiretroviral drugs to the Antiretroviral Pregnancy Registry (800-258-4263). There is increasing evidence that the use of additional retroviral agents can lower HIV transmission and is well tolerated by fetuses.[3,24]

    c. Indications for anti-*Pneumocystis* prophylaxis. These are the same as for the nonpregnant patient.

    d. Opportunistic infections. These infections should be treated aggressively because risks to the fetus are greater if the mother does not receive timely therapy for her infection.

    e. Women with late-onset prenatal care. Zidovudine can reduce the vertical transmission of HIV-1 even if it is introduced for the first time during the intrapartum period or to the infant of an untreated mother.[20,25]

    f. Confidentiality issues. This is a very challenging and important issue for clinicians and their patients. Whenever possible, attempts to maintain

TABLE 2.   Pediatric AIDS Clinical Trials Group (PACTG) 076 Zidovudine (ZDV) Regimen

Time of ZDV Administration	Regimen
Antepartum	Oral administration of 100 mg ZDV five times daily, initiated at 14–34 weeks' gestation and continued throughout the pregnancy.
Intrapartum	During labor, intravenous administration of ZDV in a 1-hour initial dose of 2 mg/kg body weight, followed by a continuous infusion of 1 mg/kg body weight/hour until delivery.
Postpartum	Oral administration of ZDV to the newborn (ZDV syrup at 2 mg/kg body weight/dose every 6 hours) for the first 6 weeks of life, beginning at 8–12 hours after birth (note: intravenous dosage for infants who cannot tolerate oral intake is 1.5 mg/kg body weight intravenously every 6 hours)

From Public Health Service Task Force Recommendations for Use of Antiretroviral Drugs in Pregnant HIV-1-Infected Women for Maternal Health and Interventions to Reduce Perinatal HIV-1 Transmission in the United States, November 3, 2000.

TABLE 3. Rate of Perinatal Transmission According to Receipt of Zidovudine (ZDV) during Pregnancy and Mode of Delivery

Study Design (Reference)	Therapy	Transmission Rate with Cesarean Section	Transmission with Other Modes of Delivery	Odds Ratio (95% CI)
Observational Data (International HIV HIV Data Source)[11]	No ZDV	58/599 (10.4%)	1021/5385 (19%)	0.49 (0.29–0.7)
	ZDV	9/196 (2%)	92/1255 (7.3%)	0.26 (0.07–0.70)
Randomized trial (European Mode of Delivery)[9]	No ZDV	2/51 (4%)	16/82 (20%)	0.20 (0–0.8)
	ZDV	1/199 (1%)	5/177 (4%)	0.20 (0–1.7)

From Public Health Service Task Force Recommendations for Use of Antiretroviral Drugs in Pregnant HIV-1-Infected Women for Maternal Health and Interventions to Reduce Perinatal HIV-1 Transmission in the United States, November 3, 2000.

patient confidentiality should be made. Issues such as mandatory reporting of new HIV-positive patient as well as concern for the health and safety of the fetus, medical personnel, and sexual partners may influence the traditional patient–clinician relationship.

3. Intrapartum management

The following precautions should be undertaken.

    a. Minimize invasive procedures. These include placement of fetal scalp electrode, fetal scalp sampling, artificial rupture of membranes etc.

    b. Try to avoid episiotomy.

    c. Elective cesarean section prior to the onset of labor. There is evidence, based on prospective cohort studies[11] and RCTs,[9] that a primary cesarean section prior to the onset of labor further reduces the risk of vertical transmission (Table 3).

E. Prevention/Summary

HIV-1 disease does not have a major adverse effect on pregnancy outcome. Patients' risk factors should guide prenatal interventions designed to improve pregnancy outcomes. There has been dramatic improvement in the ability to reduce the vertical transmission of the HIV-1 virus. These steps include:

1. Recognition of HIV-1-positive women by offering universal HIV screening to all pregnant women

2. Use of zidovudine and other anti-retroviral therapies during the prenatal, intrapartum, and neonatal periods

3. Intrapartum management strategies such as avoidance of invasive procedures and use of primary cesarean intervention

4. Avoidance of breastfeeding in developed countries

References

1. American College of Obstetricians and Gynecologists Educational Bulletin: Human Immunodeficiency Virus Infections in Pregnancy. No. 232, 1997.
2. Alger L, Farley J, Robinson B, et al: Interactions of human immunodeficiency virus infection and pregnancy. Obstet Gynecol 82:787–796, 1993.
3. Augenbraun M, Minkoff HL: HIV disease in pregnancy: Antiretroviral therapy in the pregnant woman. Obstet Gynecol Clin 24:833–854, 1997.
4. Boyer PJ, Dillon M, Navaie M, et al: Factors predictive of maternal-fetal transmission of HIV-1. JAMA 271:1925–1930, 1994.
5. Chu S, Hanson D, Jones J, et al: Pregnancy rates among women infected with human immunodeficiency virus. Obstet Gynecol 87:195–198, 1996.
6. Connor E, Sperling R, Gelber R, et al: Reduction of maternal-infant transmission of human immunodeficiency virus-type 1 with zidovudine treatment. N Engl J Med 331:1173–1180, 1994.

7. Cooper E, Nugent R, Diaz C, et al: After AIDS clinical trial 076: The changing pattern of zidovudine use during pregnancy, and the subsequent reduction in the vertical transmission of human immunodeficiency virus in a cohort of infected women and their infants. J Infect Dis 174:1207–1211, 1996.
8. Culnane M, Fowler M, Lee S: Lack of long-term effects of in utero exposure to zidovudine among uninfected children born to HIV-infected women. JAMA 281:151–157, 1999.
9. European Mode of Delivery Collaboration: Elective cesarean section versus vaginal delivery in prevention of vertical HIV-1 transmission: A randomized clinical trial. Lancet 353:1035–1039, 1999.
10. Fowler M, Simonds R, Roongpisuthipong A: HIV/AIDS in infants, children and adolescents: update on perinatal HIV transmission. Pediatr Clin North Am 47:21–38, 2000.
11. International Perinatal HIV Group: The mode of delivery and the risk of vertical transmission of human immunodeficiency virus type 1—A meta-analysis of 15 prospective cohort studies. N Engl J Med 340:977–987, 1999.
12. Kotler DP: Pregnancy and gastrointestinal disorders: HIV in pregnancy. Gastroenterol Clin 27:269–280, 1998.
13. Marshall R: The HIV-positive patient. Presentation at the AAFP Family-Centered Maternity Care Conference, Seattle, July, 2000.
14. Minkoff H, Augenbraun M: Antiretroviral therapy for pregnant women. Am J Obstet Gynecol 176:478–489, 1997.
15. Newell M, Dunn D, Peckham D, et al: Caesarean section and risk of vertical transmission of HIV-1 infection. Lancet 343:1464–1467, 1994.
16. Nommsen-Rivers L, Heinig M: HIV transmission via breastfeeding: Reflections on the issues. J Hum Lact 13:179–181, 1997.
17. O'Sullivan MJ, Boyer PJ, Scott GB, et al: The pharmacokinetics and safety of zidovudine in the third trimester of pregnancy for women infected with human immunodeficiency virus and their infants: Phase I Acquired Immunodeficiency Syndrome Clinical Trials Group Study (protocol 082). Am J Obstet Gynecol 168:1510–1516, 1993.
18. Public Health Service Task Force recommendations for use of antiretroviral drugs in pregnant HIV-1-infected women for maternal health and interventions to reduce perinatal HIV-1 transmission in the United States. November 3, 2000.
19. Recommendations of the U.S. Public Health Service Task Force on the use of zidovudine to reduce perinatal transmission of human immunodeficiency virus. MMWR 43 (RR11), 1994.
20. Saba J, on behalf of the PETRA Trail Study Team: Interim analysis of early efficacy of three short ZDV/3TC combination regimens to prevent mother-to-child transmission of HIV-1: The PETRA trial. Sixth Conference on Retroviruses and Opportunistic Infections. Chicago, Illinois, 1999 (Abstract S7).
21. Sperling R, Shapiro D, Coombs R, et al: Maternal viral load, zidovudine treatment, and the risk of transmission of human immunodeficiency virus type 1 from mother to infant. N Engl J Med 335:1621–1629, 1996.
22. Temmerman M, Chomba E, Ndinya-Achola J, et al: Maternal human immunodeficiency virus-1 infection and pregnancy outcome. Obstet Gynecol 83:495–501, 1994.
23. Tuomala R: HIV in pregnancy: Prevention of transmission. Obstet Gynecol Clin 24:785–795, 1997.
24. Van Dyke R, Korber B, Popek E, et al: The Ariel project: A prospective cohort study of maternal-child transmission of human immunodeficiency virus type 1 in the era of maternal antiretroviral therapy. J Infect Dis 179:319–328, 1999.
25. Wade N, Birkhead GS, French PT: Short courses of zidovudine and perinatal transmission of HIV. N Engl J Med 340:1042–1043, 1999.

XIII. Asymptomatic Bacteriuria and Urinary Tract Infection

The diagnosis of asymptomatic bacteriuria (ASB) is made by the growth of 10^5 colonies per milliliter of a single pathogen that can be cultured from a clean-voided urinary specimen.

A. Epidemiology

The overall prevalence of asymptomatic bacteriuria (ASB) in pregnancy is 2–10%.

1. Factors that affect the prevalence of ASB[8]

The prevalence of ASB increases twofold in diabetics and is three times more common in women with a history of urinary tract infections. Other factors that can increase the prevalence of this condition include the following.

    a. Anatomic urinary tract abnormalities

    b. Low socioeconomic status (two- to threefold increase)

    c. Increased parity

    d. Sickle-cell trait

2. Causative organisms

Escherichia coli is the most common organism; others include group B streptococcus, *Klebsiella*, *Proteus*, *Enterobacter*, enterococcus, and *Staphylococcus saprophyticus*. *Gardnerella vaginalis* and *Ureaplasma urealyticum* can be found in 10–15% of urine cultures. The clinical significance of this remains unknown at this time.

B. Natural History

1. Physiologic changes in pregnancy

Pregnancy results in a number of physiologic changes that predispose a woman to urinary tract infections.[8]

    a. Hydroureter of pregnancy. This can begin as early as the 7th week of pregnancy and can progress throughout the gestation.

    b. Influence of hormonal changes. This has the effect of slowing ureteral peristalsis.

    c. Urinary retention. As pregnancy progresses the bladder can double in size, in part, due to decreased muscular tone.

2. Upper urogenital tract infections

ASB may be a marker for underlying disease, including urinary tract anomalies (20–55%) and chronic pyelonephritis (10%). There is an increased risk of ascending infection in pregnancy with increase in vesicoureteral reflux. Pyelonephritis occurs in 15–50% of pregnant women with ASB, as compared with 1–2% without.

3. Clinical correlates of urinary tract infections

Symptoms and laboratory findings of urinary infections may be misleading in pregnancy. Early in pregnancy, urinary frequency and lower abdominal or pelvic pressure are common complaints as the uterus enlarges, which causes a sensation of pressure on the bladder. Similar symptoms may recur with descent of the fetal presenting part in late pregnancy.

C. Effects on Perinatal Outcome

1. Pyelonephritis[7]

Pyelonephritis occurs in 1–2% of all pregnancies. Complications include respiratory compromise (2–8%), anemia defined as a hematocrit less than 30% (25–60%), renal insufficiency (25%, transient resolving within days), septic shock, and preterm labor. Undetected ASB in pregnancy leads to pyelonephritis 20–30% of the time.[11]

2. Preterm labor (PTL)/low-birth-weight (LBW) babies

There is a clear association between ASB and an increased incidence of PTL and LBW infants.[9] There is some controversy as to whether the ASB is a marker for low socioeconomic status and LBW or whether it is a primary determinant of these outcomes.

D. Diagnosis

The diagnosis of ASB or urinary tract infections is made based on 10^5 colonies of a single pathogen per milliliter of urine in a clean-voided specimen. Mixed gram-positive flora in colony counts less than 10^5 implies skin contaminants. Lesser colony counts are significant in catheterized specimens. Table 4 shows the sensitivity, specificity, and positive predictive values of various types of urine analyses compared to the gold standard of urine culture. Table 5 shows a cost-effectiveness analysis of these approaches.[2] It is generally preferable to obtain specimens for screening by clean-voided method rather than catheterization. Routine screening by culture is cost-effective when prevalence exceeds 2%. The U.S. Preventive Services Task Force Report has advised against the use of dipstick urinalysis for diagnosis because about 50% of patients with ASB would be missed and recommends the use of a baseline urine culture to detect ASB.[14]

TABLE 4.   Test Results of Urine Samples Obtained on Initial Visit from 1047 Pregnant Women

Test	No. of Positive Samples	No. Positive by Culture	Sensitivity (%)*	Specificity (%)*	Positive Predictive Value (%)*
Urine dipstick					
Leukocyte activity	33	4	16.7	97.2	12.1
Nitrites	14	11	45.8	99.7	78.6
Leukocyte activity or nitrites present	44	12	50.0	96.9	27.3
Leukocyte activity and nitrites present	3	3			
Gram stain					
Borderline or positive	133	33	91.7	89.2	16.5
Positive	72	20	83.3	94.9	27.8
Urinalysis					
> 10 leukocytes	16	6	25.0	99.0	37.5
> 50 leukocytes	5	2	8.3	99.7	40.0
Bacteria present	432	18	75.0	59.7	4.2
Bacteria present or leukocytes > 20	440	20	83.3	58.9	4.5
Urine culture positive	24	24	—	—	—

From Bachman JW, Heise RH, Naessens JM, Timmerman MG: A study of various tests to detect asymptomatic urinary tract infections in an obstetric population. JAMA 270:1971–1974, 1993, with permission.

* The categories presented are not all mutually exclusive. Sensitivity is the percentage of diseased patients detected by the screen, specificity, and the percentage of nondiseased patients with negative screening results; positive predictive value is the percentage of positive screen patients who actually have disease. For dipstick tests with leukocyte activity considered as positive, sensitivity was 16.7% (4/24); specificity 97.2% (994/1023); and positive predictive value 12.1% (4/23).

E. Management Guidelines for ASB and Symptomatic Lower Tract Infection

RCTs support prenatal screening on intake of all pregnant women by urine culture. Treatment of ASB reduces the incidence of preterm labor (PTL), low-birth-weight (LBW) infants and maternal morbidity such as pyelonephritis (Fig. 1).[11] The Cochrane Review of 13 trials demonstrated that the treatment of ASB was associated with a 40% decrease in PTL/LBW (OR 0.60, 95% CI 0.45—0.80, ARR 5.3%, NNT = 19).[11]

  1. Duration of treatment

Historical failure rates of single-dose therapy in pregnancy have been as high as 20–30%. RCT data indicate that single-dose therapy versus 4–7-day regimens result in comparable outcomes regarding pyelonephritis and low birth weight. Seven to ten days of the following antibiotics are also therapeutic options for ASB and symptomatic urinary tract infections.

  2. Drug regimens

    a. Ampicillin, 250–500 mg four times a day

    b. Amoxicillin, 250 mg three times a day

    c. Amoxicillin/clavulanic acid, 250 mg three times a day

    d. Nitrofurantoin, 100 mg four times a day (poor tissue coverage for upper tract infection)

    e. Trimethoprim-sulfamethoxazole, (category C, avoid in first trimester and late pregnancy, use with caution), 1 double-strength (DS) tablet twice a day

    f. Cephalexin, 250 to 500 mg four times a day

    g. Other cephalosporins.

TABLE 5. Cost-effectiveness of Screening Tests for Asymptomatic Bacteriuria in Initial Evaluation of 1047 Pregnant Women

Test	No. of Positive Samples	Total Cost ($)*	Incremental Cost per Additional Positive Culture ($)[†]	No. of "Missed" Cultures
Urine Dipstick				
Leukocyte activity	33	1872	[‡]	20
Nitrites	14	1397	—	13
Leukocyte activity or nitrites present	44	2147	750	12
Leukocyte activity and nitrites present	3	1122	[‡]	21
Gram stain				
Borderline or positive	133	19,030	1603	2
Positive	72	17,505	1790	4
Urinalysis				
> 10 leukocytes	16	16,105	[‡]	18
> 50 leukocytes	5	15,830	[‡]	22
Bacteria present	432	26,505	3587	6
Bacteria present or leukocytes > 20	440	26,705	3615	4
Urine culture positive	24	26,175	1906	

From Bachman JW, Heise RH, Naessens JM, Timmerman MG: A study of various tests to detect asymptomatic urinary tract infections in an obstetric population. JAMA 270:1971–1974, 1993, with permission.

* Total costs are based on the assumption that only that specific screening test will be used and positive screens will be assessed with urine culture. The following costs were used: dipstick urine test, $1; Gram stain, $15; urinalysis, $15; urine culture, $25. For example, using dipstick screening with all cases positive for leukocyte activity receiving urine culture results in (1047 x $1) + (33 x $25) = $1872.

† With the least costly method as a basis (i.e., urine dipstick with a positive screening result if nitrites were present), the average cost of detecting an additional positive culture was determined.

‡ This approach detects fewer positive cultures than the least costly method.

    3. Follow-up
       a. Follow-up ASB and symptomatic infection with cultures, not urinalysis.
       b. One third of patients with ASB have recurrence of bacteriuria. These patients should have repeated cultures during pregnancy.
       c. Patients with more than one relapse or reinfection should be treated with suppression therapy (half of therapeutic dose) until 2 weeks postpartum. An intravenous pyelogram should be performed after 6 weeks postpartum because of the high rate of urinary tract abnormalities. Antibiotics used in suppression include ampicillin or amoxicillin, nitrofurantoin, and cephalexin.
       d. Indications for urologic evaluation during pregnancy include a second relapse or failure to sterilize the urine.

F. Management Guidelines for Pyelonephritis
    1. Inpatient versus outpatient treatment
    Pyelonephritis during pregnancy has traditionally been treated in the inpatient setting. A recent RCT that randomized patients who were hemodynamically stable and able to take oral medications found that outcomes were comparable in both in- and outpatient settings.[6]
    2. Initial choice of antibiotics[7]
    Patients who are medically unstable should receive ampicillin or a cephalosporin plus an aminoglycoside to assure an early response. Because of the tendency for these patients to develop transient renal insufficiency, aminoglycoside drug levels should be obtained if use of these agents continues for more than 2

INFECTION
– Urinary tract
  Antibiotic vs no treatment for asymptomatic bacteriuria (12 trials reviewed)

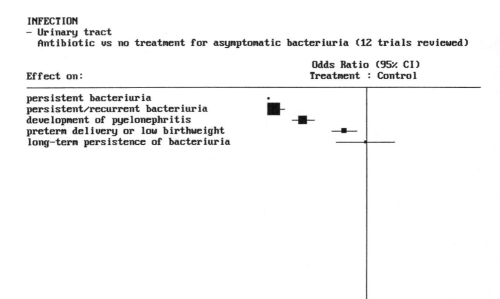

FIGURE 1. Urinary tract infection. Antibiotic versus no treatment for asymptomatic bacteriuria (12 trials reviewed). (From Smaill F: Antibiotic vs. no treatment for asymptomatic bacteriuria. In Enkin MW, Keirse MHNC, Renfrew MJ, Neilson NP [eds.]: Pregnancy and Childbirth Module. Cochrane Database of Systematic Review. Review No. 3170. Cochrane Update on Disk. Oxford, Update Software, with permission.)

days. Patients who are medically stable can be managed with single-drug regimens, including ampicillin, cefazolin, ceftriaxone, mezlocillin, or piperacillin.
3. Patient response
Patients should demonstrate improvement within 48 hours of initiation of appropriate antibiotics. Patients who fail to improve should be evaluated for obstruction, stone, or abscess. Renal ultrasound is usually sufficient, but a single-shot intravenous pyelogram may be necessary.
4. Duration of treatment
Treatment should continue with parenteral antibiotics until the patient is afebrile for 24–48 hours. Oral therapy should be continued to complete a 10–14-day course.
5. Follow-up care
After completing a course of antibiotic therapy, clinicians can opt to follow the patient expectantly with serial urine cultures or to treat with daily antibiotic suppression therapy using ampicillin, a cephalosporin, or Macrodantin. Persistent bacteriuria is less common in the prophylaxis group, although the rate of recurrent pyelonephritis is comparable (7% in prophylaxis group versus 8% in the expectant group).[5] Additional studies are required to resolve which of these management regimens are more effective.

References

1. Abyad A: Screening for asymptomatic bacteriuria in pregnancy: Urinalysis vs urine culture. J Fam Pract 33:427–429, 1991.

2. Bachman J, Heise R, Naessens J, et al: A study of various tests to detect asymptomatic urinary tract infections in an obstetric population. JAMA 270:1971–1974, 1993.
3. Hall D, Theron G, van der Horst W: Significance and treatment of asymptomatic bacteriuria during pregnancy. Internat J Gynecol Obstet 57:179–180, 1997.
4. Jakobi P, Neiger R, Merzbach D, et al: Single-dose antimicrobial therapy in the treatment of asymptomatic bacteriuria in pregnancy. Am J Obstet Gynecol 156:1148–1152, 1987.
5. Lenke R, VanDorsten J, Schifrin B: Pyelonephritis in pregnancy: A prospective randomized trial to prevent recurrent disease evaluating suppressive therapy with nitrofurantoin and close surveillance. Am J Obstet Gynecol 146:953–957, 1983.
6. Millar L, Wing D, Paul R, et al: Outpatient treatment of pyelonephritis in pregnancy: A randomized controlled trial. Obstet Gynecol 86:560–564, 1995.
7. Millar L, Cox S: Urinary tract infections complicating pregnancy. Infect Dis Clin North Am 11:13–26, 1997.
8. Patterson T, Andriole V: Detection, significance, and therapy of bacteriuria in pregnancy: Update in the managed health care era. Infect Dis Clin North Am 11:593–608, 1997.
9. Romero R, Oyarzun E, Mazor M, et al: Meta-analysis of the relationship between asymptomatic bacteriuria and preterm delivery/low birth weight. Obstet Gynecol 73:576–582, 1989.
10. Rouse D, Andrews W, Goldenberg R, et al: Screening and treatment of asymptomatic bacteriuria of pregnancy to prevent pyelonephritis: A cost-effectiveness and cost-benefit analysis. Obstet Gynecol 86:119–223, 1995.
11. Smaill F: Antibiotic versus no treatment for asymptomatic bacteriuria in pregnancy (Cochrane Review). In The Cochrane Library, Issue 4, 2000, Update Software.
12. Smaill F: Single dose vs. 4–7-day antibiotic for bacteriuria (Cochrane Review). In The Cochrane Library, Issue 4, 2000, Update Software.
13. Tincello D, Richmond D: Evaluation of reagent strips in detecting asymptomatic bacteriuria in early pregnancy: Prospective case series. BMJ 316:435–437,1998.
14. U.S. Preventive Services Task Force Guide to Clinical Preventive Services, Screening for Asymptomatic Bacteriuria, 2nd ed. Alexandria, VA, International Medical Publishing, 1996, pp 347–359.
15. Villar JK, Lydon-Rochelle MT: Duration of treatment for asymptomatic bacteriuria during pregnancy (Cochrane Review). In The Cochrane Library, Issue 4, 2000, Oxford, Update Software.

XIV. Pneumonia in Pregnancy
A. Epidemiology
1. Incidence
The incidence of pneumonia in pregnancy varies in studies from 1.5 to 2.5 per 1000 pregnancies.[9] There is some evidence that pneumonia may be increasing in some urban populations owing to increasing numbers of women with HIV infection.

2. Risk factors
Pneumonia occurs with increased frequency in women with the following risk factors.
   a. Anemia
   b. Smoking
   c. Pre-existing heart and lung disease
   d. Illicit drug use
   e. HIV infection and other immunosuppressive disease

3. Causative agents[4,9]
   a. Bacterial. The causative agents responsible for pneumonia are similar to those of the nonpregnant patient.
      i. *Streptococcus pneumoniae*. This is the cause of 30–50% of bacterial pneumonias. Clinical onset is usually abrupt and virulent. Lobar consolidation is commonly seen and pleural effusions occur in 25% of cases.
      ii. *Haemophilus influenzae*. The following risk factors or underlying risk factors are associated with an increased incidence of this bacterial infection: chronic lung disease, smoking, and pre-existing influenza infections.

      iii. *Staphylococcus aureus.* This infection often occurs as a secondary pulmonary infection after an influenza infection or occurs as a result of a bacteremia.

      iv. *Klebsiella/E coli.* These gram-negative organisms often occur as nosocomial infections in hospitalized patients. *Klebsiella* pneumonia tends to occur in women with compromised immune or nutritional states. It is a very aggressive pathogen that causes significant damage to lung tissue.

      v. Atypical infections. These include *Mycoplasma, Legionella* and chlamydia. *Mycoplasma* and chlamydia infections tend to be more gradual and less dramatic in their appearance. *Legionella* presents in a similar fashion to other bacterial pneumonias and commonly involves other organ systems (GI, renal, neurologic).

   b. Viral. Progression to pneumonia is noted more frequently in certain viral infections during pregnancy, most notably, type A influenza, varicella, rubeola, and HIV. Secondary bacterial infections, as noted above, are common.

   c. *Mycobacterium tuberculosis.* In endemic areas, the incidence of tuberculosis may approach 0.01% of all pregnancies.[5]

   d. Other agents. Other unusual pathogens, such as fungi, have been reported, along with increased rates of *Pneumocystis carinii* for patients with HIV disease.

B. Natural History

1. Altered physiology in pregnancy[8]

The tendency for infections to progress to pneumonia may be increased in pregnancy. Cell-mediated immunity appears to be somewhat diminished, especially in the second and third trimester. T helper cells are decreased, and there are altered responses to antigens. hCG, progesterone, alpha-fetoprotein, and cortisol may inhibit cell-mediated function. Functional residual capacity is decreased in pregnancy, and oxygen consumption is decreased. As a result, hypoxemia is poorly tolerated by patients with pneumonia.

2. Impact on perinatal morbidity/mortality

   a. Prenatal. Preterm labor is increased if pneumonia occurs during weeks 20 to 36 of gestation.

   b. Maternal. In the pre-antibiotic era maternal mortality for pneumonia in pregnancy approached 30%. Studies in the past two decades report mortality rates of 0–4%.[8] Women who have underlying comorbid conditions (HIV disease, chronic pulmonary or cardiac conditions, etc.) are at increased risk of serious complications such as adult respiratory distress syndrome.

   c. Fetal/neonatal. There are increased risks of prematurity that range from 4% to 44% depending on the maternal comorbidities and populations studied.[8] Various studies have noted an increased incidence of small for gestational age,[2] intrauterine fetal demise,[1] and neonatal death.[6] Varicella occurring late in pregnancy may lead to neonatal varicella (see subsection XVI).

   d. Teratogenicity. The influenza virus has not been identified as a teratogen. Varicella infections during the first 20 weeks of pregnancy are associated with a 2% risk of congenital varicella syndrome.[7]

C. Diagnosis[9]

Family physicians should use the tools available to them in the care of their general populations including shielded x-rays, sputum, and blood cultures. Other diagnostic modalities include sputum silver stains for *Pneumocystis carinii*, acid-fast stains for

Mycobacterium, and various serologic tests (direct fluorescent antibody, DNA probes, complement fixation antibody, etc.) for *Chlamydia* and *Mycoplasma pneumoniae*.

D. Management

The initial diagnosis should not be unnecessarily delayed because of physician reticence to perform a chest x-ray in the symptomatic patient. Aggressive maintenance of oxygenation is important for both the mother and the fetus. Antibiotic and antiviral therapy must be determined by clinical circumstances and the most likely causative agents. Because of the risk to the mother's life, antimicrobial therapy in the immunocompromised patient may necessitate the use of agents for which there is little experience in pregnancy. Besides standard antibiotic agents that have already been discussed, antiviral agents that can be used in pregnancy to treat pneumonia include acyclovir and amantadine. Clinicians should maintain close observation for premature labor.

E. Prevention

Clinicians should offer the influenza vaccine to all women who are pregnant during the winter months. This vaccine is safe to use during pregnancy; it decreases the risk of influenza and common complications of secondary bacterial pneumonia.

References

1. Benedetti T, Valle R, Ledger W: Antepartum pneumonia in pregnancy. Obstet Gynecol 144:413–417, 1982.
2. Berkowitz K, LaSala Al: Risk factors associated with the increasing prevalence of pneumonia during pregnancy. Am J Obstet Gynecol 163:981–985, 1990.
3. Catanzarite VA, Williams D: Adult respiratory distress syndrome in pregnancy: Report of three cases and review of the literature. Obstet Gynecol Surv 52:381–392, 1997.
4. Goodrum L: Pneumonia in pregnancy. Semin Perinatol 21:276–283, 1997.
5. Huff RW, Piper JM: Pulmonary disease in pregnancy. Int J Gynaecol Obstet 54:187–196, 1996.
6. Madinger N, Greenspoon J, Eilrodt A: Pneumonia during pregnancy: Has modern technology improved maternal and fetal outcome? Am J Obstet Gynecol 161:657–662, 1989.
7. Patuszak A, Levey M, Schick R, et al: Outcome after maternal varicella infection in the first 20 weeks of pregnancy. N Engl J Med 330:901–905, 1994.
8. Rigby F, Pastorek J: Pneumonia during pregnancy. Clin Obstet Gynecol 39:107–119, 1996.
9. Riley L: Pneumonia and tuberculosis in pregnancy. Infect Dis Clin N Amer 11:119–133, 1997.

XV. Rubella

A. Epidemiology

Maternal and fetal rubella infections were common 30 years ago. With the advent of mass rubella vaccination, the incidence of the congenital rubella syndrome has fallen to less than 10 cases per 100,000 live-births per year.[5]

B. Natural History

1. Acute rubella infection

Acute rubella infection consists of a maculopapular rash lasting up to 3 days, generalized lymphadenopathy including posterior auricular and occipital nodes, and transient arthritis and arthralgia. Fifty percent to 70% of infections are symptomatic.

2. Transmission/incubation

The incubation period is 14–21 days. Transmission occurs via respiratory droplets. Patients are most infectious in the prodromal phase preceding the rash.

3. Immunity

Immunity to rubella is documented by serology with declining complement fixation titers. This pattern is common following naturally acquired infections and vaccination. Reinfection can occur in previously infected individuals and can result in fetal transmission in about 5% of the cases that occur during the first trimester.[1]

4. Vertical transmission[3]

Rubella infections occurring during the first 11 weeks of gestation are associated with a 90% risk of congenital defects. After 16 weeks' gestation, this risk is negligible.

C. Effects on Perinatal Outcome: Congenital Rubella Syndrome[2,3,6]

1. Transient effects (newborn to 6 months old)

These include hepatosplenomegaly, pneumonia, jaundice, hemolytic anemia, and thrombocytopenic purpura.

2. Permanent abnormalities

These include sensorineural deafness (may be profound), congenital heart defects (especially patent ductus arteriosus), cataracts, microphthalmia, and encephalopathy.

3. Late-onset effects

These include endocrine dysfunction (diabetes, thyroid disease, and growth hormone deficiency), ocular and auditory damage, progressive encephalopathy, vascular sclerosis, and hypertension. Fifty to seventy percent of infants may appear normal at birth and develop late manifestations at a later time.

D. Management Guidelines

1. Routine screening

Routine screening for rubella occurs at the onset of prenatal care. A recent Canadian study indicated that routine screening for rubella during pregnancy was occurring 94% of the time.[3]

2. Potential exposure of the non-immune patient

Immediate serologic evaluation of the non-immune patient should occur with potential exposure to rubella. Hemagglutination inhibition antibodies are followed by complement-fixation antibodies within several days after onset of rash.

3. Patient with acute rubella infection during early pregnancy

Patients who have a diagnosis of acute rubella in the first 16 weeks of pregnancy should be offered counseling and consideration of termination of pregnancy. Immune globulin does not prevent congenital rubella infection but may modify its clinical course. Its use is limited to patients who do not wish to consider therapeutic abortion.

E. Prevention

The prevention of congenital rubella remains one of the most significant successful public health stories of the 20th century. About 30% of women of child-bearing age who have the two-dose MMR vaccine develop low antibody levels within 15 years of vaccination.[2] Thus, clinicians must maintain vigilance as to which of their patients should be revaccinated in the preconceptional period or during the postpartum period. Inadvertent vaccination during pregnancy is generally associated with no adverse fetal effect although subclinical neonatal rubella cases have been reported.[4]

References

1. Coulter C, Wood R, Robson J: Rubella infection in pregnancy. Commun Dis Intell 23:93–96, 1999.
2. Davidkin I, Peltola H, Leinikki P, et al: Duration of rubella immunity induced by two-dose measles, mumps and rubella (MMR) vaccination: A 15-year follow-up in Finland. J Vaccine 18:3106–3112, 2000.
3. Gyorkos TW, Tannenbaum TN, Abrahamowicz M, et al: Evaluation of rubella screening in pregnant women. CMAJ 159:1091–1097, 1998.
4. Hofmann J, Kortung M, Pustowoit B, et al: Persistent fetal rubella vaccine virus infection following inadvertent vaccination during early pregnancy. J Med Virol 61:155–158, 2000.
5. Mann JM, Preblud SR, Hoffman RE: Assessing risks of rubella infection during pregnancy. JAMA 245:1647–1651, 1981.
6. McElhaney RD, Ringer M, EdHart DJ, et al: Rubella immunity in a cohort of pregnant women. Infect Control Hosp Epidemiol 20:64–66, 1999.

7. Saltzman RL, Jordan MC: Viral infections. In Burrow GN, Ferris TF (eds): Medical Complications During Pregnancy, 3rd ed. Philadelphia, W.B. Saunders, 1988.

XVI. Varicella-Zoster
Jennifer Bell, M.D.

A. Epidemiology
1. Immune status

Most pregnant women are immune because of previous infection. History of infection is highly predictive of immunity. Eighty percent of adult women with a negative history have serologic evidence of immunity.[10] Adult immigrants from tropical countries may have a much lower rate of immunity.[9]

2. Incidence

The incidence of varicella in pregnancy is 5 to 10 in 10,000.[5]

B. Natural History
1. Transmission

Infection is transmitted by direct contact (droplet, aerosol from vesicular fluid of skin lesions) or respiratory secretions.

2. Significant exposure

This occurs by face to face contact with a case for at least 5 min, contact indoors with a case for > 1 hour, or living in the same household as a case. Infectivity extends from 1 to 2 days before onset of rash until the lesions are crusted, usually 4 to 5 days after onset of rash. The incubation period is 10 to 21 days.[9]

C. Effects on Perinatal Outcome
Prospective data from a 1998 British study[5] suggests that the varicella in gravidas may not be more severe than in nonpregnant adults.

1. Maternal pneumonia

Whether chickenpox pneumonitis is more common or severe in pregnancy remains uncertain. Retrospective data may represent reporting bias of hospitalized cases, according to the above study. Risk factors of pregnancy associated with increased severity of varicella pneumonia are: third-trimester occurrence, smoking, COPD, systemic steroids, and degree of the rash.[5]

2. Fetal varicella embryopathy

This fetal infection is similar to congenital rubella syndrome with limb hypoplasia, encephalomyelitis, cataracts, chorioretinitis, microphthalmia, and IUGR.[1] There is a 1% chance of embryopathy if infection occurs in the first trimester, 2.2% chance if between 13 and 20 weeks' gestation, and 0% if infection occurs later in pregnancy, according to prospective data from a large 1994 study.[2] Ultrasound findings for fetal infection include polyhydramnios, limb and ventricular abnormalities, fetal hydrops, and liver hyperechogenicities.[8]

3. Association with spontaneous abortion

There is no clear evidence that the rate of spontaneous abortion is increased.[2,7]

4. Vertical transmission

Perinatal transmission, and subsequent congenital disseminated varicella, is likely if maternal varicella rash occurs in the critical period between 4 days before and 2 days after delivery.[4]

  a. Infants exposed by maternal infection from 28 to 7 days before delivery. These infants receive the transplacental maternal antibody. If neonatal chickenpox ensues, it usually follows a benign course.
  b. Exposure 7 to 3 days prior to delivery. Progressively fewer newborns have varicella antibody when the mothers rash occurs 7 to 3 days before delivery.
  c. Exposure less than 3 days prior to delivery. No antibody is detected in babies born less than 3 days after onset of the mothers rash.[4]

    d. Neonatal varicella infections. Varicella infections occasionally occur in the critical period without the patient receiving the recommended immunoglobulin. The clinical attack rate in infants whose mothers developed rash between 7 days prior to and 7 days after delivery is 60%.[5]

    e. Herpes zoster in infancy. This has been reported in those born to mothers with varicella in the second half of pregnancy.[2] There is no evidence that maternal herpes zoster causes intrauterine infection.[2]

D. Management Guidelines

1. Non-immune pregnant women

These women should avoid contact with those who have varicella or zoster infections. Risk of exposure may be unavoidable in the prodromal phase (before lesions erupt).

2. Determination of immunity

Immunity is determined by enzyme-linked or latex agglutination; complement-fixation titers are not sensitive enough.[9]

3. Significant exposure in a non-immune pregnant woman

This exposure should be treated with varicella-zoster immune globulin (VZIG), 125 units/10kg. The minimum dose is 125 units, and the maximum dose is 625 units intramuscularly, given within 72 hours of exposure. Fractional doses are not recommended.[9] There is an ongoing study in which an intravenous form of VZIG is used, possibly extending this 72-hour window to a week.[3]

4. Maternal varicella infections: When to treat with antiviral therapy:

For varicella pneumonia and severe varicella in pregnancy, acyclovir has been recommended, at 10mg/kg IV three times daily for a minimum of 5 days.[5]

5. Herpes zoster

Herpes zoster does not require treatment.

6. Infants with perinatal exposure

Exposure resulting from maternal infection in which the rash occurs 5 days before until 2 days after birth should receive VZIG, 1.25 ml intramuscularly, immediately after birth. These infants must be monitored closely for 14–16 days (the end of any possible incubation period) and may still need IV or oral acyclovir at 10–15 mg/kg/dose q 8 hrs should congenital varicella ensue.[5] Maternal VZIG primarily attenuates the disease course in infants. There is some indication in a recent study that the clinical attack rate of perinatal varicella may be modified by its use.[2]

E. Prevention

1. Vaccination

This is indicated for immunocompetent persons older than 12 months without a history of varicella. In persons older than 12 years, two doses of vaccine administered 4–8 weeks apart are recommended.

2. Preconception

Question all women of childbearing age regarding chickenpox history. Those with negative replies should be offered the varicella vaccine, or serologic testing followed by vaccination of susceptibles. Pregnancy should be avoided for 1 month after each vaccine dose.[9] The Varivax manufacturer has established a Pregnancy Registry accessed by phone (800-986-8999) to monitor the outcome of women receiving the vaccine 3 months before or at any time during pregnancy.

3. Postpartum

The varicella vaccine may be considered for a nursing mother.[9] The first dose could be given upon discharge from the hospital, and the second dose at the 2 month well-child check.

References

1. Brunell PA: Fetal and neonatal varicella-zoster infections. Semin Perinatol 7:47–56, 1983.
2. Enders G, Miller E, Cradock-Watson J et al: Consequences of maternal varicella and herpes zoster in pregnancy: Prospective study of 1739 cases. Lancet 343:1547–1550, 1994.
3. Inocencion G, Loebseein R, Lalkin A, et al: Managing exposure to chickenpox during pregnancy. Can Fam Physician 44:745–747, 1998.
4. Miller E, Cradock-Watson JE, Ridehalgh MS: Outcome in newborn babies given anti-varicella-zoster immunoglobulin after perinatal maternal infection with varicella-zoster virus. Lancet 12:371–373,1989.
5. Nathwani D, Maclean A, Conway S, et al: Varicella infections in pregnancy and the newborn. Br J Infect 36:59–71,1998.
6. Paryani SG, Arvin AM: Intrauterine infection with varicella-zoster virus after maternal varicella. N Engl J Med 314:1542–1546,1986.
7. Pastuszak AL, Levy M, Schick B, et al: Outcome after maternal varicella infection in the first 20 weeks of pregnancy. N Engl J Med 330:901–905,1994.
8. Pretorius DH, Hayward I, Jones KL, et al: Sonographic evaluation of pregnancies with maternal varicella infection. J Ultrasound Med 11:459–463, 1992.
9. Prevention of varicella: Recommendations of the Advisory Committee on Immunization Practices (ACIP). MMWR 45(RR-11):1–36, 1996.
10. Rouse D, Gardner M, Allen SJ, et al: Management of the presumed susceptible varicella (chickenpox)-exposed gravida: A cost-effectiveness/cost-benefit analysis. Obstet Gynecol 87:932–936, 1996.

XVII. Cytomegalovirus

A. Epidemiology

Cytomegalovirus (CMV) is a herpes virus that commonly infects young adults. It is transmitted via respiratory droplets, urine, sexual activity, breastfeeding, and blood transfusion. Women who reside or work with young children as teachers, day care, or health care workers are at particular risk for contracting this viral infection. Young children who are infected with CMV in a day-care setting (seroprevalence 29–83%) can continue to shed this virus in urine and other secretions for up to 14 months.[8] It is estimated that up to 25% of all congenital CMV infections are related to day-care exposure.[1] Higher socioeconomic groups have a lower seroprevalence of CMV and thus are at increased risk of contracting a primary infection during pregnancy. Primary maternal infections occur in 0.7–4% of pregnancies with 30–40% of these infections resulting in congenital infection. Recurrent infection occurs more commonly (1–14%) but results in congenital infection only 0.2–2% of the time.[8] CMV is the most common congenitally acquired infection affecting approximately 45,000 fetuses per year in the U.S. (0.2–2.2% of all neonates) and causing symptomatic infections in the newborns of between 8% and 14% of these infections. Because of the subtle or asymptomatic presentation of CMV infections, clinicians underdiagnose this infection both during pregnancy and after childbirth. Congenital CMV infections are the leading infectious cause of hearing loss and developmental delay.[8]

B. Natural History

1. Maternal

CMV infections are usually subclinical, occasionally associated with a "mononucleosis"-like illness with pharyngitis, lymphadenopathy, and fever. These infections may be accompanied by hepatitis, pneumonia, and thrombocytopenia.

2. Fetal

Fetal structural effects are most pronounced after first-trimester infections and are characterized by microcephaly and intracranial calcifications. Fetal functional effects such as thrombocytopenia and hepatitis are more common with infections in latter stages of pregnancy.

3. Neonatal

a. Symptomatic (CMV inclusion disease). The newborn presents with hepatosplenomegaly (60–74%), petechiae (76–79%), jaundice (63–67%), and microcephaly (50%). Abnormal laboratory studies include thrombocytopenia, hyperbilirubinemia, abnormal liver function tests, and increased cerebrospinal fluid protein.[8] Abnormal CT findings, including ventricular enlargement and intracranial calcifications, occur in more than 50% of infected newborns. More than 90% of infants who survive the initial infection experience long-term complications such as sensorineural hearing loss, chronic neurologic dysfunction (seizures, developmental delay, mental retardation), and visual impairment.

   b. Asymptomatic. These infants have the congenital infection but are asymptomatic in the newborn period. They experience many of the long-term complications listed above but at a lower incidence. Hearing loss is the most common impairment affecting about 15% of those infected. This impairment may be detected by audio-evoked response testing as early as two to three months of age and may progress to profound hearing loss by three to four years old. Developmental delay and/or mental retardation affect about 15% of this group.

C. Effects on Perinatal Outcome[7,8]

1. Pregnancy

The majority of infections are clinically silent. Among all pregnancies, 1.2% are infected in utero with CMV. Symptomatic neonatal infection (CMV inclusion disease) may result from CMV reactivation as well as primary infection. CMV inclusion disease is more likely with first- and second-trimester infection.

2. Newborn

Ten percent of infants infected in utero develop CMV inclusion disease. Findings include hepatosplenomegaly, jaundice, thrombocytopenic purpura, chorioretinitis, cerebral calcifications, microcephaly, interstitial pneumonitis, sensorineural hearing loss, central nervous system anomalies, and mental retardation. Mortality rate is 29% in symptomatic newborns; the vast majority of newborns affected experience severe disability.

3. Post-neonatal

Ninety percent of infants infected in utero appear normal. Ten to twenty percent of these infants develop late sequelae during the first 2 years of life, including seizures, sensorineural hearing loss, psychomotor delays, ocular problems, microcephaly, and mental retardation.

D. Diagnosis

1. Prenatal

The diagnosis of maternal CMV infection is made with ELISA testing that measures a conversion from negative to positive, a fourfold or higher increase in the CMV IgG titers or the presence of CMV IgM antibodies.[10] A positive urine culture also signifies the presence of a primary or recurrent CMV infection. Women with known primary CMV infection in pregnancy have an approximate 30–40% risk of vertical transmission of the virus to their fetus. These women may opt to undergo an amniocentesis to determine if this transmission has occurred. These women need to know that only 10% of the congenital infections have a symptomatic infection at birth. Either CMV culture (sensitivity 50–69%) or polymerase chain reaction testing (sensitivity 77–100%) may be employed.[5,6] This sensitivity can be increased if there is a waiting period of at least 6 weeks between the confirmation of CMV seroconversion and performing the amniocentesis.[5] The presence of specific ultrasonographic abnormalities (abdominal calcifications, ascites, ventriculomegaly etc.) generally identify fetuses who are more severely affected.[6]

2. Neonatal

The standard diagnostic tools include culture and PCR testing of the neonatal urine. The advantage of the latter method is its more rapid reporting.

E. Management Guidelines[8]

There are currently no accepted forms of treatment of CMV during pregnancy, neonatal, or postneonatal periods. Ganciclovir has been used to treat life-threatening CMV infections in immunocompromised patients. Phase III trials are still being conducted to determine whether ganciclovir has a role in the treatment of symptomatic infection of CMV in the newborn. This agent's known teratogenicity and embryotoxicity have precluded its use during pregnancy. CMV hyperimmune gammaglobulin also has the potential to be used to treat acute neonatal infections.[6]

F. Prevention

1. Patient education

Women at increased risk of contracting CMV during pregnancy, such as daycare workers and mothers with a toddler in day care, should know their CMV antibody status. Those women who are seronegative should be counseled how to decrease the risk of acquiring this infection. This counseling should consist of frequent hand-washing and the use of gloves while changing diapers or having extensive contact with saliva. This regimen has been shown in a recent randomized controlled trial to be effective in preventing the acquisition of CMV during pregnancy.[2] Another important group at increased risk of acquiring CMV during pregnancy is the subset of young women with a history of STDs. These women should be counseled to use condoms throughout their pregnancy and to avoid new sexual partners.[1]

2. Provider education

Clinicians have not been adequately informed about the silent epidemic of CMV. The three at-risk groups identified above should undergo serologic testing for the presence of CMV IgM and IgG antibodies at the onset of pregnancy. If seronegative, they should have re-enforced counseling throughout pregnancy to minimize potential contact with sources of CMV.

3. Primary prevention: Towne vaccine

The Towne vaccine has been shown in several randomized trials to prevent transmission of CMV in kidney transplant recipients.[3] This vaccine has been tested in women of child-bearing age and has been shown to induce cellular immunity that persisted for the 6 months of monitoring.[4] This vaccine offers the potential for primary prevention of this devastating congenital infection.

References

1. Adler S: Cytomegalovirus and pregnancy. Curr Opin Obstet Gynecol 4:670–675, 1992.
2. Adler S, Finney J, Manganello A, et al: Prevention of child-to-mother transmission of cytomegalovirus by changing behaviors: A randomized controlled trial. Pediatr Infect Dis J 15:240–246, 1996.
3. Adler S: Current prospects for immunization against cytomegaloviral disease. Infect Agents Dis 5:29–35, 1996.
4. Adler S, Hempfling S, Starr S, et al: Safety and immunogenicity of the Towne strain cytomegalovirus vaccine. Pediatr Infect Dis J 17:200–206, 1998.
5. Bodeus M, Hubinont C, Bernard P, et al: Prenatal diagnosis of human cytomegalovirus by culture and polymerase chain reaction: 98 pregnancies leading to congenital infection. Prenat Diagn 19:314–317, 1999.
6. Boggess K: Perinatal viral and parasitic infections. ACOG Practice Bulletin No. 20, September 2000.
7. Brown H, Abernathy M: Cytomegalovirus infection. Semin Perinatol 22:260–266, 1998.
8. Daniel Y, Gull I, Peyser R, et al: Congenital cytomegalovirus infection. Eur J Obstet Gynaecol Reprod Biol 63:7–16, 1995.
9. Piper J, Wen T: Perinatal cytomegalovirus and toxoplasmosis: Challenges of antepartum therapy. Clin Obstet Gynecol 42:81–96, 1999.
10. Scott L, Hollier L, Dias K: Perinatal herpesvirus infections. Infect Dis Clin North Am 11:27–53, 1997.

XVIII. Toxoplasmosis
A. Epidemiology
Toxoplasma gondii is a protozoan that is commonly found in raw meat and cat feces. Its tachyzoite developmental stage is metabolically active in all mammalian species. Approximately 10–20% of women in the United States have serologic evidence of previous infection. Nevertheless, congenital toxoplasmosis is a rare occurrence in the United States, with an incidence in 1 in 10,000. The incidence is higher in countries such as France and Austria, where the consumption of undercooked meat is higher.
B. Natural History
Symptoms of infection are often mistaken for "flu" or infectious mononucleosis with pharyngitis, lymphadenopathy, fever, maculopapular rash, and lymphocytosis. Chorioretinitis can occur, with photophobia and visual blurring. Immuno-compromised individuals may experience pulmonary and central nervous system involvement.
C. Effects on Perinatal Outcome[10]
1. Timing of infection
First-trimester infections are transmitted to the fetus only 10% of the time. However, these infections tend to be more severe in more than 70% of the cases with an overall mortality rate of 5%. Third-trimester infections result in fetal infection in about 60% of cases, but the infants are generally not severely affected. A retrospective study of 564 women with toxoplasmosis in a high-risk area of France who received standard treatment showed a 29% transmission rate, with the rate sharply increasing if the infection was contracted at a later stage of pregnancy.[4] In contrast, a cohort analysis of nearly 90,000 infants in a low-risk country (Denmark) demonstrated a vertical transmission rate of 19.4% in untreated women.[9]
2. Congenital infection
Infants affected by congenital infection may demonstrate chorioretinitis, abnormal spinal fluid, anemia, splenomegaly, jaundice, fever, lymphadenopathy, intracerebral calcifications, hydrocephalus, and being small for gestational age. Most infants are asymptomatic at birth. Eighty to ninety percent of these infants develop ophthalmologic or central nervous system complications during childhood.[2]
D. Diagnosis[10]
1. Maternal infection
Diagnosis of acute toxoplasmosis in pregnancy can be made by using ELISA, hemagglutination, and immunofluorescence antibody determinations. Finding modest levels of IgG antibodies in the absence of IgM signifies remote infection and is associated with favorable outcomes. The presence of IgM antibodies probably indicates recent infection, although this antibody can linger for months. The specificity of some commercial IgM assays may be as low as 50%, resulting in an unacceptable level of false-positive tests. This erroneous test result may lead some patients with presumed toxoplasmosis early in pregnancy to terminate a pregnancy. One of the most experienced laboratories to confirm acute maternal infection is at the Palo Alto Medical Foundation (415-326-8120).
2. Fetal congenital infection
The diagnosis of fetal infection in utero required the use of fetal blood sampling for the presence of IgM antibodies or the monitoring of serial ultrasounds to detect signs of congenital infection. Suggestive sonographic findings include ventriculomegaly, microcephaly, ascites and IUGR.[2] This has now been replaced by a highly sensitive (> 98%) and specific (> 98%) polymerase chain reaction

(PCR) analysis of amniotic fluid.[5] The availability of this test can now be used to eliminate the problem of high false-positive maternal serology described above.

3. Neonatal infection

When infection is suspected in the newborn, paired maternal and neonatal blood tests looking for the presence of IgM and IgA antibodies should be done. Other viral congenital infections, notably herpes and cytomegalovirus, should be ruled out. Neonatal cerebrospinal fluid studies, head imaging, and an indirect fundoscopic exam should be undertaken.

E. Management Guidelines[2]

1. Screening

Routine screening is not recommended in the United States because of the very low prevalence of the disease. As a result, the positive predictive value (PPV) of abnormal maternal serology is less than 1%. It is recommended to screen women with HIV disease for this infection.

2. Treatment of maternal infection

Maternal infection should be treated with the macrolide spiramycin. This drug can be obtained through the Food and Drug Administration (301-4443-9553). Spiramycin (1.5 g every 12 hours) has been shown to decrease transmission rates by 60%[3] and not to cause harmful fetal effects.[12] Pyrimethamine, sulfonamides, and folic acid are added to this treatment regimen. This multidrug regimen is most effective at this time.

3. Treatment of confirmed in utero infection

A positive amniotic fluid PCR for toxoplasmosis confirms an active fetal or congenital infection. The recommended treatment regimen for this consists of pyrimethamine, sulfadiazine, and leucovorin. Clinicians should obtain pharmacologic and perinatal consultations to balance treatment efficacy with the avoidance of bone marrow suppression.

4. Treatment of newly diagnosed neonatal infection

Newborns infected with toxoplasmosis whose mothers were not treated during pregnancy benefit with treatment with drug regimens listed in this section. Improved outcomes include a reduction in hearing loss, developmental delay, and visual impairments.[8]

F. Prevention of Toxoplasmosis

In a high-prevalence area in Belgium, a risk reduction program that emphasized hygienic precautions with cats and the proper preparation of meat resulted in a 60% reduction in seroconversion.[6] In a low-prevalence country such as the U.S., family physicians should emphasize this counseling with their at-risk patients.

References

1. Bader T, Macones G, Asch D: Prenatal screening for toxoplasmosis. Obstet Gynecol 90:457–464, 1997.
2. Boyer K: Diagnosis and treatment of congenital toxoplasmosis. Advan Pediat Infect Dis 11:449–467, 1996.
3. Couvreur J, Desmonts G, Thulliez P: Prophylaxis of congenital toxoplasmosis. Effect of spiramycin on placental infections. Antimicrob Chemother 22:193–200, 1988.
4. Dunn D, Wallon M, Peyron F, et al: Mother-to-child transmission of toxoplasmosis: Risk estimates for clinical counselling. Lancet 353:1829–1833, 1999.
5. Forestier F, Hohlfeld P, Sole Y, et al: Prenatal diagnosis of congenital toxoplasmosis by PCR: Extended experience (letter). Prenat Diagn 18:405–415, 1998.
6. Foulan W, Naessens A, Derde M: Evaluation of the possibilities for preventing toxoplasmosis. Am J Perinatol 11:57–61, 1994.
7. Foulan W, Villena E, Stray-Pedersen B, et al: Treatment of toxoplasmosis during pregnancy: A multicenter study of impact on fetal transmission and children's sequelae at age 1 year. Am J Obstet Gynecol 180:410–415, 1999.

8. Guerina N, Ware J, Burbridge J, et al: Neurodevelopmental outcomes for infants with congenital *Toxoplasma* infection from a newborn serologic screening and treatment program. Pediatr Res 37:292A, 1995.
9. Lebech M, Andersen O, Christensen N, et al: Feasibility of neonatal screening for toxoplasmosis infection in the absence of prenatal treatment. Lancet 353:1834–1837, 1999.
10. Mittendorf R, Pryde P, Herschel M, et al: Is routine antenatal toxoplasmosis screening justified in the United States? Statistical considerations in the application of medical screening tests. Clin Obstet Gynecol 42:163–175, 1999.
11. Roizen N, Swisher CN, Stein MA, et al: Neurologic and developmental outcome in treated congenital toxoplasmosis. Pediatrics 95:11–29, 1995.
12. Vergani P, Ghidini A, Ceruti P, et al: Congenital toxoplasmosis: Efficacy of maternal treatment with spiramycin alone. Am J Reprod Immunol 39:335–340, 1998.

XIX. Parvovirus
A. Epidemiology
This DNA virus was first identified as a cause of non-immune hydrops fetalis in 1984.[3] This virus primarily affects children in the late winter and spring although it can occur any time of the year. Approximately 50% of women of child-bearing age are immune; thus, the other half are susceptible to contracting this illness during pregnancy.[6] Transmission of the virus occurs via contact with nasal or oral secretions. The parvovirus is hardy and appears to survive on plates and utensils. Women at highest risk of this infection include non-teaching personnel in schools (cooks, servers, etc.), day care and health care workers.[6] Other risk factors for maternal seroconversion include increasing number of children in the household, particularly if they are 6–7 years old.[9]

B. Natural History[7]
Parvovirus causes an influenza-type syndrome known as erythema infectiosum or fifth disease. Clinical signs and symptoms include the "slapped" cheek rash that spreads to the trunk and extremities in a lacy, erythematous fashion. Adults often have a symmetric polyarthralgia, most often affecting the knees and proximal interphalangeal joints. Parvovirus affects the erythroid system in the bone marrow causing both hemolysis and temporary cessation of red blood cell production. This aplastic stage can last for 7–10 days and is marked by anemia and a low reticulocyte count.

C. Effects on Perinatal Outcome
Maternal infection with parvovirus during the first half of pregnancy is associated with an increased incidence of miscarriage. Fetal infection is not associated with an increased risk of congenital anomalies. The neonatal outcome of pregnancies affected with maternal parvovirus is normal 90–95% of the time.[5,7] The major fetal complication is non-immune hydrops fetalis. This fetal complication occurs in about 3–8% of maternal infections and is thought to be a result of fetal anemia and high-output congestive heart failure.[1]

D. Diagnosis
1. Maternal infection
Diagnosis of maternal infection is made with IgM serologies that are generally positive within 3 days of the onset of symptoms. The IgM antibody remains for 1–2 months and is replaced with IgG and may be detected with ELISA, radioimmunoassay, and Western blot tests with a sensitivity of 79%.[2]
2. Fetal infection[1,2,7]
Fetal IgM antibodies only appear in the fetal circulation after 22 weeks' gestation. Therefore, it is not warranted to use this testing modality during the first 22 weeks of pregnancy. Polymerase chain reaction (PCR) testing of fetal tissue or fluids is highly sensitive but is not readily available in most settings and requires invasive fetal testing such as cordocentesis. When acute maternal infection is

confirmed with positive IgM titers, the fetus usually undergoes biweekly ultra-sounds for 8–10 weeks to see if there is any evidence of an evolving fetal hydrops situation.

E. Management[7,8]

The vast majority of maternal parvovirus infections result in normal birth outcomes. If serial ultrasounds show no evidence of fetal hydrops, no other intervention or surveillance is warranted. There are two approaches to the management of fetal hydrops. The active approach consists of repeated intrauterine fetal transfusions. The second approach is a conservative "wait and see" one that results in outcomes in retrospective studies that are comparable to the active approach. RCTs are needed to determine which approach results in the improved perinatal outcomes.

F. Prevention

Clinicians should instruct women at increased risk of exposure to parvovirus (day care, non-teacher personnel, health care workers) at preconceptional and early prenatal visits to use frequent hand-washing at their work sites. They should encourage their maternity patients to report influenza-like illnesses, especially if they are accompanied with rashes or polyarthralgias.[6]

References

1. Barron S, Pass R: Infectious causes of hydrops fetalis. Semin Perinatol 19:493–501, 1995.
2. Boggess K: Perinatal viral and parasitic infections. ADOG Practice Bulletin No. 20, September 2000.
3. Brown T, Anaud A, Ritchie L, et al: Intrauterine parvovirus infection associated with hydrops fetalis. Lancet 2:1033–1034, 1984.
4. Dieck D, Schild R, Hansmann M, et al: Prenatal diagnosis of congenital parvovirus B19 infection: Value of serological and PCR techniques in maternal and fetal serum. Prenat Diagn 19:1119–1123, 1999.
5. Guidozzi F, Ballot D, Rothberg A: Human B19 parvovirus infection in an obstetric population: A prospective study determining fetal outcome. J Reproduct Med 39:36–38, 1994.
6. Hedrick J: The effects of human parvovirus B19 and cytomegalovirus during pregnancy. J Perinat Neonat Nurs 10:30–39, 1996.
7. Levy R, Weissman, A, Blomberg G, et al: Infection by parvovirus B19 during pregnancy: A review. Obstet Gynecol Surv 52:254–259, 1997.
8. Sheikh A, Ernest J, O'Shea M: Long-term outcome in fetal hydrops from parvovirus B19 infection. Am J Obstet Gynecol 167:337–341, 1992.
9. Valeur-Jensen A, Pedersen C, Westergaard T, et al: Risk factors for parvovirus B19 infection in pregnancy. JAMA 281:1099–1105, 1999.

XX. Viral Respiratory Infections

A. Management Guidelines for the Common Cold

For decongestant purposes, pseudoephedrine appears to be the safest drug as evidenced by studies that include the Boston Collaborative Surveillance Program and the Collaborative Perinatal Project.[1,2] In addition, pseudoephedrine does not appear to alter uterine or fetal circulation.[3]

1. Oxymetazoline

Oxymetazoline is a long-acting nasal decongestant used in nasal sprays. It appears to be safe for brief use, although the tendency for tachyphylaxis is still present as in the nonpregnant state.

2. Dextromethorphan

Dextromethorphan has been found to be safe as an antitussive. Guaifenesin and terpin hydrate also appear to be safe as far as congenital malformations are concerned. Extended use of iodine-containing expectorants may be a concern as a cause of fetal goiter.

3. Combination cold preparations

If combination cold preparations are to be used, chlorpheniramine and brompheniramine appear to be safe in pregnancy.

B. Other Viral Respiratory Infections

Severe maternal infection appears to be more common in pregnant women during influenza epidemics, associated with viral pneumonia and superimposed bacterial pneumonia. Measles infection has been noted during pregnancy in epidemics, particularly among unvaccinated immigrants. Rubeola does not appear to be a teratogen but is associated with increased spontaneous abortion and perinatal mortality.[4]

References

1. Aselton PA, Jick H, Milunsky A, et al: First trimester drug use and congenital disorders. Obstet Gynecol 65:451–455, 1985.
2. Heinenon OP, Slone D, Shapiro S: Birth Defects and Drugs in Pregnancy. Littleton, MA, Publishing Sciences Group, 1977.
3. Smith CV, Rayburn WF, Anderson JC, et al: Effect of a single dose of pseudoephedrine on uterine and fetal doppler flow. Obstet Gynecol 73:803–806, 1990.
4. Stein SJ, Greenspoon JS: Rubeola during pregnancy. Obstet Gynecol 78:925–929, 1991.

SECTION B.
ABDOMINAL PAIN AND
GASTROINTESTINAL ILLNESS

Ellen L. Sakornbut, M.D.

Common obstetric-related causes of abdominal pain, such as round ligament pain and heartburn, are covered in Chapter 3. This section covers causes of abdominal pain and other gastrointestinal illnesses that are commonly seen in pregnant women.

I. Non–Trauma-Related Causes
A. Appendicitis in Pregnancy
1. Incidence and natural history

Appendicitis does not have an increased or decreased incidence during pregnancy, but delays in diagnosis and resultant increase in perforation may increase morbidity as compared with the nonpregnant state.[15] Appendicitis occurs in 0.13% (1 in 1100) of all pregnancies without predilection for any trimester. In one study, perforation occurred in 14% of cases, always if surgery occurred > 24 hours after the onset of symptoms. Accuracy of diagnosis ranges from 56–81%.

2. Effect on perinatal outcomes

Fetal mortality is about 35% with perforation. In one study, fetal losses occurred in 9% of negative laparotomies but increased to 17% if a diseased appendix was found and 75% if perforated.[1] In a series of 52 cases, fetal mortality was 10% overall with a 5% preterm birth incidence. Fetal loss was highest if appendicitis occurred in the second trimester.[30]

3. Physical findings in pregnancy

The position of the appendix usually changes during pregnancy with rotation from the right lower quadrant to the right upper quadrant as the pregnancy advances (Fig. 2). In one study, the most common symptom was right lower quadrant pain, most common physical findings were abdominal tenderness and rebound tenderness, but this was diminished in the third trimester.

4. Laboratory findings

Minor elevation of the white blood cell count is frequently seen in normal pregnancy, which may increase diagnostic difficulty.

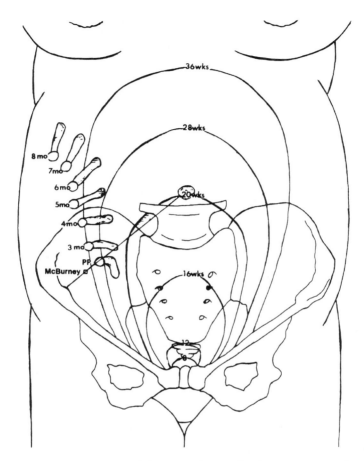

FIGURE 2. Changes in location and direction of appendix during pregnancy in relationship to McBurney's point and height of fundus at various weeks of gestation.

5. New diagnostic tests

Newer measures that have been used in diagnosis include graded-compression sonography[3] and fine catheter peritoneal cytology.[14,28] The use of these tests remains investigational.

6. Differential diagnosis

   a. Ectopic pregnancy. In the first-trimester, it is usually possible to differentiate ectopic pregnancy from appendicitis by examination and history, but a pelvic or retrocecal location of the appendix can mimic ectopic gestation. Pelvic ultrasonography and other diagnostic measures useful in the diagnosis of tubal pregnancy are discussed in Chapter 5.

   b. Rupture of a right-sided ovarian cyst. Rupture of a corpus luteal cyst may mimic appendicitis.

   c. Adnexal torsion. This may present with right-sided pain mimicking appendicitis, with tenderness and guarding present; peritoneal signs are variable. The white blood cell count may be mildly elevated. Nausea and vomiting may be present, and the location of the pain varies from adnexal or lower quadrant to upper quadrant or flank, depending on gestational age.[6]

    d. Degeneration of a uterine fibroid. This is also known as red degeneration (bionecrosis) of a uterine fibroid. This condition may present as acute pain with tenderness, vomiting, and low-grade fever. This is most common in the early second trimester. Sonography can be used to demonstrate the fibroid.

  7. Treatment options

    a. Laparoscopic appendectomy.[11] This has been successfully performed in pregnancy up to the third trimester and is limited by uterine size in late gestation.[27]

    b. Standard laparotomy and appendectomy

B. Nephrolithiasis

1. Epidemiology

The published incidence in pregnancy is about 1 in 1000.

2. Natural history

The presentation of nephrolithiasis is similar during pregnancy to the nonpregnant state with costovertebral angle, flank, or abdominal pain, which may be accompanied by hematuria, nausea, vomiting, urgency, dysuria, and frequency. Patients with renal colic may experience an increased incidence of preterm labor.[17] Nephrolithiasis most commonly presents in the third trimester.

Nephrolithiasis should be suspected if there is a previous history of renal calculi, preexisting urologic problems, fever persisting in pyelonephritis greater than 48 hours after institution of parenteral antibiotics, or more severe pain than is usually encountered with pyelonephritis.

3. Diagnosis

Ultrasonography is successful in diagnosis of stones approximately 95% of the time,[23] making intravenous pyelography necessary in complicated cases.[13,16] The intravenous pyelogram can be obtained using a minimum of films (usually a flat-plate and 3-hour post-injection).

4. Management

Conservative management is successful in most patients, but surgical interventions (including stinting, cystoscopic extraction, and more invasive procedures) may be used as necessary.[17]

C. Cholelithiasis and Cholecystitis

1. Epidemiology

The incidence of cholelithiasis is 1–2/1000 pregnancies. Pregnancy is associated with an increased risk of cholelithiasis. Elevated estrogen and progesterone levels predispose to the formation of lithogenic bile and bile stasis. The incidence of symptomatic biliary disease is not increased, although the diagnosis may be made or reported on a less frequent basis owing to numerous abdominal complaints common to pregnancy. The rate of cholecystectomy in pregnancy is between 1 and 6 per 10,000.

2. Complications of cholecystitis

Pancreatitis is a possible complication of cholelithiasis. Maternal and fetal mortality rates have been reported to be high but appear to be decreased with the use of total parenteral nutrition.

3. Options for treatment

    a. Conservative management. This is generally pursued since resolution of symptoms may occur following the pregnancy. If surgical intervention is needed, the safest time period is the second trimester.[12]

    b. Endoscopic treatment with stone extraction.[4,20] Two small case series have been published that included patients with gallstone pancreatitis and demonstrated successful resolution of symptoms without the need for pre-delivery cholecystectomy.

    c. Laparoscopic cholecystectomy.[2,8,10,19,25,32] This is performed for recurrent or intractable symptoms, including acute cholecystitis and gallstone pancreatitis and patients in the third trimester. Results of these studies have shown successful treatment without short-term or long-term consequences to mothers or babies. Its use is limited in late pregnancy because of risk of injury to the uterus.

    d. Open cholecystectomy. This operation is performed for intractable cases in which laparoscopic procedures may not be desirable.

4. Further discussion

Two larger case series totaling 89 patients demonstrated 45% and 36% of patients failing conservative therapy, respectively.[7,9] Although two patients in these series delivered prematurely, deliveries occurred 10 and 15 weeks postoperatively and appeared to be unrelated to treatment. In one series, one quarter of patients treated conservatively required cesarean cholecystectomy or cholecystectomy in the early post-partum period. No maternal or perinatal mortality or teratogenicity was noted in either series. These results suggest that biliary disease in pregnancy may be managed successfully by surgical or endoscopic methods when conservative management fails.

D. Gastroenteritis

This condition presents as in the nonpregnant patient and can be managed in a similar fashion, with oral hydration preferable if the patient tolerates fluids. The patient's hydration should be monitored more closely because of the risk of preterm labor with dehydration.

E. Acute Hepatic Disorders Related to Pregnancy

1. Intrahepatic cholestasis of pregnancy

This condition has a variable incidence depending on ethnic factors; its incidence is less than 2% in the general population in the U.S. but occurs more commonly in Chile and Sweden. This condition is characterized by intense pruritus, occasionally mild jaundice and dark urine, mild to moderate elevations of transaminases, and marked elevation of alkaline phosphatase. Serum bile acid levels and sulfated metabolites of progesterone are increased. There appears to be a disturbance of bile acid transport across the placenta. The syndrome is more common in the third trimester and resolves following delivery. It is associated with increased rates of stillbirth, fetal distress, and prematurity. There is an increased risk of maternal coagulopathy, possibly due to the use of therapies such as cholestyramine, which affects absorption of fat-soluble vitamin K.[26] Recent studies demonstrate effectiveness of ursodeoxycholic acid (UDCA) in improving bile acid transport across the placenta,[29] decrease in serum bile acids, serum bilirubin, serum transaminases, and decrease in symptoms of pruritus[5,21,22] and increased biliary excretion of sulfated progesterone metabolites.[18] Fetal outcomes appear to improve with the use of UDCA.

2. Acute fatty liver of pregnancy

This is a rare but catastrophic illness that occurs more commonly in young primiparas and multiple gestations, usually late in the third trimester.[31] The onset of the disease is heralded by anorexia, nausea, vomiting, malaise, and headache, followed by epigastric and right upper quadrant abdominal pain with jaundice, polyuria-polydipsia (in the absence of diabetes), and thrombocytopenia. The patient may become comatose with hepatic encephalopathy, bleeding diatheses, and metabolic acidosis. This illness is related to the heterozygote (carrier) state of long chain 3-hydroxyacyl-CoA-dehydrogenase deficiency in mothers carrying fetuses with this disorder of mitochondrial fatty acid oxidation. Some features are common to both acute fatty liver and preeclampsia: mild hypertension, proteinuria, and edema. Maternal mortality rates are high if diagnosis and delivery are delayed. Trends in management, including expeditious delivery of the fetus, have improved maternal mortality rates.[24]

3. Preeclampsia- and eclampsia-associated hepatic changes

These include nausea, vomiting, and epigastric and right upper quadrant pain, with liver abnormalities present in 50% of eclamptic patients. The HELLP syndrome is characterized by microangiopathic hemolytic anemia, elevated SGOT and SGPT, and thrombocytopenia. Another cause of elevated liver enzymes in pregnancy-induced hypertension is subcapsular or intrahepatic hematoma, which may lead to catastrophic rupture (see Chapter 15, section G).

4. Fulminant hepatitis

This inflammation of the liver, usually of viral origin, rarely may present with massive elevations in transaminases and bilirubin, coagulopathy, encephalopathy, and renal failure. While serologic studies are pending, there may be some difficulty in distinguishing this catastrophic illness from acute fatty liver. Delivery of the fetus is indicated in acute fatty liver and may be necessary for fetal survival in fulminant hepatitis.

References

1. Al-Mulhim AA: Acute appendicitis in pregnancy: A review of 52 cases. Int Surg 81:2995–2997, 1996.
2. Arvidsson D, Gerdin E: Laparoscopic cholecystectomy during pregnancy. Surg Laparosc Endosc 1:193–194, 1991.
3. Barloon TJ, Brown BP, Abu-Yousef MM, et al: Sonography of acute appendicitis in pregnancy. Abdom Imaging 20:149–151, 1995.
4. Barthel JS, Chowdhury T, Miedema BW: Endoscopic sphincterotomy for the treatment of gallstone pancreatitis during pregnancy. Surg Endosc 12:394–399, 1998.
5. Brites D, Rodriques CM, Oliveira N, et al: Correction of maternal serum bile acid profile during ursodeoxycholic acid therapy in cholestasis of pregnancy. J Hepatol 28:91–98, 1998.
6. Chambers JT, Thiagarajah S, Kitchin JD: Torsion of the normal fallopian tube during pregnancy. Obstet Gynecol 54:487–489, 1979.
7. Davis A, Katz VL, Cox R: Gallbladder disease in pregnancy. J Reprod Med 40:759–762, 1995.
8. Eichenberg BJ, Vandelin J, Miguel C, et al: Laparoscopic cholecystectomy in the third trimester of pregnancy. Am Surg 62:874–877, 1996.
9. Glasgow RE, Visser BC, Harris HW, et al. Changing management of gallstone disease during pregnancy. Surg Endosc 12:241–246, 1998.
10. Gouldman JW, Sticca RP, Rippon MB, et al: Laparoscopic cholecystectomy in pregnancy. Am Surg 64:93–97, 1998.
11. Gurbuz AT, Peetz ME: The acute abdomen in the pregnant patient: Is there a role for laparoscopy? Surg Endosc 11:98–102, 1997.
12. Hiatt JR, Hiatt JCG, Williams RA, et al: Biliary disease in pregnancy: Strategy for surgical management. Am J Surg 151:263–265, 1986.
13. Horowitz E, Schmidt JD: Renal calculi in pregnancy. Clin Obstet Gynecol 28:324–338, 1985.
14. Lim HK, Bae SH, Seo GS: Diagnosis of acute appendicitis in pregnant women: Value of sonography. Am J Radiol 159:539–542, 1992.
15. Mahmoodian S: Appendicitis complicating pregnancy. South Med J 85:19–24, 1992.
16. Maikranz P, Coe FL, Parks J, et al: Nephrolithiasis in pregnancy. Am J Kidney Dis 9:354–358, 1987.
17. Marlow RA: Nephrolithiasis in pregnancy. Am Fam Physician 40:185–189, 1989.
18. Meng LJ, Reyes H, Palma J, et al: Effects of ursodeoxycholic acid on conjugated bile acids and progesterone metabolites in serum and urine of patients with intrahepatic cholestasis of pregnancy. J Hepatol 27:1029–1040, 1997.
19. Morrell D, Mullins JR, Harrison PB: Laparoscopic cholecystectomy during pregnancy in symptomatic patients. Surgery 112:856–859, 1992.
20. Nesbitt TH, Kay HH, McCoy MC, et al: Endoscopic management of biliary disease in pregnancy. Obstet Gynecol 87:806–809, 1996.
21. Nicastri Pl, Diaferia A, Tartagni M, et al: A randomized placebo-controlled trial of ursodeoxycholic acid and S-adenosylmethionine in the treatment intrahepatic cholestasis of pregnancy. Br J Obstet Gynaecol 105:1205–1207, 1998.

22. Palma J, Reyes H, Ribalta J, et al: Ursodeoxycholic acid in the treatment of cholestasis of pregnancy: A randomized, double-blind study controlled with placebo. J Hepatol 27:1022–1028, 1997.
23. Parulkar BG, Hopkins TB, Wollin MR, et al: Renal colic in pregnancy: A case for conservative management. J Urol 159:365–348, 1998.
24. Pereira SP, O'Donohue J, Wendon J, et al: Maternal and perinatal outcome in severe pregnancy-related liver disease. Hepatology 26:1258–1262, 1997.
25. Pucci RO, Seed RW: Case report of laparoscopic cholecystectomy in the third trimester of pregnancy. Am J Obstet Gynecol 165:401–402, 1991.
26. Reyes H: The enigma of intrahepatic cholestasis of pregnancy: Lessons from Chile. Hepatology 2:87–90, 1982.
27. Schreiber JH: Laparoscopic appendectomy in pregnancy. Surg Endosc 4:100–102, 1990.
28. Scott-Coombes DM, Vipond MN, Thompson JN: Acute right iliac fossa pain in pregnancy: The role of fine-catheter peritoneal cytology. Br J Surg 79:110–115, 1992.
29. Serrano MA, Brites D, Larena MG, et al: Beneficial effects of ursodeoxycholic acid on alterations induced by cholestasis of pregnancy in bile acid transport across the human placenta. J Hepatol 25:829–839, 1998.
30. To WW, Ngai CS, Ma HK: Pregnancies complicated by acute appendicitis. Aust N Z J Surg 65:799–803, 1995.
31. Werner CJ, Zoller DP, Baskin WN, et al: Acute fatty liver of pregnancy associated with maternal and fetal acidosis. J Fam Pract 26:198–203, 1988.
32. Wischner JD, Zolfaghari D, Wohlgemuth SD, et al: Laparoscopic cholecystectomy in pregnancy: A report of six cases and review of the literature. Surg Endosc 10:314–318, 1996.

SECTION C.
TRAUMA IN PREGNANCY

Mark Deutchman, M.D.

This section addresses diagnostic and management issues of trauma in pregnancy, with special attention to blunt abdominal trauma.

I. Scope of the Problem
Trauma is the leading non-obstetric cause of maternal death in the childbearing age group.[7] Six to seven percent of pregnant women suffer some type of trauma during pregnancy. Maternal survival is a good predictor of fetal survival, but does not guarantee fetal survival. Fetal death rates in pregnancy exceed maternal death rates three- to nine-fold.[13]

II. Causes
A. Motor Vehicle Accidents
Most trauma in pregnancy occurs as a result of motor vehicle accidents. Pregnant women may mistakenly assume that it is inadvisable for them to wear seatbelts or may wear them improperly. Both lap and shoulder belts should be worn during all trimesters of pregnancy. Airbags should not be disabled during pregnancy.[3]
B. Domestic Violence
Physical abuse has been reported in 3–29% of pregnant women depending on population and study method.[14] Depression, substance abuse, and frequent emergency room visits are common indicators of domestic violence; however, this problem spans all ages, races, and socioeconomic groups.[17] Victims frequently conceal their situation. A history of abuse must be sought out by clinicians and victims encouraged to seek help. Pregnant women who have been victims of domestic violence have an increased incidence of preterm labor and chorioamnionitis.[4]
C. Falls
Awkwardness of movement as pregnancy progresses and orthostatic hypotensive episodes increase the risk of falls during pregnancy.

III. Clinical Outcomes
A. Complications Associated with Trauma
One series of trauma patients included only two abruptions in 84 patients. The most common complication in this series was preterm labor, occurring in 20% of patients. Motor vehicle accidents constituted only 35% of the trauma seen, and both patients with abruption were injured in motor vehicle accidents.[20]
B. Fetal Outcomes
The leading cause of fetal death is maternal death, usually due to head and chest injuries. The leading cause of fetal death in trauma in which the mother survives is abruption. Poor pregnancy outcome in trauma patients is directly correlated with the severity of injuries.[12] Maternal pelvic fracture is highly correlated with poor fetal outcome and can result in massive maternal retroperitoneal hemorrhage.

IV. Trauma and the Physiologic Effects of Pregnancy
The uterus becomes an abdominal organ, making it susceptible to direct injury. Signs of peritoneal irritation are diminished. Plasma volume, cardiac output, heart rate, fibrinogen, white blood cell count, and arterial pH increase. Blood pressure, hematocrit, serum bicarbonate, and pCO_2 decrease. Thirty percent of blood volume may be lost before clinical signs of hypovolemia appear.

V. Effects of Maternal Trauma on the Fetus
Maternal blood flow is maintained at the expense of uteroplacental blood flow.[10]
The fetus may be severely compromised even when maternal vital signs are normal.
A. Preterm Labor/Preterm Premature Rupture of Membranes (PPROM)
Preterm labor can accompany even minor trauma. The presence of contractions should increase the clinical suspicion of abruption.[18] Premature rupture of membranes may occur.
B. Placental Abruption
Placental abruption may occur as the result of direct injury and shearing forces or as a result of the effects of maternal shock.[12] Abruption can occur up to 4 or 5 days after trauma.[11] All injuries, even very minor ones, can produce abruption; therefore, all patients should be evaluated.
C. Uterine Rupture
Uterine rupture is rare but is associated with nearly 100% fetal mortality.[16]
D. Penetrating Trauma
Direct fetal injury is most likely in cases of penetrating trauma, such as stab or gunshot wounds, and with maternal pelvic fracture.
E. Fetomaternal Hemorrhage
Fetomaternal hemorrhage may result in fetal anemia, fetal death, and maternal isoimmunization.

VI. Fetal Outcomes as a Result of Maternal Injury
A. Major Trauma
Major trauma resulting in long bone fractures, rib fractures, and life-threatening maternal injury is associated with a 40% incidence of fetal death.
B. Minor Maternal Injury
The fetal death rate in cases of minor maternal injury is less than 2%.
C. Maternal Hypoperfusion
Sensitive indicators of tissue hypoperfusion include serum bicarbonate levels < 19 to 24 mEq/L and elevated serum lactate levels. This has been correlated with poor fetal outcome, as has fluid resuscitation with large amounts of intravenous fluids and decreased maternal pH and pO_2.[8]

VII. Assessment of the Traumatized Mother and Fetus

Initial assessment of the severely injured pregnant trauma patient is the same as that of any trauma patient.
- Airway: secure the airway
- Breathing: administer oxygen and assist ventilation
- Circulation: control bleeding, establish IV access and administer volume replacement
- Disability or neurologic deficits
- Exposure—environment

VIII. Special Considerations in the Resuscitation of Pregnant Patients[5]

A. Aspiration

Aspiration of vomited stomach contents is an increased risk. Rapid sequence intubation and gastric emptying are preferred.

B. Vena Cava Compression

Position the patient in the left lateral position rather than supine to avoid vena cava compression and resultant maternal supine hypotension. Avoid lower extremity IV lines because vena cava compression by the gravid uterus may prevent infused fluids from reaching the maternal central circulation.

C. Fluid Resuscitation

Replace estimated blood loss 3:1 with lactated Ringer's solution

D. Use of Vasopressors

The vasopressors norepinephrine and epinephrine should be avoided because they decrease uterine blood flow. Ephedrine increases both maternal BP and uterine blood flow. Dopamine increases uterine blood flow in dosage up to 5 µg/kg/min.

E. Placement of Chest Tubes

Chest tubes placement should be higher than usual because of diaphragm elevation in pregnancy.

IX. Diagnostic Tests/Physical Findings—Maternal

Any clinically indicated diagnostic tests usually used in trauma evaluation should be performed including x-rays, blood counts and typing, and peritoneal lavage or ultrasound to rule out intraperitoneal hemorrhage. The threshold for sonographic diagnosis of hemoperitoneum is probably about 200 ml in nonpregnant patients; the threshold in pregnant patients is unknown.

A. Indicators of Hypoperfusion

A low maternal serum bicarbonate level (below 19–24 mEq/L) or an elevated serum lactate level has been shown to be a sensitive indicator of tissue hypoperfusion even when vital signs are normal.[8]

B. Fetomaternal Hemorrhage

Routine use of coagulation tests and testing for fetomaternal hemorrhage using the Kleihauer-Betke (K-B) test (except in Rh-negative mothers) has not been shown to help in evaluation or management,[6] but K-B testing is still recommended for all patients by some authors.[9,16]

C. Maternal Hemorrhage

If vaginal examination reveals bleeding, abruption or another severe event such as uterine rupture should be assumed. Ultrasonography may be used to examine for abruption, but a negative test does not rule out a placental abruption. The absence of vaginal bleeding does not rule out abruption because concealed hemorrhage has been found to be more likely in abruption caused by trauma.[6,12]

D. Assessing for Rupture of the Membranes

If vaginal examination reveals fluid, fern testing and pH testing (Nitrazine testing) for amniotic fluid should be performed to determine if membranes have been ruptured.

E. Maternal/Fetal Surveillance

Electronic uterine activity monitoring should be initiated on mothers at or beyond 20 weeks' gestation. Patients with minor trauma may be monitored for four hours[16] while those with more severe trauma should be monitored for 24 hours.[18] Uterine contractions occurring at a frequency of 6 to 8 per hour or more indicate increased risk for abruption and premature delivery.

Subjective reports of abdominal pain and objective findings of abdominal tenderness have not been shown to help predict which patients are at higher risk for preterm delivery.[15]

X. Diagnostic Tests—Fetal

Electronic fetal monitoring may detect fetal heart rate abnormalities with or without accompanying uterine contractions. Late fetal heart decelerations should be assumed to represent fetal compromise. A sinusoidal fetal heart rate pattern is associated with fetal anemia from fetomaternal hemorrhage or abruption. Ultrasonography may provide significant amounts of information, including gestational age, placental location, assistance in diagnosing abruption, and presence of uterine rupture. Placental abruption remains a clinical diagnosis and cannot be ruled out by ultrasonography if the clinical presentation suggests that abruption is present.

XI. Therapeutic Decisions and Dilemmas

These include duration of monitoring, use of tocolysis for preterm labor, discharge criteria, and use of $Rh_o(D)$ immune globulin.[1]

A. Duration of Monitoring for Minor Trauma

In the case of minor trauma, a short period of monitoring (nonstress test) is recommended.[9,18] A prospective series found that a 4-hour monitoring period and a Kleihauer-Betke test were able to detect all patients with trauma-related poor pregnancy outcome who would not otherwise have been hospitalized owing to the severity of their trauma. Frequent preterm contractions (> 8/hour) were associated with abruption.[16] Extended monitoring or more extensive evaluation is not warranted unless there is evidence of abruption, fetal compromise, or frequent preterm contractions.[18]

B. Duration of Monitoring for Major Trauma

In the case of major trauma, some authors recommend 24 hours of continuous electronic fetal monitoring to detect placental abruption and preterm labor.[20]

C. Evidence of Placental Abruption

Most abruptions are evident using fetal monitoring in the first few hours. Signs and findings associated with abruption include:[6,16]
1. More than 6–8 uterine contractions per hour
2. Vaginal bleeding
3. Uterine tenderness
4. Signs of maternal hypovolemia
5. Fetal heart rate pattern abnormalities

D. Role of Tocolysis

Some authors believe it is justifiable if the fetus is stable and note that it is usually successful.[20] If tocolysis is to be used, magnesium sulfate is preferable to beta-mimetics since the latter cause both maternal and fetal tachycardia and may mask signs of shock.

E. Rh Immune Gobulin

The $Rh_o(D)$ immune globulin (Rhogam) dosage for Rh-negative mothers is based on Kleihauer-Betke testing. One fetal cell per 1000 maternal cells represents a 5-ml hemorrhage (assuming a maternal blood volume of 5 liters). Rh-negative mothers can be sensitized by as few as 1–3 fetal cells per 500,000 maternal cells. Rh-negative mothers should receive 300 micrograms of $Rh_o(D)$ immune globulin (Rhogam) for each 15 ml of estimated fetal cells in their circulation. The minimum Rho(D) immune globulin (Rhogam) dosage should be 300 µg.

F. Discharge Criteria

The duration of observation and period of monitoring continue to be a matter of physician judgment. These discharge criteria are prudent based on available evidence:

1. Resolution of uterine contractions
2. Reassuring fetal heart rate pattern
3. Confirmation that membranes are not ruptured
4. No vaginal bleeding or uterine tenderness
5. If patient is Rh negative, appropriate dose of $Rh_o(D)$ immune globulin (Rhogam) has been given.
6. Patient understands discharge instructions and follow-up plans.

XII. Perimortem Cesarean Delivery

Fetal survival is impossible for more than a few minutes after maternal death. In its Advanced Cardiac Life Support program, the American Heart Association recommends that all physicians be prepared to perform perimortem cesarean delivery of a viable fetus whose mother has not responded to 4–5 minutes of cardiopulmonary resuscitation.[3] This procedure is also recommended by the American College of Obstetricians and Gynecologists although no time criteria are specified.[2] Longer arrest-to-delivery times are associated with increased neurologic deficits in surviving infants. Perimortem cesarean delivery is also recommended as an aid to maternal resuscitation since emptying the uterus dramatically increases cardiac output by relieving uterine compression of the aorta and vena cava. When perimortem cesarean delivery is performed, the attending team should be prepared to provide resuscitation care for the newborn.

References

1. Agnoli FL, Deutchman ME: Trauma in pregnancy. J Fam Pract 37:588–592, 1993.
2. American College of Obstetricians and Gynecologists. Obstetric Aspects of Trauma Management. ACOG Technical Bulletin No. 251, Washington, DC, American College of Obstetricians and Gynecologists, September 1998.
3. American Heart Association: Advanced Cardiac Life Support 1997–1999: Cardiac Arrest Associated with Pregnancy. Dallas, TX, American Heart Association.
4. Berenson AB, Wiemann CM, Wilkinson GS, et al: Perinatal morbidity associated with violence experienced by pregnant women. Am J Obstet Gynecol 170:760-769, 1994.
5. Coleman MT, Trianfo VA, Rund DA: Nonobstetric emergencies in pregnancy: Trauma and surgical conditions. Am J Obstet Gynecol 177:497–502, 1997.
6. Dahmus MA, Sibai BM: Blunt abdominal trauma: Are there any predictive factors for abruptio placentae or maternal-fetal distress? Am J Obstet Gynecol 169:1054–1059, 1993.
7. Fildes J, Reed L, Jones N, et al: Trauma: The leading cause of maternal death. J Trauma 32:643–645, 1992.
8. George ER, Vanderkwaak T, Scholten DJ: Factors influencing pregnancy outcome after trauma. Am Surg 58:594–598, 1992.
9. Goodwin TM, Breen MT: Pregnancy outcome and fetomaternal hemorrhage after noncatastrophic trauma. Am J Obstet Gynecol 162:665–671, 1990.
10. Greiss FC: Uterine vascular response to hemorrhage during pregnancy. Obstet Gynecol 27:549–554, 1966.
11. Higgins SD, Garite TJ: Late abruptio placentae in trauma patients: Implications for monitoring. Obstet Gynecol 63(3 Suppl):10S–12S, 1984.
12. Kettel LM, Branch DW, Scott JR: Occult placental abruption after maternal trauma. Obstet Gynecol 71:449–453, 1988.
13. Kissinger DP, Rozycki GS, Morris JA, et al: Trauma in pregnancy: Predicting pregnancy outcome. Arch Surg 126:1079–1086, 1991.
14. McFarlane J, Parker B, Soeken K, et al: Assessing for abuse during pregnancy: Severity and frequency of injuries and associated entry into prenatal care. JAMA 267:3176–3178, 1992.

15. Pak LL, Reece EA, Chan L: Is adverse pregnancy outcome predictable after blunt abdominal trauma? Am J Obstet Gynecol 179:1140–1144, 1998.
16. Pearleman MD, Tintinalli JE, Lorenz RP: A prospective, controlled study of outcome after trauma during pregnancy. Am J Obstet Gynecol 162:1502–1510, 1990.
17. Poole GV, Martin JN, Perry KG, et al: Trauma in pregnancy: The role of interpersonal violence. Am J Obstet Gynecol 174:1873–1876, 1996.
18. Rosenfeld JA: Abdominal trauma in pregnancy: When is fetal monitoring necessary? Postgrad Med 88:89–94, 1990.
19. Trauma in Pregnancy: Advanced Trauma Life Support, American College of Surgeons, 1992, pp 283–292.
20. Williams JK, McClain L, Rosemurgy AS, et al: Evaluation of blunt abdominal trauma in the third trimester of pregnancy: Maternal and fetal considerations. Obstet Gynecol 75:33–37, 1990.

SECTION D.
DERMATOSES OF PREGNANCY

Ellen L. Sakornbut, M.D.

I. Classification
Some confusion exists because of uncommon conditions that have been described by different authors over a period of many years in the medical literature. Several entities may represent the same condition. More recent descriptions of these entities use immunofluorescent studies. Several conditions that have been described as unique dermatoses of pregnancy probably represent other dermatologic diseases presenting in pregnancy or dermatologic manifestations of other pregnancy syndromes. A classification scheme is presented:
   A. Pruritic Urticarial Papules and Plaques of Pregnancy (PUPPP)
   B. Herpes Gestationis
   C. Pruritus Gravidarum
   D. Impetigo Herpetiformis
   E. Other Variants

II. Description of Dermatoses
   ### A. PUPPP (Pruritic Urticarial Papules and Plaques of Pregnancy)
   Other diagnoses that are probably the same condition include Bourne's toxemic rash and the late form of prurigo of pregnancy. Another suggested name for this condition is polymorphic eruption of pregnancy.
   1. PUPPP
   This is the most common dermatologic condition occurring in 1 out of 200 to 300 pregnancies. Three fourths of patients are primigravidas. This condition usually presents late in the third trimester and is a benign nuisance condition.
      a. Distribution. PUPPP often begins in periumbilical striae, then spreads to buttocks, thighs, inner arms, lower back, and sometimes breasts, hands, and feet.
      b. Appearance. Lesions appear as erythematous papules and urticarial plaques. Halos may present around lesions, which are occasionally vesicular (Fig. 3).
      c. Laboratory findings. No laboratory abnormalities are seen. Histopathologic findings are nonspecific. PUPPP is not clearly associated with pregnancy complications.[1]
   ### B. Pemphigoid Gestationis (formerly Herpes Gestationis)
   1. Epidemiology
   This is a rare condition (1 in 40,000) that usually starts in the second trimester. It is correlated with certain HLA types and may recur in subsequent pregnancies.

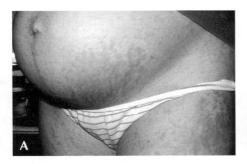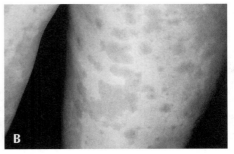

FIGURE 3.   Pruritic urticarial papules and plaques of pregnancy (PUPPP). *A,* Erythematous papules in the striae of a 21-year-old primigravida woman. *B,* Urticarial papules and plaques that are not associated with striae on the thighs of a woman with PUPPP. (From Fitzpatrick JE, Aeling JL (eds): Dermatology Secrets in Color, 2nd ed. Philadelphia, Hanley & Belfus, 2001, with permission.)

2. Clinical presentation/natural history

The eruptions begin on the abdomen, especially around the umbilicus, and then spread to the buttocks, trunk, and extremities, sparing the oral mucosa. Herpes gestationis begins with a systemic prodromal phase, which consists of fever, malaise, nausea, and a burning sensation or pruritus of the skin. Papules, vesicles, and bullae develop, resembling bullous pemphigoid. There is a possible association between this condition and preterm delivery.[4]

3. Laboratory findings

The major laboratory abnormality is a leukocytosis with an associated eosinophilia. Histopathologic features include a linear band of complement or immunoglobulins at the dermoepidermal junction. This is related to an autoimmune reaction to a placental matrix antigen.[3]

4. Treatment

Systemic steroids may be used for treatment.

C. Pruritus Gravidarum

This condition is characterized by generalized pruritus, sometimes resulting in diffuse excoriations. Pruritus gravidarum may represent a mild form of cholestasis of pregnancy.

Prurigo of pregnancy is a condition with eczematous plaques that may be due to cholestasis in an atopic patient.

D. Impetigo Herpetiformis

This is a rare condition with onset usually in the third trimester. Impetigo herpetiformis probably represents severe pustular psoriasis occurring in pregnancy. Common systemic manifestations include fever, nausea, vomiting, diarrhea, dehydration, hypocalcemia, and tetany.

E. Other Variants

Other entities have been named that probably represent variants of the aforementioned conditions or extremely rare conditions.[2]

References

1. Aronson IK, Bond S, Fiedler VC, et al: Pruritic urticarial papules and plaques of pregnancy: Clinical and immunopathologic observations in 57 patients. J Am Acad Dermatol 39:933–939, 1998.
2. Erickson CV, Matus NR: Skin disorders of pregnancy. Am Fam Physician 49:605–610, 1994.
3. Kelly SE, Black MM: Pemphigoid gestations. Semin Dermatol 8:12–17, 1989.
4. Mascaro JM Jr, Lecha M, Mascaro JM: Fetal morbidity in herpes gestationis. Arch Dermatol 131:1209–1210, 1995.

SECTION E.
ACUTE NEUROLOGIC CONDITIONS

Ellen L. Sakornbut, M.D.

I. Carpal Tunnel Syndrome (CTS)

A. Epidemiology/Natural History

Two to twenty five per cent of pregnant women experience nocturnal hand pain, but a much smaller percentage demonstrates nerve conduction or EMG abnormalities. Symptoms are more common in older primiparous women with generalized edema.[3]

B. Differential Diagnosis

This should include acroparesthesia caused by kinking of blood vessels in the thoracic outlet. Median nerve distribution is important in making the diagnosis.

C. Treatment

Treatment is usually successful with wrist splints, reducing pain and improving grip strength.[2] If symptoms are more persistent, steroid injection into the carpal tunnel may be used. The majority of cases resolve postpartum. If the onset of carpal tunnel symptoms occurs in the first two trimesters of pregnancy or if the patient has a positive Phalen test within 30 seconds and abnormal two-point discrimination at the fingertips (> 6 mm), she is more likely to fail conservative therapy and require surgery post-partum.[5] Patients with CTS in pregnancy are more likely to develop CTS in the nonpregnant state.[1]

II. Bell's Palsy[6]

Bell's palsy is three times more common during pregnancy than in nonpregnant women of the same age. It is most common in the third trimester. Treatment with steroids is indicated if onset is earlier than the late third trimester and facial nerve paralysis is complete. Prognosis is good in most cases.

III. Meralgia Paresthetica

Entrapment of the lateral femoral cutaneous nerve beneath the inguinal ligament causes painful paresthesias along the lateral thigh. This peripheral nerve entrapment is caused by rapid weight gain and the enlarging uterus and usually occurs in the third trimester.[4] No treatment is necessary because the condition resolves spontaneously postpartum.

IV. Obstetric Palsy

A. Pathophysiology

An obstetric palsy is caused by compression of lumbosacral nerve plexus and individual nerves against the pelvic bones by the fetal head. Alternatively, nerve compression may occur with forceps rotation. The incidence of obstetric palsy has decreased because of modern obstetric practices.

B. At-Risk Patients

The patients at increased risk for an obstetric palsy are short primigravidas with cephalopelvic disproportion or patients with occiput posterior presentation or other reasons for midforceps delivery. The patient may have experienced a protracted second stage. The patient may remember onset of sharp pain during the second stage.

C. Footdrop Palsy

The most common palsy is footdrop associated with compression of the L4 and L5 roots against the sacrum.[7] L4, L5, and S1 roots may be compressed in the pelvis close to the sciatic notch presenting a picture similar to typical sciatica. Footdrop palsy may also be caused by peroneal nerve compression between leg holders and the head of the fibula. Most patients recover within 8 weeks because the injury usually involves only distortion of the myelin sheath (neurapraxic lesion). If recovery takes longer, an EMG can be performed to diagnose axonal degeneration.

V. Pseudotumor Cerebri
This condition occurs when there is increased intracranial pressure occurring in the absence of mass lesion or hydrocephalus. This condition is associated with obese and pregnant women and rarely women on oral contraceptives. It usually begins in the second trimester and lasts 1–3 months or may last until the postpartum period. Pseudotumor cerebri usually responds to repeated lumbar puncture and may require corticosteroid therapy.

References
1. Al-Qattan MM, Manktelow RT, Bowen CV: Pregnancy-induced carpal tunnel syndrome requiring surgical release longer than 2 years after delivery. Obstet Gynecol 84:249–251, 1994.
2. Courts RB: Splinting for symptoms of carpal tunnel syndrome during pregnancy. J Hand Ther 8:31–34, 1995.
3. Ekman-Ordeberg G, Salgeback S, Ordeberg G: Carpal tunnel syndrome in pregnancy: A prospective study. Acta Obstet Gynaecol Scand 66:233–235, 1987.
4. Jones RK: Meralgia paresthetica as a cause of leg discomfort. Can Med Assoc J 111:541–542, 1974.
5. Stahl S, Blumenfeld Z, Yarnitsky D: Carpal tunnel syndrome in pregnancy: Indications for early surgery. J Neurol Sci 136:182–184, 1996.
6. Walling A: Bell's palsy in pregnancy and the puerperium. J Fam Pract 36:559–563, 1993.
7. Whittaker WG: Injuries to the sacral plexus in obstetrics. J Can Med Assoc 79:622–627, 1978.

SECTION F.
CERVICAL DYSPLASIA IN PREGNANCY

Elizabeth G. Baxley, M.D.

The risk of cervical dysplasia in pregnant women is similar to that of nonpregnant women, with an incidence on Papanicolaou (Pap) smear screening of 1.2–2.2%. Cervical biopsy specimens find histologically proven cervical intraepithelial neoplasia in 0.19–53% of pregnant patients,[9,15] but carcinoma of the cervix is uncommon, occurring in only 2 to 10 of every 10,000.[3,4,12] Pregnancy itself appears to have no influence on the course of patients with carcinoma of the cervix.[3,4] Rather, clinical stage is the most important predictor of prognosis.

The evaluation and management of the abnormal Pap smear during pregnancy present unique challenges to the clinician because of changes that occur in the cervix during pregnancy, and concern for the well-being of the fetus and continuation of the pregnancy. Cervical glands and stroma undergo normal physiologic changes with pregnancy, including squamous metaplasia and endocervical gland hyperplasia. Decidual cells with variably staining cytoplasm and large nuclei may mimic a high-grade squamous intraepithelial lesion (HGSIL) as they degenerate and shed from the endometrium.[11] Hormonal changes of pregnancy cause increased edema and vascularity of the cervix and other pelvic structures, creating potential technical difficulties for even the most experienced colposcopist.[6] Physiologic or metaplastic changes of the cervix during pregnancy can easily resemble cervical intraepithelial neoplasia (CIN), and the enhanced vascularity may accentuate existing vascular patterns, suggesting that the lesions are of a higher grade than in reality.[2,3]

I. Colposcopy During Pregnancy

A. Indications

The goal in evaluating abnormal cervical cytology during pregnancy is to rule out the presence of invasive cervical cancer.[8] A colposcopic examination, with biopsies when indicated, is recommended when dysplasia is discovered during pregnancy. Other indications for colposcopy are similar to those in the nonpregnant state and include the presence of human papillomavirus, genital condyloma, or a clinically suspicious lesion regardless of normal cytology.

B. Technique

The progressive physiologic changes in the cervix during pregnancy render the transformation zone easily accessible for satisfactory colposcopic examination, particularly after 16–18 weeks' gestation.[5] The technique is the same as in a non-pregnant woman, with the exception that the endocervical curettage is contraindicated as it may induce premature pregnancy loss or rupture of membranes. The examination should be gentle because tissue fragility is more common in pregnancy. Acetic acid may be applied by using a spray bottle, providing a more gentle mechanism of staining.[2] Excessive mucus secretion may take more time to clear before the examination.

Cervical biopsy during pregnancy is often accompanied by brisk bleeding, but should not be omitted based on concern of complications, as the risk of true hemorrhage is low and no adverse birth outcomes have been associated with colposcopic biopsy. When bleeding does occur, simple pressure should be applied for several minutes as long as bleeding is not excessive despite pressure. Monsel's solution almost always stops bleeding that is not controlled with pressure, but occasionally a suture is required.

During late gestation, the examination may become even more difficult. Edema, smooth muscle hypertrophy, and softening of connective tissue result in greater vaginal distensibility, which predisposes to the vaginal walls collapsing on the speculum, hindering visualization of the cervix. A condom with the tip cut off may be slipped over the speculum to aid in visualization, or a clear plastic speculum may be used. The cervix may also be displaced posteriorly, and the presenting part of the fetus may be deep into the pelvis.

II. Management of Abnormal Cytology during Pregnancy

A. Progression of Dysplasia during Pregnancy

Histologically proven progression to a higher grade of dysplasia during pregnancy has been shown to be as low as 7%, with few to no women developing microinvasive or invasive cancer between antenatal and postpartum evaluation.[7,14] Because progression of low-grade dysplasia to carcinoma is unusual during a normal gestation, recent recommendations have suggested that squamous atypia, atypical squamous cells of undetermined significance, or low-grade intraepithelial lesions on a Pap smear do not require colposcopic examination during pregnancy.[7]

B. The Role of Colposcopy during Pregnancy

Even when colposcopic examination is done, biopsy may be safely omitted when the cytology and clinical impression do not suggest a high-grade lesion or invasive cancer.[3]

Because some patients with mild or moderate dysplasia on cytologic screening are discovered to have invasive cancer on colposcopy with biopsy, others recommend that this step not be omitted based on a low-grade lesion on Pap smear.[12] Colposcopy alone, without directed biopsy, also carries a significant risk of underestimating the severity of the lesion.[5]

C. Management of Low-Grade Lesions

After the initial exam, women with low-grade lesions may be examined each trimester with Pap smear screening and colposcopy, performing a biopsy only if clinical findings suggest a higher-grade lesion. Definitive evaluation should occur 12 weeks postpartum, the time it takes for the cervix to return to a normal physiologic state. Colposcopically directed biopsies (including endocervical curettage) should occur early during the postpartum period even if the postpartum Pap smear is negative, as 11.1% of histologically proven cervical intraepithelial neoplasia cases have normal postpartum cytology.[8] The postpartum diagnosis rarely exceeds the diagnosis during pregnancy.

D. Management of Suspected Microinvasive Disease

In cases of suspected microinvasive disease, a large wedge biopsy or conization is often needed to rule out frankly invasive cancer. Conization is reported to have complication rates (post-procedure bleeding, preterm delivery, pregnancy loss) ranging from 29% to 32%.[5] Thus, its use should be limited to situations in which microinvasion is suspected on colposcopy and biopsy, or to cases in which malignant cytology is discovered and colposcopy fails to eliminate the possibility of invasive disease.[8]

LOOP excision has not been shown to consistently produce diagnostic specimens and has been associated with a significant rate of residual disease.[13] Morbidity is similar to that of cone biopsy, and occurs more often when the procedure is performed in the third trimester. Use of LOOP excision, like conization, is best reserved for limited indications. Pregnancy may be allowed to continue if the diagnostic biopsy or cone specimen shows complete excision of the lesion.[2]

E. Invasive Cervical Carcinoma

When frankly invasive carcinoma of the cervix is discovered during pregnancy, optimal treatment may require termination or result in pregnancy loss. If the lesion is discovered at a stage close to fetal viability, the pregnancy may be allowed to safely continue.[2]

III. Mode of Delivery

There is no contraindication to vaginal delivery in women with cervical intraepithelial neoplasia; in fact, a healing effect of vaginal delivery has been suggested. Disease regression has been reported in women with antepartum cervical dysplasia.[2,15] In one study, 60% of women who delivered vaginally experienced disease regression, as compared to none of the women who delivered by cesarean section (p < 0.0002).[1] Disruption and destruction of tissue from the trauma of a vaginal delivery has been postulated as a reason for these observed differences.[15]

IV. Patient Education

Health care providers should be sensitive to the psychosocial aspects of the evaluation of an abnormal Pap smear during pregnancy. The pregnant woman in this situation faces realistic fears about her own health and the health of her baby, particularly if she has preinvasive or invasive disease. She may be faced with a decision of pregnancy continuation versus termination, and may also have concerns about future fertility. The anxiety resulting from these concerns should be addressed and reassurance given appropriate to the findings, so that the pregnancy may continue without stress and interruption in daily routines and relationships.[10]

V. Summary

Cytologic screening of the uterine cervix is an important part of prenatal care. In the majority of women, cervical dysplasia can be evaluated and observed during pregnancy and treated postpartum without adversely affecting the pregnancy, disease progression, or mode of delivery. Colposcopy and directed biopsy in pregnancy represent a safe, accurate means of assessing the pregnant woman with abnormal cervical cytology.

References

1. Ahdoot D, Van Nostrand KM, Nguyen NJ, et al: The effect of route of delivery on regression of abnormal cervical cytologic findings in the postpartum period. Am J Obstet Gynecol 178:1116–1120, 1998.
2. Anderson MC, Jordan JA, Morse AR, et al: Pregnancy. In A Text and Atlas of Integrated Colposcopy. Chicago, Mosby-Year Book, 1991, pp 202–210.
3. Apgar BS, Zoschnick LB: Triage of the abnormal Papanicolaou smear in pregnancy. Prim Care 25:483–500, 1998.
4. Baltzer J, Regenbrecht ME, Kopcke W, et al: Carcinoma of the cervix and pregnancy. Int J Gynaecol Obstet 31:317–323, 1990.
5. Economos K, Veridiano NP, Delke I, et al: Abnormal cervical cytology in pregnancy: A 17-year experience. Obstet Gynecol 81:915–918, 1993.
6. Fowler WC, Walton LA, Edelman DA: Cervical intraepithelial neoplasia during pregnancy. South Med J 73:1180–1185, 1980.
7. Jain AG, Higgins RV, Boyle MJ: Management of low-grade squamous intraepithelial lesions during pregnancy. Am J Obstet Gynecol 177:298–302, 1997.
8. LaPolla JP, O'Neill C, Wetrich D: Colposcopic management of abnormal cervical cytology in pregnancy. J Reprod Med 33:301–306, 1988.
9. Lurain JR, Gallup DG: Management of abnormal Papanicolaou smears in pregnancy. Obstet Gynecol 53:484–488, 1979.
10. McGee JE: Management of cervical dysplasia in pregnancy. Nurse Pract 12:34–42, 1987.
11. Michael CW, Esfahani FM: Pregnancy-related changes: A retrospective review of 278 cervical smears. Diagn Cytopathol 17:99–107, 1997.
12. Patsner B: Management of low-grade cervical dysplasia during pregnancy. South Med J 83:1405–1412, 1990.
13. Robinson WR, Webb S, Tirpack J, et al: Management of cervical intraepithelial neoplasia during pregnancy with LOOP excision. Gynecol Oncol 64:153–155, 1997.
14. Woodrow N, Permezel M, Butterfield L, et al: Abnormal cervical cytology in pregnancy: Experience of 811 cases. Aust N Z J Obstet Gynaecol 38: 161–165, 1998.
15. Yoonessi M, Wieckowska W, Mariniello D, et al: Cervical intra-epithelial neoplasia in pregnancy. Int J Gynaecol Obstet 20:111–118, 1982.

CHAPTER 9

Treatment of Psychiatric Disorders in Pregnancy

Ellen L. Sakornbut, M.D., and James Sloan Manning, M.D.

Emotional and psychiatric disorders are some of the most common problems encountered by caregivers of women during the reproductive years. This chapter examines common psychiatric disorders from the prospective of the well-being of the pregnant woman and fetus, nonpharmacologic treatment, medication safety, and the impact of treatment on pregnancy issues. The discussion of major diagnostic criteria or the use of psychological instruments is beyond the scope of this chapter.

SECTION A.
AFFECTIVE DISORDERS

I. Unipolar Depression
The epidemiology, natural history, diagnosis, and management of unipolar depression are discussed below.

A. Epidemiology and Natural History of Depression in Pregnancy
While the incidence of depression is cited to be as common as 1 in 10 people, the prevalence of women with this diagnosis is higher. Depression during pregnancy has been associated with poor pregnancy outcome, including low birth weight, premature birth, and delivery of a small-for-gestational-age infant.[31,35] In the past, clinicians considered pregnancy a period of relative quiescence for women and mood disorders. More recent studies, however, document a significant prevalence of depressive episodes and a high rate of relapse during pregnancy for women with depression who discontinue treatment prior to conception or at discovery of pregnancy.[6,40]

Some authors cite the incidence of depression to be unchanged from that of nonpregnant women in the reproductive age group.[17] However, special groups of patients deserve consideration for continuance of medication or treatment of affective disorder if diagnosed. The rate of recurrence of bipolar disorder during pregnancy with discontinuance of lithium is greater than 50%, similar to nonpregnant controls observed over a 40-week period. The rate of recurrence of bipolar disorder is even higher (relative risk 2.9) in women postpartum compared with nonpregnant controls followed in weeks 41–64 after discontinuance of lithium.[40] In addition, some studies have found increased rates of depression in pregnant women being treated for substance abuse,[15] those who have been victims of sexual, verbal, or physical abuse,[16] and assault victims.[28] Whether depressive symptoms represent normal grieving or clinical depression, women who have experienced stillbirth in the previous pregnancy are at greater risk than controls for depressive symptoms during and after the next pregnancy, especially in pregnancies occurring less than 1 year after the stillbirth.[19]

If untreated, clinical depression will generally not improve in the postpartum period, when the incidence of depressive disorders increases. During the postpartum period, the mother-infant dyad may be further at risk for poor bonding and other difficulties in adaptation to family life (see Chapter 20, section A).

B. Diagnosis of Depression

The diagnostic criteria for depression during pregnancy do not differ from the nonpregnant state. Clinicians may feel more comfortable in using screening instruments, such as the Beck Depression Inventory or Zung Depression Scale, to identify patients who warrant further assessment. They should recognize that screening instruments have a 20% false-positive rate and application of standard diagnostic criteria is advisable. The DSM-IV is the current U.S. standard for psychiatric diagnosis. A primary care version has been developed that focuses on symptomatic presentations common in this setting.[2] The DSM-IV PC uses the same symptom-driven diagnostic criteria as the original DSM-IV.

C. Nonpharmacologic Treatment

Psychotherapy may be chosen for women with mild to moderate depression, particularly those who are reluctant to try medication during pregnancy or the postpartum period. Two forms of psychotherapy have emerged as particularly beneficial in the treatment of depression. **Cognitive-behavioral therapy (CBT)** focuses on the negativistic, self-defeating thoughts common in depressive states. It theorizes that negative thoughts (often experienced as automatic and self-deprecating) often give rise to feelings of depression and have as their enduring source irrational beliefs about self, surroundings, and the future. Patients using CBT learn to monitor themselves and stop automatic thoughts with negative affective valence (e.g, "I'm so stupid," "I can't do anything right," "Nothing will ever change") and rationally examine the evidence for these thoughts as truth statements. Patients then learn to substitute rational thinking for irrational thoughts. In this way they restructure the inaccurate and usually negative, pessimistic, and devaluing beliefs that serve as sources or reinforcers of the negative thinking.[44] **Interpersonal therapy (IPT)** focuses on role identity, transitions, and conflicts that often surround the psychosocial triggers of syndromes or episodes of illness. IPT has been shown to be effective in the maintenance treatment of major depression alone and in combination with medication.[10,11]

D. Indications for Pharmacologic Treatment

While some physicians may hesitate to use antidepressant medication during pregnancy, the risk of untreated depression often outweighs the risks of medication. As many as 75% of women who attempt to discontinue antidepressants during pregnancy experience relapse. The use of medication to treat depression during pregnancy involves an informed consent process weighing risks and benefits. Similarly informed women may make widely divergent decisions. Fortunately, the current information for the safety of antidepressant use during pregnancy, labor, and postpartum periods is reassuring.

E. Pharmacologic Treatment during Pregnancy

1. Tricyclic antidepressants (FDA category D)

Tricyclic antidepressants (TCAs) do not appear to increase the rate of fetal malformations, intrauterine death, or alter postnatal development, although the quality and quantity of studies are insufficient.[29,43]

2. Selective serotonin reuptake inhibitors (SSRIs) (FDA category C)

A prospective, controlled cohort study of 228 women exposed to fluoxetine during pregnancy demonstrated no increase in miscarriage or major fetal malformations. This study found an increase in minor malformations in fluoxetine-exposed infants and an increase in poor neonatal adaptation, prematurity, admission to special-care nurseries, and lower birth weights in infants with third-trimester fluoxetine exposure.[5] Approximately 30% of these women were taking other psychotropic medications during pregnancy, but regression analysis eliminated the effects of benzodiazepine use in these findings. A later study of 115 pregnancies found no clear pattern of neonatal complications with third-trimester fluoxetine use.[14] These data were extracted from a larger prospective study of 796 women exposed to fluoxetine during the first trimester of pregnancy that demonstrated no increase in miscarriage or malformations.[13] There are currently more than 2000 patients in the fluoxetine in pregnancy registry; about 1600 of these women have been followed prospectively. Neurobehavioral testing of infants exposed to fluoxetine failed to demonstrate neurologic or behavioral differences between exposed and control groups.[29]

A prospective, controlled, cohort study of 267 women exposed to other SSRIs (sertraline, fluvoxamine, and paroxetine) during pregnancy demonstrated no increase in malformations, stillbirth, miscarriage, or prematurity. Birth weights were similar in the study and control group.[22] In spite of these reassuring data, it must be remembered that the numbers of patients in this study for individual compounds are small and lack the statistical power necessary to make generalizations. The SSRIs are widely divergent in chemical structure and no assumptions about class safety can be made.

II. Bipolar Disorder
A. Bipolar Disorder and Pregnancy
Patients with bipolar illness, whether type I or II, may experience acute worsening during pregnancy or in the immediate postpartum period. Bipolar women are at greater risk of reproductive cycle events triggering symptomatic episodes. Women with a history of bipolar disorder should be strongly considered for prophylaxis with a mood-stabilizing agent in the immediate postpartum period based on a high rate of relapse in untreated women.[8,28] Postpartum psychosis, rare compared to postpartum depression, is considered by many authorities to be a bipolar spectrum condition. Dysphoric manias accompanied by Schneiderian first-rank psychotic symptoms (hallucinations, thought broadcasting, etc.) may be seen.

B. Diagnosis of Bipolar I and Bipolar II Disorder
Bipolar I disorder is differentiated from bipolar II disorder by the presence of mania. Bipolar II illness (hypomania with major depression) is considered the most common presentation of the illness. The current DSM-IV criteria for hypomanic episodes require 4 days of expanded mood. However, 1–3-day episodes are more typical. Thus, the DSM-IV criteria lack sensitivity for the diagnosis. National Institute of Mental Health prospective data point to several temperamental/personality determinants that may be more associated with bipolar (usually bipolar II) outcome.[1] These are mood lability, the presence of mental or physical energy/activity existing concurrently with the depressed mood, social anxiety, and intense daydreaming. Clinicians may be less comfortable making a diagnosis of bipolar illness. Its prevalence is higher than previously believed, and hypomanic episodes are recurrent (to be distinguished from normal happiness that does not occur in this recurrent manner). Clinicians also fail to consider family history, longitudinal course, and problematic treatment responses to antidepressant therapy (refractory, erratic, premature, or short-lived).[25] Affected children of bipolar I patients pursue a predominantly depressive course, and cyclic temperamental presentations often precede syndromal episodes.

C. Nonpharmacologic Treatment
Psychotherapy may be chosen by patients with mild to moderate symptoms. Sleep hygiene as well as avoidance of mood-altering substances (including caffeine) and third-shift work may be very helpful.

D. Pharmacologic Treatment
Risk-benefit decisions regarding the treatment of bipolar illness during pregnancy are similar to those in unipolar depression, with the exception that mood stabilizers such as lithium, valproate, and carbamazepine are known risks as teratogens in first-trimester exposures. These are discussed below.

E. Impact of Pharmacologic Treatment on Pregnancy
Three mood-stabilizing agents are summarized below with respect to their use in pregnancy.

1. Lithium (FDA category D)
Early studies suggested a strong link between Ebstein's anomaly of the heart and lithium exposure.[34,45] While the relative risk of this rare defect calculated in these studies was estimated to be as much as 400, more recent prospective and retrospective cohort studies demonstrate a relative risk of 1.5–3.0 and 1.2–7.7 for cardiac malformations.[7,20] Furthermore, during an 8-year regional study of congenital heart disease in the Baltimore-Washington area, approximately 1% of children with congenital heart disease had Ebstein's anomaly, with a prevalence of 5.2 per 100,000 births. Of the 47 children with Ebstein's anomaly, the only factor that was associated with this anomaly was benzodiazepine exposure.[9]

2. Valproic acid (FDA category D)
Fetal levels are the same or higher than maternal levels. Neural tube defects (especially spina bifida) occur in 2.5% of infants exposed to valproic acid during the first trimester. Maternal serum alpha-fetoprotein and targeted ultrasound examinations are indicated. Recent information suggests that valproate teratogenicity is dose-related. Doses greater than 1000 mg/day are associated with greater risk of major congenital malformations than pregnancies exposed to lower daily doses.[4] Other malformations include cardiac, oral clefts, hypospadias, and limb reduction defects.[4] The overall risk for fetal defects appears to be between 5% and 8%. Breast milk levels are 2% of maternal serum levels; hence, there are no contraindications to breastfeeding.

3. Carbamazepine (FDA category C)
Carbamazepine has been associated with craniofacial defects, fingernail hypoplasia, and developmental delays.[21,23] Breast milk levels are 40% of maternal serum levels and there are no contraindications to breastfeeding.

F. Electroconvulsive Therapy
Refractory and psychotic depression has been treated with electroconvulsive therapy (ECT) in all trimesters of pregnancy. A review of 300 case reports covering 5 decades found a complication rate of less than 10%. Complications included transient fetal arrhythmias, uterine contractions, abdominal pain, and mild vaginal bleeding.[27] An additional report of abdominal pain, maternal hypertension, and vaginal bleeding with recurrent ECT speculates that these episodes represented recurrent mild abruption.[33]

Recommendations for precautions with ECT during pregnancy include pelvic examination, discontinuance of nonessential anticholinergic medication, uterine and fetal monitoring, intravenous hydration and administration of a nonparticulate antacid prior to the procedure, intubation during the procedure, and elevation of the pregnant woman's right hip to reduce caval compression.[27] Additionally, since it appears that abruption may occur with ECT,[33] the authors recommend that the procedure not be performed in women with hypertensive disorders, and that it be discontinued if the procedure results in vaginal bleeding, severe hypertension, or abdominal pain.

SECTION B.
ANXIETY DISORDERS

The anxiety disorders addressed in this section include panic attacks, generalized anxiety disorder (GAD), agoraphobia and obsessive compulsive disorder (OCD).

I. Panic Attacks
Evidence about panic disorder in pregnancy comes from retrospective studies, with some women experiencing relief of panic symptoms during pregnancy and others experiencing exacerbation or onset in the postpartum period.[18]

A. Nonpharmacologic Treatment
Psychotherapy of panic disorder is generally cognitive-based with particular attention to exposure-response control strategies, controlled breathing techniques, etc.

B. Pharmacologic Treatment
1. Antidepressants
Case reports of low-dose imipramine for treatment of panic disorder indicate successful use of this agent during pregnancy.[41] (See earlier discussion for comments on tricyclic antidepressants and SSRIs in pregnancy.)
2. Benzodiazepines (FDA category D)
Although some earlier studies suggested a possible link of benzodiazepine use and congenital defects, an Israeli study including approximately 600 women using benzodiazepines during pregnancy did not find any increase in congenital defects.[30] Neonatal abstinence syndrome (NAS) and "floppy baby" may occur in infants who received benzodiazepines during the third trimester with withdrawal symptoms, sedation, hypotonia, poor suck, apneic spells, and impaired response to cold stress.[26] Studies of cord blood levels of diazepam administered to women in labor demonstrate almost double the concentration in cord blood as compared to maternal levels, resulting in significant increases in respiratory depression and muscle tone inhibition.[32] Neurobehavioral effects have been studied up to 4 years of age with variable results.[30,39]

This information suggests considerable caution be exercised if benzodiazepines are administered extensively during the end of the third trimester or during labor.

II. Generalized Anxiety Disorder
Generalized anxiety disorder responds to TCAs, SSRIs, buspirone, and venlafaxine. TCAs and SSRIs have been summarized previously. There are no published reports of buspirone use in humans during pregnancy. Venlafaxine has not been widely studied in pregnancy, but no adverse events have been associated with its use.[22]

III. Agoraphobia
The treatment of agoraphobia entails control of panic attacks and anticipatory anxiety with psychotherapy (cognitive) aimed at regaining a sense of mastery of one's environment.

IV. Obsessive-Compulsive Disorder
Prospective studies are lacking on the influence of pregnancy and postpartum events as a result of OCD. Some women with postpartum flares of OCD have reported aggressive obsessions directed toward the newborn,[24] and another retrospective interview study reported 29% of women with worsening in the postpartum period, but the majority of women remained stable during pregnancy.[42] Treatment options finclude the use of SSRIs and clomipramine.

SECTION C.
SCHIZOPHRENIA

Schizophrenia occurs in approximately 1–1.5% of the general population. Community mental health centers treat many of these patients living in the community setting. While fertility rates may be diminished among patients with anovulatory cycles due to neuroleptic medication, functional issues diminish the ability of patients with schizophrenia to effectively use contraception.

I. Effect of Schizophrenia on Pregnancy

Limited numbers of studies are available looking at pregnancy complications in this chronically ill population. Available evidence suggests that schizophrenic women are at increased risk for delivery of low-birth-weight infants.[3] The interpretation of this study is difficult because of the heterogeneity of populations studied and small study size. A retrospective, descriptive study included psychiatric diagnoses as diverse as schizophrenia, depression, and nonpsychiatric diagnoses of epilepsy.[36] This study that spanned nearly a decade found an increased risk of operative and assisted delivery with uncontrolled psychotic symptoms in labor. This study also found that symptoms of schizophrenia worsened significantly during (30%) and immediately after birth (50%).

II. Schizophrenia with Intellectual Disability

Schizophrenia also may coexist with intellectual disability. The incidence of schizophrenia in an intellectually disabled population is approximately 3%. In this population, high rates of pregnancy and birth complications have been noted, including preeclampsia, dysmaturity, and labor abnormalities.[37] Confounding factors include an increased rate of smoking, substance abuse, and low socioeconomic status.

III. Treatment of Schizophrenia in Pregnancy

The majority of patients carrying a diagnosis of schizophrenia or schizophreniform-like psychosis need adequate pharmacologic management during pregnancy to allow normal function in activities of daily living and cooperation with pregnancy care.

The minimum effective dose should be used, keeping in mind the possibility of exacerbation during the intra- and postpartum period. High-potency agents appear to be the first-line choice in pregnancy, with little information available on newer agents, such as clozapine, a category B agent.[37]

IV. Effect of Pharmacologic Treatment on Pregnancy
A. Teratogenicity
Studies of children born to schizophrenic mothers with neuroleptic exposures during pregnancy do not suggest an increased risk of fetal defects.[12]
B. Effects on Fetal Monitoring
Neuroleptic agents may diminish fetal heart rate reactivity and may confound interpretation of antepartum testing.

SECTION D.
SUMMARY

The presence of acute or chronic psychiatric illness during pregnancy may necessitate the continuance of prepregnancy medication or the institution of pharmacotherapy during pregnancy. The presence of untreated or poorly controlled psychiatric illness during pregnancy has been associated in some instances with adverse pregnancy outcome and perinatal morbidity. Psychiatric illness may diminish the ability of the patient to participate in pregnancy care.

Some clinicians and patients may opt for nonpharmacologic therapy, but clinicians should be aware of high-risk conditions that make relapse more likely. In addition, the failure of nonpharmacologic therapy to control symptoms sufficiently may make the addition of pharmacotherapy critical to the overall well-being of the pregnant woman and to her ability to function with the increasing stressors of late pregnancy and the postpartum period.

There is fair evidence from prospective cohort studies that major depressive illness may be safely treated with SSRIs during pregnancy. For women with serious, long-term psychiatric disability such as schizophrenia, pharmacologic management should be continued with the realization that some psychoactive medications alter fetal reactivity in antepartum testing. Infants exposed to benzodiazepines during late pregnancy and labor should be observed for untoward effects in the newborn period.

References

1. Akiskal HS, Maser JD, Zeller PJ, et al: Switching from "unipolar" to bipolar II: An 11-year prospective study of clinical and temperamental predictors in 559 patients. Arch Gen Psychiatry 52:114–123, 1995
2. American Psychiatric Association: Diagnostic and Statistical Manual of Mental Disorders, Primary Care Version, 4th ed. Washington, DC, 1995.
3. Bennedsen BE: Adverse pregnancy outcome in schizophrenic women: Occurrence and risk factors. Schizophr Res 33:1–26,1998.
4. Bradai R, Robert E: Prenatal ultrasonographic diagnosis in epileptic mother on valproic acid: Retrospective study of 161 cases in central eastern France register of congenital malformations. J Gynecol Obstet Biol Reprod (Paris) 27:413–419,1998.
5. Chambers CD, Johnson KA, Dick LM, et al: Birth outcomes in pregnant women taking fluoxetine. N Engl J Med 335:1010–1015, 1996.
6. Cohen LS, et al: Biological Psychiatry (in press).
7. Cohen LS, Friedman JM, Jefferson JW, et al: A re-evaluation of risk of in utero exposure to lithium. JAMA 271:146–150, 1994.
8. Cohen LS, Sichel DA, Robertson LM, et al: Postpartum prophylaxis for women with bipolar disorder. Am J Psychiatry 152:1641–1645, 1995.
9. Correa-Villasenor A, Ferenz C, Neill CA, et al: Epstein's anomaly of the tricuspid valve: Genetic and environmental factors. The Baltimore-Washington Infant Study Group. Teratology 50:137–147, 1994.
10. Frank E, Grochocinski VJ, Spanier CA, et al: Interpersonal psychotherapy and antidepressant medication: Evaluation of a sequential treatment strategy in women with recurrent major depression. J Clin Psychiatry 61:51–57, 2000.
11. Frank E, Kupfer DJ, Wagner EF, et al: Efficacy of interpersonal psychotherapy as a maintenance treatment of recurrent depression: Contributing factors. Arch Gen Psychiatry 48:1053–1059, 1991.
12. Godet PF, Marie-Cardine M: Neuroleptics, schizophrenia, and pregnancy: Epidemiologic and teratologic study. Encephale 17:543–547, 1991.
13. Goldstein DJ, Corbin LA, Sundell KL: Effects of first-trimester fluoxetine exposure on the newborn. Obstet Gynecol 89:713–718, 1997.
14. Goldstein DJ: Effects of third trimester fluoxetine exposure on the newborn. J Clin Psychopharmacol 15:417–420, 1995.
15. Hans SL: Demographic and psychological characteristics of substance-abusing pregnant women. Clin Perinatol 26:55–74, 1999.
16. Hedin LW, Janson PO: The invisible wounds: The occurrence of psychological abuse and anxiety compared with previous experience of physical abuse during the child-bearing years. J Psychosom Obstet Gynecol 20:136–144, 1999.
17. Hendrick V, Altshuler L, Cohen L, et al: Evaluation of mental health and depression during pregnancy: Position paper. Psychopharmacology Bull 34:297–299, 1998.
18. Hertzberg T, Wahlbeck K: The impact of pregnancy and puerperium on panic disorder: A review. J Psychosom Obstet Gynaecol 20:59–64, 1999.
19. Hughes PM, Turton P, Evans CD: Stillbirth as risk factor for depression and anxiety in the subsequent pregnancy: A cohort study. BMJ 318:1721–1724, 1999.
20. Jacobson SJ, Jones K, Johnson K, et al: Prospective multicentre study of pregnancy outcome after lithium exposure during the first trimester. Lancet 339:530–533, 1992.

21. Jones KL, Lacro RV, Johnson BA, et al: Pattern of malformations in children of women treated with carbemazepine during pregnancy. N Engl J Med 320:1661–1666, 1989.
22. Kulin NA, Pastuszak A, Sage SR, et al: Pregnancy outcome following maternal use of the new selective serotonin reuptake inhibitors: A prospective controlled multicenter study. JAMA 279:609–610, 1998.
23. Lindhout D, Hoppener RJ, Meinhard H: Teratogenicity of antiepileptic drug combinations with special emphasis on epoxidation of carbemazepine. Epilepsia 25:77–83, 1984.
24. Maina G, Albert U, Bogetto F, et al: Recent life events and obsessive-compulsive disorder (OCD): The role of pregnancy/delivery. Psychiatry Res 89:49–58, 1999.
25. Manning JS, Haykal RF, Akiskal HS: The role of bipolarity in depression in the family practice setting. Psychiatric Clin North Am 22:689–703, 1999.
26. McElhatton PR: The effects of benzodiazepine use during pregnancy and lactation. Reprod Toxicol 8:461–475, 1994.
27. Miller LJ: Use of electroconvulsive therapy in pregnancy. Hosp Community Psychiatry 45:444–450, 1994.
28. Nayak MB, Al-Yattama M: Assault victim history as a factor in depression during pregnancy. Obstet Gynecol 94:204–208, 1999.
29. Nulman I, Rovet J, Stewart DE, et al: Neurodevelopment of children exposed in utero to antidepressant drugs. N Engl J Med 336:258–262, 1997.
30. Ornoy A, Arnon J, Shechtman S, et al: Is benzodiazepine use during pregnancy really teratogenic? Reprod Toxicol 12:511–515, 1998.
31. Orr ST, Miller CA: Maternal depressive symptoms and the risk of poor pregnancy outcome. J Clin Epidemiol 17:165–171, 1995.
32. Pan B, Lu Y, Wang D: Determination of diazepam concentration in maternal and fetal serum after intravenous administration during active phase of labor and its effects on neonates. Chung Hua Fu Chan Ko Tsa Chih 30:707–710, 1995.
33. Sherer DM, D'Amico ML, Warshal DP, et al: Recurrent mild abruptio placentae occurring immediately after repeated electroconvulsive therapy in pregnancy. Am J Obstet Gynecol 165:652–653, 1991.
34. Sipek A: Lithium and Ebstein's anomaly. Cor Vasa 31:149–156, 1989.
35. Steer RA, Scholl TO, Hediger ML, et al: Self-reported depression and negative pregnancy outcomes. J Clin Epidemiol 45:1093–1099, 1992.
36. Takeuchi R: Influence of maternal neuropsychiatric disorders on clinical course of pregnancy and neonatal outcome. Nippon Sanka Fujinka Gakkai Zasshi 48:1071–1078, 1996.
37. Trixler M, Tenyi T: Antipsychotic use in pregnancy. What are the best treatment options? Drug Safety 16:403–410, 1997.
38. Van Gent EM, Verhoeven WM: Bipolar illness, lithium prophylaxis, and pregnancy. Pharmacopsychiatry 25:187–191, 1992.
39. Viggedal G, Hagberg BS, Laegreid L, et al: Mental development in late infancy after prenatal exposure to benzodiazepines—a prospective study. J Child Psychol Psychiatry 34:295–305, 1993.
40. Viguera AC, Nonacs R, Cohen LS, et al: Risk of recurrence of bipolar disorder in pregnant and non-pregnant women after discontinuing lithium maintenance. Am J Psychiatry 157:179–184, 2000.
41. Ware MR, DeVane CL: Imipramine treatment of panic disorder during pregnancy. J Clin Psychiatry 51:482–484, 1990.
42. Williams KE, Koran LM: Obsessive-compulsive disorder in pregnancy, the puerperium, and the premenstruum. J Clin Psychiatry 58:330–334, 1997.
43. Wisner KL, Gelenberg AJ, Leonard H, et al: Pharmacologic treatment of depression during pregnancy. JAMA 282:1264–1269, 1999.
44. Wright JH, Beck AT: Cognitive therapy. In Hales RE, Yudofsky SC, Talbott JA (eds): Textbook of Psychiatry, 2nd ed, Washington, DC, The American Psychiatric Press, 1994, p 1083.
45. Zalstein E, Koren G, Einarson T, et al: A case-control study on the association between first trimester exposure to lithium and Ebstein's anomaly. Am J Cardiol 65:817–818, 1990.

CHAPTER 10

Antenatal Testing for Fetal Surveillance and Management of the Postterm Pregnancy

Stephen D. Ratcliffe, M.D., M.S.P.H.

This chapter describes how to use the tools available to family physicians for assessing fetal well-being during pregnancy. These tools are *screening* tests, and they should be used in a discriminating fashion. Emphasis is placed on the proper interpretation of these tests as well as on how to improve their diagnostic accuracy. Antenatal testing represents an area in which local practice standards are not well supported by the evidence of randomized, controlled trials. An attempt is made to present these testing modalities in a useful context for the family physician. This chapter also addresses the management of the post dates pregnancy.

SECTION A.
OVERVIEW OF ANTENATAL TESTING

I. Use of a Screening Instrument
Antenatal screening tests are used to assess the health of the fetus. Many factors need to be considered in interpreting the results of these tests:
- What is the condition that warrants additional fetal surveillance?
- Given this condition, what is the likelihood or probability that the fetus is at considerable risk for hypoxemia or acidosis?
- What is the gestational age?
- Are there other factors that can be causing the apparent abnormal test, such as the use of medication or the presence of maternal dehydration?

However, before clinicians begin to take these factors into account, they should strive to understand the underlying concepts that are essential to the accurate interpretation of antenatal screening tests.

A. Sensitivity
Sensitivity refers to the percentage of tests that are abnormal when the fetus is compromised (i.e., a true-positive test result). As Table 1 shows, applying the nonstress test (NST) to various maternal conditions, the sensitivity of this test to identify compromised fetuses accurately is low.[13] For example, when evaluating patients with intrauterine growth restriction (IUGR), a sensitivity of 56% means that when underlying fetal compromise is present, the NST is nonreactive in just greater than half of the cases. The NST is reactive or normal 44% of the time despite the presence of a pathologic condition that may be detected by using more sensitive tests.

B. Specificity
Specificity refers to the percentage of tests that are normal when the fetus is normal or not compromised (i.e., a true-negative result). Commonly used antenatal tests, such as NSTs and contraction stress tests (CSTs), have a high specificity (> 95%).

313

TABLE 1. Use of Nonstress Test as a Screening Test		
Condition (%)	Sensitivity (%)	Positive Predictive Value (%)
Postdatism	0.44	0.15
IUGR	0.56	0.69
Hypertension	0.31	0.44
Diabetes mellitus	0.53	0.31

IUGR = intrauterine growth restriction.
From Devoe LD: The nonstress test. Obstet Gynecol Clin North Am 17:111, 1990, with permission.

When test results are normal, an additional period of waiting is safe, depending on the condition undergoing surveillance.

C. Positive Predictive Value

The positive predictive value refers to the diagnostic accuracy of an abnormal test result to predict a compromised fetus. As the possibility or probability of a given abnormality or complication decreases, the positive predictive value of the test also decreases. For this reason, antenatal testing should be used selectively to assess high-risk pregnancies and not applied routinely to low-risk pregnancies. Using data from Table 1, the positive predictive value of a nonreactive NST in predicting a compromised fetus when assessing the postterm pregnancy is only 15%. The test has a false-positive rate of 85%. For this reason, abnormal NSTs are followed up by CSTs and biophysical profiles (BPPs), which have a higher positive predictive value.

D. Negative Predictive Value

The negative predictive value refers to the diagnostic accuracy of a normal test result to predict a healthy fetus. Antenatal testing, when used to assess the postterm pregnancy, has a negative predictive value greater than 99% in predicting fetal viability or the prevention of a fetal demise within 1 week. Table 2 summarizes the negative predictive value of four common tests of fetal well-being.[4]

II. Major Indications for Antenatal Testing

Patients who have the following *maternal* conditions are candidates for antenatal testing:[4]

- Type I diabetes mellitus
- Hypertension
- Antiphospholipid syndrome
- Hyperthyroidism (poorly controlled)
- Hemoglobinopathies
- Chronic renal disease
- Systemic lupus erythematosus
- Cyanotic heart disease
- Maternal substance abuse
  (see Chapter 4, section F)

There are also specific pregnancy-related conditions in which antenatal surveillance tests may be indicated, as follows:

TABLE 2. Reassurance of Normal Fetal Surveillance Tests: Prevention of Fetal Demise

Type of Fetal Surveillance	No. Studied in Case Series	Stillbirth Rate* Within 1 Week of Normal Test	Negative Predictive Value (%)
Nonstress test	5,861	1.9/1000	99.8
Contraction stress test	12,656	0.3/1000	99.97
Biophysical profile	44,828	0.8/1000	99.92
Modified biophysical profile	54,617	0.8/1000	99.92

* The stillbirth rate is corrected for lethal congenital anomalies and unpredictable causes of demise.
Data compiled from American College of Obstetricians and Gynecologists Practice Bulletin: No. 9, October 1999.

- Rh-sensitized pregnancy
- Pregnancy-induced hypertension
- Decreased fetal movement
- Oligohydramnios
- Polyhydramnios

- IUGR
- Postterm pregnancy
- Previous fetal demise
- Multiple gestation

III. Effect of Gestational Age on Antenatal Testing

Many situations arise in caring for the *preterm* prenatal patient in which assessment of fetal well-being is helpful before deciding if further intervention is warranted. Fetal reactivity and heart rate acceleration patterns are less pronounced in the preterm fetus. This section focuses on how to adapt antenatal testing for the preterm fetus between 24 and 34 weeks of gestation.

A. Effect of Gestational Age on Diagnostic Criteria

Castillo et al.[9] studied 30 women with prolonged nonstress testing every 2 weeks beginning at 24 weeks of gestation to compile the following normative data for the preterm fetus.

1. Baseline fetal heart rate
The baseline fetal heart rate decreases steadily as a function of advancing gestational age.
2. Frequency of fetal heart rate accelerations
Fetal heart rate accelerations occur less often at earlier gestational ages and tend to be at a lesser amplitude.
3. Frequency of fetal heart rate decelerations
Fetal heart rate decelerations remain relatively constant throughout the entire gestational period.

B. Effect of Gestational Age on Nonstress Test Interpretation

At an earlier gestational age, the clinician should extend the period of evaluation from 30 to 60 minutes and lower the amplitude of heart rate accelerations for NST reactivity from 15 beats/min to 10 beats/min.

C. Use of Antenatal Testing with Preterm Premature Rupture of the Membranes

Preterm premature rupture of the membranes (PPROM) is a particularly challenging and dangerous condition to manage (see Chapter 11, section H). The two major complications of this condition are infection (chorioamnionitis) and decreased amniotic fluid (oligohydramnios). The family physician may decide to refer the patient to a tertiary care center at an early gestational age because of availability of neonatal intensive care services. There are situations, however, when this is not feasible.

1. Monitoring for infection
Neither the NST nor the BPP has been shown to be a sensitive predictor of chorioamnionitis in the event of PPROM, although both of these tests are commonly used in this setting for this purpose.[12]
2. Monitoring for decreased amniotic fluid
Oligohydramnios, often associated with fetal distress and adverse neonatal outcome, occurs more frequently with PPROM. The clinician can monitor this condition directly by obtaining an amniotic fluid index (AFI). The AFI varies daily with PPROM. The NST, performed daily, appears to predict accurately a fetus that is being compromised secondary to oligohydramnios.[20] Clinicians should assess the NST for both its reactivity but also for the presence or lack of variable decelerations as a marker of umbilical cord compression.

IV. When to Begin Antenatal Surveillance

Antenatal fetal surveillance is initiated when a maternal or pregnancy-related condition is suspected to be exerting harmful effects on fetal health. This surveillance usually begins at 32 to 34 weeks of gestation but may start earlier or later depending on the indication for monitoring. When these tests are applied to low-risk populations in a nonselective fashion, the high percentage of false-positive results can lead to unnecessary iatrogenic interventions.

SECTION B.
TYPES OF ANTENATAL TESTING

I. Nonstress Test

The NST, developed in the early 1970s, remains a mainstay in assessing the presence or lack of fetal well-being.[18] An NST is reactive, or normal, when fetal heart rate accelerations occur in conjunction with perceived fetal movement. Accelerations take place through stimulation of the cardioaccelerator fibers from the upper thoracic spinal cord and are affected by activity in the brain stem and cortex.[13] These neurologic pathways are influenced by numerous intrinsic and extrinsic factors: sympathetic discharge and adrenergic receptors, behavioral state, circadian rhythms, gestational age and maturation, intrinsic rate and myocardial contractility, baroreceptor and chemoreceptor reflexes, exogenous dietary substrates, and drugs.

A reactive NST generally indicates that the fetal autonomic nervous system is intact and that its oxygenation status is satisfactory. A reactive NST correctly identifies a healthy fetus 99.8% of the time (see Table 2). The duration of this healthy prognosis varies depending on the maternal or fetal condition undergoing surveillance. Patients with PPROM often undergo fetal surveillance using NSTs on a daily basis, whereas the postterm pregnancy patient generally undergoes testing twice a week.

A. Technique and Interpretation

1. Indications and contraindications

The NST generally is used as the primary screening test when there is an increased index of suspicion for IUGR, fetal hypoxemia, or placental insufficiency. Lists of associated maternal and fetal conditions were presented earlier in this chapter. There are no major contraindications to the administration of the NST, although the family physician must interpret the test in light of potentially confounding situations. Concurrent maternal illnesses, use of sedative medications, and caloric deprivation are some of the conditions that can result in a nonreactive NST when the fetus is not compromised.

2. Administration of the nonstress test

The NST should be administered under stable, predictable circumstances. Factors to be considered include the following.

    a. Dietary state: NST testing preferably should be conducted 1 to 2 hours after eating.

    b. Medications: Drug usage or smoking concurrent with testing should be avoided, if possible.

    c. Maternal position: A semi-Fowler position, with hip displacement, should be used for patients.

    d. Gestational age: The clinician may use different testing criteria at a gestational age less than 34 weeks, as addressed in section A.

    e. Testing time: Testing usually requires 30 minutes but may be extended to 60 to 90 minutes.

3. Criteria for a reactive or normal nonstress test

An NST is considered to be reactive when two accelerations of greater than 15 beats/min occur in a 20-minute span. The *long* criteria state that the accelerations should remain above the 15 beats/min rate for 15 seconds; the *short* criteria suggest accelerations should initially exceed 15 beats/min and should take longer than 10 seconds to return to the baseline. The two criteria are comparable in predicting fetal compromise.[46]

4. Improving diagnostic accuracy

Depending on the condition being evaluated, Table 1 shows that the false-positive rate of a nonreactive NST varies from six out of every seven tests for the postterm pregnancy to one out of every three tests for IUGR. Many strategies have been developed for use as an adjunct to the NST to improve its accuracy.

   a. Fetal heart rate decelerations: When doing an NST, the clinician should be alerted to the presence of variable decelerations, with or without contractions. These decelerations may suggest the possibility of cord compression, which often is secondary to oligohydramnios. When feasible, an AFI should be obtained. The AFI is particularly important if a prolonged deceleration occurs (i.e., lasting > 1 minute and < 90 beats/min or 40 beats below the baseline rate).[8] Labor induction may be indicated in this situation.

   b. Amniotic fluid volume: The importance of adequate amniotic fluid has been established.[43] Some centers routinely combine the NST and AFI, particularly in the evaluation of the postterm pregnancy. This combining of these testing factors is called the *modified biophysical profile* (MBPP), detailed later in this section.

   c. Use of the nonstress test with vibroacoustic stimulation: Vibroacoustic stimulation is a method of fetal stimulation that uses a single 1- to 2-second sound stimulus applied to the lower maternal abdomen with an artificial larynx. The healthy fetus should respond to this stimulation with fetal heart rate accelerations. One group has used vibroacoustic stimulation extensively in conjunction with NST and AFI and has experienced no fetal deaths among 2628 women.[10] The main advantage of this regimen is the shortening of the testing time, which results in cost savings and a decreased need for nursing personnel. Further prospective studies are needed to substantiate this testing regimen.

B. Management of the Nonreactive Nonstress Test

The physician should take into account multiple factors in evaluating a nonreactive NST (e.g., risk status of the patient, gestational age).[17] Figure 1 presents a decision-making algorithm for this situation, the main points of which are summarized as follows:

- Assess for concurrent maternal conditions that could lead to a nonreactive NST.
- Extend the testing period, when possible, to 60–90 minutes.
- If extending the testing period is not a viable option, use vibroacoustic stimulation to attempt to obtain a reactive tracing.
- Evaluate other parameters of the fetal tracing. Obtain an AFI, particularly if variable decelerations are present.
- Conduct a CST or BPP if the NST remains nonreactive.
- Consider induction based on fetal lung maturity in the presence of oligohydramnios or a positive CST.

C. Evidence to Support Use of Nonstress Testing

Despite the widespread use of NSTs in the United States, the four randomized controlled trials that studied the efficacy of this screening test do not support its use in assessing future fetal well-being.[32] Retrospective case reviews in which the NST has been used as the initial test of fetal surveillance for high-risk pregnancies have been associated with a sixfold reduction in perinatal mortality compared with unscreened groups of low-risk patients.[13] This test conveys useful information regarding immediate fetal health and also appears to provide limited prognostic information regarding future fetal or placental reserve.[29]

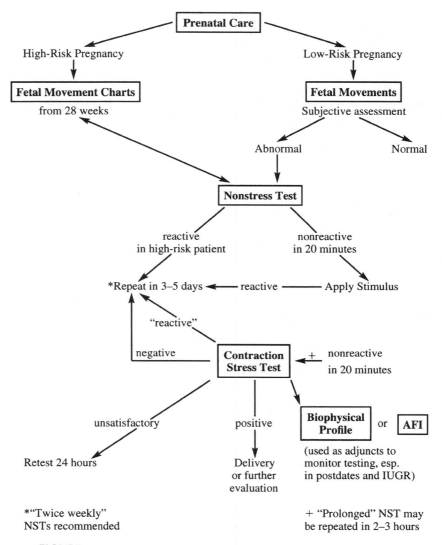

FIGURE 1. Antepartum testing. (Courtesy of Kent Petrie, MD, Vail, CO.)

II. Contraction Stress Test

The CST, developed by Ray and Freeman in the early 1970s,[39] measures the fetal response to maternal contractions. The late decelerations that occur after a contraction may indicate fetal hypoxia as a result of placental insufficiency.

A. Administration of Contraction Stress Test

Uterine contractions (three in 10 minutes) should occur with a low-dose oxytocin infusion (0.5 mU/min) or as a result of nipple stimulation. To perform the latter, the patient performs unilateral nipple stimulation to produce three contractions in a 10-minute period. The patient should remain in a semi-Fowler position for both of these techniques to prevent aortocaval compression and maternal hypotension. These techniques to achieve uterine contractions have comparable efficacy, with the nipple stimulation CST being more cost-effective.[41]

B. Indications
CSTs usually are performed when fetal compromise is suspected and the more preliminary test, the NST, has been nonreactive or nonreassuring.

C. Contraindications
CSTs should not be performed in situations in which vaginal delivery is contraindicated, including the following:
- Previous classical cesarean section
- Preterm labor (actual or threatened)
- Preterm premature rupture of membranes (PPROM)
- Known placenta previa

D. Interpretation
A CST is *positive* when greater than 50% of the contractions are followed by late decelerations. Uterine hyperstimulation (contractions occurring more often than every 2 minutes or lasting > 90 seconds) should not be present.

An *equivocal* CST occurs in the setting of hyperstimulation or when occasional late decelerations are noted.

A *negative* CST is one in which no decelerations are noted.

E. Management of a Positive Contraction Stress Test
Every attempt should be made to correct any underlying maternal condition that may be contributing to the positive CST.[4,24] Attention to the reactivity of the fetal tracing also is an important factor.

1. Nonreactive positive test

A nonreactive, positive CST generally indicates fetal compromise and should be acted on in an expeditious fashion, usually in the form of labor induction.

2. Reactive positive test

A reactive, positive CST often is a false-positive test result and may not require immediate delivery as long as a plan for further assessment is delineated. When possible, the family physician should consult an obstetrician or perinatologist to assist in developing a management plan in this situation. A BPP may be used in this situation.

3. Reactive negative test

A reactive, negative CST, a normal test result, is viewed as reassuring, and the recommended follow-up for fetal surveillance depends on the severity of the condition being monitored. If variable decelerations are noted in an otherwise reassuring test, an AFI should be done to assess for oligohydramnios.

III. Fetal Movement Counting
A. Natural History of Fetal Movement
A mother's perception of fetal movement is an age-old technique for assessing fetal well-being. Studies using real-time ultrasonography have shown that the fetus has frequent gross body movements (up to an average of 17 movements in 20 minutes).[40] A periodicity and diurnal variation in fetal body movements have been noted, with the number of fetal movements being less in the morning and more in the evening. It is common for women to perceive a slight decrease in the total amount of fetal movement as pregnancy progresses, largely as a result of increasing fetal size and decreasing amniotic fluid. The number of fetal movements and overall pattern of activity should not markedly diminish as a woman approaches her due date.[40]

1. History of fetal movement counting

In the 1970s, investigators attempted to develop fetal movement counting testing regimens. None of the regimens presented in this section have been shown in randomized controlled trials to decrease perinatal mortality when applied nonselectively to low-risk populations.[15]

2. Decreased fetal movement as a presenting complaint

Expectant mothers presenting to labor and delivery with the chief complaint of decreased fetal movement have a compromised fetus 8% to 12% of the time.[1,46] The remaining patients, who have reactive NSTs and normal AFIs, do not appear to need further monitoring or other fetal surveillance, unless additional risk factors are present. It is prudent to counsel patients to be aware of fetal movements and to agree on a surveillance plan when a marked decrease in movement is noted.

B. Testing Regimens

Many different regimens for counting fetal movements have been developed. Patient convenience factors often have affected compliance with these regimens. Despite the lack of supporting evidence, the family physician may choose to use one of the methods described here on a selective basis to complement other types of antenatal tests, such as the NST.

1. Count to 10 method

The count to 10 method is popular and has a high patient acceptance rate.[45] The patient chooses a 2-hour period when she can quietly monitor fetal movements. Fetal movement is defined as any kick, flutter, swish, or roll. Moore and Piacquadio[30] found that the mean time to perceive the 10 movements was 20.9 minutes and that 99.5% of patients had counted 10 movements within 90 minutes. This study recommended fetal movement counting only in the evening because of the increased movements associated with diurnal variation, although other studies have allowed the patient to choose the best time to perform the test.[30] A variation of the count to 10 method is the Cardiff method, which has women counting the first 10 movements each morning.[38] Anytime 10 movements are not noted in a 2-hour period, the patient should report this to her care provider.

2. Other methods

Other methods use discrete time periods (i.e., 60 minutes repeated three times a week). The Sadovsky method[42] has patients counting four movements three times a day after meals. This method requires greater time and organizational commitment than the count to 10 method.

C. Management of a Perceived Decrease in Fetal Movement

Clinicians should encourage patients to develop an awareness of fetal movement and to agree on a surveillance plan if decreased fetal movement is noted. Clinicians may choose to incorporate formal fetal movement counting regimens to complement other antenatal testing, although randomized controlled trials do not support their use to improve perinatal outcomes. The count to 10 method has been most acceptable to patients.

IV. Biophysical Profile

The BPP, first reported by Manning in 1980,[25] uses a combination of high-resolution ultrasonography and the NST to assess for evidence of fetal hypoxemia or compromise. When applied to known high-risk conditions, such as IUGR, the BPP has been able to reduce perinatal mortality below that of low-risk populations.[26]

A. Indications and Contraindications

The BPP is used to assess the status of the fetus in high-risk pregnancies, usually when the primary test of surveillance, the NST, is equivocal or nonreactive.

B. Test Administration

A clinician or technician skilled at ultrasonography spends 30 minutes observing fetal breathing movements, gross body movements, and tone, using defined standards. The AFI is calculated, and an NST is performed. Some centers omit the NST if the other four testing parameters are judged to be normal. Each of these five areas of surveillance has objective criteria that must be met to arrive at a score of 2. As originally designed by Manning, each of the five areas should receive either a 0 or 2 score (i.e., no partial score of 1).[25] Although 30 minutes of observation has been allowed to complete the BPP, the average time to record the sonographic aspects of the test is 8 minutes, and fewer than 2% of tests require 30 minutes of observation.

C. Test Interpretation

BPPs that are 8 out of 8 (NST excluded) or 10 out of 10 are viewed as reassuring and have a lower false-positive rate (higher specificity) than the NST or CST. In this situation, the clinician can avoid intervention in the setting of prematurity or an immature cervix. A low BPP score of 0–2 has a strong correlation to fetal hypoxemia and should be viewed as a indication for immediate delivery with the availability of neonatal resuscitation. A score of 4 usually warrants immediate action, whereas a score of 6 is more equivocal and requires serial testing to determine the most appropriate course of action.

D. Evidence to Support Use of Biophysical Profile

There has been widespread use of the BPP as a screening test for fetal well-being. There have only been two randomized controlled trials (n = 654) that study its efficacy in improving perinatal outcomes, however.[2] These randomized controlled trials do not support its use as a superior test of fetal well-being over its counterpart, the NST. The Cochrane Library states that "the data are insufficient to reach any definite conclusion about the benefit or otherwise of the biophysical profile as a test of fetal well being."

E. Management Decisions Based on BPP Findings

1. Normal score

The BPP is used primarily to evaluate the high-risk pregnancy, particularly after a NST is nonreactive and the CST is positive or equivocal (or contraindicated). A normal BPP may allow the practitioner to wait an additional period if elective delivery is otherwise not necessary at the time.

2. Low score

A low BPP score of 0 to 4 is an indication for immediate delivery with availability of neonatal resuscitation.

3. Equivocal score

An equivocal BPP score of 6 necessitates further testing with a CST or serial BPP measurements.

V. Modified Biophysical Profile

The MBPP takes two of the most sensitive components of the BPP, the NST and AFI, to create a relatively new test of fetal surveillance.[29,31] It is less time-consuming and expensive than the BPP and provides an evaluation of immediate fetal health and uteroplacental function using the NST and the AFI.

A. Indications and Contraindications

The MBPP is used in many settings as an initial test of fetal well-being for many maternal and pregnancy-related conditions. There are no contraindications, although clinicians should be aware of factors, such as maternal sedation or illness, that can result in an abnormal NST with a healthy fetus (i.e., a false-positive test).

B. Test Administration/Interpretation

The NST is administered in the manner described earlier. The AFI is determined using bedside ultrasound and is the sum of the measurements of the deepest vertical pockets of amniotic fluid found in each of the four abdominal quadrants. The measured fluid pockets must be free of umbilical cord. The MBPP is abnormal if the NST is abnormal (nonreactive, presence of deep or prolonged variable decelerations,

TABLE 3.   Positive Predictive Value of Components of the Modified Biophysical Profile for Prediction of Fetal Compromise in Labor

Components	Positive Predictive Value (%)
Nonreactive NST plus AFI > 5 plus no decelerations	50
Nonreactive NST plus AFI < 5 plus no decelerations	57
Nonreactive NST plus AFI < 5 plus decelerations	64
Complete biophysical profile < 8	59
Nonreactive NST	57
AFI < 5	37
Presence of decelerations	39
Prolonged decelerations	63
Variable decelerations	37
Late declerations	34

NST = nonstress test; AFI = amniotic fluid index.
From Miller D, Rabello Y, Paul R: The modified biophysical profile: Antepartum testing in the 1990s. Am J Obstet Gynecol 174:812–817, 1996, with permission.

presence of late decelerations) or if the AFI is less than 5 cm. AFIs of 5–8 cm are considered *low normal* and may require follow-up scanning at more frequent intervals (see Chapter 6, section H).

C. Evidence to Support the Use of Modified Biophysical Profile

The MBPP has not been studied in a randomized prospective fashion. Miller et al.[29] reported on a series of 15,482 high-risk pregnancies in which 54,617 MBPPs were performed as an initial test of fetal surveillance. This elegant study provides evidence of how this test can be viewed with respect to other forms of antenatal testing.

1. Positive predictive value of modified biophysical profile
The positive predictive values in Table 3 were generated with the application of MBPP to selected high-risk conditions. When this test is applied to low-risk patients, the positive predictive value of this test falls dramatically. The combination of the NST and AFI decreases the false-positive rate when both are abnormal.

2. Negative predictive value of modified biophysical profile
The negative predictive value of the MBPP is comparable to that of the BPP and CST and is higher than the NST alone (see Table 1).

D. Clinical Application of Modified Biophysical Profile

The evidence to date suggests that the use of the MBPP instead of the NST in assessing the postterm pregnancy results in a 50% decrease in rate of fetal demise in the week after a normal test result (0.8 fetal deaths per 1000 versus 1.9 fetal deaths per 1000).

VI. Umbilical Artery Doppler Velocimetry

Umbilical artery Doppler velocimetry is a test of antenatal surveillance that became available in university and many community hospitals in the 1990s. It uses ultrasound technology to observe umbilical artery blood flow during diastole, which in normal fetuses is a high-velocity state. Fetuses developing uteroplacental insufficiency show decreased velocity, absent flow, or, in severely affected states, a reversal of flow. This new technology has been studied using randomized controlled trials more than any other form of fetal surveillance.[33–35]

A. Indications and Contraindications

The only indication for Doppler velocimetry is to evaluate the umbilical vascular status in pregnancies complicated by IUGR. Doppler velocimetry has been studied in other pregnancy-related and maternal conditions, such as postterm pregnancy, and has not been found to be superior to other existing forms of fetal surveillance.[27,37] There are no contraindications for performing this noninvasive test.

B. Test Administration and Interpretation

Doppler velocimetry measures flow indices of the umbilical artery peak waveform during systole (S), the end-diastolic frequency shift (D), and the mean peak frequency shift over the cardiac cycle (A) that result in the following measurements:[4]

- Systolic/diastolic ratio (S/D)
- Resistance index (S-D/S)
- Pulsatility index (S-D/A)

Abnormal DV has been defined as absent end-diastolic flow or a flow index greater than 2 standard deviations above the mean for gestational age. Reversed end-diastolic flow, an uncommon finding, is associated with poor perinatal outcomes and is viewed as an ominous finding.[22]

C. Evidence to Support the Use of DV

A previous meta-analysis published in the Cochrane Library concluded that the use of Doppler velocimetry as a means of surveillance in pregnancies complicated by IUGR was associated with a decrease in perinatal mortality.[33] Concern has arisen over the veracity of the data of one of the trials included in the previous meta-analysis. The current Cochrane Review excludes this study, and as a result the outcome of improved perinatal mortality narrowly misses statistical significance (odds ratio, 0.71; confidence interval, 0.50 to 1.01).[33] Eleven trials are included with 6965 participants (Fig. 2). The Cochrane editor states that there is currently insufficient power in the number of study participants to make a definitive statement about the ability of Doppler velocimetry

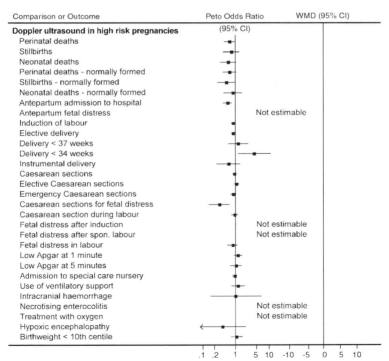

FIGURE 2. Screening and diagnosis in fetal compromise. Doppler ultrasound in high-risk pregnancies (Cochrane Review). The Cochrane Libarary, Issue 4. Oxford, Update Software, 2000, with permission.)

to improve perinatal mortality. The outcomes that are improved with the use of Doppler velocimetry versus NST in the evaluation of IUGR include the following:

- Decreased number of antenatal admissions (odds ratio, 0.56; confidence interval, 0.43 to 0.72; number needed to treat [NNT] = 8)
- Decreased number of inductions (odds ratio, 0.83; confidence interval 0.74 to 0.93; NNT = 25)
- Decreased number of elective deliveries (inductions plus elective cesarean sections) (odds ratio, 0.86; confidence interval, 0.77 to 0.96; NNT = 30)
- Decreased number of cesarean section for fetal distress (odds ratio, 0.42; confidence interval, 0.24 to 0.71; NNT = 14)

D. Clinical Application

Doppler velocimetry is a technology associated with many important clinical outcomes. It is probably associated with a 29% decrease in the relative risk of perinatal mortality (absolute risk reduction of perinatal mortality, 0.4%; NNT = 250). Further trials are needed to confirm this association. Doppler velocimetry is a tool primarily used by perinatologists to manage patients with IUGR. Family physicians who use this tool should do so in concert with a high-risk obstetric consultant. This test is a more accurate predictor of fetal compromise because its higher positive predictive value results in fewer false-positive tests and an improvement in the patient-oriented outcomes listed previously.

SECTION C.
MANAGEMENT OF
THE POSTTERM PREGNANCY

I. Definitions

A. Postterm Pregnancy

The postterm pregnancy, defined as one lasting longer than 294 days (42 weeks) from the onset of the last menstrual period, occurs in 3.5% to 12% of patients. Problems with inaccurate dating appear to explain the variance in this incidence.

B. Prolonged Pregnancy

The prolonged pregnancy is defined as one lasting longer than 287 days (41 weeks) from the onset of the last menstrual period.

II. Natural History

Before the advent of antenatal fetal surveillance, McClure-Brown[28] found that perinatal mortality increased with gestational age such that by 42 weeks of gestation, there was a doubling of the baseline rate (10.0/1000), and by 44 weeks of gestation, there was a four-fold increase. Although these rates are much lower in the 1990s, there is still a fetal mortality rate in the general population (fetal malformations excluded) of about 2 per 1000 in pregnancies lasting longer than 290 days despite optimal antenatal testing regimens.[16] A review of perinatal mortality in London confirmed that the rate of stillbirths at 43 weeks gestation was 2 per 1000.[21] Perinatal morbidity also is influenced by postdatism. Sources of increased perinatal morbidity with this condition include the following:

A. Dysmaturity

Dysmaturity occurs in 20% of postterm pregnancies because of chronic uteroplacental insufficiency.

B. Meconium

There is an increased incidence of meconium passage and meconium aspiration syndrome in the postterm pregnancy.

C. Fetal Macrosomia

Increased incidence of macrosomia in the postterm fetus may contribute to an increased cesarean section rate or complications of shoulder dystocia.

D. Oligohydramnios

The incidence of oligohydramnios increases with the postterm pregnancy. This increased incidence occurs, in part, secondary to decreased placental function.[43]

III. Management Issues

A. Importance of Accurate Dating

The large variation in the incidence of postterm pregnancy most likely is due to inaccurate dating of the pregnancy. Every maternity care provider knows the challenges of trying to date a pregnancy accurately. Many patients or health care systems cannot afford to provide routine dating ultrasound scans as described subsequently. Kramer et al.[23] described the following parameters to assist the clinician in establishing an accurate estimated date of confinement:

- Positive human chorionic gonadotropin by 5 weeks of gestation. A positive urine human chorionic gonadotropin now can be obtained beginning at about 10 days' postconception because of the increased sensitivity of this test.
- Fetal heart tones (determined by electronic Doppler) by 11–12 weeks
- Fetal heart tones (determined by fetoscope) by 19–20 weeks
- Quickening for primigravida at 19 weeks and for multigravida by 17 weeks
- Fundal height at the umbilicus by 20 weeks

Unfortunately, many patients present for initial prenatal care after 12 weeks of gestation, rendering some of the above-listed criteria unattainable. Additional relevant information that should be obtained at the initial prenatal visit is that related to the last menstrual period, including the onset and relative normalcy as compared with typical periods for that patient. The intermenstrual frequency should be elicited.

B. Evidence to Reduce the Need for Induction of Postterm Pregnancy

1. Routine ultrasound scans to establish accurate dating

The Cochrane Library has analyzed the data of the four randomized trials that looked at routine versus indicated ultrasound in pregnancy. "Routine early pregnancy ultrasound reduces the number of women who require induction of labor for apparently post-term pregnancy" (odds ratio, 0.68; confidence interval, 0.57 to 0.82; NNT = 100; absolute risk reduction = 1%). Clinicians must balance the benefit of performing one less induction for every 100 early ultrasound examinations versus the cost associated with ultrasound examinations and labor induction.

2. Routine stripping or sweeping of the membranes

Sweeping of the membranes is a procedure that clinicians perform beginning at 38 to 40 weeks by placing their gloved index finger approximately 2 cm into the cervix and making a circular, sweeping motion. This maneuver is performed on a weekly basis in an attempt to reduce the number of patients who develop postterm pregnancy, requiring induction. The Cochrane Library has analyzed 12 randomized controlled trials of this intervention. Table 4 shows the significant outcomes. The procedure results in a shortening of pregnancy and 9% absolute risk reduction in inductions for postdatism, without increasing the risk of rupture of membranes or other untoward neonatal complications. For every 11 patients undergoing sweeping of the membranes, one induction is averted. Patient discomfort was measured in only one study, but results indicate that this is an important factor for the practitioner to weigh.

C. Antenatal Testing Regimens

1. When to begin antenatal surveillance

There is no evidence to begin antenatal surveillance until the pregnancy becomes prolonged at greater than 41 weeks of gestation.[6]

2. Types of fetal surveillance

The two major tests used to monitor postterm pregnancy are the NST and MBPP (combination of the NST and AFI). The reported stillbirth rate associated with

TABLE 4. Outcomes Associated with Sweeping of the Membranes

Clinical Outcome	Odds Ratio	Confidence Interval	NNT	Absolute Risk Reduction (%)
Patient delivered within 48 h	0.43	0.30–0.61	6	16
Patient delivered within 1 wk	0.52	0.41–0.67	7	14
Patient delivered before 41 weeks	0.59	0.41–0.85	11	9
Patient delivered before 42 weeks	0.28	0.12–0.65	20	5
Patient did not require formal induction	0.58	0.43–0.79	11	9
Patient stated that vaginal examinations were painful	3.78	2.07–6.90	3 (no. needed to harm)	30 absolute increase

NNT = number needed to treat.
From Boulvain M, Irion O: Stripping/sweeping of the membranes for inducing labour or preventing post-term pregnancy. Cochrane Review. The Cochrane Library, Issue 4. Oxford, Update Software, 1999, with permission.

NSTs to monitor postterm surveillance has been reported at 2.13 to 2.72 per 1000.[5,44] These studies in the 1980s were doing weekly NST monitoring. A fetal mortality rate of 1.12 per 1000 was reported on 8038 consecutive postterm pregnancies using the MBPP once during the 42nd week and twice weekly thereafter.[16] In the absence of randomized controlled trial data comparing the two methods, it appears that the MBPP has a lower false-negative rate or higher negative predictive value and is the test of choice.

D. Induction at 41 or Greater Weeks of Gestation Versus Expectant Management
Induction of labor at 41 to 42 weeks of gestation results in lower cesarean rates than for patients managed expectantly (Fig. 3).[11,19] The approximate 2 per 1000 antepartum

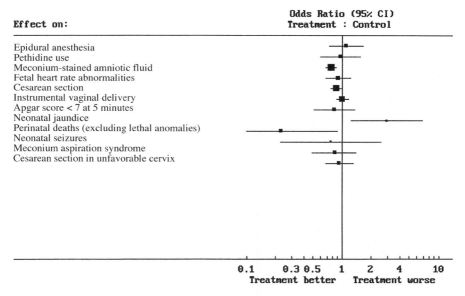

FIGURE 3. Postterm pregnancy. Elective induction of labor at > 41 weeks of gestation (13 trials reviewed). (From Crowley P: Elective induction of labour at 41 + weeks' gestation. In Enkin MW, Keirse MJNC, Renfrew MJ, Neilson JP (eds): Pregnancy and Childbirth Module. Cochrane Database of Systematic Reviews: Review No. 04144. Cochrane Updates on Disk. Oxford, Update Software, 1994, with permission.)

fetal death per week using NST fetal surveillance appears now to be 1 per 1000 using the MBPP. The number needed to induce to prevent one stillborn outcome is 500 based on studies compiled over 20 years. A more realistic number needed to induce is closer to 1000 based on the data presented here. Clinicians performing twice-weekly MBPP at greater than 41 weeks of gestation can provide this information to their patients in deciding when to start an induction. The bulletin by ACOG addressing the management of postterm pregnancy stated that induction at 42 weeks is recommended with a favorable cervix.[3] Expectant management until 43 weeks of gestation with an unfavorable cervix and reassuring fetal surveillance is appropriate. The availability of cervical ripening agents has prompted many clinicians to induce at 42 weeks of gestation despite the presence of cervical immaturity.

IV. Summary

Accurate dating of pregnancy is vital so that patients and practitioners can deal appropriately with the postterm pregnancy and its attendant risks. Based on randomized controlled trials, effective strategies to reduce the number of postterm inductions include routine early ultrasound scans to establish accurate estimated dates of confinement and weekly sweeping of the membranes beginning at 38 to 40 weeks of gestation.

Nonrandomized studies suggest that antenatal surveillance should begin at greater than 41 weeks of gestation and should be continued on a biweekly basis. The MBPP is the recommended screening test.

Induction of labor at greater than 41 weeks of gestation compared with expectant management has been shown in multiple randomized controlled trials to lower cesarean section rates and is associated with a reduction in perinatal mortality. Between 500 and 1000 inductions are required to occur to avert a fetal demise.

References

1. Ahn M, Phelan J, Smith C, et al: Antepartum fetal surveillance in the patient with decreased fetal movement. Am J Obstet Gynecol 157:860–863, 1987.
2. Alfirevic Z, Neilson J: Biophysical profile for fetal assessment in high risk pregnancies. Cochrane Review The Cochrane Library, Issue 4. 2000, Oxford, Update Software.
3. American College of Obstetricians and Gynecologists Criteria Set: Posterm pregnancy. No. 10, August 1995.
4. American College of Obstetricians and Gynecologists Practice Bulletin: Antepartum fetal surveillance. No. 9, October 1999.
5. Barss V, Frigoletto F, Diamond F: Stillbirth after nonstress testing. Obstet Gynecol 65:541–544, 1985.
6. Bochner C, Williams J, Castro L, et al: The efficacy of starting postterm antenatal testing at 41 weeks as compared with 42 weeks of gestational age. Am J Obstet Gynecol 159:550–554,1988.
7. Boulvain M, Irion O: Stripping/sweeping of the membranes to induce labour or to prevent post-term pregnancy. Cochrane Review. The Cochrane Library, Issue 3. Oxford, Update Software, 2000.
8. Bourgeois F, Thiagarajah S, Harbert G: The significance of fetal heart rate decelerations during nonstress testing. Am J Obstet Gynecol 150:213–216, 1984.
9. Castillo R, Devoe L, Arthur M, et al: The preterm nonstress test: Effects of gestational age and length of study. Am J Obstet Gynecol 160:172–175, 1989.
10. Clark S, Sabey P, Jolley K: Nonstress testing with acoustic stimulation and amniotic fluid volume assessment: 5973 tests without unexpected fetal death. Am J Obstet Gynecol 160:694–697, 1989.
11. Crowley P: Interventions for preventing or improving outcomes of delivery at or beyond term. Cochrane Review The Cochrane Libary, Issue 4. Oxford, Update Software, 2000.
12. Del Valle G, Joffe G, Izquierdo L, et al: The biophysical profile and the nonstress test: Poor predictors of chorioamnionitis and fetal infection in prolonged preterm premature rupture of membranes. Obstet Gynecol 80:106–110, 1992.
13. Devoe L: The nonstress test. Obstet Gynecol Clin North Am 17:111–128, 1990.
14. Freeman R, Anderson G, Dorchester W: A prospective multi-institutional study of antepartum fetal heart rate monitoring: I. Risk of perinatal mortality and morbidity according to antepartum fetal heart rate test results. Am J Obstet Gynecol 143:771–777, 1982.
15. Grant A, Elbourne D, Valentin L, Alexander A: Routine formal fetal movement counting and risk of antepartum late death in normally formed singletons. Lancet 2(8659):345–349, 1989.

16. Grubb D, Rabello Y, Paul R: Post-term pregnancy: fetal death rate with antepartum surveillance Obstet Gynecol 79:1024–1026, 1992.
17. Grundy H, Freeman R, Lederman S, Dorchester W: Nonreactive contraction stress test: Clinical significance. Obstet Gynecol 64:338–342, 1984.
18. Hammacher K: The clinical significance of cardiotography. In Huntingford P, Hunter M, Saling E (eds): Perinatal Medicine. New York, Academic Press, 1970, pp 80–93.
19. Hannah M, Hannah W, Hellman J, et al: Induction of labor as compared with serial antenatal monitoring in post-term pregnancy. N Engl J Med 326:1587–1592, 1992.
20. Harding J, Jackson D, Lewis D, et al: Correlation of amniotic fluid index and nonstress test in patients with preterm premature rupture of membranes. Am J Obstet Gynecol 165:1088–1094, 1991.
21. Hilder L, Costeloe K, Thilaganathan B: Prolonged pregnancy: evaluating gestation-specific risks of fetal and infant mortality. Br J Obstet Gynaecol 105:169–173, 1998.
22. Karsdorp V, van Vugt J, van Geijn H, et al: Clinical significance of absent or reversed end diastolic velocity waveforms in umbilical artery. Lancet 344:1664–1668, 1994.
23. Kramer M, McLean F, Boyd M, et al: The validity of gestational age estimation by menstrual dating in term, preterm, and postterm gestations. JAMA 260:3306–3308, 1988.
24. Lagrew D: The contraction stress test. Clin Obstet Gynecol 38:11–25, 1995.
25. Manning F: The fetal biophysical profile score: Current status. Obstet Gynecol Clin N Amer 17:147–162, 1990.
26. Manning F, Morrison I, Harman C, et al: Fetal assessment based on fetal biophysical profile scoring: Experience in 19,221 referred high-risk pregnancies. Am J Obstet Gynecol 157:880–884, 1987.
27. Mason G, Lilford R, Porter J, et al: Randomised comparison of routine versus highly selective use of Doppler ultrasound in low risk pregnancies. Br J Obstet Gynaecol 100:130–133, 1993.
28. McClure-Brown J: Postmaturity. Am J Obstet Gynecol 85:73–78, 1963.
29. Miller D, Rabello Y, Paul R: The modified biophysical profile: Antepartum testing in the 1990s. Am J Obstet Gynecol 174:812–817, 1996.
30. Moore T, Piacquadio K: A prospective evaluation of fetal movement screening to reduce the incidence of antepartum fetal death. Am J Obstet Gynecol 160:1075–1079, 1989.
31. Nageotte M, Towers C, Asrat T, et al: Perinatal outcome with the modified biophysical profile. Am J Obstet Gynecol 170:1672–1676, 1994.
32. Neilson JP: Cardiotocography for antepartum fetal assessment. In Enkin MW, Keirse MJNC, Renfrew MJ, Neilson JP (eds): Pregnancy and Childbirth Module. Cochrane Database of Systematic Reviews: Review No. 03881. Cochrane Updates on Disk. Oxford, Update Software, 1994.
33. Neilson JP: Doppler ultrasound in high risk pregnancies. In Enkin MW, Keirse MJNC, Renfrew MJ, Neilson JP (eds): Pregnancy and Childbirth Module. Cochrane Database of Systematic Reviews: Review No. 03881. Cochrane Updates on Disk. Oxford, Update Software, 1994.
34. Neilson JP, Alfirevic Z: Doppler ultrasound in high risk pregnancies (Cochrane Review). The Cochrane Library, Issue 4. Oxford, Update Software, 2000.
35. Newnham J, O'Dea M, Reid K, et al: Doppler flow velocity waveform analysis in high risk pregnancies: A randomized controlled trial. Br J Obstet Gynaecol 98:956–963, 1991.
36. Nienhuis S, Vles J, Gerver W, et al: Doppler ultrasonography in suspected intrauterine growth retardation: A randomized clinical trial. Ultrasound Obstet Gynecol 9:6–13, 1997.
37. Pearce J, McFarland P: A comparison of Doppler flow velocity waveforms, amniotic fluid columns, and the nonstress test as a means of monitoring post-dates pregnancies. Obstet Gynecol 77:204–208, 1991.
38. Pearson J, Weaver J: Fetal activity and fetal wellbeing: An evaluation. BMJ 1:1305–1307, 1976.
39. Ray M, Freeman R: Clinical experience with the oxytocin challenge test. Am J Obstet Gynecol 114:1–8, 1972.
40. Rayburn W: Fetal body movement monitoring. Obstet Gynecol Clin North Am 17:129–145, 1990.
41. Rosenzweig B, Levy J, Schipiour P, et al: Comparison of nipple stimulation and exogenous oxytocin contraction stress tests: A randomized prospective study. J Reprod Med 34:950–954, 1989.
42. Sadovsky E, et al: Monitoring fetal movement: a useful screening test. Contemp Ob/Gyn 1–6, 1985.
43. Sarno A, Ahn M, Phelan J: Intrapartum amniotic fluid volume at term: Association of ruptured membranes, oligohydramnios and increased fetal risk. J Reprod Med 35:719–723, 1990.
44. Small M, Phelan J, Smith C, et al: An active management approach to the postdate fetus with a reactive nonstress test and fetal heart rate decelerations. Obstet Gynecol 70:636–640, 1987.
45. Smith C, Davis S, Rayburn W: Patients' acceptance of monitoring fetal movement: A randomized comparison of charting techniques. J Reprod Med 37:144–146, 1992.
46. Whitty J, Garfinkel D, Divon M: Maternal perception of decreased fetal movement as an indication of antepartum testing in a low-risk population. Am J Obstet Gynecol 165:1084–1088, 1991.
47. Willis D, Blanco J, Hamblen K, Stovall D: The nonstress test: Criteria for the duration of fetal heart rate acceleration. J Reprod Med 35:901–903, 1990.

CHAPTER 11

Preterm Labor

William Sayres, Jr., M.D.

Preterm labor (PTL) and subsequent preterm delivery (PTD) of infants before 37 weeks of gestation are among the most vexing problems in obstetrics. Although neonatal mortality and morbidity have improved with advances in neonatal medicine, the incidence of PTD in the United States has increased from 9.4% of births in 1984 to 11% in 1995.[51] Complications of prematurity are responsible for more than 60% of neonatal morbidity and mortality.[44] The results of large-scale programs for the reduction of PTD have been inconsistent at best.

Birth weight is an important predictor of neonatal outcome. Low-birth-weight (< 2500 g) infants account for two thirds of U.S. neonatal deaths. Very low–birth-weight infants (< 1500 g) account for one half of neonatal deaths. Very low–birth-weight infants have a 95 times greater risk of death than infants born weighing greater than 2500 g at birth and a 7 times greater risk of death than infants weighing 1500 to 2499 g at birth. Intrauterine growth restriction accounts for a significant percentage of low-birth-weight infants and may lower the birth weight of 30% of infants born prematurely.[44]

This chapter advocates a clinical approach that seeks to identify patients who are most likely to deliver prematurely and to identify interventions aimed to decrease these risks. Once a patient presents with symptoms suggestive of PTL, rapid diagnosis of this disorder is important. Using the best evidence available, the clinician first must decide if treatment is indicated, then decide on therapy.

SECTION A.
RISK FACTORS FOR PRETERM LABOR

One half of PTDs are the result of spontaneous onset of labor with intact membranes. One fourth of PTDs are considered medically indicated. Neonatal outcomes for indicated PTDs are no different than outcomes for spontaneous PTD.[52] One fourth of PTDs follow preterm premature rupture of the fetal membranes (PPROM).

I. Demographic and Historical Risk Factors
Multiple demographic and historical risk factors for preterm delivery have been identified. Table 1 lists patient characteristics frequently associated with PTD. The impact of individual risk factors varies among populations and individuals. Previous PTD is the most predictive historical risk factor. Women with a history of one previous PTD carry a 17% to 37% risk of recurrence.[2] Risk increases with subsequent PTDs. The effect of stress is greatest if there is an increase during the pregnancy.[62] Physically strenuous work worsens the prognosis of low socioeconomic groups in particular.[58]

II. Maternal Infection
An evolving but consistent literature points to the important impact of maternal genitourinary infection on the pathogenesis of PTL.[45,46]

TABLE 1.   Risk Factors for Preterm Delivery

Demographic and Psychosocial	Pregnancy History	Medical/Gynecologic History	Current Pregnancy
Low SES	History of PTD	Uterine anomalies:	Maternal infection:
Maternal age < 18 and > 35		Bicornuate uterus	Bacteriuria
Black race		Cervical changes	Syphilis, gonorrhea,
Psychosocial stress		resulting from DES	chlamydia
Physically strenuous work		exposure	GBS
Substance abuse		Cervical incompetence:	Bacterial vaginosis
Tobacco		History of cervical	First or second trimester
Cocaine		conization or multiple	vaginal bleeding
Alcohol		abortions	Uterine enlargement:
Poor nutritional status			Multiple pregnancy
BMI < 19.8			Polyhydramnios
Poor pregnancy			Cervical change
weight gain			Uterine activity

SES, socioeconomic status; BMI, body-mass index; PTD, preterm delivery; DES, diethylstilbestrol; GBS, group B streptococcus.

A. Asymptomatic Bacteriuria

Asymptomatic bacteriuria, as an antecedent to pyelonephritis, has been strongly associated with PTL.[59]

B. Lower Genitourinary Infection

Infections with syphilis, gonorrhea, and chlamydia are all associated with PTD and low birth weight.

C. Maternal Group B Streptococcal Infection

Maternal group B streptococcal infection is significantly associated with increased neonatal morbidity and mortality. There is an inconsistent association of maternal group B streptococcal infection with PTL, although it appears to be associated with PPROM.[56]

D. Bacterial Vaginosis

Bacterial vaginosis is a polymicrobial infection by anaerobic bacteria, *Gardnerella vaginalis* and *Mycoplasma hominis* replacing the normal lactobacillus-predominant flora of the vagina. Bacterial vaginosis is associated with an increased risk of PTD (odds ratio, 1.4 to 1.8).[17,24,26,46]

SECTION B.
ESTABLISHMENT OF RISK ASSESSMENT AND ANTENATAL INTERVENTIONS FOR THE PREVENTION OF PRETERM DELIVERY

I. Establishment of Risk

Accurate assessment of risk for PTD allows for the focusing of resources and interventions on patients most likely to benefit. The variable results of carefully studied PTD prevention programs may be the result of inaccurate antenatal risk assessment or ineffective interventions.[28] Table 2 presents odds ratios associated with selected antenatal screening tests for PTD. Rather than presenting the opportunity for primary prevention of PTL, some of these tests may reflect a pathologic process that has already begun.

A. Risk Scoring

Many risk-scoring systems have been developed, usually within the context of global PTD prevention programs. Table 3 presents the system developed for a successful family practice-based program in a rural setting.[63] Patients in this program underwent risk assessment at the onset of care and at 28 and 32 weeks of gestation. Most risk assessment tools have low positive predictive values.[1,48]

TABLE 2. Performance of Clinical Indicators in Anticipation of PTD/PTL

Test or Symptom	Odds Ratio	Reference
BMI < 19.8	Nullipara 2.31 Multipara 1.76	42
History of PTD	2.01	42
Manual cervical exam	1.43 per unit Bishop score	42
Cervical ultrasound	For cervical length at or below: 40 mm/1.98 35 mm/2.35 30 mm/3.79 26 mm/6.19 22 mm/9.49 13 mm/13.99	25
Fetal fibronectin		
Threatened PTL	Positive test: 5.0 for delivery within one week Negative test: 0.2	6
Asymptomatic low risk	Positive test: 3.2 Negative test: 0.8	6
Asymptomatic high risk	Positive test: 2.0 Negative test: 0.4	6
1st- or 2nd-trimester vaginal bleeding	1.61	42
Bacterial vaginosis	1.84	41

B. Manual Cervical Examination

Safe and inexpensive, a digital cervical examination offers an immediate assessment of risk. A *cervical score* (cervical length [cm] – cervical dilation [cm]) of less than 0 is predictive of PTD. A Bishop score of greater than or equal to 6 indicates high risk.[29] Cervical dilation greater than or equal to 1 and effacement greater than or equal to 30% also indicates risk.[60]

C. Ultrasound Examination of the Cervix

Because the results of the cervical examination vary between examiners, ultrasound has been advocated as offering a more reproducible cervical evaluation. As ultrasound cervical length shortens to less than 30 mm at 24 and 28 weeks of gestation, risk for PTD progressively increases.[29] Table 2 quantifies these risks.

TABLE 3. Preterm Labor Risk Assessment*

Factors	History	This Pregnancy

≥ 1 Major Factors	Previous preterm labor and delivery
	Previous cone biopsy
	Uterine anomaly
	DES exposure in utero
	> 1 second trimester abortion
		Multiple gestation
		Cervical cerclage
		Polyhydramnios
		Cervix dilated > 1cm at 28- or
		  32-week exam
		Cervix effaced > 80% at 28- or
		  32-week exam
		Uterine irritability
		Abdominal surgery

≥ 2 Minor Factors	1 second trimester abortion > 2 first trimester abortions	Bleeding after week 12 Pyelonephritis Smoking > 10 cigarettes per day Febrile illness (T > 39°C)

* Patient is considered "high-risk" for PTL when the following conditions are present.
Data from Yawn BP, Yawn RA: Preterm birth prevention in rural practice. JAMA 262:230–233, 1989.

D. Fetal Fibronectin Testing

Fetal fibronectin is a fetal basement membrane protein. This protein is found in cervicovaginal secretions and indicates disruption of the fetal-maternal interface. In high-risk patients, such as those with prior PTD, the presence of cervical fetal fibronectin is predictive of PTD.[28] Predictive values fall in low-risk populations.[10] Low likelihood of PTD with a negative result may make the test useful for ruling out PTL. Table 2 quantifies these risks.

II. Psychosocial Interventions for the Prevention of Preterm Delivery

A. Antenatal Education

The primary focus of antenatal education efforts is on the early recognition of symptoms of PTL. The premise behind this educational effort is that women who recognize their contractions present to their providers in earlier stages of PTL and have a higher likelihood of successful tocolysis.[63] Educational programs also have been aimed at the providers of prenatal care, particularly the varied personnel interacting with the patient as she negotiates the system. Before evaluation by her provider, the patient encounters medical receptionists, telephone triage personnel, nursing staff, and others. If these staff members are not alerted to the symptoms of PTL, inappropriate delay between onset of symptoms and clinical evaluation may occur. Prenatal providers are challenged by the variability of symptoms that may precede PTL, including vaginal discharge, bleeding, backache, and diarrhea.[31] Not only do patients often present with atypical symptoms, but also the literature suggests that 50% of women do not feel their contractions at all or do not perceive them as painful.[31] It is critical to the success of education-based programs that clinicians and their support staff maintain a high level of suspicion when the patient presents with these symptoms.

B. Psychosocial Support

An enhanced social and emotional environment has positive psychological and behavioral effects and also may be reflected in better physical health. A meta-analysis of prospective studies of social support in pregnancy failed to show a decrease in the low-birth-weight rate, however.[27] A high suspicion for psychosocial duress should be maintained and these issues explored with the patient. Women who suffer a drastic increase in personal stress during pregnancy should be identified as having greater potential for adverse pregnancy outcome (see Chapter 4, section B).[62]

C. Lifestyle Modification

Educational and behavior modification efforts should focus on at-risk aspects of a patient's lifestyle. Smoking and other substance abuse should be addressed aggressively. Continued smoking in the face of active counseling may serve as an indicator of other psychosocial stresses (see Chapter 4, section F).

D. Nutritional Support

Nutritional support has been studied among large groups of pregnant women from lower socioeconomic groups. Patients who present with low weight and experience poor weight gain during pregnancy are at high risk for PTD.[21] Among these women, many of whom may be malnourished and at risk for PTL and low birth weight, dietary supplements of calories and protein increase birth weights 40–60 g on the average but do not extend gestations.[41] Although gestations may not be extended by dietary supplements, increasing birth weight can be expected to improve prognosis (see Chapter 3, section A). Calcium supplementation (2.0 g/d) in at-risk populations (low socioeconomic status, lactose intolerance) has been associated with a lower incidence of PTD as well as with lower rates of hypertension and proteinuric preeclampsia.[4]

E. Activity Restriction

The use of prophylactic bed rest has not been shown to prevent PTD in high-risk pregnancies and in one trial of twin pregnancies was associated with an increased rate of PTD.[57] Once a diagnosis of PTL or early cervical change has been established, however, activity restriction becomes important. For various reasons, many patients are poorly compliant with activity restriction. It is critical that the patient's psychosocial background be explored carefully in the context of PTD. Creative use of community and family resources may be required for compliance.

F. Sexual Activity

Sexual activity in itself does not increase the risk of PTD.[55] Self-palpation for uterine contractions after sexual activity is recommended for patients thought to be at increased risk for PTL. Patients diagnosed with PTL or early cervical change should maintain pelvic rest.

G. Regular Nursing Contact

Patients at increased risk for PTL and PTD have benefited from intense nursing contact.[16]

III. Medical Interventions
A. Screening for Infection

1. Gonorrhea, syphilis, and chlamydia

Clinicians should perform routine screening for gonorrhea, syphilis, and chlamydia at the onset of prenatal care. Patients who have positive results should undergo a test of cure at a subsequent appointment. The Centers for Disease Control and Prevention recommends that clinicians consider re-screening patients considered at increased risk of contracting one of these sexually transmitted diseases during pregnancy at the beginning of the third trimester (see Chapter 8, section A).

2. Group B streptococcus

Guidelines for universal prenatal screening versus *risk-based* management are discussed in Chapter 8, section A. For patients at risk for PTD, screening could be considered at earlier than 35 to 37 gestational weeks, although evidence to support this is lacking.[9]

3. Bacterial vaginosis

The incidence of PTD is reduced by screening for and treatment of BV in patients already considered high-risk for PTD because of previous PTD or low prepregnancy weight (BMI < 19.8).[24,26,46] Clinicians should screen these high-risk women for BV at the onset of prenatal care and again at 24 to 28 weeks of gestation.

A recent RCT demonstrated that screening and treatment of BV in asymptomatic low-risk women did *not* reduce the incidence of PTD.[8] Although many screening tests are possible, reliable office-based tests include vaginal pH greater than 4.5, wet mount for clue cells, and amine odor (positive whiff test). Treatment of diagnosed infection includes either clindamycin, 300 mg orally twice daily for 7 days[42] or metronidazole, 500 mg orally twice daily for 7 days.[24]

4. Home uterine activity monitoring

Patients may not experience contractions that may presage the onset of PTL. Asymptomatic uterine contractions may be detected with a home uterine activity monitor. Women considered high risk for PTD typically are monitored for 1 hour twice daily from gestational weeks 24 to 36. Monitor recordings are then transmitted electronically to a central location, possibly hundreds of miles away. Patients are contacted daily by a nurse.

Controversy surrounds the application of home uterine activity monitoring to clinical practice. Although contractions are associated with an increased risk of PTD, outcomes of monitored patients do not show a consistent beneficial effect, whereas use of prophylactic tocolytics and unscheduled visits increase.[13,16,38]

SECTION C.
DIAGNOSIS OF PRETERM LABOR

Early diagnosis of PTL is critical to tocolytic success. Tocolysis is less effective when initiated after the cervix has reached 3 cm dilation and 50% effacement.[63] Distinguishing true PTL from clinically unimportant symptoms often is difficult. Use of contractions as the sole criterion for diagnosis may result in error in 40% to 70% of cases. Contractions cease spontaneously in 30% of patients; the diagnosis of true PTL can be a difficult one.[25]

I. Definition of Preterm Labor
Labor is defined as regular uterine contractions accompanied by descent of the presenting fetal part and progressive dilation and effacement of the cervix. Cervical effacement of 80% or dilation of greater than or equal to 2 cm in the presence of regular uterine contractions would indicate PTL. Patients often present without all the features mentioned previously. The clinician is then faced with the difficult task of identifying women who will progress into full-blown PTL, while avoiding inappropriate treatment of those in false labor.

A. Gestational Age
Knowledge of the patient's gestational age plays an important role in PTL management.

B. Rupture of the Fetal Membranes
The clinician should use a sterile speculum examination to evaluate pooling, ferning, and nitrazine reaction. In this setting, the risk of PPROM is large so that an initial digital cervical examination should be avoided.

C. Infectious Disease Surveillance
Cervical cultures for gonorrhea and chlamydia are indicated, if not already done. Unless the patient is a known carrier, perineal and perirectal culture for group B streptococcus should be obtained. The clinician should consider evaluation for bacterial vaginosis.

D. Urinalysis
A urinalysis is indicated to rule out infection, renal disease, and hypertensive disorders.

E. Fetal Fibronectin
Women presenting with painful, regular contractions can undergo fetal fibronectin testing before having a digital cervical examination. For symptomatic patients, the presence of fetal fibronectin indicates a higher risk for subsequent PTD. The high negative predictive value of the test is also of use in terms of clinical decision making. A digital cervical examination results in an increased number of false-positive results. This test is not readily available for many family physicians at this time.

F. Serial Digital Cervical Examinations
Serial cervical examinations are required to detect progressive changes in cervical effacement and dilation. Having one clinician perform these examinations tends to minimize differences in examination techniques.

G. Ultrasound Examination
Ultrasound examinations are useful for confirmation of gestational age, follow-up fetal growth, amniotic fluid volume, and placental location. The dating accuracy of a third-trimester ultrasound is ± 3 weeks. A detailed screen for fetal anomalies, if not already available, also should be considered.[50]

H. Other Medical Conditions
Other concurrent conditions, such as cholecystitis, appendicitis, and viral gastroenteritis, may precipitate PTL. A thorough review of systems and physical examination should identify these conditions.

II. Distinguishing False From True Labor

For the symptomatic patient who presents *without cervical changes* noted earlier, tocolytic therapy should be delayed until true labor is diagnosed.

A. Hydration

Oral or careful intravenous hydration (< 500 ml) may reduce symptoms of uterine irritability. Maternal hydration status may be assessed with urine specific gravity. Sedation and rest may be used along with hydration.

B. Serial Examinations

Repeated gentle digital cervical examinations, after intact fetal membranes have been established, provide the clinician with the necessary information to make a diagnosis of true PTL.

III. Fetal Prognosis

A decision to treat PTL reflects the clinician's assessment that the risk to the fetus being delivered immediately is greater than the risk to fetus and mother of tocolysis. Tocolysis may delay delivery only 24 to 48 hours, time enough for glucocorticoid administration and potential maternal transport. With advancing gestational age, fetal prognosis improves, and incremental gains in prognosis decrease. Neonatal survival improves to 90% at 29 weeks, after which mortality decreases by 1% per week gained. Morbidity improves significantly until 35 weeks, after which delaying delivery exerts less of an effect.[12] The birth weight at which mortality ceases to improve significantly is 1600 gm, whereas morbidity improves significantly until 1900 g.[20]

SECTION D.
PHARMACOLOGIC MANAGEMENT
OF PRETERM LABOR

Once the diagnosis of PTL has been established and expected improvement in fetal prognosis is believed to justify medical interventions to delay delivery, tocolysis should be considered. The data supporting the use of tocolytics are equivocal, whereas potentially severe side effects of these agents affecting mother and fetus are well documented.

I. Contraindications to Tocolysis

Contraindications are presented in the Table 4 as well as contraindications to individual tocolytic agents. Clinicians must consider conditions that may predispose the mother to complications of pharmacologic tocolysis. Conditions of pregnancy threatening fetal viability also must be considered.

II. Laboratory Studies

If use of tocolytics is to be considered, admission laboratory studies should include complete blood counts, serum electrolytes, glucose, and urinalysis. An admission electrocardiogram also may be considered for patients who have a history of organic heart disease.

TABLE 4. Contraindications to Tocolysis

General	Relative	Beta-Sympathomimetics	Magnesium Sulfate
Fetal distress	PPROM	Maternal organic heart disease	Hypocalcemia
Chorioamnionitis		Poorly controlled diabetes,	Myasthenia gravis
Maternal medical instability		thyrotoxicosis, hypertension	Renal failure

PPROM, preterm premature rupture of membranes.

III. Beta-Sympathomimetics
A. Mechanism of Action
Beta-Sympathomimetics cause smooth muscle relaxation through activation of uterine β_2-receptors. Intracellular cyclic adenosine monophosphate levels are increased, reducing availability of intracellular free calcium. The affinity of myosin light-chain kinase for calmodulin also is decreased, reducing the sensitivity of the myosin-actin contractile unit for calcium.[7]
B. Metabolism
Excretion occurs primarily through the kidney. Half-life varies greatly among patients. Terbutaline and ritodrine cross the placenta.[7]
C. Efficacy
The efficacy of beta-mimetic tocolytics remains a highly debated topic despite approval of ritodrine by the U.S. Food and Drug Administration since 1980. The use of these agents delays delivery of patients in PTL for approximately 48 hours. Outcome studies that measure neonatal morbidity (respiratory distress syndrome) and mortality have shown inconsistent results, however (Fig. 1).[34] Once labor has been stopped successfully with the parenteral administration of beta-mimetic agents, oral agents commonly are prescribed, although inconsistent support for this practice is found in the literature.[43] There is no demonstrated benefit for the prophylactic use of beta-mimetics for patients judged to be *at risk* for PTL.[34]

The use of these drugs has done little to reduce the national rates of premature delivery. This lack of consistent research support for the use of beta-mimetic agents provides a contrast to well-documented adverse drug effects, described subsequently, and indicates a thoughtful and considered approach to their use. Use of these drugs for tocolysis of multiple pregnancy has been associated with higher morbidity, and administration of steroids has not been shown to improve neonatal

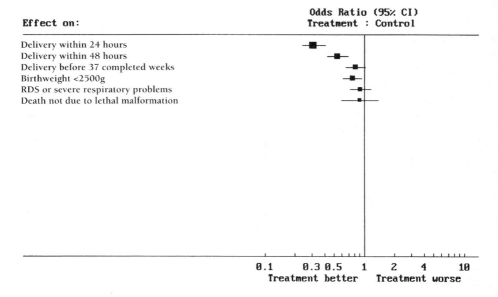

FIGURE 1.   Beta-sympathomimetic tocolytics in treatment of preterm labor (16 trials reviewed). RDS = Respiratory distress syndrome. (From Keirse MJNC: Betamimetic tocolytics in preterm labour. In Enkin MW, Keirse MJNC, Renfrew MJ, Neilson JP (eds): Pregnancy and Childbirth Module. Cochrane Database of Systematic Reviews, Review No. 03237. Cochrane Updates on Disk. Oxford, Update Software, 1994, with permission.)

prognosis.[50] The use of these agents may prolong a pregnancy long enough to transport the patient to a center that is better equipped to handle a premature neonate. Another use of these agents is to prolong a pregnancy such that corticosteroids may be administered prior to 34 weeks gestation.

D. Adverse Drug Effects
1. Maternal
   a. Cardiovascular:[32] The hemodynamic changes of pregnancy exacerbate the cardiovascular side effects of beta-mimetic drugs. In particular, maternal plasma volume is increased (especially in multiple gestations, which present more frequently in PTL). Baseline cardiac output is increased in pregnancy. The more severe side effects generally occur during parenteral therapy. Patients with preexisting heart disease (i.e., valvular heart disease, coronary heart disease and hypertension) are at particular risk for potentially disastrous complications, such as congestive heart failure and myocardial ischemia.

      Maternal tachycardia (average maximum increase in pulse of 40 beats/min) occurs in more than 80% of patients. Increase in maternal pulse is predictable enough that it can be used as a basis for dosage of tocolytics. Hypertension, hypotension, and an increase in pulse pressure may occur with beta-mimetic agents. Nodal and ventricular cardiac arrhythmias may occur in 2% of patients treated parenterally.

      Congestive heart failure is the most common serious cardiovascular side effect of these agents.[25] Predisposing conditions include multiple gestation, persistent tachycardia (> 130 beats/min), maternal infection, and iatrogenic fluid overload. There may be an association between antepartum glucocorticoid use and maternal congestive heart failure as well.[7]
   b. Metabolic effects: Glucose intolerance is believed to be secondary to increased gluconeogenesis. The use of beta-mimetic drugs should be avoided in women with insulin dependent diabetes because frank diabetic ketoacidosis may occur.[7] Hypokalemia occurs secondary to potassium influx into cells and does not represent overall depletion of stores. Potassium therapy is not necessary unless levels fall to less than 2.5 mEq/L.[7]
   c. Symptomatic side effects: Women frequently suffer from nervousness, restlessness, and anxiety. Although not necessarily medically significant, these symptoms may lead to noncompliance. Nausea, vomiting, and flushing may occur.

2. Fetal Side Effects
Effects on the fetus appear to be less drastic than maternal effects and consist of tachycardia, hypoglycemia, hypocalcemia, and hypotension.[7]

E. Dosage and Monitoring of Therapy
For dosage and monitoring of therapy, see Table 5.

IV. Magnesium Sulfate
A. Mechanism of Action
Smooth muscle relaxation occurs secondary to the reduction of acetylcholine released at the motor end plate or by direct effects through competition with calcium at the motor end plate or in the cell membrane.[7]

B. Metabolism
The kidney primarily excretes magnesium. Caution is indicated for patients with potential renal disease.[7]

C. Efficacy
Although in widespread use as a tocolytic, there are few data available to support the efficacy of magnesium sulfate as a tocolytic. Meta-analysis of available randomized

TABLE 5. Administration and Dosage of Tocolytics

Tocolytic	Infusion Rate	Oral Dosage	Comments
Ritodrine	Initiate at 50–100 µg/min Increase infusion by 50 µg/min every 15–20 min until labor is inhibited, side effects occur, or a maximal infusion rate of 350 µg/min is reached Sustain infusion for 12–24 hrs	Initial dose of 10 mg 30 min before stopping infusion, then 10 mg every 2 hrs or 20 mg every 5 hrs for 24 hrs Maintenance: 10–20 mg every 4–6 hrs Maximum dose is 120 mg/day	Use with caution Assess for maternal-fetal contraindications Monitor for maternal adverse effects, such as CHF
Terbutaline	Continuous infusion: 250 µg loading dose IV over 1–2 min 10–25 µg/min for 12 or more hours Intermittent subcutaneous dosage: 250 µg SC every 4 hrs	2.5–5.0 mg every 4 hrs	Same precautions as with ritodrine
Magnesium sulfate	Loading dose: 4–6 g IV over 20 min Maintenance: 1–4 g/hr for 8–12 hrs		Efficacy in prolonging gestation in question
Nifedipine		Loading dose: 10–20 mg sublingually every 20 min for up to 3 doses Maintenance: 10–20 mg orally every 6 hrs	Use is investigational at this point
Indomethacin		Loading dose: 50 mg orally or 50–100 mg rectally Maintenance: 25–50 mg orally every 4–6 hrs	Secondary agent used in gestations < 34 weeks Duration of use not to exceed 24–48 hours
Glucocorticoids	Betamethasone phosphate or acetate: 12 mg IM, repeat in 24 hrs Dexamethasone phosphate: 6 mg IM every 12 hrs up to maximum dose of 24 mg		Evidence strongly supports its use with PTL or PPROM prior to 4 weeks of gestation to reduce RDS and neonatal mortality

IV, intravenously; IM, intramuscularly; SC, subcutaneously; PPROM, preterm premature rupture of membranes; CHF, congestive heart failure; RDS, respiratory distress syndrome.

controlled trials showed no effect on prolonging pregnancy, decreasing neonatal respiratory distress syndrome, or improving neonatal survival.[37] Compared with beta-mimetics, however, side effects are less severe, and therapeutic drug levels can be monitored. Addition of this agent to ritodrine may increase the efficacy of the former, but the risk of side effects, in particular pulmonary edema, may be increased.[7] Magnesium levels of 4 to 8 mEq/L are thought to be associated with tocolysis.[25] Oral magnesium is ineffective in the treatment and prevention of PTL, and it is ineffective for maintenance therapy after acute treatment.

D. Adverse Drug Effects

1. Maternal

Magnesium toxicity is dose dependent and can be anticipated by monitoring maternal magnesium levels and neurological examination. With proper precautions, magnesium is probably safer for tocolysis than ritodrine or terbutaline. Calcium is available for reversal of magnesium toxicity.[7]

2. Fetal
Newborns do not appear to excrete magnesium as rapidly as adults and may
show drowsiness and hypotonia. These effects are more pronounced when mag-
nesium is administered for longer than 24 hours.[7]
E. Dosage
Table 5 provides dosage information.

V. Calcium Channel Blockers
A. Mechanism of Action
Through the blockade of membrane-bound calcium channels, influx of calcium
ions, which usually occurs with cell excitation, does not occur, and contraction is inhibited. Nifedipine, which has few cardiac side effects, has been the agent primarily
studied.[35]
B. Efficacy
Only a few studies of efficacy are available and should be considered preliminary.
Nifedipine appears to have a similar efficacy to ritodrine.[35]
C. Side Effects
Maternal flushing, headache, dizziness, and nausea are due to transient hypotension, which might be severe with sublingual administration of nifedipine. Animal
studies have shown a decrease in uterine blood flow with a corresponding drop in
fetal arterial oxygen pressure and oxygen saturation. These effects have not been
shown in the small number of humans studied. Blood pressure must be monitored
closely.[7,25]
D. Dosage
Table 5 provides dosage information.

VI. Prostaglandin Synthetase Inhibitors
A. Mechanism
Prostaglandins appear to play a role in the processes of cervical ripening, gap junction formation, and uterine contractions, all of which are necessary for labor.
Prostaglandin synthetase allows the conversion of arachidonic acid to active
metabolites, including prostaglandin $F_{2\alpha}$ and prostaglandin E. By blocking this conversion, it is postulated, PTL may be stopped.[25]
B. Efficacy
As with calcium channel blockers, large prospective studies of efficacy are not
available for analysis. In the published randomized controlled trials, however, indomethacin and sulindac appear to be as effective as ritodrine in the treatment of
PTL.[36]
C. Adverse Drug Effects
Maternal effects are mild and consist mainly of gastritis. Renal effects must be kept
in mind, especially in the presence of dehydration. Fetal effects are most concerning. Premature closure of the ductus arteriosus has been shown. It appears to be reversible and more significant at more mature gestations. Oligohydramnios can occur
secondary to decreased fetal urine output and resolves with discontinuation of the
drug. Primary fetal pulmonary hypertension and necrotizing enterocolitis have been
noted with therapy of greater than 2 days' duration.[7,25]
Because of these potential adverse side effects, family physicians should use
these agents to treat PTL in gestations less than 34 weeks and for periods not to
exceed 24 to 48 hours. The decision to use these agents should be done with obstetric or perinatal consultation, whenever possible.
D. Dosage
Table 5 provides dosage information.

VII. Antibiotics
A. Mechanism of Action
Maternal upper genital tract infection may be associated with 20% of preterm deliveries. Occult chorioamnionitis has been shown in 5% to 10% of women with PTL and intact membranes. Specific organisms identified in the amniotic fluid of women in PTL include *Fusobacterium*, *Bacteroides ureolyticus*, and *Ureaplasma urealyticum*. Ascending infection is thought to be the mechanism by which bacterial vaginosis is associated with PTD. Cervical and amniotic infections may initiate uterine contractions through the inappropriate production of prostaglandins E_2 and $F_{2\alpha}$. Prostaglandin production may be stimulated by the metabolic byproducts of infecting organisms and by the host inflammatory response to infection.[3,40]
B. Efficacy
Specific organisms that have been targeted in prospective randomized trials of antibiotics in the prevention and treatment of PTL include *M. hominis*, *U. urealyticum*, *Chlamydia trachomatis*, and group B streptococcus. Although ascending genital tract infection has been clearly implicated in the pathogenesis of PTL, intrapartum use of antibiotics does not appear to prolong pregnancy or improve neonatal morbidity and mortality.[40]
C. Group B Streptococcal Prophylaxis
PTL is an indication for group B streptococcal antibiotic prophylaxis.[9] Assuming a maternal colonization rate of 19%, the overall risk of early-onset neonatal group B streptococcal disease is 1:100 in infants delivered before 35 weeks' gestation.[56]

VIII. Glucocorticoids for Fetal Lung Maturation
A. Mechanism
Fetal lung maturation appears to be accelerated through the stimulation of surfactant release in alveoli.
B. Efficacy
Evidence from large, prospective, randomized trials is strong that glucocorticoids given before 34 weeks of gestation, at least 24 hours and not longer than 7 days before delivery improve neonatal outcomes.[14,42] No data are available on repeat administration of glucocorticoids after the 7-day therapeutic window. This intervention decreases the incidence and severity of respiratory distress syndrome and improves neonatal survival rates (Figure 2). Glucocorticoid administration also improves neonatal morbidity in the setting of PTL with ruptured membranes before 34 weeks of gestation.[14] Table 6 shows the number needed to treat with glucocorticoids to prevent these devastating neonatal outcomes. Data on efficacy at less than 27 weeks of gestation are scant.[50] In one retrospective study, repeat administration of glucocorticoids after the initial 7-day window was associated with no improvement in neonatal outcome along with increased mortality, decreased fetal growth, and prolonged adrenal supression.
C. Side Effects
Maternal diabetes and hypertension may potentially deteriorate with glucocorticoid administration.[14] Betamethasone used in conjunction with beta-sympathomimetic

TABLE 6.   Corticosteroids Prior to Preterm Delivery[14]

Improved Perinatal Outcomes	Number Needed to Treat (NNT) to Achieve Outcome
Decreased incidence of respiratory distress syndrome	11
Decreased incidence of neonatal intraventricular hemorrhage	9
Decreased incidence of neonatal death	25

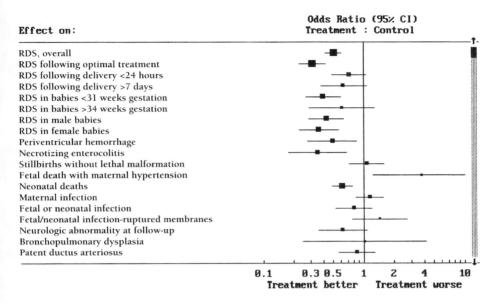

FIGURE 2.   Effect of corticosteroids on fetal maturation given before preterm delivery (15 trials reviewed). RDS = Respiratory distress syndrome. (From Crowley P: Corticosteroids prior to preterm delivery. In Enkin MW, Keirse MNC, Renfrew MJ, Neilson JP (eds): Pregnancy and Childbirth Module. Cochrane Database of Systematic Reviews, Review No. 02955. Cochrane Updates on Disk. Oxford, Update Software, 1994, with permission.)

agents has been associated with maternal pulmonary edema, although it (and dexamethasone) has minimal mineralocorticoid activity.[22]

D. Dosage

See Table 5 for dosage information.

SECTION E.
INCOMPETENT CERVIX

I. Epidemiology

Cervical incompetence plays an independent but related role with uterine contractions in PTD. The incidence of incompetent cervix has been reported to be 1:500 to 1:2000 pregnancies.[53] Although this area has not been studied thoroughly, it is likely that this condition does not exist as a single entity. Many other factors (i.e., preterm contractions) contribute to the premature dilation of the cervix. The diagnostic challenge is assessing the contribution of cervical incompetence to PTD along with the contribution of other factors. The role of other factors in this disorder explains the high rate (70%) of pregnancy success without intervention in women with a previous diagnosis of an incompetent cervix and the failure of some trials to show a benefit from cervical cerclage.[23] Because surgical intervention often is the treatment of choice, correct diagnosis is crucial.

II. Pathophysiology

The cause of this disorder can be divided into congenital conditions and cervical trauma. *In utero* exposure to diethylstilbestrol (DES) is most commonly associated with congenital incompetent cervix as well as with other female reproductive tract abnormalities. Visible abnormalities, such as the coxcomb or hood appearance of the cervix, should raise the suspicion of cervical incompetence resulting from DES exposure.[33] Trauma to the cervix may result in incompetence, although the effects are highly variable and depend on extent of trauma and maternal factors. Common sources of cervical trauma include precipitous delivery, overzealous mechanical dilation, recurrent induced abortions, and cervical conization.[30]

III. Diagnosis of Incompetent Cervix
A. Preconception
Although incompetent cervix may be suggested by the above-mentioned historical factors, diagnosis is made on a functional basis. As cervical cerclage is commonly used; it is crucial to exclude other reasons for preterm cervical dilation (e.g., preterm contractions or infection) before making this diagnosis. Recurrent second trimester pregnancy loss, especially with a history of rapid, painless cervical effacement and dilation, strongly suggests an incompetent cervix. Preconceptual diagnosis remains problematic because cervical anatomy and function are different in the pregnant state. A hysterosalpingogram may show cervical abnormalities and other reproductive tract abnormalities, which might explain recurrent second-trimester pregnancy loss.
B. Prenatal
Once pregnancy has been established, this diagnosis can be made on the basis of preterm cervical effacement and dilatation without other causes (i.e. uterine contractions or infection).

IV. Management
Treatment of incompetent cervix is bed rest, along with close monitoring of cervical status and uterine activity. Elimination of risk factors for PTL should be pursued as much as possible. Some centers use ultrasound to follow cervical status. Application of this technology depends on local expertise. Trials evaluating the efficacy of cerclage placement for women judged to be at high risk of PTL and PTD have had variable results.[23] There has been a statistically nonsignificant trend to prolong pregnancies but with an accompanying increase in hospital admissions, frequency of tocolysis, and puerperal sepsis. The decision to place a cerclage should be made carefully.

SECTION F.
MANAGEMENT OF PRETERM DELIVERY

I. Maternal Transfer
Intensive perinatal and neonatal care has improved the prognosis of preterm infants, especially those born before 32 weeks of gestation.[21] Maternal transfer is a necessary consideration when preterm delivery is considered unavoidable and neonatal intensive care services are not available.

II. Fetal Surveillance
The decision to monitor the preterm fetus should be made with the consideration that the low-birth-weight infant is more susceptible to the deleterious effects of asphyxia and acidosis. In particular, asphyxia leads to a higher incidence of respiratory disorders and intraventricular hemorrhage.[61] Given the catastrophic consequences of prolonged asphyxia before delivery of the preterm infant, continuous direct fetal monitoring is recommended. Preterm fetal heart tracings are more likely to appear nonreactive than those of term gestations, presumably because of fetal central nervous system immaturity. Diagnosis of fetal asphyxia indicates immediate delivery.

III. Route and Method of Delivery

The debate surrounding the method of delivery of the preterm infant centers on the risk of intraventricular hemorrhage from decompression of the fetal head as it is delivered over the perineum. It is not entirely clear if such a mechanism for intraventricular hemorrhage exists. The greatest influence on intraventricular hemorrhage is the birth weight and gestational age of the infant.[6] Prophylactic cesarean delivery of the vertex infant does not necessarily allow for a wider route of delivery in the preterm gestation and has potentially more complications than cesarean at term. Prophylactic forceps has been advocated as a way to avoid trauma to the fetal head but appears to have little therapeutic effect on the basis of retrospective studies.[54] *Generous* episiotomy has been recommended but also has failed to show improved outcomes in retrospective studies.[6] The lack of prospective randomized trials in this area calls for a commonsense approach. Prophylactic forceps cannot be recommended. Vacuum extraction is contraindicated in premature delivery. Use of episiotomy can be justified when obstruction at the perineum significantly delays delivery.

IV. Anesthesia

Management of pain in the PTL is complicated by the enormous psychosocial stress the laboring mother might be experiencing. Because of potential depression of the neonate, narcotic analgesia should be used with caution, just as in a term delivery. Epidural anesthesia may offer the theoretic advantage of a *relaxed* perineum, although the potential fetal malposition and increased rates of forceps deliveries also must be considered. No prospective trials are available to recommend one method of anesthesia over another.

SECTION G.
PROGRAMS AIMED AT IDENTIFYING PATIENTS
AT RISK FOR PRETERM LABOR
AND SUBSEQUENT PATIENT CARE

I. Background

Women who fail to seek prenatal care are at significant risk of PTD. Provision of routine prenatal care, however, does not prevent those poor outcomes. Modeled after programs developed in France by Papiernik and later adopted by Creasy and colleagues, *enhanced*[21] prenatal care seeks first to identify patients at highest risk for PTD. Patients then are followed closely in hopes of diagnosing PTL in its early stages and improving the chance of delaying delivery.[63] These programs have met with mixed results but overall have not been shown to reduce the incidence of preterm births. At a minimum, the adoption of a system such as presented subsequently would provide a framework in which newer developments might be adopted.

II. Provider Education

All hospital, paramedical, and office personnel (i.e., receptionists, nurses, paramedics) with potential contact with pregnant patients receive an educational program aimed at improving knowledge of PTL. The purpose of this education is to streamline the evaluation and treatment of patients potentially suffering from PTL. Depending on the scope of the educational program and the community in which it is developed, community-wide awareness of PTL is increased as well.

III. Risk Assessment

To focus medical and psychosocial attention on patients most likely to benefit from that attention, each patient is evaluated using a risk-scoring system.[63] Recognizing that risk may change over time, patients are evaluated for risk at presentation for care, 28 weeks, and 32 weeks. Low-risk patients with symptoms of PTL are transferred to the high-risk group. Risk scoring may lead to an increase in interventions and has not been shown to decrease the incidence of PTD.[1] It is recommended that providers evaluate risk-scoring systems and modify them to fit individual practices. The imperfections of risk-scoring systems warrant a low threshold of suspicion for PTL in low-risk patients as well.

IV. Prenatal Screening
A. Baseline Urine Culture
A baseline urine culture is obtained to screen for asymptomatic bacteriuria.
B. Sexually Transmitted Disease Screening
Screening for sexually transmitted diseases should be repeated at 28 weeks for high-risk individuals.
C. Bacterial Vaginosis Screening
Bacterial vaginosis screening should be done at onset of care and 24 to 28 weeks for patients with previous history of PTD or with body mass index less than 19.
D. Drug Screening
Drug screening should be considered for high-risk individuals.
E. Fetal Fibronectin
Although fetal fibronectin may have some use in the assessment of the symptomatic patient (see Table 2), there is no evidence to support routine antenatal fibronectin testing.
F. Ultrasound Assessment of Cervical Length
See Table 2 to determine utility in high-risk conditions.

V. Patient Management
Low-risk and high-risk patients receive individual education on signs and symptoms of PTL. High-risk patients are seen weekly or biweekly from 24 to 34 weeks of gestation. Yawn et al.'s PTL prevention program had providers doing screening cervical checks on all patients at 24 and 28 weeks of gestation.[63] There are no prospective trials that support this particular intervention. Patients with symptoms of uterine contractions or less specific symptoms of lower backache, pelvic pressure, or increased vaginal discharge undergo an evaluation for the presence of PTL. This evaluation may include a period of fetal monitoring. The intent of this *low-threshold* evaluation is to arrive at an diagnosis of PTL at an earlier point.

SECTION H.
PRETERM PREMATURE RUPTURE
OF THE MEMBRANES

I. Definition
PPROM is the rupture of the fetal membranes before the onset of labor before 37 weeks of gestation.

II. Epidemiology
The incidence of PPROM is about 1% and may account for one third of preterm deliveries. Table 1 lists risk factors associated with PPROM.[2]

III. Natural History
The later in pregnancy the membranes rupture, the greater likelihood that delivery will ensue within 24 hours. Although the principal threat to the fetus in PPROM is prematurity, infection contributes to fetal and maternal morbidity, while playing a role in the initiation of labor.

IV. Management

A. Diagnosis and Initial Assessment

During the initial examination of the patient with PPROM, the clinician should never perform a digital cervical examination. Manual vaginal examination shortens the latency between rupture of membranes and onset of labor and increases the chance of intrauterine infection.

1. Sterile speculum examination

Direct observation of fluid flowing from the cervical canal is the most reliable method of diagnosis. Having the patient cough or the application of fundal pressure may promote flow of fluid. Fluid in the vaginal vault may be tested for ferning and reaction with nitrazine paper, although the test loses accuracy if the fluid is contaminated by blood, urine, or antiseptic solutions. Observation of blue fluid after amnioinfusion of indigocarmine dye confirms diagnosis.

2. Accurate dating of the pregnancy must be obtained

Ultrasound evaluation should be considered in all cases of PPROM. Oligohydramnios supports the diagnosis of PPROM. Dating of the pregnancy and estimated fetal weight and presentation are important information obtained as well, although these estimates are likely to be affected by oligohydramnios.

3. Testing for fetal lung maturity

Amniotic fluid may be used to assess fetal lung maturity using the **phosphatidyl glycerol test**. Routine amniocentesis remains controversial, but it allows a more complete fetal lung evaluation as well as a chance to culture the amniotic fluid.

4. Screening for infection

Cervical cultures for *C. trachomatis* and *Neisseria gonorrhoeae* as well as distal vaginal and anal cultures for group B streptococcus should be obtained.

5. Fetal monitoring

Umbilical cord compression and infection may lead to fetal compromise. Nonstress tests and amniotic fluid indices are the mainstays of fetal surveillance (see Chapter 10, section A).

B. Management

As in the management of PTL, the clinician is faced with balancing the risks and benefits of pregnancy prolongation versus early delivery. Risks of prolonged ruptured membranes include chorioamnionitis and umbilical cord compression. Delay of delivery may allow for fetal lung maturation and administration of corticosteroids. The benefits of expectant management versus active induction of labor can be expected to be greater earlier in the gestation.

1. Fetal monitoring

Nonstress testing is performed to measure any immediate evidence of fetal hypoxemia or acidosis. Amniotic fluid index is done to assess for oligohydramnios (see Chapter 10, section A).

2. Monitoring for infection

Maternal temperature and fetal heart rate should be followed. Routine leukocyte counts or other parameters (such as C-reactive protein) have not been found to offer consistently any advantage in early diagnosis (see Chapter 15, section C).

3. Antibiotic therapy

Antibiotic therapy has been shown to prolong pregnancy and decrease perinatal infections, neonatal intraventricular hemorrhage, and respiratory distress syndrome, while not reducing perinatal mortality (Table 7). Ampicillin and erythromycin given intravenously for 48 hours followed by an additional 5 days of oral therapy was used in one large trial.[49]

TABLE 7. Antimicrobial Therapy in Expectant Management
of Preterm Premature Rupture of the Membranes[39]

Improved outcome	Number Needed to Treat (NNT) to Achieve Outcome
Prolonged gestation more than 48 hours	9
Prolonged gestation more than one week	7.5
Decreased incidence of chorioamnionitis	12.5
Decreased incidence of neonatal infection	20
Decreased incidence of neonatal RDS	25
Decreased incidence of neonatal ventilation for more than 28 days	14

4. Group B streptococcus prophylaxis
Unless cultures are negative and there is no previous history of group B streptococcus infection, intrapartum prophylactic antibiotics should be given.
5. Corticosteroids
Corticosteroids result in a decrease in respiratory distress syndrome and intraventricular hemorrhage in infants born prematurely as a result of PPROM.[14] Repeated courses of corticosteroids in the treatment of PPROM are not associated with an increased risk of chorioamnionitis.[18]
6. Tocolysis
Tocolysis does not improve pregnancy outcome. The potential benefit of pregnancy prolongation for the administration of corticosteroids has not been studied in prospective trials.

SECTION I.
CONCLUSION

The prevention of the premature birth of low-birth-weight infants is the major challenge of obstetric care in the United States. Scientific advances have led to a greater understanding of the cause of PTL. In a significant subgroup of patients, infection appears to play an important role in pathogenesis. Improvement in early diagnosis of PTL and identification of patients most at risk for PTD would improve the efficacy of antenatal interventions. Interventions for the primary prevention of PTD are lacking, as are effective and safe agents for tocolysis. Given current understanding, PTD has a complex, multifactorial cause and is clearly influenced by psychosocial factors. Family physicians are uniquely positioned to intervene at all levels of the natural history of PTD, from preconception care to the posthospital care of the premature infant.

References

1. Alexander S, Keirse MJ: Formal risk scoring during pregnancy. In Chalmers I, Wilkin MW, Keirse MJ (eds): Effective Care in Pregnancy and Childbirth. Vol I. Oxford University Press, 1989, pp 633–646.
2. American College of Obstetricians and Gynecologists: Preterm Labor. Technical bulletin No. 206. Washington, DC, ACOG, 1995.
3. Andrews WW, Goldenberg RL, Hauth JC: Preterm labor: Emerging role of genital tract infections. Infect Agents Dis 4:196–211, 1995.
4. Attallah AN, Hofmeyr GJ, Luley L: Calcium supplementation during pregnancy to prevent hypertensive disorders and related adverse outcomes (Cochrane Review). In The Cochrane Library, Issue 4, Oxford, Software, 2000.
5. Banks BA, Cnaan A, Morgan MA, et al: Multiple courses of antenatal corticosteroids and outcome of premature neonates. North American Thyrotropin-Releasing Hormone Study Group. Am J Obstet Gynecol 181:709–717, 1999.

6. Barrett JM, Boehm FH, Vaughn WK: The effect of type of delivery on neonatal outcome in singleton infants of birth weight of 1000 gm or less. JAMA 250:625–629, 1983.
7. Besinger RE, Niebyl JR: The safety and efficacy of tocolytic agents for the treatment of preterm labor. Obstet Gynecol Surv 45:415–439, 1990.
8. Carey JC, Klebanoff MA, Hauth JC, et al: Metronidazole to prevent preterm delivery in pregnant women with asymptomatic bacterial vaginosis. N Engl J Med 342:534–540, 2000.
9. Centers for Disease Control and Prevention: Prevention of perinatal group B streptococcal disease: A public health perspective. MMWR 45(RR-7), 1996.
10. Chien PFN, Khan KS, et al: The diagnostic accuracy of cervico-vaginal fetal fibronectin in predicting preterm delivery: An overview. Br J Obstet Gynaecol 104:436–444, 1997.
11. Cnattingius S, Granath F, Petersson G, Harlow BL: The influence of gestational age and smoking habits on the risk of subsequent preterm deliveries. N Engl J Med 341:943–948, 1999.
12. Copper RL, Goldenberg RL, et al: A multicenter study of preterm birth weight and gestational age-specific neonatal mortality. Am J Obstet Gynecol 168:78–84, 1993.
13. Corwin MJ, Mou SM, Sunderji SG, et al: Multicenter randomized clinical trial of home uterine activity monitoring: Pregnancy outcomes for all women randomized. Am J Obstet Gynecol 175:1281–1285, 1996.
14. Crowley P: Corticosteroids prior to preterm delivery. In The Cochrane Library, 2000, Issue 4. Oxford, Update Software.
15. Dinsmoor MJ, Irons SJ, Christmas JT, et al: Premature rupture of the membranes associated with recent cocaine use. Am J Obstet Gynecol 171:305–308, 1994.
16. Dyson DC, Danbe KH, et al: Monitoring women at high risk for preterm labor. N Engl J Med 338:15–19, 1998.
17. Flynn CA, Helwig AL, Meurer LN: Bacterial vaginosis in pregnancy and role of prematurity: A meta-analysis. J Fam Pract 48:885–892, 1999.
18. Ghidini A, Salafia C, Minior V: Repeated courses of steroids in preterm membrane rupture do not increase the risk of histologic chorioamnionitis. Am J Perinatol 14:309–313, 1997.
19. Gjerdingen DK: Premature labor, part I: Risk assessment, etiologic factors, and diagnosis. J Am Board Fam Pract 5:495–509, 1992.
20. Goldenberg RL, Nelson KG, Davis RO, et al: Delay in delivery: influence of gestational age and the duration of delay on perinatal outcome. Obstet Gynecol 64:480–484, 1984.
21. Goldenberg RL, Rouse DJ: Prevention of premature birth. N Engl J Med 339:313–320, 1998.
22. Gonik B, Creasy RK: Preterm labor: Its diagnosis and management. Am J Obstet Gynecol 154:3–8, 1986.
23. Grant AM: Cervical cerclage (all trials). In Chalmers I (ed): Oxford Database of Perinatal Trials. Version 1.3, Disk Issue 8, Autumn 1992. Record 4135.
24. Hauth JC, Goldenberg RL, et al: Reduced incidence of preterm delivery with metronidazole and erythromycin in women with bacterial vaginosis. N Engl J Med 333:1732–1736, 1995.
25. Higby K, Xenakis EM-J, Pauerstein CJ: Do tocolytic agents stop preterm labor? A critical and comprehensive review of efficacy and safety. Am J Obstet Gynecol 168:1247–1259, 1993.
26. Hillier SL, Nugent RP, et al: Association between bacterial vaginosis and preterm delivery of a low-birth-weight infant. N Engl J Med 333:1737–1742, 1995.
27. Hodnett ED: Support from caregivers during at-risk pregnancy. In Cochrane Library, Issue 4, Oxford, Update Software, 2000.
28. Iams JD, Goldenberg RL, et al: The preterm prediction study: Recurrence risk of spontaneous preterm birth. Am J Obstet Gynecol 178:1035–1040, 1998.
29. Iams JD, Goldenberg RL, et al: The length of the cervix and the risk of spontaneous premature delivery. N Engl J Med 334:567–572, 1996.
30. Jones JM, Sweetnam P, Hibbard BM: The outcome of pregnancy after cone biopsy of the cervix: A case-control study. Br J Obstet Gynaecol 86:913–916, 1979.
31. Katz M, Goodyear K, Creasy RK: Early signs and symptoms of preterm labor. Am J Obstet Gynecol 162:1150–1153, 1990.
32. Katz M, Robertson PA, Creasy RK: Cardiovascular complications associated with terbutaline treatment for preterm labor. Am J Obstet Gynecol 139:605–608, 1981.
33. Kaufman RH, Adam E, Binder GL, Gerthoffer E: Upper genital tract changes and pregnancy outcome in offspring exposed in utero to diethylstilbestrol. Am J Obstet Gynecol 137:299–306, 1980.
34. Keirse MJNC: Betamimetic tocolytics in preterm labour. In Chalmers I (ed): Oxford Database of Perinatal Trials. Version 1.3, Disk Issue 8, Autumn 1992. Record 3237.
35. Keirse MJNC: Calcium antagonists versus beta-mimetics in preterm labour. In Chalmers I (ed): Oxford Database of Perinatal Trials. Version 1.3, Disk Issue 8, Autumn 1992. Record 6195.
36. Keirse MJNC: Indomethacin tocolysis in preterm labour. In Chalmers I (ed): Oxford Database of Perinatal Trials. Version 1.3, Disk Issue 8, Autumn 1992.
37. Keirse MJNC: Magnesium sulfate in preterm labour. In Chalmers T (ed): Oxford Database of Perinatal Trials. Version 1.3, Disk Issue 8, Autumn 1992. Record 6192.

38. Keirse MJNC: Home uterine activity monitoring for preventing preterm deliveries. In Enkin MW, Keirse MJNC, Renfrew MJ, Neilson JP (eds): Pregnancy and Childbirth Module. Cochrane Database of Systematic Reviews, Review # 06656. Cochrane Updates on Disk. Oxford Update Software, 1994.
39. Kenyon S, Boulvan M: Antibiotics for preterm premature rupture of the fetal membranes. In The Cochrane Library, Issue 4, 2000.
40. King J, Flenady V: Antibiotics in preterm labor with intact membranes. In The Cochrane Library, Issue 4, 1999. Oxford, Update Software, 2000.
41. Kramer MS: High protein supplementation In pregnancy. In The Cochrane Library, Issue 4, 2000. Oxford, Update Software, 2000.
42. Liggins GC, Howie RN: A controlled trial of antepartum glucocorticoid treatment for prevention of the respiratory distress syndrome on premature infants. Pediatrics 50:515–525, 1972.
43. Macones GA, Berlin M, Berlin JA: Efficacy of oral beta-agonist maintenance therapy in preterm labor: A meta-analysis. Obstet Gynecol 85:313–317, 1995.
44. McCormick MC: The contribution of low birth weight to infant mortality and childhood morbidity. N Engl J Med 312:82–90, 1985.
45. McGregor JA, French JI, et al: Prevention of premature birth by screening and treatment for common genital tract infections: Results of a prospective controlled trial. Am J Obstet Gynecol 173:157–167, 1995.
46. Meis PJ, Goldenberg RL, et al: The preterm prediction study: Significance of vaginal infections. Am J Obstet Gynecol 173:1231–1235, 1995.
47. Mercer B, Arheart K: Antimicrobial therapy in the expectant management of preterm premature rupture of the membranes. Lancet 346:1271–1279, 1995.
48. Mercer BM, Goldenberg RL, et al: The preterm prediction study: A clinical risk assessment system. Am J Obstet Gynecol 174:1885–1895, 1996.
49. Mercer BM, Miodovnik M, Thurnau GR, et al: Antibiotic therapy for reduction of infant morbidity after preterm rupture of the membranes: A randomized trial. JAMA 278:989–995, 1997.
50. Morrison JJ, Rennie JM: Clinical, scientific and ethical aspects of fetal and neonatal care at extremely preterm periods of gestation. Br J Obstet Gynaecol 104:1341–1350, 1997.
51. National Center for Health Statistics: Monthly vital statistics report. Vol 45, No 11, June 10, 1997.
52. Owen J, Baker SL, Hauth JL: Is indicated or spontaneous preterm delivery more advantageous for the fetus? Am J Obstet Gynecol 163:868–872, 1990.
53. Parisi VM: Cervical incompetence and preterm labor. Clin Obstet Gynecol 31:585–598, 1988.
54. Platek D, Chazotte C, Schulman M: Episiotomy does not protect against intraventricular hemorrhage in the very-low-birth-weight neonate. Am J Obstet Gynecol 168:371–376, 1993.
55. Read JS, Klebanoff MA: Sexual intercourse during pregnancy and preterm delivery: Effects of vaginal microorganisms. Am J Obstet Gynecol 163:514–519, 1993.
56. Regan J, Klebanoff M, Nugent R, et al: Colonization with group B streptococci in pregnancy and adverse outcome: VIP Study Group. Am J Obstet Gynecol 174:1354–1360, 1996.
57. Sanders MC, Dick JS, Brown I: The effects of hospital admission for bedrest on the duration of twin pregnancy: A randomized trial. Lancet i:793–795, 1985.
58. Simpson JL: Are physical activity and employment related to preterm birth and low birth weight? Am J Obstet Gynecol 168:1231–1238, 1993.
59. Smaill F: Antibiotic versus no treatment for asymptomatic bacteriuria in pregnancy (Cochrane Review). In The Cochrane Library, Issue 4, 2000. Oxford, Update Software, 2000.
60. Stubbs TM, Van Dorsten JP, Miller MC: The preterm cervix and preterm labor: Relative risks, predictive values, and change over time. Am J Obstet Gynecol 155:829–834, 1986.
61. Westgren LM, Malcus P, Svenningsen N: Intrauterine asphyxia and long-term outcome in preterm fetuses. Obstet Gynecol 67:512–516, 1986.
62. Williamson HA, LeFevre M, Hector M: Association between life stress and serious perinatal complications. J Fam Pract 29:489–496, 1989.
63. Yawn BP, Yawn RA: Preterm birth prevention in a rural practice. JAMA 262:230–233, 1989.

CHAPTER 12

Birth Crisis: Caring for the Family Experiencing Perinatal Death or the Birth of a Child with Medical Complications

Ita M. Killeen, M.D.

For most people, the birth of a child is eagerly anticipated. Each family member is eager to see the perfect miracle that has been created and is likely to have developed expectations that the infant will be in good physical condition. Any significant variation from a healthy birth outcome is likely to trigger feelings of loss. In these situations, parents, family members, friends, and health care providers all grieve the loss of the healthy child they were expecting. Each individual goes through a separate and distinct process of emotional adaptation to accept any deformities or limitations that are part of this new life. This chapter discusses strategies that health care providers can use to support families who experience the birth of a child who is stillborn, is premature, or has congenital anomalies or other significant medical problems. A perinatal crisis can occur any time after the period of viability. Although issues of grief related to miscarriage earlier in pregnancy are relevant, they are discussed elsewhere (see Chapter 5).

I. Preparation for a Birth Crisis
Perinatal death and the birth of infants with significant problems are inevitable aspects of maternity care. Preplanning for these types of crises by hospital staff is essential so that families receive optimal care and support when complications occur. Many factors affect how a birth crisis is handled. If parents are aware of complications during the pregnancy and have had some opportunity—even a few hours—to prepare for the possibility of an adverse outcome, they are likely to deal with it more successfully than if the problem comes as a complete surprise at the time of birth. A woman and her partner who have gone through a relatively short and easy labor may have a different perspective on the issues surrounding perinatal loss than parents who have experienced an arduous and prolonged labor or a cesarean section. The social supports available to the delivering woman and the woman's cultural background affect substantially the manner in which the family experiences grief after a perinatal tragedy.

II. Impact on Families
A. Maternal Reactions
Prenatal experiences often influence the intensity of the grief that a mother feels in the event of an adverse pregnancy outcome. This influence is related to the strength of the prenatal attachment that the mother has experienced. Lederman[11] defines behaviors indicative of attachment as "recognizing the individuality and attributes of the fetus, imaginative role rehearsal, thoughts about giving of oneself to the child, and fantasy about interactions with the child." Many mothers have a specific sense of the child after quickening and often indicate this through use of affectionate names for the fetus.

Women typically are concerned about the health of their child during pregnancy and may feel responsible for a fetal demise or the birth of a child with significant disabilities. This feeling of responsibility is enhanced when there are preexisting conditions that may have affected the pregnancy, such as hypertension or diabetes, or if the mother made lifestyle choices (e.g., smoking, alcohol or substance use, poor nutrition) that are associated with poor birth outcomes. Remorse about lack of commitment to prenatal care or adherence to regularly scheduled appointments may play a role in feelings of grief.

When the birthing experience results in an infant with a medical problem or disability, it precipitates a state of crisis in both parents, but often this is more prominent in the mother. Mothers often perceive the infant to be a part of their physical selves. As such, there is a significant emotional reaction to the loss of the child that had been envisioned.[16] The fact that this psychological bereavement occurs simultaneously with the physiologic recovery from pregnancy and delivery can complicate the postpartum course further.

Risk factors for more intense or complicated grief reactions include loss at a later gestational age, preloss feelings of low self-esteem and a sense of inadequacy, preexisting psychiatric symptoms, and absence of other living children. Women with these risk factors will often benefit from referral for professional support at the time of as well as after a pregnancy loss.[8]

When a diagnosis of a severe anomaly is made during pregnancy, many women are faced with the heartbreaking decision of whether to continue or terminate the pregnancy. This situation often prompts a reevaluation of values and religious beliefs. A decision to terminate a pregnancy often is associated with feelings of guilt in addition to the grief of losing a wanted child. Because of the controversial nature of such a decision, many women keep the termination a secret outside of a trusted few family members and friends. This secrecy may lead to a feeling of profound isolation during the grief period.[1] When a prenatal diagnosis is made that is incompatible with life, a perinatal hospice approach may provide a meaningful alternative to termination of pregnancy for some women.[2]

B. Paternal Reactions

Fathers experience a sense of loss and responsibility at the time of a perinatal crisis, the severity of which may be influenced by their involvement in the pregnancy, the mental image they had of the infant and its future, or their perception of how the situation will affect their partner and their relationship.[16] Many men are involved in the pregnancy from the outset, anticipating the new baby, accompanying the mother to ultrasound appointments, hearing fetal heart tones at prenatal visits, feeling fetal movements, and participating in preparations for the nursery at home. Fathers report that the social support they receive is markedly different than that directed toward the mother. Expressions of sympathy from family members, employers, or friends that occur during the immediate bereavement period are frequently directed at how the mother is doing. Fathers often experience a lack of social acceptance for their own grieving, even though they may experience difficulty returning to their normal work and family routines. They report feeling a mixture of need for isolation as well as opportunities for appropriate support in their grieving. They often try to develop face-saving composure.[7]

Although fathers experience sadness, they also feel that they have to be strong to support their wives. Fathers typically find a role in handling the concrete tasks of caring for siblings, notifying family and friends of the crisis, and making funeral arrangements when necessary.[18] Many men feel a sense of powerlessness to help their partner or infant at the time of birth crisis, which may be manifest in their becoming critical of or angry with medical personnel caring for their partners.[9] Some fathers experience a *double-bind* situation, worrying that discussing their feelings with their partner will upset her, yet being aware that not sharing feelings makes them appear uncaring.[15]

C. Siblings

The grieving response of siblings may vary, depending on the meaning of the newborn and his or her death to the sibling and the family. The intensity of sibling grief often correlates with the level of parental distress. Grieving parents may have decreased ability to be emotionally available to their remaining children. They may be uncertain as to how to discuss the loss with surviving children. Some may believe they should shield siblings from their sadness and pain. A reluctance to talk about the dead infant may then be interpreted as an indication of blame by young children.

Young children do not have a clear concept of time, and they have difficulty understanding the permanency of death. Their feelings of separation, abandonment, and threat to security may be problematic as they experience grief in the family. Toddlers through early school-age children may have concrete questions about death (i.e., "How can Johnny eat when he is dead?"). Preadolescents and teenagers may act out their feelings through behavior changes.[5]

D. Staff Reactions

Physicians have characterized their response to a fetal demise or birth of a child with significant handicapping conditions as following the same continuum of grief as that experienced by parents.[12] Throughout the pregnancy, physicians and nurses have been developing close relationships with the patient, her family or support persons, and the unborn fetus. As such, they may share in feelings of grief when a loss occurs.

Complicating this normal grief response, health care providers also are faced with questioning their own care and management decisions during the pregnancy and labor. This questioning often leads them to feeling some measure of responsibility for the outcome, whether or not it is warranted. Physicians caring for patients for whom there is a sudden, unexpected death of an infant report fear that they "had missed something and might be blamed for the death." Nurses have reported similar concerns while caring for the laboring patient and wondered if quicker recognition of potential problems may have resulted in a better outcome. Health care providers' personal experiences with life, childbearing, and family interactions have a significant impact on their grief experience and the empathy they feel with the affected family.

E. Extended Family

Extended family may include aunts, uncles, grandparents, and close friends of the expectant couple. These individuals often share an eagerness with the parents for the new infant to be incorporated into the family. The loss of an infant through fetal demise or the perceived inability of the child to participate in usual family activities because of a disability may generate expressions of loss and grief. As with fathers, working through this grief process can be submerged or delayed in family members as they support the parents of the deceased or handicapped child.[14] Often, expressions of grief or a loss are not expressed fully until several months have passed.

For all parties, the grief process is a necessary step in the healing process and, as such, is psychologically adaptive. Individuals move through a range of emotional responses based on their own individual needs. Recognition of these needs may affect the medical management and follow-up of these families. Variables that affect individual grief reactions relate to previous losses experienced (alone and as a couple), the meaning of this pregnancy to each family member, cultural influences that dictate accepted patterns of mourning behaviors, and the inner strength of the individuals grieving and their extended family.

III. Medical Management

Medical management of the birth crisis focuses first on the medical stability of the infant and the mother. If an intensive resuscitation effort is required, some member of the staff should be assigned to provide support and information to the parents. It is essential that parents have the opportunity to see and, preferably, to touch their infant before it is taken from the birthing room. Only in cases of absolute emergency should this step be omitted. Absence of contact with the infant only generates more fear and anxiety and opens the door for questions about the veracity of the care providers. If the infant has to be moved to another unit, at least one family member should be invited to accompany the infant, recognizing that families may deal with this situation differently. For example, fathers may feel torn between staying with their partner at this time of mutual crisis and leaving to be with the newborn.

IV. Psychological Management

A. Timing, Location, and Participants

As soon as possible, the health care provider needs to meet with the parents. It is important that the meeting be held in a quiet, private room without interruptions from other staff, so that parents and care provider can focus on the issues being discussed. Anyone whom the couple wishes to be present should be included in the discussion, including older siblings of the infant, extended family members, and other social supports as identified. Parents should never be placed in the position of solo decision making on issues that may have long-term implications. Grief reactions can become more complicated if the clinician unwittingly separates the parents. Talking with the couple together starts the process of open communication between the couple that can continue in the future. Parents usually report knowing that there is a problem with their infant before or at the same time as the health care providers. A sensitive, open, and direct approach to communication is most likely to be successful.

B. Conveying Information

Trout[17] suggests that the first aspect of this interaction be the "facilitation of the love relationship between this baby and the parents." During the meeting with the parents, it is important to maintain a positive tone that emphasizes the infant's personhood and positive attributes, while realistically portraying the problems that exist. Information about the child's death or about the diagnosis of a child with a significant medical problem should be conveyed in a nonjudgmental, empathic tone. It is necessary to balance conveying complete information to the parents at the initial encounter with not overwhelming them. Although it is essential that complete information about the infant's condition, treatment, and prognosis be given, parents may not retain fully some, or even most, of what is said at the initial meeting. Care providers should acknowledge this early in the conversation and assure parents that they will return later to answer additional questions that arise.

Parents may differ in the ways that they process information and make decisions. Some are more comfortable with thorough explanations that include all the possible outcomes. These parents often are immediately prepared to take an active role in decision making. Others may wish the provider to emphasize what is most likely to happen without exploration of every conceivable occurrence. They may wish to defer to the physician or health care provider's judgment in most or all decisions. Care providers should avoid making assumptions about what people prefer but instead should inquire about the level of information that is desired at the initial meeting. Addressing the process of communication early makes this an open topic for future discussions as parents adapt over time.

One of the most challenging things for parents to deal with is the uncertainty that typically exists in these situations. Care providers need to be sensitive to the conflicting information that parents may receive from other professionals and from family members about what has occurred and what should be done. The quality and amount of education provided to a family involved in a birth crisis is a major factor in determining which families go on to function well and which families experience chaos and dysfunction.[3] Decisions that must be made should be framed in terms of the parents' own family values, whenever possible. Important principles to remember when communicating with families include the following:

1. Avoid use of nedical jargon

Understanding can be facilitated by avoiding the use of medical jargon and abbreviations as well as by physically demonstrating equipment or showing pictures that depict relevant findings. It often is helpful to review the labor and delivery process and to give positive feedback to the parents for their own actions and decisions when appropriate. When describing known medical syndromes, using common lay terms in conjunction with technical language is a helpful educational technique.

2. Provide written information

Whenever possible, parents should be provided with written information about what they have experienced, the normal grief response, and any medical or social information that would help them deal with ongoing disabilities in the newborn. Preprinted materials, diagrams, and videotapes can help parents to process complex information accurately after a discussion has taken place.

3. Be realistic and hopeful

In their discussion, providers should balance presentation of a realistic picture without eliminating hope for the best possible outcome. They should be willing to say, "I don't know" when this is an appropriate response. Predictions always should be avoided because an individual infant's course often can prove these predictions wrong.

C. Examination

Parents need to be appraised of any anomalies, even when a fetal demise has occurred. When family members view the body of an infant who has obvious physical abnormalities, it is suggested that the infant be dressed or draped initially in a manner that focuses on the more normal-appearing body parts. Subsequently the care provider can examine the infant in the presence of the parents, gradually revealing and explaining areas of deformity. Positive comments on the normal aspects of the infant are important at this time, with statements such as "what perfect little hands." Postmortem examination is recommended when there is no obvious cause of demise, and chromosomal studies should be obtained when there is a physical anomaly. The option of having an autopsy always should be presented in a respectful way that emphasizes the care that the body will receive and the benefits of this procedure to surviving and future family members.

For the infant who has died, it is important to suggest that family members see and hold the deceased infant for as long as they wish. If the parents refuse or are reluctant to see or hold the infant, ask them what they would like to hear about the infant. Many hospitals photograph the infant, and some offer a lock of hair or newborn cap for the family to keep in memory of the lost child. The ability to hold, see, and touch the dead infant or the infant with disabilities often decreases parental fears and fantasies about infant abnormalities. Positive regard for the individual child and family can be communicated by calling the child by name or, if the child has not yet been named, using the terms "your daughter" or "your son." In the case of a child with disabilities, hearing that the infant has strong lungs, a lusty cry, or beautiful eyes helps the parents focus on their child as an individual.

D. Emotional Issues

During the first meeting, it is important to review emotionally laden issues with parents. Physicians must be willing to hear a range of emotions, including anger, sadness, disbelief, or denial that parents may express at the time of crisis. This catharsis is important in enabling them to proceed through the remainder of the grief process and to adapt to the situation. Mothers often wonder if their actions were responsible for the outcome and express guilt about perinatal problems but may be reluctant to voice those concerns aloud. A gentle open-ended inquiry (i.e., "Is there anything you are wondering about that might have caused, or contributed to, this?") is helpful in getting parents to air their concerns and allowing an opportunity for the provider to reassure parents that they did not cause the poor outcome. Parents should be counseled about the range of emotional responses they may experience over time and be assured that the feelings that they have are normal and can be managed realistically.

Virtually every parent asks the question "why me?" This question should be understood as a complex expression of emotion in addition to being a request for information. Health care providers should take care when responding to this question by considering both levels. Medical explanations should be labeled as offering a scientific answer to the question, and providers should differentiate between what is well-established factual information and what is informed judgment or conjecture. At the same time, providers should acknowledge that such explanations do not address fully the range of emotions that parents usually have and should ask about personal, spiritual, or religious beliefs. Parents should be encouraged to explore their values with trusted family members, friends, clergy, or professionals as a key element of working through grief. The acknowledgment that "you didn't deserve this" and "this isn't fair" can be a helpful initial response to the existential question of "Why me?"[10]

E. Available Resources

Parents face significant adaptive tasks in caring for infants with medical problems or disabilities.[3] As the integral caregivers for the child, parents must have a sense of competence and strength before the child leaves the hospital. If a child is born with significant disabilities, parents may express concerns about the child's future independence. Realism, without eliminating hope, is appropriate here. Information should be given about the varieties of social supports and services available for a child with handicapping conditions. Helping parents to realize that a disability may not be as much of an impediment to future independence as initially perceived can help in their acceptance of the disability. Interactions always should end with a review of the information presented, a mutually agreed-on plan of action, and a specifically scheduled time to meet again.

Health care providers need to be knowledgeable about key community resources so that they can make prompt, appropriate referrals. Parent-to-parent support services can be particularly useful. Families consistently report that contact with other parents who have been in similar situations or have children with similar diagnoses is extraordinarily helpful in providing emotional support, technical information, and resource guidance. Experienced parents fill a role that complements the work of professionals. Some hospitals and community organizations have established formal parent-matching systems. In other settings, this is done on a more informal basis. Names of parents should not be given to infant bereavement groups without permission, however. Likewise, professional or paraprofessional support agencies should not be contacted before receiving parental approval.

F. Coping

Parents frequently seek reassurance about the impact of perinatal crisis on marital and family relationships. Parents may feel a sense of personal failure and fear that both they and their child will not be accepted as integral components of the family structure. They may worry that there will be extraordinary stresses within their marriage. These fears may be realistic, in that marital and family disruption often occurs in this situation. Support and assistance in dealing with family issues should be offered, while avoiding false reassurance. This support is best accomplished by not assuming how parents or family members will react to such a situation but rather by being forthright and inquiring directly about such concerns.

Parents who have a child with a disability or chronic illness often struggle to accept and incorporate that child into their lives. They need to develop a sense of control in dealing with the child's needs and the changes necessary in their own lives. There is a potential for recurrent or chronic feelings of grief among parents and other family members, which can occur unexpectedly and be manifest in many different emotional forms. These are normal aspects of coping with the many challenges that families experience in these situations and should not be characterized otherwise, unless significant mental health problems develop. The coping process required in adapting to the birth of a child with a medical complication or disability requires the adjustment of internal values to allow reattachment after the loss of the idealized child. This adjustment typically takes place as family members strive to normalize life and progress through the child's developmental milestones.

Different strategies may be necessary to support individual family members over time. For the family experiencing the death of a child, the continuity provider plays an important role in sharing prenatal memories of the early excitement and, later, the heartache of the pregnancy loss. It is important for the provider to refer to the child by name and to give some anticipatory guidance to the parents about what to expect as they proceed through the grief process. Discussion of these feelings and the importance of being open to the support of others can be helpful. Informing couples that it is common for partners to be at different stages of grief at different times may reduce conflict and misunderstanding in the relationship.

G. Siblings

Children need open and direct communication when faced with a death in the family. In the setting of fetal demise, young children need to hear clearly that the fetus or infant has died, avoiding the confusion that can accompany euphemisms such as "God took the baby away" or "The baby is in an eternal sleep." Encouraging siblings of all ages to discuss their understanding of and feelings about the death of the infant is important in helping children deal with the experience of loss. Books and stories about the death of pets or animals can be helpful in explaining the concept of death and associated feelings that can occur. Well-intentioned statements to older children that they must be strong for their parents may encourage them to deny their own feelings of sadness and should be avoided.[5]

H. Discharge Planning

Families who have a child with special health care needs need to have well-organized plans developed before hospital discharge. Parents should leave the hospital with concrete information provided about professional services, in-home supports, parent-to-parent contacts, and access to emergency care. Isolation often is the most significant factor in poor parental adaptation. As part of the emergence of empowerment, parents need to develop a sense of confidence about their ability to meet their child's needs before they leave the hospital.

Early and frequent follow-up must be scheduled at the time of discharge to assist in the family's ongoing adaptation. Postpartum depression is a possible manifestation of family stresses and inadequate supportive relationships.[13] Referrals to family-centered services in the community, including early intervention programs, parent organizations, and other resources, can be an effective way of ensuring that families receive the support they need.

Couples often inquire about how long they should wait before attempting another pregnancy. Although time should be allowed for parents to grieve the pregnancy loss, at least one prospective study has shown that early repeat pregnancy after a *miscarriage* significantly lessened feelings of grief for many women. Rather than giving advice on the ideal timing of the next pregnancy, it is prudent for the provider to explore with parents their own feelings about timing of subsequent pregnancies, to answer questions they may have, and to relay information on feelings that might arise in a subsequent pregnancy. These feelings include happiness and fear or anxiety. Exploring ways of coping with these feelings in advance may be useful. The risk of viewing the new infant as a *replacement child* can be discussed.[4]

I. Practitioner Feelings

It is important for the practitioner to be aware of his or her own feelings of loss when a birth crisis occurs. It is unreasonable to expect that professionals do not react emotionally to difficult situations. Families generally are quite accepting of care providers' expressions of emotion.

Professionals should look to colleagues, friends, and their own family for continuing support rather than to parents. One study reviewed ethical decision-making processes among nurses and physicians and found that there are significant differences in values, motivations, and expectations.[6] These differences may lead to communication gaps among professional colleagues. Nurses often place the highest value on a caring perspective, which entails responsiveness and sensitivity to the patient's wishes. Physicians may place a higher emphasis on a patient's rights and a scientific approach that implies a major concern with disease and its cure. It is important to understand this potential difference in thinking and approach between nurses and physicians because this has the potential to interfere unnecessarily with the support provided to parents or families in crisis situations. Professionals need to communicate openly with each other to ensure that this interference does not occur.

Fears about malpractice litigation or professional review when unfavorable birth outcomes occur may undermine open and honest communication at a time when it is most important. Fear of being blamed, anxiety over the medical management of a case, or identification with a parent's grief must not result in provider avoidance of parents. A commitment to being *present* for parents at the time of and after a birth crisis is an important role for the primary care provider.

V. Conclusion

Considerable work has been done on the general principles of crisis intervention. The basic tenets include providing care based on individuals' needs; breaking down large problems into smaller, more manageable components; pointing out assets as well as problems; focusing on short-term goals; linking people in crisis with reliable supports; and planning frequent follow-up contacts. These principles apply well to the management of birth crisis.

Acknowledgments

The author acknowledges significant contributions from Maureen Van Dinter, R.N., F.N.P., C.P.N.P., and William E. Schwab, M.D.

References

1. Bryar SH: One day you're pregnant and one day you're not: Pregnancy interruption for fetal anomalies. JOGGN 25:560–566, 1997.
2. Calhoun BC, Reitman JS, Hoeldtke NJ: Perinatal hospice: A response to partial birth abortion for infants with congenital defects. Issues Law Med 13:125–143, 1997.

3. Canam C: Common adaptive tasks facing parents of children with chronic conditions. J Adv Nurs 18:46–53, 1993.
4. Cuisinier M, Janssen H, de Graauw C, et al: Pregnancy following miscarriage: Course of grief and some determining factors. J Psychosom Obstet Gynecol 17:168–174, 1966.
5. Gibbons MB: A child dies, a child survives: The impact of sibling loss. J Pediatr Health Care 6, 1992.
6. Grundstein-Amado R: Differences in ethical decision-making processes among doctors and nurses. J Adv Nurs 17:129–137, 1992.
7. Honig AS: Working in partnership with parents of handicapped infants. Early Child Dev Care 14:13–36, 1984.
8. Hunfeld JAM, Wladimiroff JW, Passchier J: The grief of late pregnancy loss. Patient Education and Counseling 31:57–64, 1997.
9. Johnson MP, Puddifoot JE: The grief response in the partners of women who miscarry. Br J Med Psychol 69:313–327, 1966.
10. Kushner HS: When Bad Things Happen to Good People. New York, Avon, 1981.
11. Lederman RP: Psychosocial Adaptation in Pregnancy: Assessment of Seven Dimensions of Maternal Development. Englewood Cliffs, NJ, Prentice-Hall, 1984, p 21.
12. Mandell F, McCain M, Reece R: Sudden and unexpected death. Am J Dis Child 141:748–750, 1987.
13. O'Sullivan SB: Infant-caregiver interaction and the social development of handicapped infants. Phys Occup Ther Pediatr 5:1–12, 1985–86.
14. Parks RM: Parental reactions to the birth of a handicapped child. Health Soc Work 2:51–66, 1977.
15. Puddifoot JE, Johnson MP: The legitimacy of grieving: The partner's experience at miscarriage. Soc Sci Med 45:837–845, 1997.
16. Theut SK, Pedersen FA, Zaslow MJ, et al: Perinatal loss and parental bereavement. Am J Psychiatry 146:635–639, 1989.
17. Trout MD: Birth of a sick or handicapped infant: Impact on the family. Child Welfare 62:337–348, 1983.
18. Worth NJ: Becoming a father to a stillborn child. Clin Nurs Res 6:71–89, 1997.

CHAPTER 13

Management of Labor

Walter L. Larimore, M.D., and Kent Petrie, M.D.

Family-centered birthing defines the birth process as a normal physiologic process that should be managed expectantly, positively, and conservatively with the expectation of a good outcome until proved otherwise and with the understanding that birth is a vital life event for the family experiencing it. The World Health Organization (WHO) defines normal birth as "spontaneous in onset, low-risk at the start of labour and remaining so throughout labour and delivery . . . the infant is born spontaneously in the vertex position between 37 and 42 completed weeks of pregnancy . . . after birth the mother and infant are in good condition."[97] The aim of care in normal birth is "to achieve a healthy mother and child with the least possible level of intervention that is compatible with safety."[97]

This chapter assumes that there must be a valid, evidence-based reason to interfere in any way with the normal, natural, physiologic process of birth. Birth attendants who practice evidence-based maternity care need to review critically the potential risks, benefits, safety, and cost of each tradition, practice, procedure, or intervention selected by them or the family. The effect on the encouragement and empowerment of the childbearing family unit, particularly the woman giving birth, must be assessed critically. Each intervention must be evaluated as part of the entire birth event, with the understanding that small, seemingly insignificant interventions may have a cascade effect on the entire birth and family.

Family-centered and person-centered providers must understand that the *maximin* strategy and worst-case scenario practiced by many obstetric providers,[11] when applied to low-risk labors, may not be as safe or satisfying for the mother, unborn child, or birth attendant as is a less interventional approach. The goal of family-centered birthing must include not only safety for the mother and child, but also the provision of the birthing experience as a positive steppingstone into parenthood and family life. Whether childbirth is experienced as a natural physiologic family-oriented event or as a *high-tech* medical procedure has much more to do with the attitude and approach of the parturient's medical and nursing attendants than with her clinical condition. In most low-risk populations, more than 90% of women should be able to have a healthy birthing outcome without medical intervention.[84] The approach to the miracle of birth discussed in this chapter is one that should foster the normal physiologic processes and gain maximum benefit from the childbearing couple's inherent physical, psychosocial, and spiritual resources. Any balanced approach to the birth process requires attentiveness to possible complications and an ability to respond to them appropriately.

This chapter bases its recommendations, whenever possible, on randomized controlled trial data but, secondary to space constraints, references only the most important studies. When lacking firm evidence on which to base beliefs or practices, birth attendants should allow their patients to decide among the available options for the aspects of their birth care for which safety benefits are not proved. The reader is referred in particular to *Care in Normal Birth: A Practical Guide. Report of a Technical Working*

Group, by the WHO[97]; *A Guide to Effective Care in Pregnancy and Childbirth* by Enkin et al.[26]; and the *Cochrane Library*,[15] a registry of randomized controlled trials organized into systematic reviews using rigorous meta-analyses, updated on a quarterly basis.

This chapter uses the WHO classification of practices in normal birth, which rates birthing interventions from category A to category D, [97] as follows:

Category A.   Practices that are demonstrably useful and should be encouraged
Category B.   Practices that are clearly harmful or ineffective and should be eliminated
Category C.   Practices for which insufficient evidence exists to support a clear recommendation and that should be used with caution while further research clarifies the issue
Category D.   Practices that frequently are used inappropriately

See Table 1 for a summary of the recommendations. The WHO report addresses issues of care in normal birth regardless of the setting, level of care, or type of birth attendant. It makes recommendations that are not tied to a particular country, culture, or region.

TABLE 1.   The WHO Classification of Practices in Normal Birth*

Category A. Practices That Are Demonstrably Useful and Should Be Encouraged
  1. A personal plan determining where and by whom birth will be attended, made with the woman during pregnancy and made known to her husband/partner and, if applicable, to the family
  2. Risk assessment of pregnancy during prenatal care, reevaluated at each contact with the health system and at the time of the first contact with the caregiver during labor, and throughout labor
  3. Monitoring the woman's physical and emotional well-being throughout labor and delivery and at the conclusion of the birth process
  4. Offering oral fluids during labor and delivery
  5. Respecting women's informed choice of place and birth
  6. Providing care in labor and delivery at the most peripheral level where birth is feasible and safe and where the woman feels safe and confident
  7. Respecting the right of women to privacy in the birthing place
  8. Empathetic support by caregivers during labor and delivery
  9. Respecting women's choice of companions during labor and birth
 10. Giving women as much information and explanation as they desire
 11. Noninvasive, nonpharmacologic methods of pain relief during labor, such as massage and relaxation techniques
 12. Fetal monitoring with intermittent auscultation
 13. Single use of disposable materials and appropriate decontamination of reusable materials throughout labor and delivery
 14. Use of gloves in vaginal examination, during delivery of the infant, and in handling the placenta
 15. Freedom in position and movement throughout labor
 16. Encouragement of nonsupine position in labor
 17. Careful monitoring of the progress of labor, for instance by the use of the WHO partograph
 18. Prophylactic oxytocin in the third stage of labor in women with a risk of postpartum hemorrhage or endangered by a small amount of blood loss
 19. Sterility in cutting of the cord
 20. Prevention of hypothermia of the infant
 21. Early skin-to-skin contact between the mother and infant and support of the initiation of breast-feeding within 1 hour postpartum in accordance with the WHO guideline on breast-feeding
 22. Routine examination of the placenta and membranes

Category B: Practices That Are Clearly Harmful or Ineffective and Should Be Eliminated
  1. Routine use of enema
  2. Routine use of pubic shaving
  3. Routine intravenous infusion in labor
  4. Routine prophylactic insertion of intravenous cannula
  5. Routine use of the supine position in labor
  6. Rectal examination
  7. Use of x-ray pelvimetry

(Table continued on next page.)

TABLE 1. The WHO Classification of Practices in Normal Birth* *(Continued)*

Category B: Practices That Are Clearly Harmful or Ineffective and Should Be Eliminated *(Cont.)*
8. Administration of oxytocics at any time before delivery in such a way that their effect cannot be controlled
9. Routine use of lithotomy position with or without stirrups during labor
10. Sustained, directed bearing down efforts (Valsalva maneuver) during the second stage of labor
11. Massaging and stretching the perineum during the second stage of labor
12. Use of oral tablets of ergometrine in the third stage of labor to prevent or control hemorrhage
13. Routine use of parenteral ergometrine in the third stage of labor
14. Routine lavage of the uterus after delivery
15. Routine revision (manual exploration) of the uterus after delivery

Category C. Practices for Which Insufficient Evidence Exists to Support a Clear Recommendation and That Should Be Used With Caution While Further Research Clarifies the Issue
1. Nonpharmacologic methods of pain relief during labor, such as herbs, immersion in water, and nerve stimulation
2. Routine early amniotomy in the first stage of labor.
3. Fundal pressure during labor
4. Maneuvers related to protecting the perineum and the management of the fetal head at the moment of birth
5. Active manipulation of the fetus at the moment of birth
6. Routine oxytocin, controlled cord traction, or combination of the two during the third stage of labor
7. Early clamping of the umbilical cord
8. Nipple stimulation to increase uterine contractions during the third stage of labor

Category D: Practices That Are Frequently Used Inappropriately
1. Restriction of foods and fluids in labor
2. Pain control by systemic agents
3. Pain control by epidural analgesia
4. Electronic fetal monitoring
5. Wearing masks and gowns during labor attendance
6. Repeated or frequent vaginal examinations, especially by more than one caregiver
7. Oxytocin augmentation
8. Routinely moving the laboring woman to a different room at the onset of the second stage
9. Bladder catheterization
10. Encouraging the woman to push when full dilation or nearly full dilation of the cervix has been diagnosed, before the woman feels the urge to bear down herself
11. Rigid adherence to a stipulated duration of the second stage of labor, such as 1 hour, if maternal and fetal conditions are good and if there is progress of labor
12. Liberal or routine use of episiotomy
13. Manual exploration of the uterus after delivery.

* The evidence and documentation for the classification are detailed in the report: World Health Organization: Care in Normal Birth: A Practical Guide. Report of a Technical Working Group. Publication No. WHO/FRH/HSM/96.24. Geneva, WHO, 1996. Can be ordered by writing: WHO Publications Centre, 49 Sheridan Avenue, Albany, NY, 12210; phone 518-436-9686; fax 518-436-7433.

SECTION A.
NORMAL LABOR

I. Definitions

Labor is a process by which contractions of the pregnant uterus progressively dilate the cervix, then expel the fetus. *Term pregnancy* is 37 to 42 weeks of gestation. *Preterm labor* occurs before 37 weeks of gestation. *Abortion* is either spontaneous or iatrogenic termination of pregnancy before 20 weeks of gestation. A *prolonged pregnancy* occurs after 41 weeks of gestation. Pregnancy is considered *postterm* or *postdates* after 42 weeks of gestation.

II. Causes of Labor

The precise physiologic cause of labor is not completely understood. Decreased secretion of progesterone by the placenta appears to be one factor. As the placenta shifts from producing more progesterone to producing more estrogen, prostaglandin production (prostaglandin $F_{2\alpha}$ and prostaglandin E_2) appears to be stimulated, and these prostaglandins, produced by the uterine endometrium, decidua, and fetal membranes, are strong stimulants of uterine contractions. It seems less likely that oxytocin of maternal or fetal origin plays an active or essential role in the spontaneous onset of labor. The most potent stimulant to the myometrium during labor appears to be prostaglandin $F_{2\alpha}$ from the decidua.[17,62]

III. Onset of Labor

True labor is defined as progressive dilation of the cervix with uterine contractions. *False labor* is defined as uterine contractions that do not lead to cervical dilation. False labor contractions are often, but not always, irregular, of brief duration, and limited in discomfort to the lower abdomen or back. *Show* or *bloody show* is a small amount of blood-tinged mucus from the vagina and is thought to represent the extrusion of the mucus plug from the cervical canal and to be a dependable sign of the impending onset of labor, provided that the patient has not been examined. The blood loss is minimal; more significant bleeding must be considered an abnormal condition.

Labor may be difficult to define in the early stages, particularly in primigravid patients if dilation or effacement is difficult to detect. O'Driscoll et al.[71] stated that a diagnosis of labor with the nulliparous patient is confirmed or rejected depending on objective evidence of the passage of blood-stained mucus (show), spontaneous rupture of membranes, or complete effacement of the cervix (not necessarily with any dilation). Painful contractions alone are not sufficient evidence to make the diagnosis of true labor.

IV. Stages of Labor

A. Dilation

Dilation of the cervix describes the degree of opening of the cervical os. The cervix can be described as undilated or closed (0 cm), fully dilated (10 cm), or any point in between.

B. Effacement

Effacement of the cervix describes the process of thinning (or decreasing thickness) that the cervix undergoes before and during labor. The normal nonpregnant cervix is approximately 2 to 3 cm long (or thick) and is said to be uneffaced or to have 0% effacement. A 3-cm-thick cervix that has thinned to 2 cm thick would be said to be about 30% effaced, thinning to 1.5 cm thick would be 50% effaced, and so forth. With complete, or 100%, effacement, the cervix is paper-thin. Effacement is said to occur from above downward, as the internal os muscle fibers are drawn upward toward the lower uterine segment. As a general rule, nulliparas undergo nearly complete cervical effacement before dilation begins. In contrast, multiparas can undergo dilation before significant effacement begins (Fig. 1).

C. Bishop Scores

The Bishop and Modified Bishop cervical scoring systems (Table 2) are quantitative measurements for cervical dilation, effacement, station, consistency, and position. In 1964, Bishop developed this scoring system, which quantified that the state of the cervix is closely related to the success of induction of labor. Bishop concluded that a score of greater than 9 indicated that the chance of a vaginal delivery after induction was not statistically different from that observed with spontaneous labor. The American College of Obstetricians and Gynecologists (ACOG) determined subsequently that a Bishop score of at least 6 is considered favorable and likely to be associated with successful labor induction.[17]

D. Stages of Labor

Traditionally, labor has been defined as having three stages.

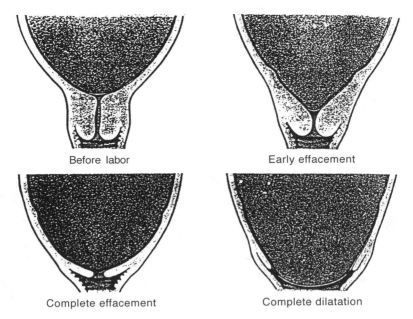

Before labor

Early effacement

Complete effacement

Complete dilatation

FIGURE 1. Cervical effacement and dilation in the primigravida. (From Mechanism of Normal Labor, Ross Clinical Education Aid, No. 13. Columbus, OH, Ross Laboratories, 1975, with permission.)

1. First stage

Prelabor is a term used by some clinicians as a period of increased uterine activity that occurs for a few weeks before labor. This uterine activity is believed to initiate softening of the cervix, some cervical effacement, or some cervical dilation. The first stage of labor begins when uterine contractions are of sufficient frequency, intensity, and duration to initiate and sustain cervical effacement and dilation and ends when the cervix is fully dilated. The first stage of labor is divided into latent (prodromal) and active phases.

   a. Latent phase: The latent phase, first described by Friedman,[30] precedes active labor by a variable duration (1 to 20 hours) and usually is characterized by less intense and less regular contractions of shorter duration

TABLE 2. Bishop Scoring of Inducibility of Labor

Factor	Score			
	0	1	2	3
Dilatation (cm)	Closed	1–2	3–4	≥ 5
Effacement (%) *or*	0–30	40–50	60–70	≥ 80
Length (cm)*	4	2–4	1–2	< 1
Station of head from spines (cm)	−3	−2	−1, 0	+1, +2
Consistency	Firm	Medium	Soft	
Position of os	Posterior	Mild	Anterior	

Note. A score of 0–13 indicates increasing ease of inducibility
* Use either effacement or length but not both.
Modified from Romney SL: Gynecology and Obstetrics: The Health Care of Women, 2nd ed. New York, McGraw-Hill, 1981.

and can be difficult to distinguish from false labor. A prolonged latent phase is defined as being greater than or equal to 20 hours in primigravidas and greater than or equal to 14 hours in multigravidas.

b. Active phase: The active phase of labor is characterized by regular, intense contractions, lasting at least 60 seconds. The active phase of labor is more rapid and predictable than the latent phase, yet there is still considerable individual variation. In general, the active phase begins when the cervix is dilated to 4 or 5 cm. The 95th percentile for the minimum slope of cervical dilation for active labor in primigravidas is 1.2 cm dilation per hour and in multigravidas is 1.5 cm per hour. During the active phase, the fetal head should descend progressively in the pelvis; however, failure for the fetal head to descend should not be considered abnormal until the cervix is fully dilated.

The average duration of first-stage labor in primigravidas is 8 hours and in multigravidas 5 hours. The duration of the latent phase varies considerably, with little impact on the prognosis for delivery. The rate of cervical dilatation in the active phase correlates with the outcome of labor.

From observation of the progress of normal labors, Friedman described a graphic representation of progressive cervical dilation (Fig. 2). Friedman divided the active phase of the first stage of labor into three stages: (1) acceleration phase, (2) phase of maximum slope, and (3) deceleration phase

Composite Curves of Abnormal Labor Progress

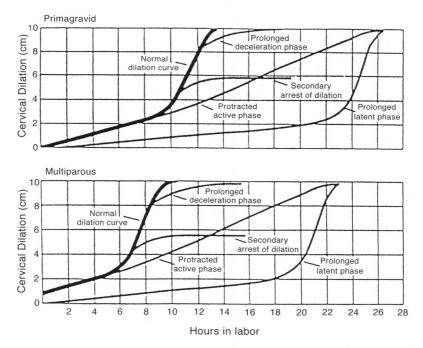

FIGURE 2. Composite curves of abnormal labor progress. (Adapted from Friedman EA: Disordered labor: Objective evaluation and management. J Fam Pract 2:167–172, 1975, with permission.)

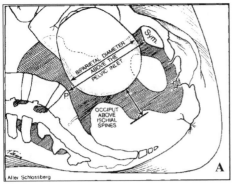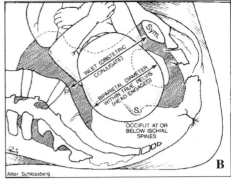

FIGURE 3. **A,** When the lowermost portion of the fetal head is above the ischial spines, the biparietal diameter of the head is not likely to have passed through the pelvic inlet and is not engaged. (P = sacral promontory; Sym = symphysis pubis.) **B,** When the lowermost portion of the fetal head is at or below the ischial spines, it is usually engaged. Exceptions occur when there is considerable molding or caput formation or both. (P = sacral promontory; Sym = symphysis pubis; S = ischial spine.)

     c. Engagement. The fetal head can become engaged before or during labor. Practically speaking, engagement occurs when the presenting part has reached the ischial spines (0 station). Engagement in the vertex presentation refers to the descent of the biparietal diameter, the greatest transverse diameter of the fetal head to or through the pelvic inlet (Fig. 3).

     d. Transition phase: Transition is the period of active labor just before the cervix reaches full dilation. Contraction pains tend to be most intense at this time and may be most difficult to handle. Transition often is associated with nausea and a premature urge to push.

2. Second stage

Second-stage labor begins when dilation of the cervix is complete and ends with the birth of the infant. Average duration is 50 minutes in primiparous women and 20 minutes in multiparous women. Second stage is considered prolonged at or beyond 2 hours for primiparas and at or beyond 1 hour for multiparas, if no regional anesthesia is being used. Second stage involving the use of regional anesthesia can be 1 hour longer (3 hours for primiparas and 2 hours for multiparas). If progress is being made, most family physicians do not intervene during a prolonged second stage, provided that the mother and fetus are stable, except to monitor the situation carefully and to encourage position changes.

     a. Cardinal movements of labor: The cardinal movements of labor, occurring in the first and second stage of labor are shown in Figure 4.

     b. Engagement and flexion of the head
- Internal rotation
- Delivery by extension of the head
- External rotation
- Delivery of the anterior shoulder
- Delivery of the posterior shoulder

3. Third stage

The third stage of labor begins after delivery and ends when the placenta is expelled. The third stage has been divided into the phase of placental separation and the phase of placental extrusion.

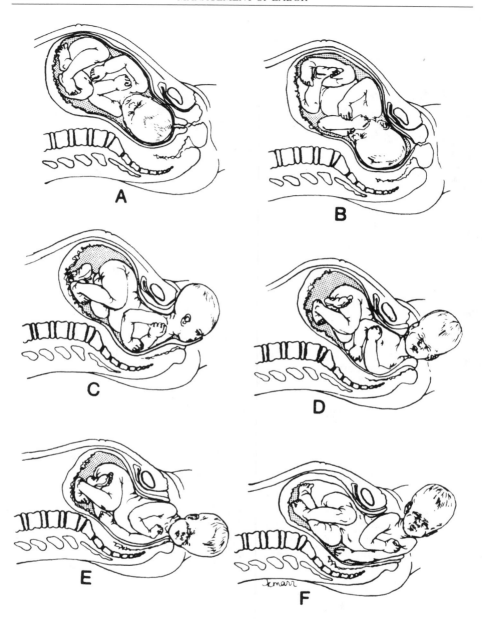

FIGURE 4. Mechanism of labor in the left occiput anterior position. **A**, Engagement and flexion of the head. **B**, Internal rotation. **C**, Delivery by extension of the head. **D**, External rotation. **E**, Delivery of the anterior shoulder. **F**, Delivery of the posterior shoulder. (From Niswander K: Obstetric and Gynecologic Disorders: A Practitioner's Guide. Flushing, NY, Medical Examination, 1975, with permission.)

4. Fourth stage

Some authorities define a fourth stage of labor as being the period of time after expulsion of the placenta. The length of time for the fourth stage is variable, depending on the authority discussing the stage.

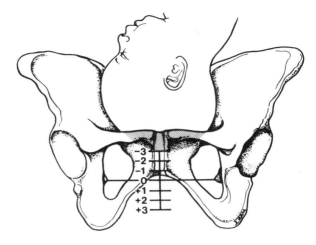

FIGURE 5. Estimation of descent of fetal head into the pelvis. Zero station is diagnosed when the fetal vertex has reached the level of the ischial spines. (From Niswander K: Obstetrics: Essentials of Clinical Practice, 2nd ed. Boston, Little, Brown, 1981, with permission.)

E. Palpation of the Presenting Part

1. Identification

On initial assessment of the cervix, the presentation of the infant should be identified. Initial palpation of the cervix is contraindicated if there is a history of bleeding or rupture of membranes without labor. Vertex presentation usually is confirmed by palpation of suture lines or fontanel. Palpation that cannot confirm the identity of the presenting part with reasonable certainty should cause one to consider a transabdominal ultrasound examination.

2. Station

The relationship between the fetal presenting part and the pelvic landmarks is defined by station. When the presenting part is at 0 station, it is at the level of the ischial spines (the major landmarks for the midpelvis). If the presenting part is 1 or 2 cm below the spines, it is described as +1 or +2 station. If it is 1 or 2 cm above the spines, it is described as −1 or −2 station. The presenting part is defined as floating when it is palpated at −3 station or above. The presenting part is said to be ballotable when it can be pressed easily out of the pelvis and *float* up into the uterus. At +3 station, the presenting part is typically *crowning* (distending the perineum during contractions) (Fig. 5).

3. Position

The position of the presenting part describes the relationship between a certain portion of the presenting part and the surrounding pelvis. Anterior is closest to the symphysis, posterior is closest to the coccyx, and transverse is closest to the sidewall (Fig. 6). The index landmark for the vertex presentation is the occiput, for the breech presentation is the sacrum, and for a face presentation is the mentum (or chin). For example, *occiput posterior* defines the occiput as being closest to the maternal coccyx, and *left occiput anterior* implies that the occiput is directed toward the left side of the maternal symphysis (Fig. 7).

4. Asynclitism

Although the fetal head tends to rest in the transverse axis of the pelvic inlet during labor, the sagittal suture, although remaining parallel to that axis, may not lie midway between the sacral promontory and the symphysis pubis. The lateral deflection of the fetal head anteriorly or posteriorly is called *asynclitism*. Posterior asynclitism is deflection of the sagittal suture toward the sacrum or coccyx. Anterior asynclitism is deflection toward the symphysis. Moderate degrees of asynclitism can result in dysfunctional labor, and position changes in

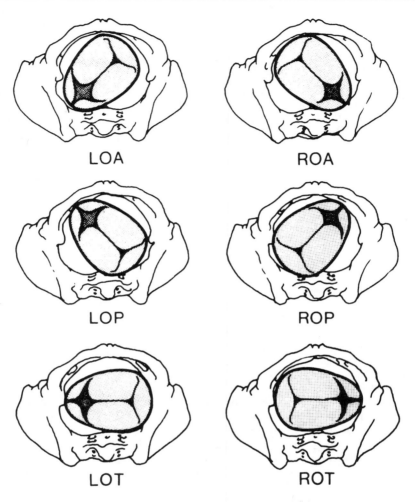

FIGURE 6. Vaginal palpation of the large and small fontanels and the frontal, sagittal, and lambdoidal sutures determines the position of the vertex. (LOA = left occiput anterior; ROA = right occiput anterior; LOP = left occiput posterior; ROP = right occiput posterior; LOT = left occiput transverse; ROT = right occiput transverse. (From Niswander K: Obstetric and Gynecologic Disorders: A Practitioner's Guide. Flushing, NY, Medical Examination, 1975, with permission.)

labor that reduce the degree of asynclitism are those positions that allow the fetal head to find or take advantage of the roomiest areas of the pelvic cavity.
5. Fetal head changes
   a. Caput succedaneum: During normal labor, the fetal head undergoes a variety of changes when in the vertex position. If the part of the fetal scalp overlying the cervical os becomes edematous before the complete dilation of the cervix, this swelling is known as *caput* or *caput succedaneum*.
   b. Molding: Movement of the fetal skull secondary to the flexibility of the suture lines is critical to the fetus during labor and delivery. Usually the margins of the occipital bones (and less frequently the margins of the frontal bone) are pressed under the margins of the parietal bones, or

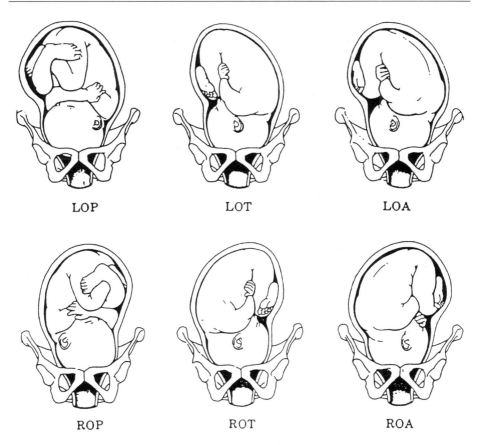

LOP   LOT   LOA

ROP   ROT   ROA

FIGURE 7. Various vertex presentations. (LOP = left occiput posterior; LOT = left occiput transverse; LOA = left occiput anterior; ROP = right occiput posterior; ROT = right occiput transverse; ROA = right occiput anterior.) (From Obstetrical Presentation and Position. Columbus, OH, Ross Laboratories, 1975, with permission.)

the parietal bones may overlap one another. This process, called *molding*, is quite important, especially in the contracted pelvis, because it may account for a reduction in the biparietal diameter of the fetal skull by 0.5–1.0 cm.

F. Evaluation of Pelvic Adequacy

Even in the most experienced hands, clinical pelvimetry and x-ray pelvimetry have limited application. Pelvic adequacy is proved only by a trial of labor.

1. Clinical pelvimetry

Clinical pelvimetry is the clinical estimation of pelvic adequacy. Clinically the anterior-posterior diameter of the inlet of the true pelvis is estimated by determining the diagonal conjugate measurement, the distance from the sacral promontory to the inner inferior surface of the pubis, which is measured clinically (Fig 8). A measurement of greater than 11.5 cm suggests but does not confirm adequacy. The interspinous diameter is estimated by palpating the distance between the ischial spines (Fig. 9). This clinical estimate of the midpelvis requires experience. A distance of 9 cm or less suggests possible contracture. The arch of the pubis is the clinical measurement of use in determining the pelvic

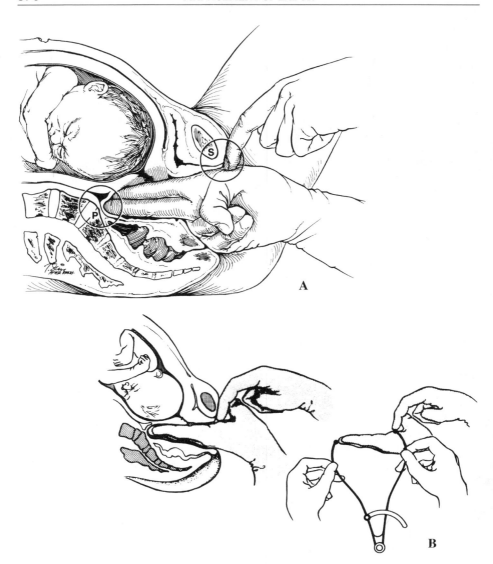

FIGURE 8. **A**, Vaginal examination to determine the diagonal conjugate. (P = sacral promontory; S = symphysis pubis.) **B**, Estimation of diagonal conjugate measurement. Vaginal fingers reach for the promontory of the sacrum, with note taken of the point at which the symphysis pubis touches the metacarpal bone (left). The distance is measured with the calipers (right). (From Niswander K: Obstetrics: Essentials of Clinical Practice, 2nd ed. Boston, Little, Brown, 1981, with permission.)

outlet. Pelvic angles less than 90 degrees may increase the risk of vaginal tearing or the need for episiotomy, particularly in primiparas. Pubic angles greater than 90 degrees may decrease these risks.

G. Care in Early Labor
1. Maximin approach
Birth attendants trained in high-risk tertiary centers often develop a *maximin approach*[11] to labor, whereby they "choose the alternative that makes the best of

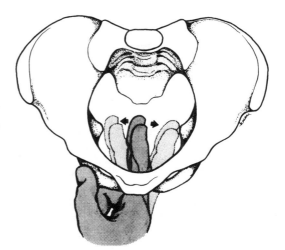

FIGURE 9. Palpation of ischial spines to estimate interspinous diameter. (From Niswander K: Obstetrics: Essentials of Clinical Practice, 2nd ed. Boston, Little, Brown, 1981, with permission.)

the worst possible outcome, regardless of the probability that that outcome will occur." This is also called the *worst-case analysis*, whereby "one accepts the least favorable interpretation of intelligence reports concerning the enemy's forces and intentions, and directs one's own strategy toward the worst possible contingencies."[11] In the hands of clinicians who care for low-risk women, however, this strategy may be illogical, unsatisfying, expensive, and potentially harmful. The evolution of the management of normal labor in the U.S. into one that is increasingly interventional appears more often than not to have occurred without the support of randomized controlled trial data. This chapter examines the data that support or refute many traditional labor and delivery interventions, practices, and procedures used to manage normal labor.

2. Family-centered birthing

Many birth attendants approach the management of labor using principles of family-centered birthing and following a philosophy of avoiding unnecessary medical interventions and of fostering maximum involvement of patients in decisions about their care.[84] The elements of family-centered birthing are discussed in this chapter. The major goal of family-centered birthing is safe childbirth for the mother and the infant. Secondary goals include enhancement of the childbearing woman's social support systems, facilitation of parent-child bonding, and equipping and empowering the childbearing family.[58–61]

3. The Ps

In the past, many physicians viewed labor as a process that can and must be managed for pregnant patients. Standard maternal care text books discuss the three Ps of labor management: *p*ower, *p*assage, and *p*assenger. Some have expanded these basic three to include a fourth *P*: either *p*ositions (meaning position changes during labor and delivery) or *p*syche (meaning psychosocial preparation and support).

Increasing comment is appearing in the literature that most labor does not need to be interventionally managed and that knowing when and how not to intervene may be an higher order skill than routinely intervening.[67] Said another way: "if you mess around with a process that works well 98% of the time, there is potential for much harm."[45] "In populations where medical intervention is used only when clearly necessary, more than 90% of women will have a healthy birth outcome without any intervention."[82] Asking the question: "What then can maternity care providers do to keep normal labor normal?" has led to the development of the 10 *P*s of keeping normal labor normal: (1) *p*hilosophy, (2) *p*artners, (3) *p*roviders, (4) *p*ain control, (5) *p*rocedures, (6) *p*atience, (7) *p*reparation, (8) *p*ositions, (9) *p*ayment mechanisms, and (10) *p*rayer or spirituality.[57]

A considerable and growing literature suggests that there are interventions and noninterventions that maternity caregivers, payers, and institutions could consider, delete, or provide that would increase their likelihood of keeping normal labor normal. Many of these are discussed in this chapter.

4. Sterile vaginal examination on admission

Use of sterile gloves during all vaginal examinations during pregnancy, labor, and delivery is a WHO category A recommendation. Repeated or frequent vaginal examinations, especially by more than one caregiver carries a WHO category D rating and should be avoided as much as possible. Rectal examinations have virtually no place in the birth setting and carry a WHO category B rating as a practice that should be eliminated.

If rupture of the membranes is suspected in the patient at term but cannot be confirmed with perineal observation, the cervix can be visualized by using a sterile speculum, carefully inserted, so as to visualize any fluid in the posterior vaginal fornix. A digital examination should not be performed under these circumstances. Vernix or meconium, when observed, confirms the rupture of the membranes and the presence of amniotic fluid. If the fluid present is still in question, a sample may be collected for testing. If no fluid is seen, the fetus may be pushed out of the pelvis with a hand placed above the pubis, externally, by an assistant, and the cervix visualized during this process for leakage of fluid. If none is seen, fluid from the os can be collected for testing.

    a. Nitrazine test: The basis for the nitrazine test is the fact that the normal pH of the vaginal secretions is 2.5 to 4.5, and the pH of the amniotic fluid is usually 7.0 to 7.5. Nitrazine test papers can be used to evaluate secretion pH colorimetrically. A sterile swab can be used to collect the secretions or fluid, which is touched to the nitrazine paper, and the color obtained is compared with a color chart. Ruptured membranes can be indicated by a pH of 6.5 to 7.5 (blue/green, blue/gray, or deep blue). Intact membranes can be indicated by a pH of less than 4.5 (yellow, olive/yellow, or olive/green). False-positive nitrazine readings may occur with a bloody show, with cervical mucus, or in the presence of semen.

    b. Ferning: Amniotic fluid if placed on a microscope slide and allowed to air dry can be examined under a microscope and is seen to look like the fronds of a Boston fern. Normal vaginal secretions produce a granular pattern when dried on a microscope slide.

5. Digital vaginal examination on admission

Unless there has been abnormal bleeding, prolonged rupture of membranes, or a question of whether the membranes have ruptured or not, a digital vaginal examination should be performed to obtain information on the following.

    a. Cervix: Dilation, effacement (length), softness, and location of the cervix should be noted. The relationship of the cervix to the presenting part can be described as being anterior, midposition, or posterior. A premature cervix usually is posterior and begins the process of moving anteriorly as the cervix ripens.

    b. Presenting part: The presenting part and its position should be determined if possible.

    c. Station: The station should be determined.

d. Pelvic anatomy: The pelvic architecture, pubic angle, ischial spine prominence, and coccyx or sacral position may be determined because each of these clinical pelvimetric assessments can be useful in selecting labor interventions. For example, a pubic angle less than 90° may result in a longer second stage for birth attendants attempting delivery over an intact perineum because the fetal head is directed more posteriorly, and additional time for delivery may be needed.

H. Labor Interventions

1. NPO and intravenous fluids

Nothing by mouth (NPO), the tradition of routinely withholding food and drink during labor, has been practiced widely in the past. One obstetric textbook stated: "In essentially all circumstances, food and oral fluids should be withheld during active labor and delivery."[75] The traditional rationale is to prevent aspiration; however, the risk appears to be low, and aspiration has not been reported as a significant cause of maternal death. Birth attendants using NPO policy typically use intravenous fluids. Routine NPO and intravenous fluid policies lack supporting scientific evidence and may pose risks, such as immobilization, fluid overload, and maternal hyperglycemia.[26,84,88] When given the choice, most women prefer taking oral liquids in labor. A reasonable alternative for a woman who does not want or need intravenous fluids, but may desire intravenous access later in labor (i.e., for pain medications) is a heparin lock, even though the prophylactic use of an intravenous cannula only has a WHO category B rating. The offering of oral fluids during labor and delivery has a WHO category A classification, and the restriction of food and fluids during labor has a WHO category D classification. Further, routine intravenous fluids in labor has a WHO category B classification.

2. Enemas

Enemas in early labor have traditionally been used in the belief that they shorten labor, reduce pain, and reduce fecal contamination. No studies have shown a difference in duration of labor of women who did or did not receive an enema, however. There are no data of increased neonatal infection or increased perineal wound infections in women who do not have an enema. In fact, there is no medical evidence to support the routine use of enemas in laboring women.[88] One meta-analysis stated: "There is insufficient evidence to recommend the use of enemas during labor. Enemas generate discomfort and generate costs and unless there is evidence to promote their use, this should be discouraged."[16] Routine use of an enema has a WHO category B classification.

3. Perineal shaving

Perineal shaves or shaving the pubic hair in labor is commonly used in some settings. Traditionally, shaving was performed to reduce wound infections and to improve wound approximation. Shaving the skin does not diminish surgical wound infections, however, and preoperative cleaning without shaving results in less likelihood of infection. Shaving can lead to increased postpartum discomfort. Routine shaving of the perineum in laboring women is neither desirable nor necessary.[7,26,75,78] In cases in which the perineal hair is long or dense, these hairs can be clipped shorter if necessary for laceration repair. When given the choice, most women prefer avoiding routine perineal shaving and enemas. Routine perineal shaving has a WHO category B classification.

4. Amniotomy

Amniotomy, or deliberate rupture of the fetal membranes, is a well-established tradition of labor in the U.S. Reported purposes for amniotomy include evaluation of the amniotic fluid for meconium, ease in applying internal monitoring devices, and reduction of time in labor. Potential adverse effects have been suggested, however, including cord prolapse, maternal or fetal infection, fetal laceration or scalp infection, fetal cephalohematoma, increased caput, and increased malalignment of fetal cranial bones. Animal studies report greater force of cervical dilation with the head alone than when fetal membranes are intact. Most of the randomized controlled trials show that amniotomy performed between 3 and 6 cm dilation shortens labor by 1–2 hours and show a trend toward reduction in the use of oxytocin and 5-minute Apgar score of less than 7.[29] One randomized controlled trial showed that amniotomy reduced the incidence of dystocia, defined as a period of at least 4 hours, after 3 cm dilation, with a mean rate of dilatation of less than 0.5 cm/hour.

The *Cochrane Review* states:[29]

The trend toward an increase in Caesarean section rate seen in the meta-analysis, combined with the (unpublished) evidence of an increase in the hourly rate of fetal heart abnormalities, and the increase in the frequency of Caesarean section for fetal distress observed in one multicentre trial suggest that we should temper our enthusiasm for a policy of routine early amniotomy. Adverse effects of amniotomy (on fetal heart rate tracings, and consequently, on the risk of Caesarean section for fetal distress) are likely to be greatest in centres where electronic fetal monitoring is routinely used without fetal scalp blood sampling as an adjunct. These effects would likely be attenuated by fetal blood sampling, by amnioinfusion in the presence of worrisome variable decelerations, or by a combination of both. In essence, this implies providing interventions to minimize the secondary effects of a previous routine intervention. Given the current state of knowledge, it would seem to be a reasonable approach to reserve amniotomy for labours which are progressing slowing.

Most randomized controlled trials on amniotomy occurred in centers where a large percentage of the mothers received epidural anesthesia.[29,73] Figure 10 is a

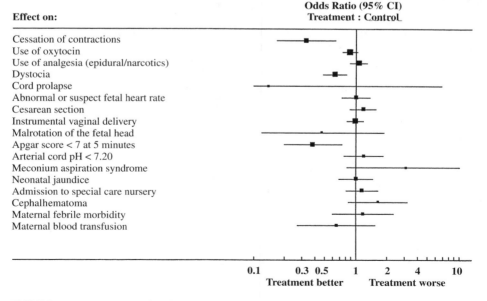

FIGURE 10. Amniotomy for shortening spontaneous labor (8 trials reviewed). (From Fraser WD, Turcot L, Krauss I, Brisson-Carrol G: Cochrane Review The Cochrane Library, Issue 1. Oxford, Update Software, 2000, with permission.)

representation of the benefits and risks of amniotomy, from several randomized, controlled trials.

If amniotomy is to be performed during labor, the following criteria should be met:
- Vertex presentation
- Engagement in the pelvis
- Adequate cervical dilatation to allow an atraumatic procedure but at least 3 cm dilatation
- Evaluation of fetal heart tones immediately before and after the procedure

Routine early amniotomy in the first stage of labor has a WHO category C classification.

5. Active management of labor

O'Driscoll et al.[71] in the early 1970s introduced the practice of active management of labor (AML) in primigravidas at National Maternity Hospital in Dublin, Ireland. (See also Chapter 14, section A.) The original goal of AML was to ensure delivery of every patient within 12 hours of admission for labor. AML now is recognized as a primigravid labor management regimen that has kept cesarean section rates low (5–7%) and stable over 30 years at the National Maternity Hospital. During this same time frame, the cesarean section rate in the U.S. has seen a fourfold increase. There has been considerable interest in adapting aspects of AML to settings in the United States.

The AML protocol applies to primiparous patients with a singleton fetus in the vertex position; in the absence of fetal distress, meconium, macrosomia, malposition, and major bleeding; includes the presence of a midwife throughout labor; and includes extensive prenatal education. Outcome data from four randomized controlled trials in the United States, at this time, do not show strong support that the routine use of active management of labor confers clear benefits for primigravid patients. Most centers in the United States using the AML protocol do not provide the labor support services listed in the Irish studies; therefore, the results obtained may not be equally beneficial. The following are the key elements of AML used at the National Maternity Hospital in Dublin, Ireland:

  a. Standard antenatal education program: Primigravid patients are taught that once a diagnosis of labor is made, they will most likely deliver within 12 hours and will receive constant supportive care by a nurse-midwife.
  b. Precise diagnosis of labor: Applying the labor criteria of regular, painful contractions in the presence of complete cervical effacement, rupture of membranes, or bloody show, an attempt is made to keep this diagnosis precise.
  c. Amniotomy: An amniotomy is performed after diagnosing labor.
  d. Continuous emotional support: A nurse-midwife provides constant nursing and emotional support throughout the labor process.
  e. Intermittent fetal auscultation and movement in labor: Patients are encouraged to ambulate during labor and are monitored on an intermittent basis using fetal auscultation.
  f. Prompt diagnosis and treatment of ineffective uterine contractions: Progress of labor that is not making approximately 1 cm per hour of cervical dilation is treated with the institution of oxytocin augmentation using an initial rate of 4 to 6 mU/min and increased in those increments until a maximum infusion rate of 34 to 40 mU/min. These doses would be considered high, excessive, or *dangerous* in most U.S. hospitals. Patients in Dublin often are allowed to be off the monitor (intermittent

auscultation is used) and out of bed while on oxytocin, likely affecting outcomes.

g. Continuous Internal Medical Audit. Every primigravid labor record is reviewed on a weekly basis to monitor for compliance with the labor management protocol.

I. Alternatives in Delivery Sites

In the U.S., the options for delivery sites have expanded from conventional hospital obstetric units to in-hospital birthing units, freestanding birth centers, home birth centers, and the family's home. Traditional labor care in the United States assumes that hospitals are the safest place for every birth. Proponents of nonhospital alternatives emphasize their ability to identify high-risk women with intrapartum complications at an early, not yet serious, stage and transfer rapidly patients who need immediate hospital care. Skeptics point to the impreciseness of risk prediction for labor, however.

Proponents of out-of-hospital delivery believe that hospital complications appear to arise without warning because few hospital care providers remain with their patients throughout the entire labor. Early signs and symptoms of complications may remain unrecognized until the *apparent-sudden* emergency. Proponents also point out the risks of being in a hospital in general, including iatrogenic complications, side effects to medications, side effects to technology, nosocomial infections, and iatrogenic cesarean birth rate.

Many reports have been published on the outcomes of nonhospital childbirth practices. Most of these have been retrospective and limited to states or intrastate regions. Accumulation of these data cannot resolve the safety questions because outpatient practices that experience poor outcomes rarely publish their results, and small retrospective studies on almost any topic skew toward success. In a 1982 Institute of Medicine report, it was concluded that there was insufficient information to determine the relative safety of any birth setting, including hospitals. In 2000, the Cochrane Library, in its meta-analysis on home versus hospital birthing, concluded: "There is no strong evidence to favour either home or hospital birth for selected, low risk pregnant women. In countries and areas where it is possible to establish a home birth service backed up by a modern hospital system, all low risk pregnant women should be offered the possibility of considering a planned home birth and they should be informed about the quality of the available evidence to guide their choice."[72] Respecting a woman's informed choice of the location of her birth is a WHO category A classification. Providing care in labor and delivery at the most peripheral level where birth is feasible and safe and where the woman feels safe and confident is also a WHO category A classification.

This chapter confines its discussion primarily to in-hospital care. The principles and practices suggested can equally be applied by the maternity caregiver in any labor setting, however.

V. Summary

After initially admitting and evaluating a woman in labor, routine procedures, protocols, or procedures that lack evidence of benefit to the mother or to the fetus should remain the choice of the childbearing family. Family physicians need to be aware of data that affect these decisions to manage laboring women with a more flexible and individual plan. Clinicians who adhere to routine plans and traditions the safety or efficacy of which is not substantiated in the medical literature do so only to comfort themselves. The low-risk laboring woman should have the right to decide the aspects of care for which safety benefits are small or unproven.

SECTION B.
AMBULATION AND POSITIONS IN LABOR

I. History and Traditions

For the last century in most industrialized nations, the labor position chosen by most physicians has been the supine position. When women are allowed to choose their own position of labor, however, they seldom choose the supine position. In latent and early active stage labor, women almost never choose the dorsal lithotomy position. One quote in the medical literature from 1882 sums up the commonsense reasons for avoiding the supine or dorsal lithotomy positions: "The care with which the parturient women of uncivilized people avoid the dorsal decubitus, the modern obstetric position at the termination of labor, is sufficient evidence that it is a most undesirable position for ordinary cases of confinement." Women choose vertical positions (sitting, standing, squatting, kneeling) or nonsupine horizontal positions (side-lying or knee chest). When women are allowed or encouraged to change or choose positions while in labor and without instruction, the average woman frequently changes positions, with an average of seven to eight position changes.

Before institutionalized labor and delivery, walking was practiced in the latent stage of labor. No studies have shown risk of fetal compromise in women allowed to ambulate during labor. Several case studies have shown that encouraging women to ambulate in labor and to assume a variety of positions in labor and delivery increases maternal satisfaction, reduces the rates of episiotomy, and increases the incidence of spontaneous delivery.

II. Position in Labor

No evidence in the literature suggests that the supine position in labor is advantageous, and much evidence suggests that the dorsal position may result in a cascade effect of problems (Fig. 11). Encouragement of a nonsupine position in labor has a WHO category A classification, and routine use of the supine position has a WHO category B classification. Further, routine use of lithotomy position with or without stirrups during labor also has a WHO Category B classification.

Some women are adversely affected in the supine position because of decreased blood pressure, decreased uterine flow, and increased catecholamines. These problems often can be prevented or alleviated by position changes and avoidance, whenever possible, of the supine position.[80,87] The effect of position on maternal and fetal condition has been investigated in several randomized controlled trials. Women's reports of pain in labor seem consistently less with vertical or side-lying positions, but measures of analgesic use are conflicting. Randomized cotrolled trials suggest that the upright position in the first stage of labor, when compared with the recumbent position, results in decreased use of epidural anesthesia and oxytocin; reduced risk of fetal heart rate abnormalities; reduced diagnoses of fetal distress; a trend toward improved Apgar scores; and reduced postpartum hemorrhage, caput, and cephalhematoma. Many studies have evaluated the effect of position on uterine contractility and labor duration. Four of seven randomized controlled trials and several case study series have shown shorter labor duration and greater uterine contraction intensity in vertical positions. The side-lying position has been shown to result in greater contraction intensity and shorter labor duration.

One recent randomized controlled trial on the effect of walking on labor and delivery concluded that it did not provide any particular benefit or negative consequence.[10] This study was done in an institution with an epidural rate of approximately 6%, a cesarean rate of approximately 6%, and a forcep rate of approximately 4%. It is likely that these rates are not going to be improved by ". . . walking, talking, partying, jumping up and

Adverse consequences of dorsal position

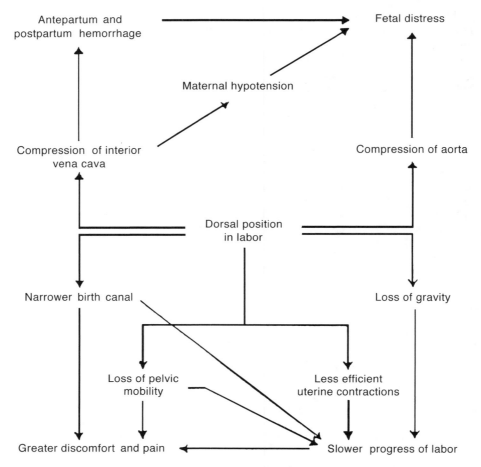

FIGURE 11. Dorsal recumbency, although convenient for vaginal examinations, intravenous fluids, and electronic fetal monitoring, does not hasten labor. (From McKay S, Mahart CS: Laboring patients need more freedom to move. Contemp OB/GYN July:90–119, 1984, with permission.)

down, or whatever. There is almost no room to demonstrate the study effect."[54] Position change may be more important than any single *best* position.[27]

III. Advantages of Position Change in Labor

Because the positions chosen by women to relieve pain may improve the progress of labor, pain may be a biologically useful stimulus to their seeking the most advantageous labor position. Position change has been reported to make labor more comfortable and efficient through a variety of mechanisms, as follows:

• Uterine contractions are often stronger in intensity but lower in pain.
• Positions other than the dorsal supine may improve the uterospinal axis.
• Position change away from the dorsal lithotomy may improve maternal blood pressure and placental flow.

- Multiple positions present a variety of head angles to the pelvis.
- The uterine drive axis may be improved with position changes.
- The pelvis can be physically enlarged in certain positions. For example, the squatting position may open the pelvic outlet by as much as 28%.

IV. Labor in Water
See the discussion on nonpharmacologic pain control and the discussion on delivery in water later.

IV. Summary
If women are to use the many positions available to them in labor successfully to maximize comfort and improve labor progress and efficiency, they must be instructed in these types of positions by their care provider and encouraged to practice them. Family physicians need to gain comfort and experience with different labor positions to provide maximum assistance to laboring patients.

SECTION C.
INTRAPARTUM PAIN MANAGEMENT

Relief of pain in labor provides the patient with the comfort needed to experience her birth process as positively as possible, while avoiding fetal compromise or causing other harm. Options available in the United States include psychoprophylaxis, narcotic analgesics, nitrous oxide, and regional analgesia. Any medication given during labor has potential side effects for the mother or infant; therefore, none should be administered as a matter of routine.[28] Ideal pain relief should provide good analgesia, be safe for the mother and infant, be predictable and constant in its effects, be reversible if necessary, be easy to administer, and be under the control of the mother. It should not interfere with uterine contractions or interfere with the mother's mobility. A method that fulfills all of these criteria does not yet exist.[28]

I. Psychoprophylaxis
A. History
In the 1940s, physicians recognized the relationship between fear and the intensity of pain in labor. Since the 1970s, a variety of psychoprophylactic methods have been used by laboring patients.[19,27] These techniques of relaxation, positive imagery, and breathing generally are mastered by the patient during the prenatal period. Prenatal education that includes relaxation skills and focusing on positive outcomes has been shown to be more successful than those that solely teach breathing techniques. The effect of prenatal education can vary depending on the teaching ability of the individual instructor.
B. Prenatal Education Classes
Increasing numbers of women use non–drug-centered methods, possibly to maintain control, a matter of great importance to some. The least formal of these methods is the removal of anxiety through educating the woman and a trusted companion who will be present at the birth. The Lamaze and Bradley methods are two popular examples of techniques or methods that commonly are taught in prenatal education classes that use psychoprophylaxis to control fear and anxiety and increase tolerance to pain. Women routinely should be encouraged to participate in classes offering education in these techniques.[26,87]
C. Nonpharmacologic Pain Control
Noninvasive, nonpharmacologic methods of pain relief during labor, such as massage and relaxation techniques, are a WHO category A classification. Nonpharmacologic

techniques are received well by laboring women and have virtually no demonstrated adverse effects.[87] Few data exist regarding the efficacy of hypnosis, physical touching, or biofeedback. Other nonpharmacologic methods, discussed elsewhere in this chapter, include support from labor attendants, position changes, physical contact, and ambulation. Approximately 90% of women find relaxation and massage to be good for pain relief. Its effectiveness depends on the compliance of the woman, the stage of labor at which it is used, and the availability of the partner to help.[28]

Transcutaneous electrical nerve stimulator (TENS) units do not seem to be helpful and are problematic for many women.[47] In the British Isles, about 5.5% of women use TENS in labor. A quarter of these women thought that it gave good pain relief, but another quarter did not find it helpful.[28] Other surveys have confirmed that TENS provides no or limited benefits.[14] Modifications of equipment or technique may increase the usefulness of this technique.

Herbal and alternative natural remedies increasingly are used in pregnancy and labor and are discussed in depth in Chapter 2, section H. Nonpharmacologic methods of pain relief during labor, such as herbs and nerve stimulation, have a WHO category C classification.

Studies of hydrotherapy in labor have investigated only immersion in warm water, not showers.[70] Although the professionals may be divided about hydrotherapy, women in labor like to use warm water baths in the first and early second stages of labor.[70] Women report that the heat is analgesic, and the buoyancy of water is relaxing. One randomized controlled trial of hydrotherapy showed an association with a slower increase in pain, quicker increases in the Bishop score, less labor augmentation, and higher patient satisfaction.[12] When data from the few randomized controlled trials are combined, however, there is no significant evidence of any benefit or risk of the use of water immersion during labor.[70] The Cochrane Library cautions, "It is recommended that the routine use of immersion in water during labour should be used with care. Although no significant adverse effects have been reported, the possibility of adverse outcome for the neonate should not be ignored. Until good evidence is available on the possible benefits and harmful effects, it is suggested that labour in water be limited to controlled trials or situations with ongoing audit of possible complications."[70] Immersion in water during labor has a WHO category C classification.

A promising technique for first-stage back labor is four 0.1 ml intradermal injections of sterile water with a 25G or 27G needle to form small blebs in the skin. Two injection sites are over the posterior superior iliac spines; two are 2 to 3 cm below and 1 to 2 cm medial to the first points.[79] The injections cause intense stinging for 15 to 30 seconds, followed within 2 minutes by partial to complete relief of back pain lasting 45 to 90 minutes. The injections can be repeated as needed. At least three published randomized controlled trials have reported similar results.[3,64,95]

Women who strongly expect that psychoprophylaxis, when performed correctly, will prevent all pain may respond with disappointment, anger, or guilt if the pain is greater than expected. Although decreasing anxiety and fear does increase tolerance for labor pain, it is important to realize that there are women who benefit from pain medication during labor.[4,9,87]

II. Analgesia and Anesthesia
A. Narcotic Pain Control
Narcotics are popular and commonly used labor analgesics that can be given by oral, intramuscular, or intravenous routes.[25,87] They are used by about 5% of women in Britian.[28] The side effects include sedation and respiratory depression of the mother or neonate as well as reduced newborn sucking reflex and reduced newborn social

interaction. The oncologic (but not obstetric) literature discusses the buildup of narcotic metabolites with prolonged use of narcotics. Caution may need to be exercised when using narcotics in prolonged labors. Other potential adverse effects of narcotics include maternal hypotension, nausea, vomiting, dizziness, and decreased gastric motility. These effects can be accentuated in an acidotic fetus because all narcotics are weak bases. Naloxone (Narcan) is a parenteral narcotic antagonist that can reverse narcotic respiratory depression but may only partially reverse this effect. As a potent narcotic antagonist, it has the potential to stimulate cardiorespiratory arrest or seizures in narcotic-addicted patients—mother or neonate.

When compared with epidural anesthesia, women receiving opioid analgesia are more likely to have a shorter first and second stage of labor, have a reduced risk of cesarean delivery or operative vaginal delivery, and have a dramatically reduced risk of fever during labor. (see discussion of epidural analgesia later). Pain control by systemic agents has a WHO category D classification.

B. Inhaled Analgesia

Inhaled gaseous analgesics have been used in the United States for more than 50 years.[87] A nitrous oxide and oxygen mixture is described as being easy to use and appears to be relatively safe. It is used in about 60% of deliveries in Great Britain where about 85% of users find it helpful.[28] One report suggested that nitrous oxide shortened labor. Excellent pain relief is reported nearly 75% of the time, but a major disadvantage is occasional nausea and vomiting[87] Physicians in the United States seem concerned about nitrous oxide because to obtain adequate analgesia may require doses that risk aspiration.[9,25,87]

C. Regional Analgesia

A variety of techniques and anesthetic agents are available for peripheral or regional blocks. Each approach has risks and benefits, which should be reviewed with the childbearing couple preferably during prenatal counseling.

1. Pudendal block

Pudendal block usually is helpful only for the final stage of labor and spontaneous delivery because it provides anesthesia only to the lower portion of the vagina and the introitus (see Chapter 17, section B).

2. Paracervical block

Paracervical block is effective in relieving the discomfort of uterine contractions during the first stage of labor.[4,9] Practiced much more commonly in the 1950s and 1960s, its use decreased with reports of fetal bradycardia and fetal death. A review of 70,000 patients treated with paracervical block has shown that the transient fetal bradycardia associated with paracervical block did not indicate fetal distress, however. Others have found a significantly higher incidence of post–paracervical block fetal bradycardia when the fetal heart rate pattern was abnormal before the block. Some recommend restricting the use of paracervical blocks to patients with normal heart rate patterns.[87]

The technique of applying the paracervical block appears to affect the incidence of fetal bradycardia. Submucous applications of local anesthetics result in significantly fewer bradycardia episodes than deeper injections. Once fetal bradycardia occurs, the effect may last 90 minutes; however, bradycardia occurs on average 7 minutes after paracervical block is administered and usually lasts 8 minutes. Paracervical anesthesia is easy to learn, is easy to administer, and results in good analgesia but should be administered in a shallow injection. See Chapter 17, section B, for further details.

3. Epidural block

Compared with other methods, epidural block provides the most effective relief in labor. It may not confer greater satisfaction with the birth experience, however,

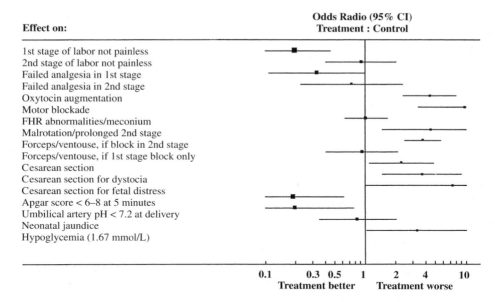

Odds Radio (95% CI)
Treatment : Control

Effect on:

1st stage of labor not painless
2nd stage of labor not painless
Failed analgesia in 1st stage
Failed analgesia in 2nd stage
Oxytocin augmentation
Motor blockade
FHR abnormalities/meconium
Malrotation/prolonged 2nd stage
Forceps/ventouse, if block in 2nd stage
Forceps/ventouse, if 1st stage block only
Cesarean section
Cesarean section for dystocia
Cesarean section for fetal distress
Apgar score < 6–8 at 5 minutes
Umbilical artery pH < 7.2 at delivery
Neonatal jaundice
Hypoglycemia (1.67 mmol/L)

0.1   0.3 0.5   1   2   4   10
Treatment better   Treatment worse

FIGURE 12. Epidural versus nonepidural analgesia in labor (9 trials reviewed). (From Howell CJ: Cochrane Review The Cochrane Library, Issue 1. Oxford, Update Software, 2000, with permission.)

and it involves many risks.[46,48] Epidural analgesia has a high acceptance rate, greater than 90% of women reporting it to be good or very good and 85% indicating they would choose it again.[28] One meta-analysis showed less patient satisfaction in epidural patients compared with patients receiving opioids (odds ratio [OR], 0.25; number needed to treat [NNT], 4).[40] Randomized controlled trial data on some of the risks and benefits of epidural anesthesia are shown in Figure 12. Pain control by epidural analgesia has a WHO category D classification.

    a. Risks of epidural block: Epidural blocks require the services of an individual skilled and practiced in the technique and significantly increase the cost of labor and delivery. Multiple potential maternal-fetal complications can occur. Because of the following potential adverse effects on labor progress and morbidity, the maternity caregiver should be prepared to intervene as necessary with oxytocin or operative delivery:

- Sudden hypotension and resultant fetal stress
- Spinal headache
- Epidural space hematoma or infection
- Inadvertent intravascular injection of anesthetic resulting in maternal seizures or cardiac arrest
- Maternal respiratory depression resulting from "high" spinal block.
- Urinary retention.

    Rates of instrumental delivery may be higher among women using an epidural block because in the more painful prolonged labors with malpositions women are more likely to receive epidural analgesia. Given the widespread use of epidural block during labor, however, there are few data from randomized trials concerning the short-term and long-term effects on women and infants.

    Meta-analysis data indicate that epidural block is likely to provide more effective pain relief during labor than alternative methods and is less likely to cause depressed infants than opioids. Epidural anesthesia is associated with lengthened labors (an average of about 1 hour, 42 minutes in the first stage and 14 minutes in the second stage), results in an increased use of oxytocin (OR, 1.5; 45% versus 32%), and causes an increased risk of maternal fever (OR, 5.35; 23% versus 5%) when compared with opioids.[40] This meta-analysis also showed that epidural anesthesia, when compared with opioids, resulted in an increased rate of cesareans (OR, 1.50; 8.2% versus 5.6%) and instrumented deliveries (OR, 2.19; NNT, 17). One review concluded that there are insufficient data to support the conclusion that epidural block does or does not affect operative vaginal delivery or cesarean delivery rates.[63]

It is particularly concerning that there are so few data on long-term follow-up of the women involved in these studies. Analyses of observational data have suggested that epidural block may increase the incidence of chronic backache, chronic headache, bladder problems, tingling and numbness, and *sensory confusion*.[9] Further randomized controlled trials are needed to investigate these possibilities. Another reviewer has stated: "Given evidence of the effects of epidural analgesia on the dynamics of labour, a mother receiving epidural analgesia may not be considered to be having a 'normal' labour."[48]

The data on the effects of epidural analgesia on infants are somewhat scanty, apart from gross measures, such as Apgar scores and blood gases. In particular, longer term follow-up of infants has been conducted in only one study. Part of the difficulty may lie in the failure to identify measurable, clinically relevant outcomes, such as feeding and mother-infant interaction. It would be helpful to have well-established outcomes that could be sought in future studies.

b. Avoiding or decreasing the risk of epidural anesthesia: Epidural anesthesia has become almost routine in many hospitals and is requested by many women. Rates of epidural anesthesia use can be decreased with increased prenatal education, increased support during labor, and management of the birthing environment. Low-dose continuous or patient-controlled epidural anesthesia may decrease the problems associated with epidural analgesia. Continuous low-dose epidural anesthesia may be discontinued or decreased before or during the second stage of labor and may decrease the risk of some of the side effects mentioned previously.[48]

The *walking epidural* (discussed subsequently) is gaining popularity in some areas of the United States. Epidural agents, such as fentanyl, provide primarily sensory blocks and may allow limited ambulation, frequent position changes, and more effective pushing at delivery. Although randomized controlled trial data are lacking on this intervention, it has several theoretic advantages over routine epidural anesthesia. Obstetric anesthetists using alternative regimens of drug type, dosage, and method of administration that could be superior to current methods used in most randomized controlled trials, need to investigate, in randomized trials, the influence of these new regimens on the progress of labor, compared with nonepidural methods of pain relief. Only then can women who wish to use these forms of pain relief be informed fully of the likely effects on the progress of their labors.

c. Contraindications to epidural
   i. Absolute
      • Infection in the area of the puncture
      • Untreated febrile illness or maternal septicemia

- Coagulation defects (acquired or inherited) or active maternal bleeding
- Uncooperative patients or patient that refuses epidural

ii. Relative or controversial
- Anticipated serious maternal hemorrhage
- Overt hypertension
- Neurologic disease
- Previous back surgery
- History of chronic low back pain

4. Spinal anesthesia

Spinal anaesthesia is used increasingly for operative procedures, including cesarean section, instrumental delivery, and manual removal of the placenta. The local anesthetic is injected into the cerebrospinal fluid through a fine (25G) atraumatic needle. The onset of action is rapid, and the effect lasts for about 2 hours. Indications, complications, and contraindications are similar to those for epidural block discussed previously, with the exception that the risk of spinal headache is higher than with epidural anesthesia.

5. Intrathecal narcotics for labor analgesia

Intrathecal analgesia is an effective technique for relief of first-stage labor pain. The procedure is safe and can be learned easily by family physicians currently performing diagnostic lumbar puncture. It is particularly useful in practices where continuous lumbar epidural anesthesia is not available.

a. Actions of intrathecal narcotics

Small doses of narcotic injected into the subarachnoid space bind selectively with opioid receptors, promoting effective analgesia (not anesthesia) without significant motor or autonomic blockade.

Intrathecal narcotics provide more effective analgesia for visceral pain than somatic pain and are more useful in early first-stage labor than in the second stage of labor. A pudendal block or local infiltration may be needed for second-stage perineal pain and repair of episiotomy or tears. Intrathecal narcotics do not prolong first-stage or second-stage labor.

The more water-soluble narcotics (morphine) are slower in onset (15 to 60 minutes) but longer acting (6 to 10 hours). They remain in the cerebrospinal fluid longer and are more likely to circulate to higher centers and cause side effects.

The more lipid-soluble narcotics (fentanyl and sufentanil) are faster in onset (5 to 10 minutes) and shorter in duration of activity (1.5 to 3.5 hours).

b. Procedure for intrathecal narcotic administration[52]

Position the patient near the edge of the bed in the lateral recumbent or sitting position determined by comfort. Flex spine anteriorly as much as possible.

Identify the L3–4 interspace at the level of the iliac crests.

Prepare and drape the L3–4 interspace area and anesthetize the skin and interspinous ligament with 1% lidocaine.

Perform lumbar puncture with a narrow gauge spinal needle (24G to 27G) using an introducer (18G to 19G), and document free flow of cerebrospinal fluid.

Inject intrathecal narcotic mixture. Common preservative-free preparations include:
- Fentanyl citrate (Sublimaze), 15-25 mcg
- Sufentanil citrate (Sufenta), 3-15 mcg
- Morphine sulfate (Duramorph), 0.2-0.5 mg

- Combination of fentanyl or sufentanil plus morphine is commonly administered.

    Remove needle and monitor maternal blood pressure and fetal heart rate for 30-60 minutes.

    The patient may ambulate when stable.

  c. Side effects of intrathecal narcotics
    - Pruritus (50%)
    - Nausea and vomiting (30% to 50%)
    - Urinary retention (30%)
    - Delayed respiratory depression (rare but more common with morphine)
    - Spinal headache (related to technique)

       Side effects can be minimized or treated with:
       i. Naltrexone (ReVia). A single dose of 12.5 to 50 mg orally is given immediately after delivery.
       ii. Nalbuphine (Nubain). This is a synthetic narcotic agonist-antagonist analgesic. A dose of 5 to 10 mg intravenously is given immediately after delivery.
       iii. Naloxone (Narcan). A dose of 0.4 mg bolus or 0.6 mg/h infusion is given for more serious side effects (e.g., urinary retention and respiratory depression).

5. Combined spinal epidurals (CSE)

Combined spinal epidurals have a rapid onset compared with epidural anesthesia alone and are believed to be more effective by some anesthesiologists.[8] Others argue that traditional epidurals are better and more effective than combined spinal epidurals.[18] Early data indicate no difference in fetal bradycardia for the two techniques. There are few data to compare combined spinal epidurals with intrathecal narcotics or standard epidurals; however, newer multiorifice catheters may produce better results than the more standard single-orifice catheters.

SECTION D.
SUPPORT IN LABOR

Randomized controlled trials consistently have shown that the presence of a companion during labor results in many favorable outcomes, including a decrease in the incidence of meconium-stained amniotic fluid, reduced use of oxytocin, and reduced cesarean birth. A reduction in low Apgar scores, fetal and maternal morbidity, and operative deliveries has been noted.[42,43,87] Figure 13 shows some of the combined outcome data from the randomized controlled trials on labor support. Respecting a woman's choice of companions during labor and birth and empathetic support by caregivers during labor and birth both have a WHO category A classification.

I. Doula Model

One of the most remarkable developments in continuous birthing support is the development of doula services. Doulas are women who are trained and experienced in childbirth, although they may or may not have given birth themselves. The doula's role is to provide physical, emotional, and informational support to women and their partners during labor and birth. The doula offers help and advice on comfort measures, such as breathing, relaxation, movement, and positioning. She assists families to gather information about the course of their labor and their options. The most crucial role of the doula is providing continuous emotional reassurance and comfort.

Doulas specialize in nonmedical skills and do not perform clinical tasks, diagnose medical conditions, offer second opinions, or give medical advice. The doula's goal is

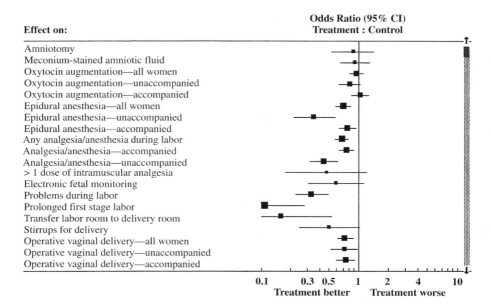

FIGURE 13. Caregiver support for women during childbirth (13 trials reviewed). (From Hodnett ED: Cochrane Review The Cochrane Library, Issue 1. Oxford, Update Software, 2000, with permission.)

to help the woman have a safe and satisfying childbirth as the woman defines it. When a doula is present, some women feel less need for pain medications or may postpone them until later in labor. It is not the role of the doula to discourage the mother from her choices. The doula helps the mother become informed about various options, including the risks, benefits, and accompanying precautions or interventions for safety. Doulas can help maximize the benefits of pain medications, while minimizing their undesirable side effects. The comfort and reassurance offered by the doula are beneficial regardless of the use of pain medications.

According to the Doulas of North America (DONA):[86]

The terminology describing labor support can be confusing. When a person uses any of the terms below to describe herself, she may need to clarify what she means by the term. "Doula"—a Greek word meaning "woman's servant." In labor support terminology, "doula" refers to a supportive companion (not a friend or loved one) professionally trained to provide labor support. "Doula" also refers to lay women who are trained or experienced in providing postpartum care (mother and newborn care, breastfeeding support and advice, cooking, childcare, errands, and light cleaning) for the new family. To distinguish between the two types of doulas, one may refer to "birth doulas" and "postpartum doulas." "Monitrice"—a French word originally used by Fernand Lamaze to refer to a specially trained nurse or midwife who provides nursing care and assessment, in addition to labor support. Today, "monitrice" is often used as a synonym for "birth assistant" or "labor assistant." "Labor Support Professional," "Labor Support Specialist," "Labor Companion"—synonyms of "birth doula." "Birth Assistant," "Labor Assistant"—sometimes these terms are used as synonyms for "doula," but also may refer to lay women who are trained to assist a midwife (vaginal exams, set up for the birth, fetal heart checks, etc.) as well as to provide some labor support.

Doula support in labor has been shown to reduce the likelihood of medication for pain relief, operative vaginal delivery, cesarean delivery, and a 5-minute Apgar score less than 7. In the trials in which hospital policy did not permit the presence of husbands, family, or friends during labour, continuous support was associated with a reduced likelihood of oxytocin augmentation. Two trials have shown that women with continuous labor support were more likely to be fully breast-feeding at 4 to 6 weeks postpartum.[76] Six trials have shown that a doula's support improves a mother's view of the childbirth experience, including more overall satisfaction, less failure to cope well during labor, less likelihood of finding labor to be worse than expected, and a higher level of personal control during childbirth.[41,42]

The effects of labor support on labor length are slight in meta-analysis.[42] Individual trials have shown decreases in problems during labor, prolonged first-stage labor, episiotomy, transfer to a separate room for delivery, and in the number of unsatisfactory father/midwife relationships. Longer term benefits found in individual trials include decreases in postpartum depression at 6 weeks after childbirth and in finding motherhood difficult.[42]

It is now considered inappropriate for hospitals to exclude any category of support person from labor and birth. If women have preferences for who should be with them at this time, these preferences should be respected and, if possible, accommodated. Maternity care providers and facilities that do not now provide continuous labor support may be wise to consider training or supporting a doula program. The national organization, Doulas of North America, is located in Seattle, Washington (Phone 206-325-1419).

The Cochrane evaluation of labor support says, "Given the clear benefits and no known risks associated with intrapartum support, every effort should be made to ensure that all labouring women receive continuous support. This support should include continuous presence, the provision of hands-on comfort, and encouragement." Depending on the circumstances, ensuring the provision of continuous support may require the following:
• Alterations in the current work activities of midwives and nurses, such that they are able to spend less time on ineffective activities and more time providing support
• Continuing education programs that teach the art and science of labour support
• Changes to more flexible methods of staffing labor wards, which permit the staff census to match more closely the patient census
• Adoption of hospital policies encouraging the presence of experienced laywomen, including female relatives

The constant attendance provided by midwives may represent a doula effect. It has been suggested that the constant or increased attendance of a labor nurse may render a doula effect. One study comparing family physicians and midwives found few differences in the management of labor and delivery; however, primiparous women managed by family physicians were more likely to undergo cesarean birth (14% versus 8%; P, .05) resulting from a diagnosis of dystocia. The authors hypothesized that the time spent in continuous support provided by the midwives, as opposed to the physicians, may have explained this observed difference. At the very least, in situations in which continuous family or nursing support is not available, the provision of a female companion would be likely to improve maternal well-being. Family physicians would be wise to consider such an intervention.

II. The Father or Significant Other
The presence of the father during labor and delivery, based on randomized controlled trials, appears to increase strongly the mother's satisfaction with the birthing experience. No evidence of harm exists from allowing fathers to be involved actively in labor and delivery or to attend cesarean births with an awake mother.[87] In multivariate models, emotional support from a mate during labor and delivery accounts for the largest portion of variance.[41] As compared with labor nurses, fathers are significantly more likely to be present in the labor room, offer comforting items, and touch their

partner. Mothers consistently rate the father's presence as significantly more helpful than that of the nurses.

Additional studies show that the impact of fathers who attend labor and delivery is greater than that of fathers who attend only early labor. Women whose partners were involved in the entire birth process report less pain, receive less medication, and report more positive experiences. The higher the level of support from the father, the less likely women were to use epidural anesthesia. A caution concerning these findings would be that preexisting differences or selection criteria may exist between the groups of fathers studied. There appears to be no risk associated with the father's attendance at labor and delivery and several positive benefits; every effort should be made to encourage and allow the father to participate actively in the labor and delivery.[60a]

III. Siblings

Allowing and encouraging the presence of siblings at all or part of their mother's labor and delivery is a more recent and growing trend. The few reports available represent self-selected families. No significant negative effects have been shown in any children studied who have attended labor or delivery. Reports by parents indicate a significant increase in care-taking and mothering behaviors in the birth-attending group, but no studies to date have controlled for selection or reporting bias.[87] The scant evidence existing concerning sibling presence at labor or delivery indicates no short-term harm to the children and suggests the possibility of increased nurturing behavior.

IV. Summary

Randomized controlled trials show multiple clear benefits and no significant risks associated with labor support (see Fig. 13). Every effort should be made to ensure that all laboring women receive support. This is especially true for trained support personnel and should include the provision of encouragement, hands-on care, position change, and ambulation assistance.

SECTION E.
INTRAPARTUM FETAL HEART RATE MONITORING

Fetal compromise resulting in intrapartum fetal asphyxia or fetal demise can be reduced with appropriate evaluation of fetal well-being. The goal of fetal heart rate monitoring should be to detect with the highest predictive value possible signs that warn of fetal compromise in time to prevent or correct adverse outcome, causing as little unnecessary intervention as possible. Continuous electronic fetal monitoring (EFM), with or without fetal scalp pH sampling, fetal scalp stimulation, or fetal vibroacoustic stimulation, and intermittent auscultation of the fetal heart are the methods most commonly used. Fetal monitoring with intermittent auscultation has a WHO category A classification, whereas EFM has a category D rating.

I. Continuous Electronic Fetal Monitoring
A. Background

Continuous EFM is a technology that dates back to the 1960s and became routine in most labor units before evidence from randomized controlled trials showed efficacy or safety. EFM is the most prevalent maternity care procedure in the U.S. In 1997, 83% of all live births had EFM, and according to the National Vital Statistics Report, this number likely is underreported.[69] EFM is routinely performed without informed consent taking place.[57]

Randomized controlled trials in a variety of delivery settings for low-risk mothers show no improvement in neonatal outcome with EFM.[5] The use of EFM increased from 44.6% of live births in 1980 to 62.2% in 1988, however. By 1992, 73.7% of pregnancies were monitored electronically in the United States.

Expert panels in the United States and Canada have advised against routine EFM in low-risk pregnancies and have found weak evidence for inclusion or exclusion for routine use in high-risk pregnancies.[86] This change in attitude among policy makers in clinical medicine was the result primarily of a series of randomized controlled trials that documented the benefits and risks of EFM. By the end of the 1990s, the ACOG stated that although all women in labor needed some form of fetal monitoring, the choice of technique (EFM or intermittent auscultation) was based on a variety of factors and should be left to the judgment of the individual physician.

Technologies such as EFM need to be developed carefully and tested in limited settings, usually academic centers, before widespread diffusion. Their efficacy and safety need to be shown before they become routine practice. As is evident from the experience with EFM, widespread diffusion of a technology before efficacy and safety are determined can lead to misuse, misunderstanding, and unnecessary concerns with malpractice and litigation.

B. Study Results

Early large retrospective studies using historical controls suggested that EFM resulted in fewer infants with low Apgar scores, reduced neonatal mortality, and improved neurologic outcome.[87,88] It had been assumed that continuous EFM would be more accurate than intermittent auscultation in detecting fetal heart rate patterns, which would be sensitive in predicting the potential for actual fetal compromise. This assumption led to many experts recommending or urging continuous EFM for all women in labor; however, this hypothesis has not been supported by most of the randomized controlled trials.

The Cochrane Library has summarized the data from nine randomized controlled trials and found that, with the exception of a small reduction in the rate of neonatal seizures in high-risk subgroups, the use of routine EFM has no measurable impact on morbidity and mortality[94] The only two follow-up studies to date have indicated that the long-term neurologic effects of these seizures have been minimal. The most serious complications of EFM use include an increased rate of cesarean births and operative vaginal deliveries.[94]

Of the randomized controlled trials that have now investigated EFM, seven have compared EFM with intermittent auscultation. One multicenter trial compared intermittent auscultation with EFM plus optional fetal scalp pH sampling in preterm labor and reported no differences in perinatal outcomes, cesarean birth rate, or 18-month psychomotor development. Another study compared a monitored group with an intermittent auscultated group and a third group with EFM and optional fetal scalp pH sampling. Although fetal scalp pH sampling reduced the increased frequency of cesarean birth, no differences in perinatal morbidity or mortality could be detected in any of the groups.

At least six randomized controlled trials have compared EFM plus scalp pH sampling with intermittent auscultation (Fig. 14). These data suggest no benefit to EFM on neonatal outcome other than the measure of neonatal seizure when EFM is backed by scalp pH. Secondary review of these data shows that the reduced risk of seizures was limited to induced, augmented, or prolonged labors.[86] This effect has not been shown in trials with premature infants, EFM without scalp pH, and liberal versus restricted EFM.[31–36]

Nine randomized controlled trials of EFM have been conducted in low-risk populations. All show clearly no difference in neonatal outcome except that assisted deliveries were more common in the EFM group. These studies revealed inconsistent results on the influence of EFM on the frequency of cesarean birth. A large

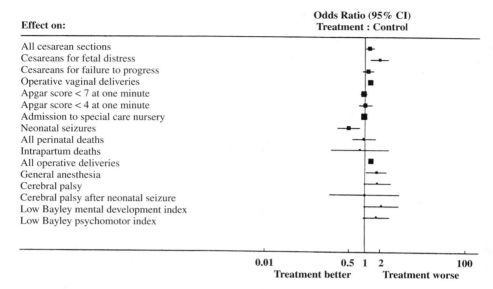

FIGURE 14. Continuous electronic heart rate monitoring for fetal assessment during labor (10 trials reviewed). (From Thacker SB, Stroup DF: Cochrane Review The Cochrane Library, Issue 1. Oxford, Update Software, 2000, with permission.)

multicenter study using multivariate analysis found an association between EFM and higher cesarean birth rates, however. One randomized controlled trial examined liberal versus restrictive use of EFM in labor and showed no significant difference in the outcomes measured.

C. Electronic Fetal Monitoring as a Screening Test

Statistically the predictive value of abnormal fetal heart rate patterns is low with continuous EFM. Only about 20% of *abnormal* EFM tracings are associated with a low 5-minute Apgar score. Multiple studies have shown that normal fetal heart rate tracings predict good 5-minute Apgar scores in more than 99% of monitored pregnancies, however, having a high negative predictive value (ability to predict the absence of disease). When applied to the population of laboring women in most family practices with a low incidence of uteroplacental insufficiency, EFM has a high incidence of false-positive results with a resulting low positive predictive value. EFM is, by itself, a poor screening test. In addition, it is not a diagnostic test. A diagnostic test should confirm or reject a possible diagnosis, a criterion not met by EFM alone.

D. Indications for Electronic Fetal Monitoring

Although current standards in many hospital settings dictate the use of continuous EFM for most high-risk patients (including thick meconium staining, oxytocin use, twins, medically complicated pregnancies, use of prostaglandin gel, abnormal fetal heart rate by auscultation, dysfunctional labor, vaginal breech delivery), ACOG recommendations state "that intermittent auscultation of the fetal heart . . . is equivalent to continuous EFM in the assessment of fetal condition."[5] The recommendations recognize, however, that "intrapartum fetal assessment by monitoring of the heart rate is only one parameter of fetal well-being" and that in certain situations "the limited number of nurses available may preclude the capacity to monitor the fetal heart rate by auscultation."[5] In addition, the individual physician's medicolegal concerns, the physician's skills in using and interpreting the technology, and the community standard of practice each contribute to an individual clinician's decision to use EFM despite the data or the risks of using EFM.

E. Medicolegal Considerations

Physicians often cite malpractice fears as a reason to continue using EFM, despite a lack of demonstrated effectiveness. It is paradoxic that monitor strips are as easily *overread* in the courtroom as the labor room. Interrater reliability is variable. EFM recordings have the potential to become more harmful than helpful during malpractice litigation defense and may increase the malpractice suit risk for providers.

F. Risks of Electronic Fetal Monitoring

EFM has the tendency to keep the mother in a supine position (WHO category B) with the potential result of a *cascade effect* secondary to aortocaval compression and poor labor mechanics (Fig. 11).

Abnormal fetal heart rate tracings have a low positive predictive value, which often leads to a cascade of unnecessary interventions and accompanying morbidities to the mother and infant.

A less common complication of internal EFM (occurring in < 2% of the deliveries) is scalp infection secondary to the scalp electrode.

Rarer complications include sepsis, cerebrospinal fluid leakage, meningitis, and cranial osteomyelitis.

The most dramatic risk of EFM is inaccurate pattern interpretation, allowing a true fetal distress to go unrecognized or causing unneeded intervention for a healthy fetus.

II. Fetal Scalp Blood pH Sampling

Sampling of the fetal scalp blood pH by micropipette is not universally available, particularly in small community or rural hospitals. Because the reliability of interpretation of fetal heart rate patterns is poor (even among experts), the addition of scalp pH sampling can be used to confirm the conservative management of labor by reducing the false-positive rate of EFM. A fetal scalp pH of less than 7.20 is an indication to intervene by having diagnosed fetal acidemia. Scalp pH results between 7.20 and 7.25 are an indication to monitor closely the fetal heart rate tracing and to repeat the scalp testing if there is any progressive deterioration. Scalp pHs of greater than 7.30 are reassuring for that point in time. Data evaluating EFM plus scalp pH compared with EFM alone or intermittent auscultation have been discussed earlier.

III. Fetal Scalp Stimulation

The use of a variety of scalp stimulation techniques is a noninvasive method that seeks to show a nonstress test acceleratory response in the fetal heart pattern of a sleepy or otherwise unresponsive fetus. The reactive nonstress test has been shown to predict accurately a nonacidotic fetus in laboring and nonlaboring women. Before labor, walking, eating, exercise, gentle rocking or shaking of the abdomen, acoustic vibrators, or acoustic sound generators all have been shown to result in acceleratory fetal heart rate patterns. During labor, stimulating the scalp with a mild pinch with an Allis or sponge forceps, poking the scalp head with an amniotomy hook, and pushing on the scalp with the distal portion of a gloved finger are types of fetal scalp stimulation that are predictive of a nonacidotic fetus if an acceleratory fetal heart rate response is achieved. A heart rate acceleration of 15 beats/min, lasting 15 seconds, has been shown to be strongly associated with a fetal scalp pH of greater than 7.20. The use of stimulation during labor to assess fetal well-being has not been well studied using randomized controlled trials.

Randomized controlled trial data are not available for fetal vibroacoustic stimulation, although a Cochrane evaluation of existing data is ongoing.[93] This relatively new, noninvasive technique to assess fetal well-being uses a fetal vibrating and sound-producing stimulator that is placed on the mother's abdomen. The response sought to the stimulation is similar to fetal movement in nonstress testing or fetal scalp stimulation. Suggestions of long-lasting (2 hours) disturbances in the fetal heart rate have been reported. Controlled trials are in order before this technique can be adopted as a routine clinical tool.

IV. Intermittent Auscultation of the Fetal Heart Rate

Randomized controlled trials have shown that intermittent auscultation is at least as effective as EFM in detecting fetuses in need of medical intervention. It imparts no direct risk to the fetus. Although it has been alleged that significant variable decelerations and evidence of uteroplacental insufficiency could escape diagnosis using periodic auscultation, no studies have yet confirmed this fear. Randomized controlled trials comparing EFM with intermittent auscultation show no clear effect on analgesic use or the mother's perception of pain, but some differences in maternal perceptions do surface. The EFM group felt too restricted in labor. Although these women tended to be left alone more often, there was no apparent difference in their perceptions of the labor as being unpleasant. In two randomized controlled trials, the method of monitoring was less important to women than was the support they receive from staff and companions. Regular auscultation by a personal attendant, as used in these studies, seems to be the practice of choice for the physiologic labor.

Many institutions that use intermittent auscultation include an initial continuous EFM period of 15 to 20 minutes. If the initial strip is normal, the patient has the option of continuous or intermittent fetal heart rate monitoring. ACOG guidelines do not mention the concept of an *admission test strip*, and the Society of Obstetrics and Gynecology of Canada guidelines specifically discourage its use. The ACOG has issued guidelines for intermittent fetal heart rate monitoring when risk factors are present during labor or when intensified monitoring is deemed to be appropriate. These guidelines, although not evidence based, are as follows.[5] During the active phase of the first stage of labor, when intermittent auscultation is used, the fetal heart rate should be evaluated every 15 minutes, preferably following a uterine contraction. During the second stage of labor, the fetal heart rate should be evaluated and recorded at least every 5 minutes.

The guidelines also state: "For low-risk patients in labor, the fetal heart rate may be monitored by either method (intermittent auscultation or continuous EFM). For such patients there are no data to demonstrate optimal time intervals for intermittent auscultation. The standard practice is to evaluate and record the fetal heart rate at least every 30 minutes following a contraction in the active stage of labor and at least every 15 minutes in the second stage of labor."[5] The auscultation is performed during a contraction and for at least 30 seconds thereafter.[5] Intermittent auscultation is (said to be) more personnel intensive than machine intensive.

If fetal heart rate auscultation is to be used as the primary method of fetal monitoring in labor, a 1:1 nurse-to-patient ratio is required, at least during the second stage of labor. It has been suggested that this staffing requirement is too vigorous for some labor and delivery units. ACOG guidelines for continuous EFM recommend that "the fetal heart rate record should be evaluated at least every 5 minutes when electronic fetal monitoring is used."[5] The staffing needs for either method, based on these guidelines, may be similar.

V. Summary

Continuous EFM alone is not a good screening tool for the population of laboring women in most family practices regardless of risk status. It offers no advantage over standard nursing care and intermittent auscultation of the fetal heart rate for most low-risk laboring women. The routine use of continuous EFM for all women in labor appears to increase the risk for instrumental and cesarean delivery with no improvement in fetal outcome. Although EFM provides reassurance for some women and many birth attendants, it is no substitute for the personal support and attendance of laboring women by supportive and caring health care personnel. All childbearing women need some form of fetal monitoring to detect developing problems. The monitoring type to be used should be individualized for each childbearing family, based on a variety of location, resource, medicolegal, and practitioner factors. The benefits once claimed for EFM are minimal. The risks associated with the use of EFM, especially the risk of cesarean delivery, warrant the critical scrutiny of each clinician as how best to use this form of fetal surveillance. The ACOG's current position, which leaves the decision to the woman and her birth attendant, is appropriate.[5]

SECTION F.
NORMAL DELIVERY AND BIRTHING POSITIONS

I. Preparation for Delivery

The delivery most often attended by family physicians is the spontaneous vaginal delivery. Before delivery and toward the end of the second stage of labor, preparation should be made for delivery. Most birth attendants begin these preparations when the multiparous patient is at near or complete dilation or when the nulliparous patient begins to crown.

Crowning is the term used to describe the appearance of the fetal scalp between the dilating introitus. As the second stage begins to near its end, the perineum bulges with each contraction and each time the woman bears down. The vaginal opening becomes more dilated by the fetal head with each contraction. During this process, the perineum begins a thinning process.

Some birth attendants assist the process with perineal massage. The birth attendant may place his or her thumb on the outside of the perineum and the pointer or pointer and middle finger on the inside of the perineum, gently massaging the perineum from midline laterally on each side. The method has been described in case studies as being soothing to the patient and the maternity caregiver, reducing the length and depth of perineal tears, reducing the need for episiotomy, and by some authors, being pain relieving.[27] Only one randomized controlled trial has looked at perineal massage, and it concluded: "Perineal massage is an effective approach to increasing the chance of delivery with an intact perineum for women with a first vaginal delivery but not for women with a previous vaginal birth."[56] Massaging and stretching the perineum during the second stage of labor is a WHO category B classification.

A large, prospective Canadian trial (the Canadian Perineal Massage Trial) reported that regular prenatal perineal massage was helpful in many ways. In this randomized controlled trial, the intervention group of pregnant women was instructed in the daily manual stretching of the perineal muscles for 10 minutes, starting at 34–35 weeks of gestation. Patients or their partners were advised to insert their thumbs into the vaginal opening and gently pull down for 2 minutes at each of the 4, 6, and 8 o'clock positions. The study showed that the prenatal perineal massage helped preserve an intact perineum without damaging a gravida's future sexual satisfaction or increasing her risk of urinary incontinence. Of the intervention group, 24% of primiparas delivered over an intact perineum compared with 15% of the control group.[56a]

II. Positioning for Delivery

The patient is placed in a delivery position or, preferably, allowed to assume the most comfortable delivery position for her delivery. The traditional dorsal lithotomy position on the delivery room table was developed almost primarily to benefit the delivering physician by allowing *adequate access to the perineum* for operational delivery.

Increasing numbers of family physicians are avoiding this delivery position, however, which has been implicated in increased delivery pain, increased perineal tears, increased extensions of episiotomies, and possibly increased fetal distress. At least 11 randomized controlled trials have evaluated delivery positions.[91] The combined data suggest that an upright position during the second stage reduces intolerable pain, difficulty bearing down, instrumented vaginal delivery, and episiotomy rate.[87,88]

The literature indicates an increasing interest in the lateral side-lying or Sims' position for delivery. This position adapts readily to almost any hospital bed, delivery bed, or delivery table (with the exception of the birthing chair) and has been reported in several case series to be associated with reduced blood loss, reduced hypotension, reduced fetal distress, decreased perceived maternal pain, and reduced numbers of episiotomies when compared with the lithotomy position. The side-lying position may not be adequate for deliveries requiring large episiotomies, operative deliveries, or regional anesthesia.[89]

Regarding the hands and knees position, the Cochrane Library suggests that: "Until evidence concerning substantive outcomes such as progress of labour and method of delivery is available, use of hands and knees position cannot be recommended as an intervention. This is not to suggest that women should not adopt this position if they find it comfortable . . . ,"[44] as has been reported in several case series.

Many of the management paradigms traditionally used with the delivering woman include positions, policies, protocols, and procedures that lack evidence of benefit to the mother or the fetus. The birth attendant needs to be aware of these data and to become more comfortable with an individualized, flexible delivery plan. Labor and delivery positions, policies, or protocols with no proven scientific basis and no indication of clear superiority for the mother or fetus should be left to the discretion of the delivering parents.

III. The Birthing Bed

Birthing beds are gaining increasing popularity and use in the United States. These beds combine the advantages of the birthing chair (mobility, ease of position change, decreased pain in second stage, improved bearing down) with the advantages of a traditional delivery table (at least for the birth attendant), while being much more comfortable than either the chair or the table. Although expensive to purchase, they are increasingly incorporated into birthing units in hospital and nonhospital settings. These multipositionable beds allow a delivering patient to assume a variety of positions. They have the advantage of equal usability for nontraditional as well as traditional or operative deliveries.

IV. Immersion in Water During Delivery

Delivery in water is a controversial issue.[66] On one hand, midwives and other maternity caregivers report that it is a relaxing and satisfying environment in which to birth.[53] On the other hand, there is a dearth of evidence as to the safety and effectiveness of this option. Its promotion as a therapeutic tool for laboring women began to appear in the English medical literature in the 1980s. The first published account of a birth in water in the United Kingdom occurred in 1987.[92] Although much more commonly practiced in the United Kingdom than the United States, its use in the United States appears to be growing.[28,70] Labor and birth in water is actively promoted as helpful and safe. Birthing pools for hire or for institutional purchase are widely advertised. It is not known how widespread water labor and delivery is in the United States. Some birthing centers and hospitals are responding to this demand by providing pools in birthing suites, whereas others allow pool rental. Many of these centers have developed guidelines for this practice; however, opinions differ as to what constitutes safe practice.

Many possible benefits are suggested for the mother and infant including nonpharmacologic pain relief, acceleration of labor, reduction of maternal blood pressure, increased maternal control over the birth environment, reduced perineal trauma, improved psychosocial outcomes, improved maternal satisfaction with labor and delivery, and avoidance of nonindicated interventions.[12,28,70]

Possible hazards that have been suggested for the mother include increased risk of infection, reduction of effective contractions, increased perineal trauma, increased risk of postpartum hemorrhage, risk of water embolism, and restriction of mobility. Possible hazards that have been suggested for the infant include increased risk of infection, increased admission to special care nurseries, risk of trauma resulting from inability to breath at birth, and water aspiration.[12,28,70]

Limited data are available from two published and two ongoing randomized controlled trials and three nonrandomized cohort studies as well as several case series. These data indicate that water labor is prolonged compared with traditional care (690 minutes versus 552 minutes) and most marked in primiparas (767 minutes versus 632 minutes); women more likely to have second-degree tears but are less likely to need augmentation. No differences were seen in episiotomy use, Apgar scores, perineal infection, or postpartum fever.[12,66]

There have been case reports of infant deaths after delivery in water, but few details have been published. In most of these cases, the infant was held under water for some considerable time after birth.[52]

Given past maternity care experiences with interventions becoming widely accepted before being adequately evaluated (i.e., continuous EFM, routine intravenous lines in labor, routine episiotomy) it seems reasonable for evidence-based maternity caregivers to insist on adequate evaluation of labor and birth in water before widespread implementation.

V. Delivery Maneuvers

As crowning progresses and after the delivery position has been achieved, appropriate drapes may be placed under the woman and the perineum prepared. Most birth attendants use an iodine solution and attempt to cleanse the vulvovaginal and rectal areas, despite any randomized controlled trial data concerning the safety or risk of doing so. Delivery anesthesia, if used, is chosen at this time; most deliveries can be performed without anesthesia if that is the patient and physician's preference.

A. Delivery of the Head

Many physicians have been taught to perform the modified Ritgen maneuver to deliver the fetal head (Fig. 15). This maneuver consists of exerting pressure on the chin of the fetus through the perineum, just in front of the coccyx, with one hand, while the other hand exerts pressure superiorly against the occiput. Historically the Ritgen maneuver accomplished the same maneuver by inserting a finger into the rectum. Classically, these maneuvers have been thought to control delivery and extend the head to allow it to be delivered through the smallest diameter. It is now recognized that extending the head on the perineum presents not the smallest diameter (the occipitobregmatic) but the largest diameter (the occipitofrontal) to the perineum (Fig. 16). The Ritgen maneuver or modified Ritgen maneuver may increase the risk of tearing or episiotomy. Although the Ritgen or modified Ritgen maneuvers can accelerate the delivery process, they may be considerably more traumatic to the maternal perineum.

Midwives have practiced the exact opposite for several centuries. As the flexed head passes through the vaginal introitus, the smallest head diameter (the occipitobregmatic) is preserved if the vertex is maintained in a state of flexion. As flexion is maintained, the perineum can be massaged slowly over the face, under the chin and

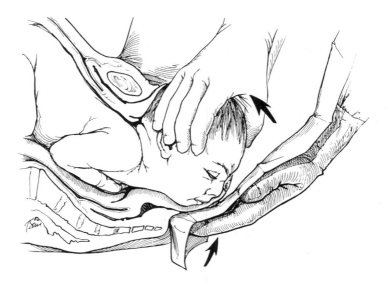

FIGURE 15. Near completion of the delivery of the fetal head by the modified Ritgen maneuver. Moderate upward pressure is applied to the fetal chin by the posterior hand, while the suboccipital area of the fetal head is held against the symphysis.

around the ears, before the head is allowed to extend. This method is less traumatic to the maternal perineum and reduces the need for episiotomy or resultant perineal tearing.

Only one randomized controlled trial has tested this hypothesis. The HOOP trial (Hands On Or Poised) in England was designed to compare the effect of two methods of perineal management used during spontaneous vaginal delivery on the prevalence of perineal pain reported at 10 days after birth. At the end of the second stage of labor, women were allocated to either the *hands on* method, in which the midwife's hands put pressure on the infant's head and support (*guard*) the perineum,

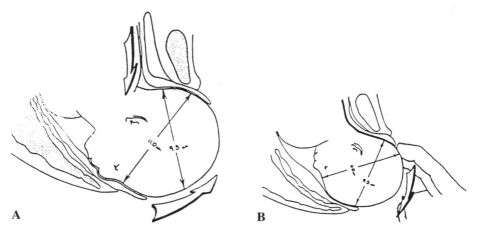

FIGURE 16. **A,** In occipitoanterior positions, pushing extends the head, causing it to present a greater (occipitofrontal) diameter. **B,** Flexing of head presents the smallest (suboccipito-bregmatic) diameter.

and then lateral flexion was used to facilitate delivery of the shoulders, or the *hands poised* method, in which the midwife kept her hands poised, not touching the head or perineum and allowing spontaneous delivery of the shoulders.[65] Of the women in the *hands poised* group, 34% reported pain in the previous 24 hours compared with 31% in the hands on group (RR, 1.10; 95% confidence interval [CI] 1.01 to 1.18; P = .02). The rate of episiotomy was significantly lower in the hands poised group (RR, 0.79; 99% CI, 0.65 to 0.96; P = .008), but the rate of manual removal of placenta was significantly higher (RR, 1.69; 99% CI, 1.02 to 2.78; P = .008). The researchers concluded that the reduction in pain observed in the hands on group potentially could affect a substantial number of women. Pending further research, maneuvers related to protecting the perineum and the management of the fetal head at the moment of birth and the active manipulation of the fetus at the moment of birth both carry a WHO category C classification.

B. Pushing at Delivery

Tradition in the U.S. is to have the mother use Valsalva pushing at the end of the second stage of labor, wherein the mother holds her breath and bears down to *push the baby out*, as opposed to expiration pushing or exhalatory bearing down, wherein the mother breathes (*breathes the baby out*) while bearing down in the second stage of labor, which is practiced by many midwives. The available data from randomized controlled trials suggest that second-stage pushing or bearing-down efforts involving the Valsalva maneuver, although resulting in a slightly shorter second stage of labor, may compromise maternal-fetal gas exchange, which can result in fetal heart rate abnormalities or reduced Apgar scores. Randomized controlled trials suggest that the practice of sustained (Valsalva) bearing down at delivery may have a deleterious fetal effect unless any potential shortening of the second stage is mandatory.[90] Sustained, directed bearing-down efforts (Valsalva pushing) during the second stage of labor has a WHO category B classification.

Another age-old pushing tradition is for the birth attendant to ask a labor attendant to apply fundal pressure at the end of the second stage. This is a practice for which insufficient evidence exists to support a clear recommendation supporting or opposing the practice. It should be used with caution until further research clarifies the issue and the practice carries a WHO category C classification. Encouraging a woman to push when full dilation or nearly full dilation of the cervix has been diagnosed, before the woman feels the urge to bear down herself, carries a WHO category D classification.

C. Oropharyngeal Suctioning

After the delivery of the head, the nostrils and mouth usually are suctioned. A finger may be passed over the neck of the fetus to determine whether it is encircled by the umbilical cord. A nuchal cord or cord around the neck occurs in 10% to 15% of all deliveries. If the cord is loose, it may be slipped over the infant's head. If extremely tight, the cord may be cut between two clamps and released or, alternatively, the infant delivered between the nuchal loop.

D. Meconium Staining

If meconium staining was present during labor or delivery, the naso-oropharynx may be suctioned thoroughly with a DeLee suction device, using a suction apparatus or wall suction instead of oral suction, before delivery of the shoulders. This technique has been shown to reduce the incidence of meconium aspiration or pneumonitis; however, care must be taken to reduce stimulation to the posterior pharynx. If the posterior pharynx is stimulated too vigorously, a vagal response may be stimulated, resulting in fetal bradycardia.

Some birth attendants differentiate between thick meconium and thin meconium. The presumption clinically is that thin meconium is *watered down* with amniotic fluid or reduced in amount when compared with thick meconium and less caustic to the fetal lung if aspirated. Many nonrandomized studies have suggested that aspiration of the upper and lower airways of infants with significant meconium staining is associated with improved outcomes. Infants in these studies included those who were depressed at birth and those who were relatively vigorous. Most neonatal textbooks continue to recommend aspiration of the upper and lower airways in cases of thick or particulate meconium staining of the amniotic fluid.

Four randomized controlled trials have addressed the problem of endotracheal intubation of vigorous meconium-stained infants born at term. There is no evidence from these data that endotracheal intubation and aspiration of the airways in nonasphyxiated meconium-stained infants is of any benefit. One review suggests that this procedure is associated with a 1.2% increased risk of developing meconium aspiration syndrome or that for every 83 vigorous meconium-stained infants born at term who are exposed to routine endotracheal intubation and aspiration at birth, one case of meconium aspiration syndrome is caused. The Cochrane Review concludes: "Until further evidence is available routine intubation of vigorous term meconium stained babies should be abandoned."[39]

E. Delivery of the Shoulders

After the head is born, it typically turns toward one of the maternal thighs, assuming a transverse position. Often the shoulders are born spontaneously, with little effort. If not, the sides of the head may be grasped between two hands. With gentle downward traction, only in the vertical plane, the anterior shoulder typically can be delivered easily. Often, clinicians then attempt to deliver the posterior shoulder before completely delivering the anterior arm (Fig. 17). Midwives have long taught that after delivering the anterior shoulder, failure to deliver completely the anterior arm may increase periurethral and vaginal tearing. Although tested in no randomized controlled trials to date, some recommend that birth attendants, after delivering the anterior shoulder, attempt to deliver the anterior arm completely.

After delivery of the anterior shoulder and arm, an upward movement of the head typically accomplishes delivery of the posterior shoulder and arm. The movements to deliver the shoulders by applying traction to the fetal head are only in a vertical plane, with as little traction as possible, to reduce any increased risk for brachial plexus, neck, or clavicle injury.

F. Delivery of the Body

After delivery of both shoulders through the introitus, the remainder of the delivery requires little or no assistance. At this point, the birth attendant can allow the parents to reach down to the perineum, grasping the infant under the arms, around the trunk, and facilitating the parent's *completing the birth* of the baby onto the maternal abdomen.

G. After Delivery

The infant's airway should be cleared completely and the umbilical cord clamped after delivery. Active manipulation of the infant at the moment of birth has a WHO category C classification. At this point, one of the labor support persons may wish to cut the cord. Sterility in cutting the cord has a WHO category A rating. Several randomized controlled trials evaluated early versus late cord clamping in the third stage of labor; however, only two employed true random allocation.[23] There is no evidence from these studies of a significant effect in the timing of cord clamping on the incidence of postpartal hemorrhage or fetomaternal transfusion. The effects on neonatal grunting, neonatal respiratory distress, or neonatal jaundice are not conclusive. Early cord clamping of the umbilical cord has a WHO category C classification.

The infant should be dried, wrapped warmly, and, if stable, allowed to bond with the mother (or parents). An exception to drying off the infant is often made for mothers who desire that the infant be delivered to their chest for bonding or breast-feeding.

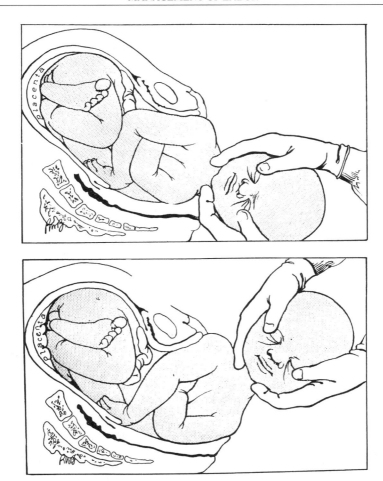

FIGURE 17. Gentle downward traction to bring about descent of anterior shoulder (top). Delivery of anterior shoulder is completed; gentle upward traction is applied to deliver the posterior shoulder (bottom).

These infants can be covered with warm blankets. No randomized controlled trial data speak against this approach, and some anecdotal data speak to increased breast-feeding success with this maneuver. Early skin-to-skin contact between the mother and child, support of the initiation of breast-feeding within 1 hour postpartum, and prevention of hypothermia of the infant all have a WHO category A classification.

H. Bonding
Although few data exist to document a maternal-infant bonding effect, no data indicate any harm from this time together, and several case series document increased maternal satisfaction with this time of bonding. A time of bonding, similar to so many other labor and delivery traditions, may be left to the discretion of the mother and should not be discouraged or prevented without indication.

VI. Episiotomy
The incision of the perineum to enlarge the vaginal introitus at the time of delivery may occur by a medial episiotomy or mediolateral episiotomy. Episiotomy is the most

commonly performed surgical procedure in the U.S. that is performed without formal informed consent.

A. Traditionally Taught Advantages

1. Myths of episiotomies

Purported advantages for episiotomy include the following:

Episiotomies are easy to repair and more likely to heal than tears.

Episiotomies are less likely to result in third-degree or fourth-degree tears.

Episiotomies reduce the risk of cystocele, rectocele, uterine prolapse, and urinary stress incontinence.

Episiotomies reduce the length of the second stage of labor.

Episiotomies protect the fetal head.

2. Evidence

Four European randomized controlled trials show that the liberal use of episiotomy results in fewer perineal tears but increased posterior trauma, while showing no reduction in urinary incontinence.[55,77] The only North American randomized controlled trial[55] suggested that restricted use of episiotomy in primiparous women was associated with an increase in birth over an intact perineum and a reduction in third-degree and fourth-degree tears. Virtually all severe perineal trauma was associated with routine episiotomy, and the episiotomy group had similar electromyogram results of the perineal muscles and similar urinary and pelvic floor symptoms to the nonepisiotomy group.

The *Cochrane Review* suggests:[13]

The primary question is whether or not to use an episiotomy routinely. The answer is clear. There is evidence to support the restrictive use of episiotomy compared with routine use of episiotomy. . . In the light of the available evidence restrictive use of episiotomy is recommended. What type of episiotomy is more beneficial, midline or mediolateral? To date there are only two published trials available, both of which . . . are of poor methodological quality, making their results uninterpretable. The evidence to support what kind of episiotomy technique to recommend, therefore, remains unanswered.

B. Risks of Episiotomy

Case studies have shown that episiotomy can result in prolonged perineal pain, prolonged sexual dysfunction, and increased risk of third-degree or fourth-degree extension lacerations. Pain and edema are the most frequent postepisiotomy complaints; however, dyspareunia and infection may be serious complications leading to significant morbidity.[87,88]

C. Randomized, Controlled Trials

In the 1970s, criticism of routine episiotomies was seen in the medical literature. Randomized controlled trials showed no difference between episiotomy and nonepisiotomy patients regarding neonatal outcome or maternal pain or urinary symptoms; however, women who avoid episiotomies seem to be more likely to have resumed sexual intercourse within 1 month of delivery and to have quicker reduction of their postpartal perineal pain scores. Studies have indicated that "routine episiotomy is no longer justified,"[13,55] and "routine episiotomy for uncomplicated spontaneous vertex vaginal deliveries is not indicated."[13,55] Data suggest a greater amount of rectal injury with the use of midline episiotomy compared with no episiotomy.[13]

D. Summary

Because women with an intact perineum have the best short-term morbidity experiences, and comparable experiences are found in women with episiotomies and tears, it is reasonable to conclude that the short-term morbidity experience is better when routine episiotomy is not performed.

SECTION G.
MANAGEMENT OF THIRD-STAGE LABOR

Third-stage labor begins after delivery of the fetus and ends with delivery of the placenta and membranes. After delivery of the infant and cutting of the umbilical cord, the placenta usually separates spontaneously from the uterine wall within 5 to 10 minutes.

There are two different approaches to the clinical management of the third stage—expectant management and active management—and these have been the subject of many reviews. *Expectant management* involves waiting for signs of separation and allowing the placenta to deliver spontaneously or be aided by gravity or nipple stimulation (although nipple stimulation to increase uterine contractions during the third stage of labor carries a WHO category D classification). Expectant management is also known as conservative or physiologic management and is popular in some northern European countries and in some units in the United States and Canada. It also is the usual practice in home deliveries.

In contrast, with *active management*, the birth attendant chooses to intervene in this process by using one or more of the following interventions:
• Administration of a prophylactic oxytocic after delivery of the infant
• Early cord clamping and cutting
• Free bleeding of the end of the cord
• Controlled cord traction of the umbilical cord
The active management of the third stage is virtually standard practice in the United Kingdom, Australia, and several other countries.

I. Delivery of the Placenta
A. Free Bleeding of the Cord
Three trials have evaluated allowing free bleeding from the placental end of the umbilical cord.[21] Although not true randomized controlled trials, when taken together, these three trials provide evidence that allowing free bleeding or free drainage from the placental end of the umbilical cord reduces the risk of fetomaternal transfusion. One active intervention during the third stage, while waiting for the placenta to separate, is to allow the umbilical cord to drain freely. This is easy to accomplish during the bonding process described previously.

B. Spontaneous Placental Separation
While waiting for the placenta to separate, the fundus may be checked frequently to ensure that the uterus does not become atonic and filled with blood. It is important to wait for signs of placental separation before applying any traction to the umbilical cord. Undue or excessive traction on the umbilical cord, before placental separation, may result in tearing of the umbilical cord, tearing of the placenta, or inversion of the uterus.

Although placental separation typically occurs within 5 to 10 minutes after delivery, 30 minutes is considered normal. Classically, separation of the placenta is indicated when
• The uterus becomes globular shaped.
• The fundus changes to a firm consistency.
• The uterus appears to rise in the abdomen.
• There is a sudden gush of blood.
• The umbilical cord appears to lengthen or protrude farther from the vagina.

C. Assisted Placental Separation
After partial or complete separation has occurred, gentle fundal massage and firm but gentle traction on the umbilical cord usually effects delivery of the placenta. The Brandt-Andrews maneuver, a cephalad shearing motion exerted with the abdominal hand on the uterus while applying traction to the umbilical cord simultaneously with the other hand

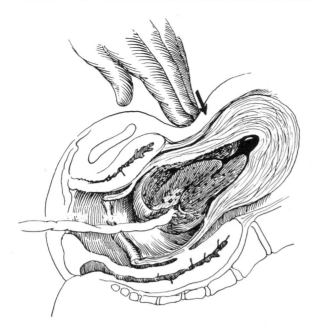

FIGURE 18. Brandt-Andrews delivery of the placenta. After the fundus is firm, moderate tension is exerted on the umbilical cord, while the other hand *shears off* the placenta from the uterine wall by upward kneading pressure on the anterior uterine wall. (From Wilson JR: Atlas of Obstetric Technic, 2nd ed. St. Louis, Mosby, 1969. Daisy Stilwell, medical illustrator, with permission.)

(Fig. 18), has been said to effect removal of the placenta easily without increasing risk of uterine inversion. Only two randomized controlled trials examined the comparison of cord traction versus fundal pressure in the third stage.[22] Both studies considered postpartum hemorrhage and manual placental removal. Both studies suggest that controlled cord traction may be preferable. These findings are reflected in lower mean blood loss and shorter third stages in the controlled traction group. One study found a greater proportion of cord rupture in the controlled traction group, however. Based on these limited data, an appropriate clinical protocol is to wait at least 5 to 10 minutes after delivery of the infant for spontaneous separation of the placenta. Gentle cord traction, fundal massage, or the Brandt-Andrews maneuver could be incorporated. If these maneuvers fail, manual extraction of the placenta may be needed. If needed and to prevent manual extraction of the placenta, 1 ml of oxytocin diluted in 9 ml of normal saline and injected into the umbilical vein through an intracath often facilitates placenta separation and is supported by randomized controlled trials (NNT = 8).[13a]

D. Manual Extraction of the Placenta

If the placenta has not separated after 20–30 minutes and cannot be removed by the maneuvers described previously, and if the patient is appropriately anesthetized, manual removal or extraction of the placenta may be performed to reduce potential excessive blood loss. Intrauterine bacterial contamination and postpartum abscess are rare complications of this procedure.

The procedure is accomplished by using one hand abdominally to grasp the fundus and hold it downward firmly. The other hand reaches into the uterine cavity to gently peel off the placenta using a *rotatory or circumferential sweep* of the hands to separate the placenta (Fig. 19). One must be assured of achieving a clean plane of separation. The placenta, after separation, may normally be easily removed. After removal, vigorous fundal massage minimizes subsequent bleeding.

E. Active Third-Stage Management of the Placenta

Randomized controlled trials of active versus conservative third-stage management have shown that active management of the third stage of labor is associated with

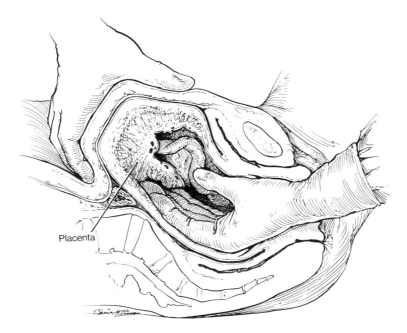

Placenta

FIGURE 19. Manual removal of the placenta. The fingers are alternately abducted, adducted, and advanced until the placenta is detached completely.

reductions in clinically estimated postpartal blood loss, increases in postpartal he-moglobin levels, reductions in postpartal blood transfusions, significant reduction in the length of the third stage, and reduced use of postpartum therapeutic oxytocics (Fig. 20). Adverse effects of active management include increased nausea, increased vomiting, increased headache, increased postpartum endometritis, increased pain in the third stage, and increased postpartum hypertension. Neonatal outcomes, when assessed, revealed no clinically important differences between the approach to the third stage with the exception that the rate of breast-feeding at hospital discharge and at 6 weeks was higher in the active management group.

The implications of these data on practice depend on the relative weight the ma-ternity caregiver places on the different outcomes. If reducing blood loss and short-ening the third stage is important, active management could be considered. If patient comfort and blood pressure control are important and the risk of excessive bleeding is not high, the conservative approach seems rational. The *Cochrane Review* meta-analysis concludes, "Routine 'active management' is superior to 'expectant manage-ment' in terms of blood loss, post partum haemorrhage and severe post partum haemorrhage and other serious complications of the third stage of labour... Active management should be routine for women expecting a singleton vaginal delivery in a maternity hospital."[74]

F. Examination of the Placenta

After removal of the placenta, the placenta, its membranes, and the umbilical cord should be examined (WHO category A recommendation). If missing cotyledons of the placenta are noted, manual exploration of the placenta is indicated. There are no data to support routine manual exploration of the uterus after delivery (WHO cate-gory D), and there are data that routine uterine lavage after delivery is harmful (WHO category B).

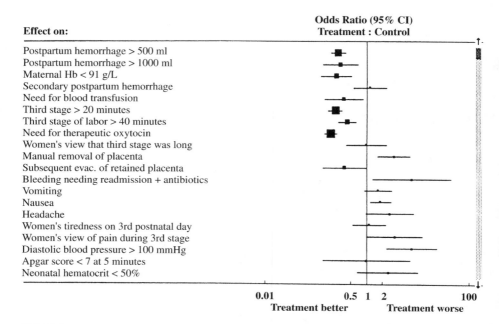

FIGURE 20. Active versus expectant management in the third stage of labor (3 trials reviewed). (From Prendiville WJ, Elbourne D, McDonald S: Cochrane Review The Cochrane Library, Issue 1. Oxford, Update Software, 2000, with permission.)

The membranes should be evaluated for vessels that end blindly at the edge of membranes. Such a finding may suggest a succenturiate lobe, which may need to be removed manually from the placenta. The umbilical cord should be examined for the presence of two arteries and a vein. The absence of one umbilical artery may suggest congenital abnormalities of the newborn. Whenever abnormalities of the placenta are suspected, pathologic evaluation of the placenta is indicated.

II. Active Prophylaxis of Postpartum Atony and Hemorrhage

Oxytocics are widely used during the normal third stage, after delivery of the placenta, to avoid excessive postpartum hemorrhage secondary to uterine atony.[68] Gentle fundal massage or checking for fundal firmness should always be a part of postpartal management. Randomized clinical trials indicate that the prophylactic use of oxytocics reduces the risk of postpartum hemorrhage by about 60%.[24] Ten randomized controlled trials compared oxytocin with ergot derivatives. Taken together, these trials indicate that ergot derivatives alone appear to be the least preferable drugs, whether compared with oxytocin alone or with oxytocin/ergonovine combination. There is a paucity of evidence comparing oxytocin/ergonovine with oxytocin alone, however.

Routine postpartum hemorrhage prophylaxis practice in the United States is to use 5 or 10 units of oxytocin intramuscularly or 20 units of oxytocin in 1 L run at 10 ml/min for a few minutes until bleeding is controlled, then at 1 to 2 ml/min. The intravenous drip (as opposed to intravenous bolus or intramuscular injection) generally is preferable because it allows for a more controlled third stage. Oxytocin given intravenously, by bolus, can cause marked hypotension. On occasions when oxytocin is insufficient, postpartum hemorrhage may occur. Treatment of this condition is discussed in detail in Chapter 15, section E.

III. Repair of Lacerations of the Birth Canal

Iatrogenic or spontaneous lacerations of the birth canal may be repaired before or after delivery of the placenta. The cervix, vagina, and perineum must be completely inspected after delivery. Conditions resulting in lacerations include precipitous deliveries, instrument deliveries, large infant deliveries, or upright deliveries. Lacerations that are large or do not stop bleeding spontaneously should be repaired. Abrasions or lacerations that do not bleed actively do not usually require suturing.

A. First-Degree Lacerations

First-degree lacerations normally are superficial lacerations that have minimal bleeding. These are most likely found on the fourchette, perineal skin, or vaginal mucosal membranes.

B. Second-Degree Lacerations

Second-degree tears include the subcutaneous tissues or fascia of the perineal body but not the rectal sphincter. Often, second-degree tears are repaired by birth attendants. Case studies indicate that these lacerations, if not bleeding, may heal faster if not sutured. No randomized controlled trials have evaluated this practice.

C. Third-Degree Lacerations

Third-degree lacerations extend through the skin, mucous membranes, and perineal body involving fibers of the rectal sphincter and are repaired in a standard fashion.

D. Fourth-Degree Lacerations

Fourth-degree lacerations are tears that extend through the rectal sphincter and expose the lumen of the rectum. All fourth-degree lacerations should be repaired anatomically and in layers, using interrupted sutures (Fig. 21).

E. Suture Materials

Multiple randomized controlled trials have evaluated suture materials available for perineal repairs.[37,38,50,51] Comparing absorbable versus nonabsorbable sutures for perineal repair, randomized controlled trials suggest that, on balance, absorbable materials are preferable to nonabsorbable materials. Absorbable suture is associated

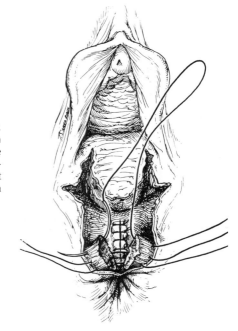

FIGURE 21. Repair of complete perineal tear. The rectal mucosa has been repaired with interrupted, fine chromic catgut sutures. The torn ends of the sphincter ani are next approximated with 2 or 3 interrupted chromic catgut sutures. The wound is then repaired, as in a second-degree laceration or an episiotomy.

with less pain in the immediate puerperium, and the need for resuturing is lessened. Randomized controlled trials evaluating continuous versus interrupted sutures suggest that a continuous, subcuticular stitch is preferable to interrupted transcutaneous sutures. The subcuticular technique is associated with less short-term pain, without any clear difference in the long-term.

Randomized controlled trials indicate that of the two most commonly used absorbable materials, polyglycolic acid is preferable to catgut or chromic suture. Based on currently available evidence, polyglycolic acid sutures (Dexon or Vicryl) should be chosen for repair of the deep layers and the perineal skin. Questions remain about the long-term consequences of this suggestion, but generally speaking, the randomized controlled trial evidence is reassuring. The frequent need to remove polyglycolic acid material in the puerperium indicates that this material is not ideal. Most of the evidence points to polyglycolic acid sutures causing less pain in the intermediate postpartum period, albeit with a tendency to cause irritation sufficient to lead to the removal of some suture material, in a few cases. The limited evidence available suggests no major differences in the long-term, with the possible exception of a greater risk of dehiscence leading to resuturing associated with catgut. Few data exist to compare tissue adhesives (such as Histoacryl) with suture for perineal skin closure.

SECTION H.
MANAGEMENT OF VAGINAL BIRTH AFTER CESAREAN BIRTH

I. Background
Vaginal birth after cesarean (VBAC) is considered an increasingly viable option for pregnant patients with previous cesarean births, and the advocacy of VBAC by practicing physicians has now made it the recommended standard of care, despite the relative lack of randomized controlled trials or quality meta-analyses on which to base this recommendation.[83,85] In the United States, the VBAC rate in 1997 was 27.4%, and in these VBACs, successful vaginal deliveries were accomplished 6% to 85% of the time. Various clinical situations appear to affect the potential success rate (Table 3). Overall the success rate is reported to be 60–70% in cases published before 1980 and 75–86% in cases published after 1980. The ACOG has published a VBAC practice guideline.[2]

II. Advantages and Disadvantages
A. Reported Advantages of VBAC (when successful)
- Lower risk of infection
- Shorter hospital stays
- Lower overall delivery costs
- Opportunity to experience family-centered birthing
- More rapid recovery
- Lower morbidity for mother and infant
- Fewer blood transfusions
- Lower mortality rate

TABLE 3. Success Rates of Vaginal Birth After Cesarean

Clinical Scenarios	Successful VBAC (%)
Induction or augmentation during labor	63
Previous cesarean birth for failure to progress	67
More than one previous vaginal delivery	75
A single previous vaginal delivery	84
Previous cesarean for breech	85

B. Reported Disadvantages of Vaginal Birth After Cesarean
- VBAC cannot be scheduled in advance
- Increased risk of incomplete or complete uterine rupture—with potential life-threatening complications for the mother or infant.
- Maternal febrile morbidity
- Cesarean birth still may be required
- Increased risk of hysterectomy with uterine rupture
- Possibility of serious perineal lacerations
- Dissatisfaction with VBAC (including maternal frustration and anger)

C. Contraindications to Vaginal Birth After Cesarean
1. Absolute contraindications

The only absolute contraindication to VBAC is a classic high vertical uterine incision because of the increased risk of uterine rupture (12% in one study). Other contraindications are other transfundal uterine surgery; medical or maternal complications that preclude vaginal delivery; a history of uterine rupture; and an inability of the institution to perform an emergency cesarean delivery because of an unavailable surgeon, anesthesiologist/anesthetist, sufficient hospital staff, or facility.

2. Relative contraindications

Relative contraindications to VBAC include lack of patient consent and a classic "low" vertical uterine incision. Although some authors consider a low vertical incision an absolute contraindication to VBAC, the overall data indicate that the risk of complete uterine rupture is no higher in women with low vertical incisions than in women with low transverse incisions.

3. Clinical situations requiring individual assessment and perhaps obstetric consultation
- Multiple gestation
- Breech presentation
- Suspected fetal macrosomia
- Unknown type of uterine incision
- Previous low vertical uterine incision
- Difficulty during trial of labor for VBAC, including the usual indications for consultation during labor

III. Clinical Scenarios
A. May Vaginal Birth After Cesarean Be Attempted If the Scar Type Cannot Be Documented?
Increasingly the medical literature indicates that VBAC is appropriate without documentation of the scar type. Authors reason that virtually every cesarean birth performed in the United States since the 1980s has used a low transverse incision, and a trial of labor in a history with an unknown scar is considered reasonable. In women who come from other countries, where classical incisions may be more common, however, documenting the scar or recommending cesarean may be the safest option. Virtually all authors recommend that the scar type be documented whenever possible.

B. Can Vaginal Birth After Cesarean Be Performed After Multiple Previous Cesarean Births?
The larger portion of the VBAC literature has studied women with a single previous cesarean. Literature that looks at women with two or more previous cesareans reveals similar success rates, however.

C. Can Vaginal Birth After Cesarean Be Attempted With Twins or Infants With Breech Presentations?

Small case studies of attempted delivery of twins by VBAC reveals success rates of 70% to 75% with no increase in maternal or neonatal morbidity or mortality, although uterine scar dehiscence occurs twice as often in multiple gestation patients as with those with single gestation. Small case studies of VBAC in infants with breech presentations show no increase in morbidity or mortality and have success rates of approximately 50%.

D. Does the Size of the Infant Affect the Vaginal Birth After Cesarean Success Rate?

As the size of the fetus increases, the chance for a successful vaginal delivery decreases, regardless of the clinical situation or history of previous cesarean birth. Case studies reveal VBAC success rates of 70% to 80% for infants weighing less than 4000 g, 50% to 60% for infants weighing 4000 to 4500 g, and 40% to 50% for infants weighing greater than 4500 g. Success rates are significantly lower in each of these groups if the patient has had a previous cesarean delivery as compared with patients without previous cesarean births. Greater infant weights do not appear to increase maternal or neonatal morbidity.

E. Can Women with Prior Cesareans Because of Cephalopelvic Disproportion Try Vaginal Birth After Cesarean?

Approximately 70% of patients experience a successful VBAC.

F. Is It Appropriate to Use Oxytocin in Patients Having a Vaginal Birth After Cesarean?

Several case studies have shown no increase in maternal or fetal morbidity with oxytocin use. One meta-analysis found no relationship between the use of oxytocin and rupture of a uterine scar.[81] Studies indicate that high infusion rates of oxytocin place VBAC patients at a higher risk for uterine rupture. The indications, protocols, and precautions for the use of low rates of infusion of oxytocin should be the same in VBAC patients as those without previous cesarean delivery. These studies indicate no increase in fetal or maternal morbidity.

G. Can Vaginal Birth After Cesarean Patients Receive Prostaglandin for Induction or Augmentation?

In general, studies indicate no increase in neonatal or maternal morbidity when indicated prostaglandin is used for induction or augmentation. There are occasional reports of uterine rupture associated with prostaglandin preparations.

H. Can Regional Anesthesia Be Used in Vaginal Birth After Cesarean Patients?

Even though there are hypothesized concerns for potentially masking the symptoms of uterine rupture, available data do not document this occurrence. Several case reports of uterine rupture in patients with epidural anesthesia reveal patients to be well aware of uterine pain despite anesthesia. In larger views of intrapartum uterine rupture in VBAC patients without regional anesthesia, more than 75% of the patients do not experience pain. No increases in morbidity of the mother or infant have been reported in several thousand patients who have been reported to receive epidural anesthesia while undergoing VBAC. VBAC is not a contraindication to epidural anesthesia. Success rates seem to be similar in VBAC candidates with and without epidural anesthesia.

I. Should Vaginal Birth After Cesarean Candidates Labor With Venous Access or Electronic Fetal Monitoring?

Despite lack of randomized controlled trial data, many centers require venous access and continuous EFM for VBAC patients because of the need to proceed to cesarean birth immediately in the event of complete uterine rupture. There are no data that support using an intravenous line with intravenous fluid rather than just a heparin lock for venous access. There are no randomized controlled trial data comparing EFM with intermittent auscultation for the VBAC patient. Most authorities recommend continuous EFM for VBAC candidates.

J. Should Family Physicians Be Restricted From Attending Vaginal Birth After Cesarean Patients?

No data show superior outcomes by, or patient preference for, one maternity caregiver over another. There are no restrictions on which caregiver should provide VBAC services.

K. Can a Vaginal Birth After Cesarean Candidate Have External Cephalic Version?

Limited data suggest that external cephalic version during the last trimester for breech presentation is as successful for women who have had a previous cesarean as in women who have not had a previous cesarean.

L. Is Delivery Different for a Vaginal Birth After Cesarean Patient?

Delivery should be no different in a VBAC patient and a patient with no uterine scar.

M. Should the Uterus Be Explored After Delivery in a Vaginal Birth After Cesarean Patient?

Whether uterine exploration after delivery should be done routinely is controversial. Most experts seem to recommend against routine exploration, however, and the WHO has classified it category D (a practice that is frequently used inappropriately). Their rationale is that virtually all asymptomatic scar dehiscences heal well, and there are no data to suggest that future pregnancy outcomes are improved by surgical repair. Excessive vaginal bleeding or signs of maternal hypovolemia require prompt evaluation of the previous scar (manual uterine exploration) and the entire genital tract.

IV. Uterine Rupture

The greatest fear clinicians have using VBAC is uterine rupture. Uterine rupture has been subclassified into complete or complete true uterine rupture, which is a through-and-through tear of the uterine wall, and incomplete uterine rupture, which is an internal and incomplete (not through-and-through) tear of the uterine wall.

A. Complete Uterine Rupture

Complete uterine rupture is accompanied classically by fetal distress and sudden blood loss, but most women with complete uterine rupture experience no pain. Incomplete uterine rupture usually is asymptomatic and does not appear to be associated with any maternal or fetal morbidity. Clinicians should be aware that much of the early VBAC literature did not distinguish between complete and incomplete uterine rupture. It may be difficult to interpret data on the incidence of uterine rupture when this distinction is not made.

Complete uterine rupture can occur in the VBAC or non-VBAC patient. Case series show strong associations between complete rupture and perinatal death or maternal morbidity. In most cases, however, maternal and fetal outcomes were good. The classically described symptoms and signs of complete uterine rupture (head recession, suprapubic bulging, maternal pain, maternal bleeding) usually are absent. If uterine rupture is to be recognized during VBAC by fetal heart tone changes, fetal distress, drop in intrauterine pressure monitor pressure with contraction, signs of hypotension or hypovolemia, or unusual uterine pain, nurses and physicians must maintain an extremely high index of suspicion. Once complete rupture is suspected, emergency cesarean delivery usually is recommended because delayed diagnosis worsens the outcome for both the mother and the infant. The ACOG currently recommends that women who have had a prior uterine rupture should undergo repeat cesarean delivery and not be candidates for VBAC.[2]

B. Incomplete Uterine Rupture

Incomplete uterine rupture in the medical literature is also called a uterine window, partial scar dehiscence, occult uterine rupture, or silent uterine rupture. In most cases reported to date, incomplete uterine rupture is asymptomatic and virtually of no clinical relevance. Some authors recommend exploration of the uterine scar routinely after delivery. The accuracy of manual exploration is unknown, however, and probably clinician dependent. Exploration is associated with increased risk of postpartum endometritis, and incomplete ruptures appear to be clinically insignificant. The recommendation to explore manually the uterus routinely post-VBAC is difficult to justify but has not yet been evaluated by randomized controlled trials.

The largest study of VBAC to date, including nearly 6000 VBACs, reported a complete uterine rupture rate of 0.18%. Other studies in the literature have published a rate of 0.17% to 1.5%. One perspective study from 1978 to 1987 reported a complete uterine rupture rate of 0.6% in VBAC patients and a 0.4% overall complete rupture rate. This study showed no serious maternal or neonatal morbidity. One meta-analysis of 31 studies of VBAC made up of more than 11,000 VBACs revealed no significant difference in the rate of complete or incomplete uterine rupture between patients undergoing VBAC and patients undergoing repeat cesarean birth. A failed trial of labor in VBAC patients has been associated with nearly a three times greater rate of incomplete or complete uterine rupture.[2,81]

V. Patient Refusal of VBAC

Studies revealed that up to 40% of VBAC candidates refuse to have VBAC.[1,6] Reported reasons have varied from serious fears about labor and delivery, fears about vaginal delivery, bodily concerns, and convenience issues. One study showed that one third of the patients with a successful VBAC regretted their decision, and 75% of the patients with an unsuccessful trial of labor were frustrated or angry.[1] When considering a VBAC, it should be remembered that a significant percentage of patients may have a strong preference for cesarean birth. Although a successful VBAC may be safer than a repeat cesarean birth, the increased morbidity associated with a cesarean after a failed trial of labor makes the overall maternal and fetal outcomes comparable. The decision of whether to attempt VBAC must be individualized. The maternity caregiver and patient must work together to determine the best choice for their situation.

VI. Summary

Virtually all women with a history of cesarean birth should be given the option of VBAC. Family physicians with obstetric privileges can manage these patients with obstetric backup when needed. The ACOG makes the following recommendations about VBAC.[2]

A. Recommendations Based on Good and Consistent Evidence

Most women with one previous cesarean delivery with a low-transverse incision are candidates for VBAC and should be counseled about VBAC and offered a trial of labor.

Epidural anesthesia may be used for VBAC.

A previous uterine incision extending into the fundus is a contraindication for VBAC.

B. Recommendations Based on Limited or Inconsistent Evidence

Women with two previous low-transverse cesarean deliveries and no contraindications who wish to attempt VBAC may be allowed a trial of labor. They should be advised that the risk of uterine rupture increases as the number of cesarean deliveries increases.

Use of oxytocin or prostaglandin gel for VBAC requires close patient monitoring.

Women with a vertical incision within the lower uterine segment that does not extend into the fundus are candidates for VBAC.

C. Recommendations Based Primarily on Consensus and Opinion

Because uterine rupture may be catastrophic, VBAC should be attempted in institutions equipped to respond to emergencies with physicians immediately available to provide emergency care.

After thorough counseling that weighs the individual benefits and risks of VBAC, the ultimate decision to attempt this procedure or undergo a repeat cesarean delivery should be made by the patient and her physician.

A superb clinical policy on VBAC has been published by the American Academy of Family Physicians: *The woman's choice: Trial of labor or elective repeat cesarean section* (to obtain, call 1-800-274-2237). An excellent overview has been published by the ACOG.[2]

References

1. Abitbol MM, Castillo I, Taylor UB, et al: Vaginal birth after cesarean section: The patient's point of view. Am Fam Physician 47:129–134, 1993.
2. ACOG Practice Bulletin: Vaginal Birth After Previous Cesarean Section. No. 5, July 1999.
3. Ader L, Hasson B, Wallin G: Parturition pain treated by intracutaneous injections of sterile water. Pain 41:133–138, 1990.
4. American College of Obstetricians and Gynecologists: Obstetric anesthesia and analgesia. American College of Obstetricians and Gynecologists Technical Bulletin No. 112. Washington, D.C., American College of Obstetricians and Gynecologists, 1988.
5. American College of Obstetricians and Gynecologists: Intrapartum fetal heart rate monitoring. American College of Obstetricians and Gynecologists Technical Bulletin No. 132. Washington, D.C., American College of Obstetricians and Gynecologists, 1989.
6. Abitbol MM: A further view on the VBAC quandary. Am Fam Physician 41:29–30, 1993.
7. Basevi V, Lavender T: Routine perineal shaving for labour. Protocol for a Cochrane Review. The Cochrane Library. Oxford, Update Software, 2001.
8. Beilin Y, Leibowitz AB, Bernstein HH, Abramovitz SE: Controversies of labor epidural analgesia. Anesth Analg 89:969–978, 1999.
9. Berman JC, Palmer SK: Obstetric anesthesia. In Fredrickson HL, Wilkins-Haug L (eds): Ob/Gyn Secrets, 2nd ed. Philadelphia, Hanley & Belfus, 1998.
10. Bloom SL, McIntire DD, Kelly MA, et al: Lack of effect of walking on labor and delivery. N Engl J Med 339:76–79, 1998.
11. Brody H, Thompson JR: The maximin strategy in modern obstetrics. J Fam Pract 12:977–985, 1981.
12. Cammu H, Clasen K, Van Wettenu L: Is having a warm bath during labor useful? Acta Obstet Gynaecol Scand 73:468–472, 1994.
13. Carroli G, Belizan J, Stamp G: Episiotomy for vaginal birth. Cochrane Review The Cochrane Library, Issue 3. Oxford, Update Software, 1999.
13a. Carroli G, Bergel E: Umbilical vein injection for the management of retained placenta. Cochrane Review. The Cochrane Library. Oxford, Update Software, 2001.
14. Carroll D, Tramer M, McQuay H, et al: Transcutaneous electrical nerve stimulation in labour pain: A systematic review. Br J Obstet Gynaecol 104:169–175, 1997.
15. Cochrane Library (database on disk and CDROM). Oxford, Update Software, 2001.
16. Cuervo LG, Rodríguez MN, Delgado MB: Enemas during labor. Cochrane Review. The Cochrane Library. Oxford, Update Software, 2001.
17. Cunningham FG (ed): Williams Obstetrics, 20th ed. Norwalk, CT, Appleton & Lange, 1996.
18. Dewan DM, Norris MC: Pro & Con: Are epidurals better than combined spinal epidurals? Fam Pract News, January 15, 1999, p. 14.
19. Dick-Read G, Wessel H, Ellis F: Childbirth Without Fear: The Original Approach to Natural Childbirth, 5th ed. New York, Harper & Row, 1984.
20. Elbourne DR: Active vs conservative third stage management. In Enkin MW, Keirse MJNC, Renfrew MJ, Neilson JP (eds): Pregnancy and Childbirth Module. Cochrane Database of Systematic Reviews, Review No. 05352. Cochrane Updates on Disk. Oxford, Update Software, 1993.
21. Elbourne DR: Active vs. conservative third-stage management—low-risk women. In Enkin MW, Keirse MJNC, Renfrew MJ, Neilson JP (eds): Pregnancy and Childbirth Module. Cochrane Database of Systematic Reviews, Review No. 05353. Cochrane Updates on Disk. Oxford, Update Software, 1993.
23. Elbourne DR: Early umbilical cord clamping in third stage of labour. In Enkin MW, Keirse MJNC, Renfrew MJ, Neilson JP (eds): Pregnancy and Childbirth Module. Cochrane Database of Systematic Reviews, Review No. 03818. Cochrane Updates on Disk. Oxford, Update Software, 1993.
24. Elbourne DR: Prophylactic oxytocics in third stage labour. In Enkin MW, Keirse MJNC, Renfrew MJ, Neilson JP (eds): Pregnancy and Childbirth Module. Cochrane Database of Systematic Reviews, Review No. 02974. Cochrane Updates on Disk. Oxford, Update Software, 1993.
25. Elbourne D, Wiseman RA. Types of intra-muscular opioids for maternal pain relief in labour. Cochrane Review. The Cochrane Library. Oxford, Update Software, 2001.

26. Enkin MW, Keirse MJNC, Renfrew MJ, Neilson J: A Guide to Effective Care in Pregnancy and Childbirth, 2nd ed. Oxford, Oxford University Press, 1995.
27. Fenwick L: Birthing: Techniques for managing the physiologic and psychosocial aspects of childbirth. Perinat Nurs May/June:51–62, 1984.
28. Findley I, Chamberlain G: ABC of labour care—Relief of pain. BMJ 318:927–930, 1999.
29. Fraser WD, Krauss I, Turcot L, Brisson-Carrol G: Amniotomy for shortening spontaneous labour. Cochrane Review. The Cochrane Library. Oxford, Update Software, 2001.
30. Friedman EA: Labor: Clinical Evaluation and Management, 2nd ed. New York, Appleton, Century, Crofts, 1978.
31. Grant AM: EFM alone vs intermittent auscultation in labour. In Enkin MW, Keirse MJNC, Renfrew MJ, Neilson JP (eds): Pregnancy and Childbirth Module. Cochrane Database of Systematic Reviews, Review No. 03298. Cochrane Updates on Disk. Oxford, Update Software, 1993.
32. Grant AM: EFM plus scalp sampling vs intermittent auscultation in labour. In Enkin MW, Keirse MJNC, Renfrew MJ, Neilson JP (eds): Pregnancy and Childbirth Module. Cochrane Database of Systematic Reviews, Review No. 03297. Cochrane Updates on Disk. Oxford, Update Software, 1993.
33. Grant AM: EFM vs intermittent auscultation in labour. In Enkin MW, Keirse MJNC, Renfrew MJ, Neilson JP (eds): Pregnancy and Childbirth Module. Cochrane Database of Systematic Reviews, Review No. 03884. Cochrane Updates on Disk. Oxford, Update Software, 1993.
34. Grant AM: Fetal blood sampling as adjunct to heart rate monitoring. In Chalmers I (ed): Oxford Database of Perinatal Trials. Oxford, Update Software, 1992.
35. Grant AM: Liberal vs restrictive use of EFM in labour. In Enkin MW, Keirse MJNC, Renfrew MJ, Neilson JP (eds): Pregnancy and Childbirth Module. Cochrane Database of Systematic Reviews, Review No. 03885. Cochrane Updates on Disk. Oxford, Update Software, 1993.
36. Grant AM: Liberal vs restrictive use of EFM in labour (low-risk labours). In Enkin MW, Keirse MJNC, Renfrew MJ, Neilson JP (eds): Pregnancy and Childbirth Module. Cochrane Database of Systematic Reviews, Review No. 03886. Cochrane Updates on Disk. Oxford, Update Software, 1993.
37. Grant AM: Polyglycolic acid vs catgut for perineal repair. In Enkin MW, Keirse MJNC, Renfrew MJ, Neilson JP (eds): Pregnancy and Childbirth Module. Cochrane Database of Systematic Reviews, Review No. 01845. Cochrane Updates on Disk. Oxford, Update Software, 1993.
38. Grant AM: Polyglycolic acid vs. silk for perineal repair. In Chalmers I (ed): Oxford Database of Perinatal Trials. Oxford, Update Software, 1992.
39. Halliday HL: Endotracheal intubation at birth for prevention of mortality and morbidity in vigorous, meconium-stained infants born at term. Cochrane Review. The Cochrane Library. Oxford, Update Software, 2001.
40. Halpern SH, Leighton BL, Ohlsson A, et al: Effect of epidural vs. parenteral opioid on the progress of labor: A meta-analysis. JAMA 280:2105–2110, 1998.
41. Hodnett ED: Support from caregivers during childbirth. In Enkin MW, Keirse MJNC, Renfrew MJ, Neilson JP (eds): Pregnancy and Childbirth Module. Cochrane Database of Systematic Reviews, Review No. 03871. Cochrane Updates on Disk. Oxford, Update Software, 1993.
42. Hodnett ED: Caregiver support for women during childbirth. Cochrane Review. The Cochrane Library. Oxford, Update Software, 2001.
43. Hodnett ED: Home-like versus conventional institutional settings for birth. Cochrane Review. The Cochrane Library. Oxford, Update Software, 2001.
44. Hofmeyr GJ, Kulier R: Hands/knees posture in late pregnancy or labour for fetal malposition (lateral or posterior). Cochrane Review. The Cochrane Library. Oxford, Update Software, 2001.
45. Hon E: In Young D (ed): Crisis in obstetrics-the management of labor. Int J Childbirth Education August: 13–15, 1987.
46. Howell CJ: Discontinuing epidural block at 8cm dilatation. In Enkin MW, Keirse MJNC, Renfrew MJ, Neilson JP (eds): Pregnancy and Childbirth Module. Cochrane Database of Systematic Reviews, Review No. 04009. Cochrane Updates on Disk. Oxford, Update Software, 1993.
47. Howell CJ: Transcutaneous nerve stimulation (TENS) in labour. In Enkin MW, Keirse MJNC, Renfrew MJ, Neilson JP (eds): Pregnancy and Childbirth Module. Cochrane Database of Systematic Reviews, Review No. 02553. Cochrane Updates on Disk. Oxford, Update Software, 1993.
48. Howell CJ: Epidural versus non-epidural analgesia for pain relief in labour. Cochrane Review. The Cochrane Library. Oxford, Update Software, 2001.
49. Johnson K: Perineal massage shown safe, beneficial in labor. Fam Pract News 29:1, 1999.
50. Kettle C, Johanson RB: Absorbable synthetic versus catgut suture material for perineal repair. Cochrane Review. The Cochrane Library. Oxford, Update Software, 2001.
51. Kettle C, Johanson RB: Continuous versus interrupted sutures for perineal repair. Cochrane Review. The Cochrane Library. Oxford, Update Software, 2001.
52. Kitzinger S: Homebirth and Other Alternatives to Hospital. London, Dorling Kindersley, 1991.
53. Kitzinger S: Sheila Kitzinger's letter from England. Birth 18:170–171, 1991.
54. Klein MC: Walking in labor. J Fam Pract 48:229, 1999.

55. Klein MC, Gauthier RJ, Jorgensen SH, et al: Does episiotomy prevent perineal trauma and pelvic floor relaxation? Online J Curr Clin Trials [serial online] (Doc No 10), 1992.
56. Labrecque M: Randomized controlled trial of prevention of perineal trauma by perineal massage during pregnancy. Am J Obstet Gynecol 180(3 pt 1):593–600, 1999.
56a. Labrecque M, Eason E, Marloux S, et al: Randomized controlled trial of prevention of perineal trauma by perineal massage during pregnancy. Am J Obstet Gynecol 180:593–600, 1999.
57. Larimore WL, Cline MK: Keeping normal labor normal. Prim Care 27:221–236, 2000.
58. Larimore WL: Family-centered birthing: History, philosophy, and need. Fam Med 27:140–146, 1995.
59. Larimore WL: Family-centered birthing: A niche for family physicians. Am Fam Physician 47:1365–1366, 1993.
60. Larimore WL: Family-centered birthing: A style of obstetrics for family physicians. Am Fam Physician 48:725–728, 1993.
60a. Larimore WL: The role of the father in childbirth. Midwifery Today, Issue 51, 1999, pp 15–17.
61. Larimore WL, Reynolds JL: Future of family practice maternity care in America: Ruminations on reproducing an endangered species—family physicians who deliver babies. J Am Bd Fam Pract 7(6):478–488, 1994.
62. Leslie KK: Physiology of labor. In Fredrickson HL, Wilkins-Haug L (eds): Ob/Gyn Secrets, 2nd ed. Philadelphia, Hanley & Belfus, 1998.
63. Lieberman E, Lang JM, Frigoletto F, Cohen A: Epidurals and cesareans: The jury is still out. Birth 26:196-199, 1999.
64. Martensson L, Wallin G: Labour pain treated with cutaneous injections of sterile water: A randomised controlled trial. Br J Obstet Gynaecol 106:633–637, 1999.
64a. Martensson L, Nyberg K, Wallin G: Subcutaneous versus intracutaneous injections of sterile water for labor analgesia: A comparison of perceived pain during administration. Br J Obstet Gynaecol 107:1248–1251, 2000.
65. McCandlish R, Bowler U, van Asten H, et al: A randomised controlled trial of care of the perineum during second stage of normal labour. Br J Obstet Gynaecol 105:1262–1272, 1998.
66. McCandlish R, Renfrew M: Immersion in water during labor and birth: The need for evaluation. Birth 20:79–85, 1993.
67. Midmer DK: Does family-centered maternity care empower women? The development of the woman-centered childbirth model. Fam Med 24:216–221, 1992.
68. Murahata SA: Third stage of labor and postpartum hemorrhage. In Fredrickson HL, Wilkins-Haug L (eds): Ob/Gyn Secrets, 2nd ed. Philadelphia, Hanley & Belfus, 1998.
69. Natl Vital Stat Rep 47:12, 1999.
70. Nikodem VC: Immersion in water during pregnancy, labour and birth. Cochrane Review The Cochrane Library, Issue 3. Oxford, Update Software, 1999.
71. O'Driscoll K, Foley M, MacDonald D: Active management of labor as an alternative to cesarean section for dystocia. Obstet Gynecol 63:485–490, 1984.
72. Olsen O, Jewell MD: Home versus hospital birth. Cochrane Review The Cochrane Library, Issue 3. Oxford, Update Software, 1999.
73. Parisi VM: Amniotomy in labor—how helpful is it? N Engl J Med 328:1193–1194, 1993.
74. Prendiville WJ, Elbourne D, McDonald S: Active versus expectant management of the third stage of labour. Cochrane Review The Cochrane Library, Issue 3. Oxford, Update Software, 1999.
75. Pritchard JA, MacDonald PC, Gant NF (eds): Williams Obstetrics, 17th ed. Norwalk, CT, Appleton-Century-Crofts, 1985.
76. Ray KL, Hodnett ED: Caregiver support for postpartum depression. Cochrane Review The Cochrane Library, Issue 3. Oxford, Update Software, 1999.
77. Renfrew MJ: Liberal use of episiotomy for spontaneous vaginal delivery. In Enkin MW, Keirse MJNC, Renfrew MJ, Neilson JP (eds): Pregnancy and Childbirth Module. Cochrane Database of Systematic Reviews, Review No. 03695. Cochrane Updates on Disk. Oxford, Update Software, 1993.
78. Renfrew MJ: Routine perineal shaving on admission in labour. In Enkin MW, Keirse MJNC, Renfrew MJ, Neilson JP (eds): Pregnancy and Childbirth Module. Cochrane Database of Systematic Reviews, Review No. 03876. Cochrane Updates on Disk. Oxford, Update Software, 1993.
79. Reynolds JL: Intracutaneous sterile water for back pain in labor. Can Fam Physician 40:1785–1792, 1994.
80. Roberts J: Maternal position during the first stage of labour. In Chalmers I, Enkin MW, Keirse MJ (eds): Effective Care in Pregnancy and Childbirth. Oxford, Oxford University Press, 1989, pp 883–892.
81. Rosen MG, Dickinson JC, Westhoff CL: Vaginal birth after cesarean: A meta-analysis of morbidity and mortality. Obstet Gynecol 77:465–470, 1991.
82. Scherger JE: Management of normal labor and birth. Primary Care 20:713–719, 1993.
83. Scherger JE: The VBAC quandary. Am Fam Physician 47:27–28, 1993.
84. Scherger JE, Levitt C, Acheson LS, et al: Teaching family-centered perinatal care in family medicine (educational research and methods). Parts I and II. Fam Med 24:288–298, 368–374, 1992.

85. Silver R: Vaginal delivery after cesarean section. In Fredrickson HL, Wilkins-Haugh L (eds): Ob/Gyn Secrets, 2nd ed. Philadelphia, Hanley & Belfus, 1998.
86. Simpkin P, Way K: The Doulas' Contribution to Modern Maternity Care. Doulas of North America Position Paper. Seattle, WA, 1998.
87. Smith MA, Acheson LS, Byrd JE, et al: A critical review of labor and birth care (clinical review). Obstetrical Interest Group of the North American Primary Care Research Group. J Fam Pract 33:281–292, 1991.
88. Smith MA, Ruffin MT, Green LA: The thoughtful management of labor. Am Fam Physician 45:1471–1481, 1993.
89. Spiby H: Lateral tilt vs. dorsal position for second stage. In Chalmers I (ed): Oxford Database of Perinatal Trials. Oxford, Update Software, 1992.
90. Spiby H: Sustained (Valsalva) vs. exhalatory bearing down in 2nd stage of labour. In Enkin MW, Keirse MJNC, Renfrew MJ, Neilson JP (eds): Pregnancy and Childbirth Module. Cochrane Database of Systematic Reviews, Review No. 03336. Cochrane Updates on Disk. Oxford, Update Software, 1993.
91. Spiby H: Upright vs recumbent position during second stage of labour. In Enkin MW, Keirse MJNC, Renfrew MJ, Neilson JP (eds): Pregnancy and Childbirth Module. Cochrane Database of Systematic Reviews, Review No. 03335. Cochrane Updates on Disk. Oxford, Update Software, 1993.
92. Stacey L: Splash baby Charlie makes medical history. Chat, November 7, 1987.
93. Tan KH, Smyth R: Fetal vibroacoustic stimulation for facilitating tests of fetal wellbeing. Protocol for a Cochrane Review. The Cochrane Library. Oxford, Update Software, 2000.
94. Thacker SB, Stroup DF: Continuous electronic heart rate monitoring versus intermittent auscultation for assessment during labor. Cochrane Review. The Cochrane Library. Oxford, Update Software, 2001.
95. Trolle B, Moller M, Kronborg H, et al: The effect of sterile water blocks on low back pain. Am J Obstet Gynecol 164:1277–1281, 1991.
96. Wildman KM, Mohl VK, Cassel JH, et al: Intrathecal analgesia for labor. J Fam Pract 44:535–540, 1997.
97. World Health Organization: Care in Normal Birth: A Practical Guide. Report of a Technical Working Group. Publication No. WHO/FRH/HSM/96.24. Geneva, WHO, 1996.

CHAPTER 14

Management of Labor Abnormalities

SECTION A.
DYSTOCIA IN THE PRIMIGRAVID PATIENT

Matthew K. Cline, M.D.

From the 1960s to the 1990s, the cesarean section rate in the United States increased over fourfold, peaking at a rate of 22.8% in 1989 and then slowly declining to 20.7% in 1997.[1] The primary cesarean section rate for 1997 was 14.6% of births, with 6.1 percent of births occurring by repeat cesarean section. While this increase is due to multiple factors, nearly 50% of cesarean sections occur due to dystocia or difficult labor in women experiencing their first labors. After reviewing the diagnosis and potential causes of dystocia, methods of prevention and treatment options will be discussed.

I. Diagnosis of Dystocia
The diagnosis of dystocia can be made when the laboring woman is not making continual progress in cervical dilatation or fetal descent during the *active* phase of labor.

II. Causes of Dystocia
A. Inaccurate Diagnosis of Labor
When a primigravid patient presents with regular, painful contractions, the clinician is faced with the question: "Is this labor?" One leading text defines labor as "progressive dilatation of the uterine cervix in association with repetitive uterine contractions."[14] The vagueness of this definition can allow the diagnosis of labor to be made when the patient is still experiencing the latent phase of labor. One of the essential components of the active management of labor, in use at National Maternity Hospital in Dublin, Ireland since the mid-1960s, is a more specific diagnosis of labor. In the Irish model, the diagnosis of labor for the primigravid patient requires not only painful, regular contractions, but also the presence of either complete cervical effacement, spontaneous rupture of membranes, or the presence of bloody show.

Another possible approach to a specific diagnosis of labor is illustrated by McNiven et al., who evaluated the use of the specific diagnosis of labor (presence of regular, painful contractions along with cervical dilatation greater than 3 cm) in nulliparous women presenting to a hospital labor and delivery unit. Patients were randomly allocated to an "early labor assessment" group (sent home with reassurance if less than 3 cm dilated) or to usual care on the labor ward. The study found that the group with the specific diagnosis of labor had a decrease in cesarean section rates from 10.6% to 7.6%, as well as lower rates of use of oxytocin augmentation, use of any pain medications or epidurals, shorter times spent in labor, and a shortened second stage of labor by nearly 20 minutes. Women in the experimental group also had significantly higher satisfaction scores.[22]

B. Dysfunctional Labor

Inadequate contractions account for greater than 80% of instances of dystocia. This condition must be appropriately managed before arriving at a diagnosis of cephalopelvic disproportion (CPD).[5] In a review of indications for cesarean section at the University of Wisconsin, over 35% of cesareans done for the diagnosis of CPD were reclassified as being done secondary to inefficient uterine contractions.[6]

C. Cephalopelvic Disproportion

In retrospect, the diagnosis of CPD is often inaccurate; 65–85% of women successfully deliver vaginally with a trial of labor after a primary cesarean section for the diagnosis of CPD.[9] Some of the reasons for a clinical diagnosis of CPD include the following:

1. Persistent occiput posterior (OP) position (see Chapter 16, section G)

OP is the most common malposition encountered in the laboring patient, with about 15% of fetuses in this position at the onset of labor. The OP malposition increases the rates of operative vaginal delivery and cesarean section, especially in the subset that remains in the OP position (about 5% of deliveries).[15]

2. Fetal macrosomia

Incidence of cesarean section increases as a function of increasing fetal weight.[28]

3. Abnormal maternal pelvis

A maternal pelvis that is narrowed in the anterior-posterior dimension (android or platypoid) is associated with an increased risk of dystocia and diagnosis of CPD. Data from the National Maternity Hospital (Dublin) support that CPD due to maternal pelvis abnormalities is uncommon, occurring in about 1 in every 250 primigravidas.

4. Other fetal malpresentations

See Chapter 16 for a discussion of other fetal malpresentations.

5. Congenital anomalies

Anomalies that distort the anatomy of the presenting part, such as hydrocephalus or a large cystic hygroma of the fetal neck, can prevent delivery of the fetus through an otherwise adequate pelvis. While this only affects a very small percentage of deliveries, it can result in CPD.

III. Factors Associated with Dystocia

A. Prolonged Latent Phase of Labor

Many authors define a prolonged latent phase as a period of regular contractions without significant cervical dilatation lasting longer than 20 hours in the primigravida and longer than 12 hours in the multipara. While previously thought to contribute only to maternal exhaustion, a retrospective study has shown that a prolonged latent phase is associated with subsequent dystocia and an increased rate of cesarean delivery.[7]

B. Contemporary Labor Management

1. Continuous electronic fetal monitoring

As discussed in Chapter 13, section E, continuous electronic fetal monitoring (EFM) became the standard before any RCTs were conducted to determine if this technology was beneficial in low-risk women in labor. Subsequent studies have revealed that the use of continuous EFM in low-risk populations is associated with an increased incidence of dystocia and cesarean section when compared to monitoring with intermittent auscultation.[27]

2. Ambulation in labor

Settings that use continuous EFM or have high rates of epidural use (see below) often restrict the freedom of the laboring mother to move about and change position during labor.

3. Use of regional anesthesia

In many obstetrical units the use of epidural (often referred to as "regional") analgesia has increased over the last two decades. During this time, an association between epidural use and increased dystocia and cesarean section rates has been noted, with one recent retrospective trial of 1733 low-risk term nulliparas with spontaneous labor showing that the risk of cesarean section was 3.7 times higher in patients who received an epidural (one additional cesarean section noted for every 7.7 epidurals).[21]

While many maternity care providers have observed a prolonged or difficult labor in the presence of an epidural, more recent meta-analyses have come to different conclusions. Halpern et al. reported on data from 10 trials (2369 patients) that showed that there was no increase in cesarean section rates associated with epidural use, though patients with epidural had longer first stages (prolonged by 42 minutes) and second stages (prolonged by 14 minutes) of labor.[18] Women with epidurals had lower pain scores during labor and had decreased rates of dissatisfaction when compared to parenteral opioids. A recent Cochrane review of 3157 patients (11 studies) found similar results, with the first stage of labor prolonged by 140 minutes, the second stage prolonged by 12 minutes, an increased use of oxytocin augmentation (odds ratio [OR] = 1.99) and instrumented vaginal delivery (OR = 1.93), but no increase in cesarean section rates associated with epidural anesthesia.[20] While these larger meta-analyses are unlikely to resolve the controversy that exists in the area of regional anesthesia and dystocia, possible methods of minimizing the effects on the progress of labor are discussed in section IV.F.

4. Premature rupture of membranes (PROM) at term without onset of labor

This entity is discussed in greater detail in section B.

5. Management of the second stage of labor

Standard management of the second stage of labor can be associated with increased dystocia. For example, the dorsal lithotomy position impairs maternal expulsive efforts and can cause vena cava compression, which impairs blood flow to the uterus. The routine initiation of maternal pushing efforts upon complete dilatation but prior to a maternal urge to push can predispose to maternal exhaustion, especially in the presence of regional anesthesia.

IV. Prevention of Dystocia

A. Antenatal Education

Expectations of labor and delivery events among primigravidas and their families can be influenced by appropriate prenatal education. In one randomized study, a 10-minute educational meeting with a clinic nurse that centered on when to come to the hospital for labor cut the rate of outpatient hospital visits for false labor from 57% of primigravidas to 30% (number needed to treat [NNT] = 3.6, meaning one patient visit to the hospital for false labor would be prevented by having 3.6 patients receive the "treatment" of an educational nurse meeting).[4]

B. Diagnosis of Labor

See above discussion of "Inaccurate Diagnosis of Labor."

C. Maternal Support during Labor

Cochrane data reveal multiple benefits of the use of an experienced labor support person (or "doula") accompanying women in labor. With the meta-analysis including 13 trials with over 4900 patients, the presence of a doula was associated with a reduced need for medication for pain relief (OR 0.60, NNT = 9.3), operative vaginal delivery (OR 0.78, NNT = 32), reduced cesarean delivery (OR 0.77, NNT = 38), and reduced number of neonates with Apgar score below 7 at 5 minutes (OR 0.50, NNT = 83). Maternal satisfaction was also improved.[19]

D. Position Changes during Labor

A recent randomized controlled trial involving 1067 women in active labor at 36 to 41 weeks' gestation concluded that there was no evidence of harm in allowing patients to ambulate throughout labor.[16] However, many authors have discussed the multiple benefits that can occur when the laboring patient is allowed to modify her position based upon comfort. "There is good evidence that position change is useful in achieving good progress in labor, is well tolerated, and can be accomplished safely. Position change may be more important than a single 'best' position."[26]

While many labor units still use the dorsal lithotomy position for delivery (mainly due to caregiver convenience), there is evidence to suggest significant benefits of other positions. Upright delivery reduces the lumbar lordosis and directs the fetal head toward the outlet of the pelvis rather than directly into the posterior aspect of the pubis. Additionally, gravity can add up to 35 mmHg to the pressure exerted by the presenting part when the mother is upright during delivery.[11]

E. Intermittent Monitoring during Labor

The Cochrane review of trials involving over 50,000 patients comparing intermittent monitoring to continuous fetal monitoring concluded the following: compared to intermittent auscultation, routine electronic fetal monitoring was associated with a decreased risk of a 1-minute Apgar score less than 4 (relative risk [RR] of 0.82; 95% confidence interval [CI] of 0.65–0.98); NNT = 167) and a decreased risk of neonatal seizures (RR = 0.50, 95% CI 0.30–0.82; NNT = 500). However, results from different studies were heterogeneous. No significant differences were seen in 1-minute Apgar scores less than 7, rate of admissions to neonatal intensive care units, and perinatal death. Electronic fetal monitoring was associated with an increased rate of cesarean delivery (RR = 1.33, 95% confidence interval 1.08 to 1.59) [NNH = 42] and total operative delivery (RR = 1.23, 95% CI 1.15–1.31; NNH = 50).[27]

F. Analgesia

The controversy that exists in the medical literature concerning epidural use and increased rates of cesarean section is discussed in section III.B.3 above. However, the meta-analyses that show no increase in the cesarean section rate with regional anesthesia do reveal that epidural use is associated with a prolonged first and second stages of labor and an increase in the rate of assisted vaginal delivery. For patients who request pharmacologic methods of pain relief, patient satisfaction is higher and pain scores during labor are lower with epidural analgesia compared to parenteral opioid analgesia.[4] With this in mind, are there specific steps that can be taken to minimize the potential for dystocia and cesarean delivery with epidural use? Lieberman et al., in a retrospective study of over 1700 nulliparas in spontaneous labor, found that the risk of cesarean section was highest in patients who received epidural anesthesia before dilating to 5 cm or descending to –1 station,[21] suggesting that delaying the use of regional anesthesia when possible may decrease the risk of dystocia. The effects of delayed initiation of epidural anesthesia on the duration of labor are uncertain.

G. Persistent OP position

Using ultrasound to determine fetal presentation revealed that while 5% of vaginal deliveries occur in the OP position, 62% of these mothers began with the fetus OA and rotation into the OP position occurred during labor. Additionally, 87% of fetuses who started labor in the OP position rotated to OA during labor.[15]

One factor identified in spontaneous rotation of the OP is the levator sling, which can enhance flexion and thus the likelihood of rotation as the fetus descends. With epidural analgesia, motor blockade can occur, thus decreasing the possibility of spontaneous rotation of the fetal head. Manual rotation techniques (see section

V.C.1.b below) generally attempt to replicate the forces provided by the levator sling and pelvic floor while adding a rotational component.

What can be done in labor to enhance spontaneous rotation? When the fetus is in the OP position, supine maternal positions encourage extension of the fetal head into the hollow of the sacrum. Having the mother curl forward at the hips will increase the force encouraging flexion of the head and present the smaller suboccipitobregmatic diameter of the fetal head to the pelvic outlet. Pelvic rocking (tilting the pelvis back and forth with the mother on her hands and knees) also can help rotate the OP fetus, as well as the use of an exaggerated lateral Sims position with the fetal spine positioned upward.[11]

V. Treatment
A. Prolonged Latent Phase
Women experiencing a prolonged latent phase (defined as over 20 hours in nulliparas) often respond best to therapeutic rest. Choices for this include morphine sulfate or other narcotics given in sufficient dose to allow the patient to sleep. The vast majority of patients will awaken in active labor, while about 10–15% will have stopped contracting and were in false labor.[8] The Irish model uses an antepartum ward where patients contracting but not in labor can be observed and treated for 12 hours before being sent home.

B. Stage One Management
1. Amniotomy
Patients treated with amniotomy early in labor have been noted to have a decreased incidence of dystocia, faster labors, and no change in neonatal outcomes. The decrease in dystocia was most pronounced in patients dilated 3 cm or more at the time of amniotomy.[12]

2. Oxytocin augmentation
Table 1 compares current low-, intermediate-, and high-dose oxytocin protocols. The low- and high-dose protocols are those suggested by ACOG in their technical bulletin[10]; the high-dose regimen is very similar to the standard oxytocin protocol used at the National Maternity Hospital in Dublin. Use of higher doses of oxytocin alone have not been shown to significantly decrease cesarean section, as an infusion rate of 8 mU/min or less is sufficient to treat dysfunctional labor 85% of the time.[23] ACOG also states that during augmentation with oxytocin, fetal well-being "should be assessed electronically or by auscultation and recorded every 15 minutes during the first stage of labor and every 5 minutes during the second stage of labor."

3. Fetal heart rate monitoring
As discussed in Chapter 13, section E, use of continuous electronic fetal monitoring in low-risk populations is associated with an increased incidence of dystocia and cesarean section. Unless there are specific indications for continuous monitoring, intermittent auscultation should be encouraged for all women in labor.

4. Monitoring the progress of labor
Most authorities consider active-phase labor arrest to occur when the cervix has not dilated despite 2 hours of active labor. This 2-hour "magic number" may

TABLE 1. Oxytocin Protocols[10,16]

Regimen	Initial Dose	Increase Increment	Dosage Interval	Maximum Dose
Low-dose	0.5–1 mU/min	1.0 mU/min	30–40 min	20 mU/min
Intermediate-dose	2 mU/min	2.0 mU/min	15 min	None
High-dose	6 mU/min	3–6 mU/min	20–40 min	42 mU/min

indeed need revision, based upon a recent study of active-phase labor arrest. Rouse et al. treated 542 women diagnosed with arrest (cervix at least 4 cm dilated with less than 1 cm of change in 2 hours) with oxytocin using a goal of obtaining at least 200 Montevideo units for at least 4 hours before considering cesarean delivery. Ninety-seven percent of parous women and 88% of nulliparas delivered vaginally (overall vaginal delivery rate 92%). In this population, the cesarean section rate would have been 26% if all patients had been operatively delivered when active-phase arrest was diagnosed. Based on the use of the 4-hour protocol, the overall cesarean section rate was 8%. In this population, the epidural rate was 96% in nulliparas and 89% in primiparas; patients were delivered by cesarean for failure to progress after the 4 hours of oxytocin, for non-vertex presentation, or for non-reassuring fetal heart tones.[23]

C. **Stage Two Management**
1. Persistent occiput posterior position
   a. Encourage position changes: This increases the chance of rotation.
   b. Attempt a manual rotation: Generally, this maneuver is attempted after the cervix is completely dilated with the presenting part on or near the pelvic floor; the goal of the operator is to recreate the forces of the levator sling while adding a slight rotational force. Selecting the appropriate hand (right hand for LOP, and left hand for ROP), the operator places the fingers of the hand together and slides them gently behind the fetal occiput. With a subsequent contraction, the patient is instructed to bear down while the fetus's head is slightly elevated, flexed, and then rotated in the appropriate direction (counterclockwise for LOP and clockwise for ROP). If the fetus rotates to OA, labor can be allowed to continue spontaneously, and a rapid delivery may follow. If partial rotation occurs, the maneuver can be repeated; if there is significant resistance to rotation, further efforts at manual rotation should not be made (see Chapter 16, section G).
   c. Vaginally assisted delivery: Attempt a vacuum-assisted or forceps-assisted delivery when the presenting part is below +2 station if maternal exhaustion occurs. Assisted vaginal deliveries can attempt to deliver the infant in an OP position (see Chapter 17, section D), although the potential for a failed operative vaginal delivery is greater than with an occiput anterior position.
   d. Rotational rorceps: Use of forceps for rotation to OA is possible, *but should be limited to operators with sufficient skill and experience with the technique of mid-forceps rotation.* Cesarean section is often the preferred method of delivery for a persistent OP in the presence of failure to descend during the second stage.
2. Pushing strategies
   a. Delay pushing until the fetal head is on the pelvic floor or until the urge to push is felt.
   b. Vary maternal pushing positions.
   c. Avoid pushing in the dorsal lithotomy position.
3. Use of oxytocin
Theoretical concerns have been raised about the ability of epidural analgesia to block certain neural reflexes that enhance pushing during the second stage (most notably Ferguson's reflex, whereby vaginal distention during the second stage increases oxytocin secretion). Observational studies using intrauterine pressure catheters have demonstrated decreased intrauterine pressures during the second stage when regional anesthesia is used.[25] In a randomized controlled trial of

starting oxytocin in the second stage of patients laboring with an epidural in place, Saunders et al. noted lower rates of operative vaginal delivery (NNT = 12) in the oxytocin group along with lower cesarean section rates (NNT = 65) and fewer second-degree lacerations. Infant outcomes were similar.[24]

D. Cephalopelvic Disproportion (CPD)

Clinicians should have a high index of suspicion for a higher incidence of dystocia with macrosomic infants, particularly if a contracted maternal pelvis is present. Neither x-ray nor computed tomography pelvimetry has been shown to be a reliable predictor of CPD. In the setting of appropriate use of oxytocin to rule out dysfunctional labor, CPD can be diagnosed when there is lack of fetal descent to a station of +1 or lower despite complete (or near-complete) cervical dilatation and in the absence of malrotation.

VI. Evidence to Support Active Management of Labor (AML)

Several early trials of various portions of active management showed decreased rates of dystocia and cesarean intervention, but did not evaluate the entire protocol. The largest U.S. trial of AML involved nearly 2000 patients and attempted to incorporate all aspects of the Irish model. This study failed to show a significant difference in cesarean section rates, although labors were nearly 2 hours shorter in the study group.[13] This study, however, did use continuous electronic fetal monitoring and epidural analgesia. A meta-analysis of the three best North American studies of AML shows a decrease in primary cesarean section rate of 34% (OR 0.66 with CI 0.54–0.81) without adverse fetal outcome. Along with subsequent decreases in patients who choose repeat cesarean rather than vaginal birth in their next pregnancy, widespread use of AML would be expected to decrease total cesarean section rate by 13%.[17]

VII. Summary

As dystocia in the primigravid is a relatively common problem, clinicians should have focused strategies for its management when it occurs. Awareness of factors that can cause dystocia can allow their avoidance in certain instances. A comprehensive understanding of the recognition, treatment and prevention of dystocia in the primigravid patient should increase the probability of a safe vaginal delivery.

References

1. Anderson RN, Ventura SJ, Peters KD, et al: Births and deaths: United States, July 1996–June 1997. Monthly Vital Statistics Report Vol. 46, No. 12, Suppl. 2. Hyattsville, MD, National Center for Health Statistics, 1998.
2. Bates RG, Helm CW, Duncan A, et al: Uterine activity in the second stage of labour and the effect of epidural analgesia. Br J Obstet Gynaecol 92:1246–1250, 1985.
3. Bloom SL, McIntire DD, Kelly MA, et al: Lack of effect of walking on labor and delivery. N Engl J Med 339:76–79, 1998.
4. Bonovich L: Recognizing the onset of labor. J Obstet Gynecol Neonat Nurs 19:141–145, 1990.
5. Boylan PC, Parisi VM: Effect of active management on latent phase labor. Am J Perinatol 7:363–365, 1990.
6. Byrd JE, Lytton DE, Vogt SC, et al: Diagnostic criteria and the management of dystocia. J Fam Pract 27:595–599, 1988.
7. Chelmow D, Kilpatrick SJ, Laros RK: Maternal and neonatal outcomes after prolonged latent phase. Obstet Gynecol 81:486–491, 1993.
8. Cohen WR, Acker DB, Friedman EA (eds): Management of Labor, 2nd ed. Rockville, MD, Aspen Publishers, 1989, pp 13–14.
9. Duff P, Southmayd K, Read JA: Outcome of trial of labor in patients with a single previous low transverse cesarean section for dystocia. Obstet Gynecol 71:380–383, 1988.
10. Dystocia and the Augmentation of Labor. ACOG Technical Bulletin Number 218, December 1995, p 5.
11. Fenwick L, Simkin P: Maternal positioning to prevent or alleviate dystocia in labor. Clin Obstet Gynecol 30:83–89, 1987.

12. Fraser WD, Marcoux S, Moutquin MM, et al: Effect of early amniotomy on the risk of dystocia in nulliparous women. N Engl J Med 328:1145–1149, 1993.

13. Frigoletto F, Leiberman E, Long J, et al: A clinical trial of active management of labor. N Engl J Med 333:745–750, 1995.

14. Gabbe SG, Niebyl JR, Simpson JL (eds): Obstetrics: Normal and Problem Pregnancies, 3rd ed. New York, Churchill Livingstone, 1996, p 371.

15. Gardberg M, Laakkonen E, Salevaara M: Intrapartum sonography and persistent occiput posterior position: A study of 408 deliveries. Obstet Gynecol 91:746–749, 1998.

16. Gerhardstein LP, Allswede MT, Sloan CT, et al: Reduction in the rate of cesarean birth with active management of labor and intermediate-dose oxytocin. J Reprod Med 40:4–8, 1995.

17. Glantz JC, McNanley TJ: Active management of labor: A meta-analysis of cesarean delivery rates for dystocia in nulliparas. Obstet Gynecol Surv 52:497–505, 1997.

18. Halpern SH, Leighton BL, Ohlsson A, et al: Effect of epidural's parenteral opioid analgesia on the progress of labor. JAMA 280:2105–2110, 1998.

19. Hodnett ED: Caregiver's support for women during childbirth (Cochrane Review). In The Cochrane Library, Issue 4, 2000. Oxford, Update Software, 1999.

20. Howell CJ: Epidural versus non-epidural analgesia for pain relief in labour (Cochrane Review). In The Cochrane Library, Issue 4, 2000. Oxford, Update Software, 1999.

21. Lieberman E, Lang JM, Cohen A, et al: Association of epidural analgesia with cesarean delivery in nulliparas. Obstet Gynecol 88:993–1000, 1996.

22. McNiven PS, Williams JI, Hodnett E, et al: An early labor assessment program: A randomized, controlled trial. Birth 25:5–10, 1998.

23. Rouse DJ, Owen J, Hauth JC: Active-phase labor arrest: Oxytocin augmentation for a least 4 hours. Obstet Gynecol 93:323–328, 1999.

24. Saunders NJ, Spiby H, Gilbert L, et al: Oxytocin infusion during second stage of labour in primiparous women using epidural analgesia: A randomised double-blind placebo controlled trial. BMJ 299:1423–1426, 1989.

25. Seitchik J, Holden AE, Castillo M: Amniotomy and oxytocin treatment of functional dystocia and the route of delivery. Am J Obstet Gynecol 155:585–592, 1986.

26. Smith MI, Acheson LS, Byrd JA, et al: A critical review of labor and birth care. J Fam Pract 33:281–292, 1991.

27. Thacker SB, Stroup DF: Continuous electronic heart rate monitoring versus intermittent auscultation for assessment during labor (Cochrane Review). In The Cochrane Library, Issue 4, 2000. Oxford, Update Software.

28. Turner MJ, Rasmussen MJ, Turner JE, et al: The influence of birth weight on labor in nulliparas. Obstet Gynecol 76:159–163, 1990.

SECTION B.
PRELABOR RUPTURE OF MEMBRANES AT TERM

Janis E. Byrd, M.D.

Spontaneous rupture of membranes before the onset of labor remains a controversial area in maternity care, with no consensus on when and how (or even if) labor should be induced. This is due both to fears of infectious morbidity, cord prolapse, increased operative delivery, and to lack of current randomized controlled trials (RCTs) that address length of the latent phase, method of induction, and use of prophylactic antibiotics.

I. Epidemiology

The incidence of ruptured membranes before labor (any gestational age) is 6–19%, occurring in about 8% of pregnancies at term. The incidence varies depending on the definition in relation to the onset of contractions, the population being studied, and whether term is defined as 36 or 37 weeks of gestation. A recent RCT found that 95% of women with term prelabor rupture of membranes (PROM) go into spontaneous labor and deliver within 28 hours.[7] Only 2% to 5% of women remain undelivered at 72 hours. Grant and Keirse[4] suggest that the latter group is probably at high risk for either underlying dystocia or deficient prostaglandin production.

II. Etiology

PROM may occur in the absence of recognized risk factors. It may often be a normal variant as the membranes undergo changes near term that lead to weakening. If a pathologic cause is present, it is most likely inflammatory or infectious in nature. Associations exist with urinary tract infection, sexually transmitted diseases (STDs), group B streptococcal colonization, bacterial vaginosis, and cigarette smoking.[1] Amniocentesis studies after PROM have shown that about one third are positive for bacteria. Eighty-eight percent are positive for bacteria after labor begins, although neither mother nor infant shows clinical signs of infection in most cases. Other associations with term PROM include polyhydramnios, multiple gestation, incompetent cervix, cerclage, prior conization, abruptio placentae, and amniocentesis.

III. Diagnosis

A. History and Physical Examination

Accurate assessment of gestational age using all available data is essential as the first step of evaluation and management. The diagnosis of rupture is based on history of passage of watery fluid and confirmed by sterile speculum examination. The cervical os may be inspected for dilatation during speculum examination, but unless immediate induction is planned, a digital examination should *not* be performed as part of the initial evaluation. Visualization of fluid in the posterior vagina is the strongest supporting evidence. The fluid may be tested with nitrazine paper for the typical blue alkaline reaction and examined under the microscope for a ferning pattern. Cervical mucus, blood, semen, bacterial vaginosis, and alkaline antiseptics are common causes of a false-positive nitrazine reaction. Care should be taken to avoid the cervical os when collecting fluid. False-positive ferning patterns can occur but are less frequent. With prolonged leakage, a pool of fluid may not be visible, and false-negative ferning and nitrazine reactions can occur. Gentle fundal pressure may produce some additional fluid. Other common causes of "leaking fluid" include urinary incontinence, vaginitis/cervicitis, cervical mucous from dilatation, bloody show, or semen. The patient also should be assessed for signs of chorioamnionitis, such as fever, uterine tenderness, or malodorous discharge (see Chapter 15, section C).

B. Electronic Fetal Heart Rate (FHR) Monitoring

Fetal heart rate (FHR) monitoring should be used to assess fetal well-being and rule out cord compression. Fetal tachycardia or loss of reactivity may precede maternal fever as indicators of chorioamnionitis.

C. Ultrasound

Ultrasound examination is not a routine part of PROM assessment but, if being done for other reasons such as a biophysical profile, may add further evidence for or against the diagnosis. In the absence of urinary tract malformation or growth restriction, a decreased amniotic fluid volume supports the diagnosis of rupture. Ultrasound also may confirm contraindications to induction such as malpresentation or placenta previa.

D. Laboratory Studies

During speculum exam cultures may be obtained for gonorrhea and chlamydia if there is any suspicion for these STDs. Group B streptococcus culture can be obtained if the carrier status of the patient is unknown. A urinalysis and urine culture are obtained in the evaluation of preterm PROM or for patients with symptoms suggestive of urinary tract infections (UTIs) or history of previous infections. Vaginal fluid may also be collected to test for pulmonary maturity if there is uncertainty that the gestational age is 37 weeks or greater. Phosphatidyl glycerol is more reliable in vaginal fluid than the lecithin-to-sphingomyelin ratio.

IV. Management

A. Induction versus Expectant Management

Active versus conservative management of the term pregnancy with PROM remains much in controversy. Grant and Keirse[4] found in their analysis of studies that were not randomized that active management with oxytocin was associated with an increase in cesarean delivery and postpartum endometritis rates without improving neonatal infectious outcomes.

B. Method of Induction

Six RCTs with acceptable methodology demonstrated that the use of prostaglandin E_2 versus oxytocin to actively manage term PROM yielded comparable results.[6] A recent meta-analysis of three management schemes compared induction by vaginal or endocervical prostaglandin E_2 versus immediate oxytocin induction versus conservative management (waiting or delayed oxytocin induction).[9] They found no differences in cesarean deliveries or neonatal infections. Vaginal prostaglandins resulted in more chorioamnionitis than immediate oxytocin (OR 1.55, 95% CI 1.09–2.21), but less chorioamnionitis than conservative management (OR 0.68, 95% CI 0.51–0.91). Immediate oxytocin induction resulted in fewer cases of chorioamnionitis (OR 0.67, 95% CI 0.52–0.85) and endometritis (OR 0.71, 95% CI 0.51–0.99) than conservative management but did not achieve significance with all measures. The Cochrane Library concludes that women with PROM at term who have labor induced with oxytocin have a lower risk of chorioamnionitis (OR 0.63, 95% CI 0.51–0.78, NNT = 37) and endometritis (OR 0.72, 95% CI 0.52–0.99, NNT = 110), and possibly a lower risk of neonatal infection (OR 0.64, 95% CI 0.44–0.95, NNT = 125) and newborn ICU admissions (OR 0.63, 95% CI 0.52–0.76, NNT = 20). Women undergoing oxytocin induction do have an increased use of epidural anesthesia and internal fetal monitoring.[10]

C. Prophylactic Antibiotics

RCTs with currently used antibiotics in term patients do not exist. The American College of Obstetricians and Gynecologists (ACOG) has recommended the use of prophylactic intrapartum antibiotics for women with PROM > 18 hours.[1] Other indications for the use of prophylactic antibiotics include documented infection with group B streptococcus or a known STD and preterm PROM (see Chapter 11, section H). Women with term PROM who undergo subsequent cesarean section also benefit from the use of prophylactic antibiotics.

D. Recommendations

If the diagnosis of term PROM is confirmed and there is no evidence of maternal infection or fetal distress, management can be either active or expectant for 24–72 hours. However, patients should undergo informed consent regarding the increased risk of maternal and neonatal infections should they opt for conservative or expectant management. Home management, if the obstetric and social situation permit, is most cost-effective. The patient should be instructed about signs of infection, daily fetal kick counts, and temperature-taking.[2,3,8] Clinicians choosing to manage term PROM expectantly should consider the use of intrapartum antibiotic prophylaxis given the current ACOG recommendation.[1] Since conservative management using prophylactic antibiotics has not been studied in RCTs, the clinician may opt for a variety of regimens including intravenous penicillin or ampicillin (that will probably require inpatient status) or the use of long-acting intramuscular cephalosporins such as ceftriaxone.

V. Prevention and Patient Education

Attempts should be made to modify risk factors, such as smoking. Routine screening for STDs should be done, infections treated, and follow-up cultures done for test of cure.

VI. Summary
Most cases of PROM occur at term. Antibiotics may be useful if there is a known or suspected cervical, vaginal, or urinary pathogen. Prophylactic antibiotics should be administered in the setting of PROM if a cesarean section occurs or labor is prolonged greater than 18 hours. Active versus expectant management in the absence of chorioamnionitis or nonreassuring fetal tracing remains an area of controversy, although expectant management results in more maternal and neonatal infections. Oxytocin induction also results in less perinatal infection than does the use of prostaglandin induction. No digital cervical examination should be performed before the onset of labor unless immediate induction is planned.

References
1. American College of Obstetricians and Gynecologists: Premature rupture of membranes. Practice Bulletin No. 1. Washington DC, American College of Obstetricians and Gynecologists, 1998.
2. Duff P, Huff RW, Gibbs RS: Management of premature rupture of membranes and unfavorable cervix in term pregnancy. Obstet Gynecol 63:597–702, 1984.
3. Fayez JA, Jasan AA, Jonas HS, et al: Management of premature rupture of the membranes. Obstet Gynecol 52:17–21, 1978.
4. Grant J, Keirse MHNC: Prelabour rupture of the membranes at term. In Chalmers I (ed): Effective Care in Pregnancy and Childbirth. Oxford, Oxford University Press, 1989, pp 1111–1117.
5. Hannah ME: Active management of prelabour rupture of membranes at 37+ weeks. In Enkin M, Keirse MJNC, Renfrew MJ, Neilson JP (eds): Pregnancy and Childbirth Module. Cochrane Database of Systematic Reviews, Review No. 03272. Cochrane Updates on Disk. Oxford, Update Software, 1994.
6. Hannah ME: Prostaglandins vs. oxytocin for prelabour rupture of membranes at 37+ weeks. In Enkin M, Keirse MJNC, Renfrew MJ, Neilson JP (eds): Pregnancy and Childbirth Module. Cochrane Database of Systematic Reviews, Review No. 03273. Cochrane Updates on Disk. Oxford, Update Software, 1994.
7. Hannah ME, Ohlsson A, Farine D, et al: Induction of labor compared with expectant management for prelabor rupture of the membranes at term. N Engl J Med 334:1005–1010, 1996.
8. Morales WJ, Lazar AJ: Expectant management of rupture of the membranes at term. South Med J 79:955–958, 1986.
9. Mozurkewich EL, Wolf FM: Premature rupture of membranes at term: A meta-analysis of three management schemes. Obstet Gynecol 89:1035–1043, 1997.
10. Tan BP, Hannah ME: Oxytocin for prelabor rupture of membranes at or near term (Cochrane Review). The Cochrane Library, Issue 4, 2000. Oxford, Update Software.

SECTION C.
INDUCTION OF LABOR

Janis E. Byrd, M.D.

The relative benefits of induction of labor versus possible adverse consequences must be addressed before a discussion of methods. Unfortunately, research is concentrated on the latter, and solid information is lacking on the relative merits versus possible harm of induction in various clinical situations. Reduction in maternal and fetal morbidity and mortality are the primary outcomes to be assessed in deciding if the procedure is indicated, but maternal and family preference, pain and discomfort, length of labor, patient and physician exhaustion, and cost also are important factors in the decision.[5,6]

I. Indications
A. Maternal Indications[1]
These indications are uncommon, but include the following:
1. Psychological distress from fetal demise
2. Severe hypertensive disease
3. Other maternal medical problems, such as diabetes mellitus or renal, pulmonary, or cardiac disease
4. Risk of precipitous labor or distance from the hospital

B. Fetal Indications

The following conditions are associated with an increased incidence of uteroplacental insufficiency. Antenatal surveillance is carried out to monitor these conditions and is discussed in Chapter 10.

1. Postterm pregnancies
2. Maternal hypertensive disease
3. Diabetes mellitus
4. Premature rupture of membranes
5. Chorioamnionitis
6. Oligohydramnios
7. Intrauterine growth restriction
8. Rh sensitization

II. Relative Contraindications to Induction of Labor[1]

A. Obstetric

1. Placenta or vasa previa
2. Abnormal lie or presentation
3. Prior classic incision
4. Pelvic abnormalities
5. Presenting part above inlet

B. Medical

1. Active genital herpes
2. Invasive cervical cancer
3. Allergy or other contraindication to the induction agent

III. Problems of Induction[10]

A. Definition of Success

Successful induction is defined as progressive cervical dilatation leading to successful vaginal delivery within 24 hours (some use 12 hours). Production of regular uterine contractions is not always synonymous with successful induction. Most studies exclude women who require subsequent cesarean section (regardless of cervical change) or those requiring a second induction.

B. Induction and Associated Outcomes

Induction of labor is not as hazardous as once thought. As Figure 1 indicates, most intermediate outcomes are not affected except for a decreased incidence of meconium-stained fluid. There is a non-significant trend for reduction in cesarean section rates. Perinatal mortality is improved only in pregnancies lasting longer than 41 weeks' gestation (see Chapter 10, section C).

IV. Cervical Readiness

A firm, rigid cervix may require 3–4 times the amount of uterine contractility to produce dilatation as a soft, compliant cervix. Therefore, the state of the cervix is the most important factor in the success or failure of induction. Bishop's (Table 2) and other scoring systems to predict inducibility are based primarily on cervical consistency, length, position, and dilatation, but these elements are interrelated and may not have the same predictive value. These systems rely on digital examination, which is highly subjective. The Bishop score was originally applied to multiparas only.

V. Cervical Ripening

The goal of cervical ripening is to prevent prolonged induction and reduce the rate of failed inductions, cesarean sections, and febrile complications. Attempts to soften the cervix pharmacologically before induction are based on the assumption that this will

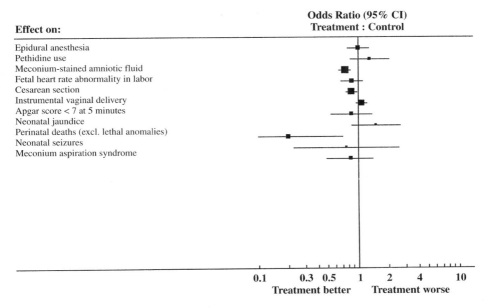

Odds Ratio (95% CI)
Treatment : Control

Effect on:

Epidural anesthesia
Pethidine use
Meconium-stained amniotic fluid
Fetal heart rate abnormality in labor
Cesarean section
Instrumental vaginal delivery
Apgar score < 7 at 5 minutes
Neonatal jaundice
Perinatal deaths (excl. lethal anomalies)
Neonatal seizures
Meconium aspiration syndrome

0.1   0.3 0.5   1   2   4   10
Treatment better   Treatment worse

FIGURE 1. Elective induction of labor at or beyond term (19 trials reviewed). (From Crowley P: Elective induction of labour at or beyond term. In Enkin MW, Keirse MJNC, Renfrew MJ, Neilson JP (eds): Pregnancy and Childbirth Module. Cochrane Database of Systematic Reviews, Review No. 04142. Cochrane Update on Disk. Oxford, Update Software, 1994, with permission.)

have the same significance as if softening occurred physiologically. Cervical changes are not merely mechanical but involve chemical changes in the collagen and proteoglycan matrix, increase in edema and vascularity, and increase in leukocytes and macrophages.

A. Prostaglandins and Cervical Ripening[10]

Prostaglandins were initially noted to soften the cervix without inducing labor when used in second-trimester terminations. At term, about half of treated patients will go into labor and deliver within 24 hours. Twenty-five of 27 trials comparing prostaglandins with placebo or no treatment found that labor occurred more frequently before induction in the group receiving prostaglandins. There was a statistically significant difference between groups with more women in the prostaglandin group having adequate cervical change.

1. Route of administration

These trials were not large enough to draw definite conclusions but seem to suggest some superiority of the endocervical route, with more women going into labor and delivering during ripening and decreased rate of cesarean birth. An advantage

TABLE 2. Bishop Scoring

	0	1	2	3
Dilatation	0	1–2	3–4	5–6
Effacement	0–30	40–50	60–70	80
Station	−3	−2	−1	+1, +2
Consistency	Firm	Medium	Soft	—
Position	Posterior	Mid	Anterior	

Inducibility: 5 = multipara, 7 = primipara.

to the vaginal insert is the ability to remove it by the tail if hyperstimulation occurs. Attempts to wash out vaginal gels are ineffective.

2. Prostaglandins and uterine hyperstimulation

Uterine hypertonus or hyperstimulation occurred more often in prostaglandin-treated women than in women with placebo or no treatment.

3. Fetal heart rate abnormalities

Fetal heart rate abnormalities occurred more frequently but did not reach statistical significance.

4. Effect on cesarean intervention

Cesarean section was performed more often during ripening in the prostaglandin-treated group.

5. Use of epidural anesthesia

The use of epidural anesthesia was lower in the prostaglandin-treated women, although few studies reported on this outcome.

6. Outcomes

Successful induction, as defined previously, was significantly better for prostaglandin-treated women.

     a. Cesarean intervention: There was also a statistically significant reduction in the cesarean birth rate with prostaglandin treatment compared with placebo or no treatment and a decrease in the instrumental vaginal delivery rate. The increased cesarean section rate during ripening was offset by a decreased rate during labor.

     b. Postpartum hemorrhage: Seven trials with 500 women did not show any influence on the incidence of postpartum hemorrhage.

     c. Data on various infant outcome measures did not show any influence of cervical ripening.

7. Vaginal versus endocervical prostaglandins

Two RCTs compared vaginal versus endocervical prostaglandins. These trials were not large enough to draw definite conclusions but suggest superiority of the endocervical route, with more women going into labor and delivering during ripening and decreased rate of cesarean birth. An advantage to the vaginal insert is the ability to remove it by the tail if hyperstimulation occurs. Attempts to wash out vaginal gels are ineffective.

8. Types of prostaglandins

Prostaglandin E_2 has replaced prostaglandin $F_{2\alpha}$ because of its increased potency and, therefore, lower dose required. Trials did not show any clinically important differences otherwise.

B. Other Methods of Cervical Ripening

Estrogen, oxytocin, relaxin, and mechanical methods, such as laminaria or tents, have not been useful approaches to ripening of the cervix.[10]

     1. Breast stimulation

This technique, when done for 3 hours a day for 3 consecutive days, in two different trials showed that women were more likely to go into labor than the control group.[10]

     2. Prostaglandin plus intracervical Foley catheter

Perry[13] found prostaglandin gel plus intracervical Foley catheter superior to intravaginal prostaglandin alone with interval to ripening of 7.5 hours versus 12 hours (p < 0.01), and delivery of 90% versus 69% in 24 hours.

VI. Methods of Induction[9]
A. Stripping/Sweeping the Membranes

This maneuver results in increased prostaglandin production proportional to the area of detachment. The Cochrane Review summarizing the results of 6 RCTs demonstrated that stripping of the membranes results in a 9% absolute risk reduction in the need for formal induction (OR 0.58, C.I. 0.43–0.79, NNT = 11).[4] A potential risk of accidental rupture of membranes or bleeding from undiagnosed previa exists with this method.

B. Amniotomy

1. High amniotomy

Amniotomy with the presenting part above the pelvic inlet has not been assessed by RCTs. The potential danger is that of umbilical cord prolapse. If the clinician decides that the increased risk of cord prolapse as a result of a high amniotomy is justified by the potential benefits, a controlled amniotomy using a pudendal block needle that is protected by a trumpet may be a safer route to pursue.

2. Low amniotomy

This procedure that ruptures the presenting forebag is the usual method. Results are variable; greater than 50% of both primiparas and multiparas are in labor within 12 hours. A disadvantage of this method is irrevocable commitment to delivery although 15–25% of women are still not in labor after 24 hours following premature rupture of the membranes (PROM). Cord prolapse can still occur with low amniotomy. Assessment of the station of the vertex and application of the head to the cervix should be done before amniotomy, and fetal heart tones should be monitored during the procedure.

C. Amniotomy plus Oxytocin

Two RCTs showed that more women delivered at both 12 and 24 hours when oxytocin was started within a few hours compared with amniotomy without oxytocin.[9] At 12 hours, 32–36.5% of the oxytocin group were delivered compared with 14–16.4% of the amniotomy-only group. There were also decreases in the cesarean and forceps delivery rates and a decreased incidence of postpartum hemorrhage when oxytocin was started early. The one RCT that compared oxytocin alone found fewer women in labor at 6 hours versus those who also had amniotomy.[9] This trial did not find differences in percentages delivered within 24 or 48 hours or in the cesarean rate.

D. Oral, Intracervical, and Vaginal Prostaglandins

1. Prostaglandin E_2 versus $F_{2\alpha}$

A number of RCTs indicate that the use of prostaglandins versus oxytocin is associated with a higher rate of successful induction and vaginal delivery within 12 hours but none as yet have FDA approval for this indication.[8] A wide range of doses,[18] vehicles, and routes of administration as well as differences in parity, cervical scoring, time for ripening and subsequent methods of induction characterize these studies. Prostaglandin E_2 has replaced prostaglandin $F_{2\alpha}$ because of its increased potency. However, the latter was used in 5 of the previously quoted studies and prostaglandin E_1 was used in one study.

2. Prostaglandin E_1 (misoprostol)

Misoprostol is an attractive agent because of its decreased cost, apparent increased efficacy, and availability of oral preparations. Increased patient satisfaction and possible decreased charting for nursing compared to oxytocin infusions also make this a favorable alternative. In September 2000, the manufacturer announced it did not intend to do further research for this indication and warned providers against off-label use. The oral form has subsequently been removed from the market.

    a. Efficacy of misoprostol: Sanchez-Ramos et al.,[14] in a meta-analysis of RCTs from 1986 to 1995 found a lower cesarean rate (15% vs. 21.5%) and a 5-hour reduction in time from first dose to delivery. Eighty-four percent of patients developed active labor with only 35% requiring oxytocin.

    b. Misoprostol (prostaglandin E_1) versus dinoprostone (E_2): Several studies[3,11,12,15,16,17] have compared vaginal misoprostol to either intracervical or intravaginal E_2 (dinoprostone). Vaginal misoprostol increased the rate of cervical ripening, decreased time in labor, and decreased use of oxytocin. All found increased rates of tachysystole but no significant differences in maternal or neonatal outcomes.

c. Oxytocin versus vaginal misoprostol: Kramer[7] compared vaginal misoprostol to oxytocin and found a decrease in cesarean section for dystocia and decreased use of epidural anesthesia.

d. Vaginal misoprostol versus conventional methods of induction: Windrim[21] compared vaginal misoprostol to various standard induction methods and found no difference in time to vaginal birth, cesarean birth rate, use of epidural anesthesia, or neonatal outcomes. There were no significant gastrointestinal side effects.

e. Vaginal versus oral misoprostol: Bennett[2] in an RCT of vaginal vs. oral administration of misoprostol found a shorter time to delivery with the vaginal route but a higher rate of fetal heart rate abnormalities. There was no difference in rates of cesarean delivery, use of epidural anesthesia, or neonatal outcomes.

f. Vaginal misoprostol and PROM at term: When used for PROM at term,[19] there was an increase of 1 hour from start of induction to onset of labor compared to oxytocin, but only 37% of the misoprostol group required oxytocin. There were no differences in vaginal delivery rates (86.7% with misoprostol vs. 85.9% with oxytocin, RR 1.17, CI 0.78–1.78). There were no differences in hyperstimulation, fetal heart rate abnormalities, meconium, Apgar scores, need for resuscitation, or admissions to neonatal intensive care. Rates of chorioamnionitis were similar (28.6% with misoprostol vs. 26.3% with oxytocin, RR 1.06 (CI 0.78–1.45).

g. Use of misoprostol for patients attempting a vaginal birth after cesarean section (VBAC): The study was terminated because of uterine rupture in 2 of 17 patients.[20]

E. Oxytocin Protocols

Until recently, protocols for the induction or augmentation of labor called for rapid increases in the oxytocin dosage at 15-minute intervals until an adequate contraction pattern was obtained. Newer studies show a possible higher rate of hyperstimulation, manifested by fetal distress, with this protocol, and studies of the in vitro activity of oxytocin have led to recommendations for lower-dose protocols with longer intervals between dose increments. These studies, however, did not find any difference in outcome in neonates who had oxytocin stopped or decreased for hyperstimulation or fetal distress. The main risks to patients identified with hypercontractility and fetal distress appeared to be an increase in the total labor time owing to stoppage and delay in the oxytocin infusion. Nevertheless, some real threat does exist, and the incidence of the diagnosis of hypercontractility and fetal distress can be decreased with 30-minute rather than 15-minute intervals. Greater dose intervals, such as 1 hour, may result in unacceptable delay in reaching a therapeutic response.

The American College of Obstetricians and Gynecologists (ACOG) guidelines currently call for oxytocin to be administered in a controlled intravenous infusion of a diluted solution by a secondary administration set into a primary infusion of physiologic electrolyte solution.[1] ACOG recommends initial doses of 0.5 to 1.0 mU/min, with increases every 30–60 minutes by increments of 1–2 mU/min, until satisfactory labor is achieved or a maximum of 20–40 mU/min is reached (noting that 90% of patients will respond with 16 mU/min or less). Local and institutional preferences should be considered in developing procedures for the administration of oxytocin. Pulsed infusions at 10-minute intervals may also decrease the amount of medication and fluid given.

ACOG recommends electronic fetal and uterine monitoring for patients receiving oxytocin. Initial and periodic examinations monitoring cervical progress are important to ongoing management of the oxytocin infusion. As with other patients in labor, maternal vital signs must be monitored carefully and appropriately modified for other complications (e.g., hypertension or infection). Attention to the amount and type of fluids that the patient receives is particularly important in any long-term administration of oxytocin. Using concentrations of 20 units of oxytocin/L (rather than 10 units/L) and limitation of the total dose to 40 to 50 units prevent complications of fluid overload.

Medical and nursing staff attending patients on oxytocin must be trained to recognize signs of maternal or fetal complications of the drug and begin emergent therapy (discontinuance of the drug, oxygen, change in maternal position) as indicated. Provision for abdominal delivery within 30 minutes should be documented before initiating oxytocin therapy, should complications necessitate this option.

V. Summary

The reduction in maternal and fetal morbidity is the primary outcome to be assessed in deciding if the induction of labor is indicated. Induction of labor is associated with a non-significant increase of cesarean intervention. The state of the cervix is the most important factor in predicting the success of induction. Cervical ripening with prostaglandin gel can decrease prolonged induction, failed induction, and operative delivery rates. Oxytocin plus amniotomy results in higher delivery rates at 12 and 24 hours and decreased operative delivery rates than either method alone. Prostaglandins used for induction may be more effective than oxytocin, but further studies are needed to confirm this preliminary evidence. There is insufficient evidence to determine differences in safety for the fetus between different induction methods.

References

1. American College of Obstetricians and Gynecologists: Induction and Augmentation of Labor. ACOG Technical Bulletin No. 217. Washington, DC, American College of Obstetricians and Gynecologists, 1995.
2. Bennett K, Butt K, Crane J, et al: A masked randomized comparison of oral and vaginal administration of misoprostol for labor induction. Obstet Gynecol 92:481–486, 1998.
3. Boulvain M, Irion O: Stripping/sweeping of the membranes to induce labour or to prevent post-term pregnancy (Cochrane Review). In The Cochrane Library, Issue 4, 2000.
4. Buser D, Mora G, Arias F: A randomized comparison between misoprostol and dinoprostone for cervical ripening and labor induction in patients with unfavorable cervices. Obstet Gynecol 89:481–485, 1997.
5. Chalmers J, Keirse M: Evaluating elective delivery. In Chalmers I (ed): Effective Care in Pregnancy and Childbirth. Oxford, Oxford University Press, 1989, pp 981–987.
6. Crowley P: Elective induction of labour at or beyond term. In Enkin MW, Keirse MJNC, Renfrew MJ, Neilson JP (eds): Pregnancy and Childbirth Module. Cochrane Database of Systematic Review, Review No. 04142. Cochrane Updates on Disk. Oxford, Update Software, 1994.
7. Kramer R, Gilson G, Morrison D, et al: A randomized trial of misoprostol and oxytocin for induction of labor: Safety and efficacy. Obstet Gynecol 89:387–391, 1997.
8. Keirse MJNC: Vaginal prostaglandins vs. oxytocin for induction of labour. In Enkin MJ, Keirse MJNC, Renfrew MJ, Neilson JP (eds): Pregnancy and Childbirth Module. Cochrane Database of Systematic Reviews, Review No. 04538. Cochrane updates on Disk 1. Oxford, Update Software, 1994.
9. Keirse M, Chalmers I: Methods for inducing labor. In Chalmers I (ed): Effective Care in Pregnancy and Childbirth. Oxford, Oxford University Press, 1989, pp 1057–1079.
10. Keirse M, Van Oppen C: Preparing the cervix for induction of labor. In Chalmers I (ed): Effective Care in Pregnancy and Childbirth. Oxford, Oxford University Press, 1989, pp 988–1056.
11. Magtibay P, Ramin K, Harris D, et al: Misoprostol as a labor induction agent. J Mat Fetal Med 7:15–18, 1998.
12. Mundle W, Young D: Vaginal misoprostol for induction of labor: A randomized controlled trial. Obstet Gynecol 88:521–525, 1996.
13. Perry K, Larmon J, May W, et al: Cervical ripening: A randomized comparison between intravaginal misoprostol and an intracervical balloon catheter combined with intravaginal dinoprostone. Am J Obstet Gynecol 178:1333–1340, 1998.

14. Sanchez-Ramos L, Kaunitz A, Wears R, et al: Misoprostol for cervical ripening and labor induction: A meta-analysis. Obstet Gynecol 89:633–642, 1997.
15. Sanchez-Ramos L, Peterson D, Delke I, et al: Labor induction with prostaglandin E_1 misoprostol compared with dinoprostone vaginal insert: a randomized trial. Obstet Gynecol 91:401–405, 1998.
16. Wing D, Jones M, Rahall A, et al: A comparison of misoprostol and prostaglandin E_2 gel for preinduction cervical ripening and labor induction. Am J Obstet Gynecol 172:1804–1810, 1995.
17. Wing D, Rahall A, Jones M, et al: Misoprostol: an effective agent for cervical ripening and labor induction. Am J Obstet Gynecol 172:1811–1816, 1995.
18. Wing D, Paul R: A comparison of differing dosing regimens of vaginally administered misoprostol for cervical ripening and labor induction. Am J Obstet Gynecol 175:158–164, 1996.
19. Wing D, Paul RP: Induction of labor with misoprostol for premature rupture of membranes beyond thirty-six weeks' gestation. Am J Obstet Gynecol 179:94–99, 1998.
20. Wing D, Lovett K, Paul R: Disruption of prior uterine incision following misoprostol for labor induction in women with previous cesarean delivery. Obstet Gynecol 91:828–830, 1998.
21. Windrim R, Bennett K, Mundle W, et al: Oral administration of misoprostol for labor induction: a randomized controlled trial. Obstet Gynecol 89:392–397, 1997.

CHAPTER 15

Intrapartum Complications

SECTION A.
FETAL INTOLERANCE OF LABOR

Kent Petrie, M.D.

I. Introduction
Continuous electronic fetal heart rate monitoring (EFM) is a technology that is commonly used to assess fetal well-being during labor. Despite lack of evidence that outcomes are improved with its use (see detailed discussion in Chapter 12), EFM is applied to 75% of laboring patients in the United States.[11] In many hospitals it is still routinely used, especially in high-risk patients. This chapter discusses definitions and standards for interpretation of EFM tracings and suggests strategies for dealing with non-reassuring fetal heart rate (FHR) patterns that should reduce unnecessary interventions.

II. EFM Protocols
In North America, both the American College of Obstetricians and Gynecologists (ACOG) and the Society of Obstetricians and Gynecologists of Canada (SOGC) have issued policy statements regarding the use of EFM.[2,15] Current recommendations do not distinguish between external and internal FHR monitoring. Modern computerized external Doppler monitor tracings have high signal quality, making the external FHR tracings as reliable as internal fetal scalp electrode tracings.

A. Admission Monitor "Test Strip"
A common practice in North American hospitals is to have patients undergo at least 20 minutes of external EFM on admission to labor and delivery, or prior to being sent home after a "courtesy check" in the emergency department or maternity ward. Several older studies correlated an admission non-reassuring FHR pattern with fetal acidosis and fetal death.[7] More recent reports have suggested adverse outcomes associated with admission non-reassuring FHR patterns. These include:
1. Meconium-stained amniotic fluid
2. Meconium aspiration
3. Apgar scores < 7 at 1 and 5 minutes
4. Seizures in the first 24 hours of life

Small numbers of non-reassuring patterns in these studies, however, make their confidence limits wide.[12] Poor positive predictive value of non-reassuring FHR patterns in RCTs makes one skeptical that an "admission strip" would be any better, prompting SOGC to discourage their use.[15] ACOG does not mention the use of admission strips.[2] If performed, the admission strip may at best serve as a baseline upon which change can be measured. A fetus showing a non-reassuring FHR pattern on initial presentation in labor may already be neurologically abnormal. Intrapartum asphyxia is suggested when the admission FHR pattern is reassuring, but subsequently becomes non-reassuring, particularly when associated with a rise in FHR baseline, or prolonged tachycardia, with absent variability (see definitions below).

B. The Low-Risk Patient

The low-risk patient may be monitored by continuous EFM or intermittent auscultation (by Doppler or DeLee stethoscope) during and for at least 1 minute after a uterine contraction every 30 minutes during the first stage of labor, and every 15 minutes during the second stage of labor. Due to intrapartum events, a low-risk patient can become high-risk at any time.

While ACOG considers intermittent auscultation an "option," SOGC makes a much stronger statement: "The preferred method of fetal health surveillance for low-risk women during labour is intermittent fetal heart auscultation with a handheld Doppler."[15]

C. The High-Risk Patient

Common high-risk conditions for which increased intrapartum surveillance is appropriate include the following:[2]

1. Oxytocin induction/augmentation
2. Twins
3. Hypertension/preeclampsia
4. Dysfunctional labor
5. Meconium staining
6. Vaginal breech
7. Diabetes
8. Prematurity
9. Premature rupture of membranes
10. Intrauterine growth restriction
11. Oligohydramnios
12. Abnormal FHR by auscultation
13. Significant vaginal bleeding and/or suspected abruption

High-risk patients may be monitored by one of the following methods.

1. Intermittent auscultation

This is evaluated and recorded during and for one minute after uterine contractions every 15 minutes during the first stage of labor, and every 5 minutes during the second stage of labor.

2. Continuous EFM (external or internal)

This should result in an evaluation of the tracing at least every 15 minutes during the first stage of labor and every 5 minutes during the second stage. Documentation of the evaluation is important.

III. Definitions of Electronic Fetal Monitor Patterns[12]

A. Fetal Heart Rate Baseline

1. Normal baseline (FHR 120–160 bpm)

The FHR is determined by a balance of inhibitory influences of the vagus nerve and excitatory influences of the sympathetic nervous system. Progressive vagal dominance occurs as the fetus reaches term, resulting in a gradual decrease in the baseline FHR.

2. Bradycardia (FHR < 120 bpm)

Bradycardia in the range 100–120 bpm is considered moderate and is common in prolonged gestations and occiput posterior and transverse presentations. Bradycardia below 100 bpm is considered severe and is more commonly associated with fetal asphyxia. Non-asphyxial causes of bradycardia include fetal bradyarrhythmias (heart block), drugs (beta-blockers and "caine" anesthetics, e.g., paracervical block anesthesia), and hypothermia.

3. Tachycardia (FHR > 160 bpm)

Tachycardia is considered moderate when between 160 and 180 bpm and severe when above 200 bpm. Non-asphyxial causes of fetal tachycardia include prematurity, maternal fever, chorioamnionitis, hyperthyroidism, maternal or fetal anemia, parasympatholytic drugs (atropine, scopolamine, hydroxyzine), and sympathomimetic agents (ritodrine, terbutaline).

B. Fetal Heart Rate Variability

Fetal heart rate baseline variability is key to the assessment of fetal well-being. It is an important index of cardiovascular function and is regulated by the fetal autonomic nervous system. The presence of normal FHR baseline variability (≥ 6 bpm) predicts a vigorous fetus at the time of measurement, even in the presence of decelerations and baseline FHR changes. FHR variability has typically been described on internal fetal scalp electrode tracings, but modern external monitors with computer autocorrelation produce tracings that mirror internal monitor quality.

1. National Institutes of Health (NIH) guidelines

The 1997 NIH Research Guidelines for the Interpretation of EFM defined categories of FHR variability to be used in describing fetal tracings.[11] The guidelines make no distinction between "short-term" (beat-to-beat) and "long-term" variability, but make the following definitions:

    a. Absent variability. This equals undetectable FHR variability.

    b. Minimal variability. This corresponds to variability ≤ 5 bpm.

    c. Moderate variability. This is variability between 6 and 25 bpm.

    d. Marked variability. This is variability > 25 bpm. This was formerly called saltatory variability, from the Latin word *saltare* = to leap.

    e. Sinusoidal variability. This is a regular sine-wave baseline pattern with absent variability that may be seen in severe fetal anemia or asphyxia. It should be distinguished from the pseudosinusoidal pattern, a benign form of long-term variability that is less regular and in which beat-to-beat variability is preserved.[16]

    f. Non-asphyxial causes of minimal or absent FHR variability. These include:

      i. Prematurity (variability should be normal after 32 weeks' gestation)

      ii. Fetal sleep state (usually transient and returns spontaneously in 30–40 minutes or with stimulation)

      iii. Absent fetal cerebral cortex (anencephaly)

      iv. Drug effects[16]

        • Central nervous system depressants (narcotics, diazepam, magnesium sulfate)

        • Parasympatholytics (atropine, scopolamine, hydroxyzine)

        • Central-acting adrenergic agents (methyldopa)

        • Beta-adrenergic agents that induce fetal tachycardia (ritodrine, terbutaline) can also decrease FHR variability.

C. Accelerations

FHR accelerations (a rise in FHR by at least 15 bpm for 15 seconds or more) are considered a reassuring sign of fetal well-being. Accelerations may occur spontaneously or in response to uterine contractions, brief umbilical cord compression, vaginal examination, fetal scalp stimulation, or external acoustic stimulation.

D. Early Decelerations

Early decelerations are due to fetal head compression during uterine contractions that result in vagal stimulation and slowing of the fetal heart rate. They are not associated with fetal asphyxia.

E. Variable Decelerations

Variable decelerations are the most common pattern of periodic change in FHR and are due to umbilical cord compression or substantial head compression (in the second stage of labor). Variable decelerations are considered severe if they drop below 60 bpm, or drop by 60 bpm below the established baseline, or last longer than 60 seconds (the rule of 60s).[12]

Variable decelerations are generally associated with favorable outcomes. However, a persistent pattern of repetitive variables is considered non-reassuring and may lead to fetal hypoxia and acidosis. Variable decelerations that are most worrisome are those that lack an initial and secondary acceleration, have a prolonged secondary acceleration ("overshoot"), show a slow or "late" recovery to baseline, or are associated with a loss of FHR variability.[12]

F. Late Decelerations

Late decelerations are associated with uteroplacental insufficiency and are provoked by uterine contractions. Maternal hypotension (especially after epidural anesthesia) and uterine hyperstimulation (with labor induction) are common transient causes of late decelerations. Correction of these problems will usually result in resolution of the pattern. Persistent late decelerations, when associated with absent or minimal FHR variability, are a potential ominous indicator of fetal asphyxia.

IV. Classification of FHR Patterns

In order to understand the current accepted classification scheme for FHR patterns, the following definitions are important.

A. Fetal Asphyxia

Asphyxia refers to the insufficiency or absence of exchange of respiratory gases within the fetal circulation. Asphyxia results in increasing degrees of hypoxemia, hypercarbia, and acidosis. Prolonged hypoxia leads to anaerobic metabolism and lactic acidemia, which aggravates the fetal acidosis.[12] Asphyxia is a term describing a physiologic state of the fetus. Although asphyxia may be reflected by certain FHR patterns, the term is best avoided in describing FHR tracings.

B. Fetal Distress

Fetal distress has been defined as a "persistent fetal asphyxia that, if not corrected or circumvented, will result in permanent neurologic damage or death."[13] Fetal distress is an imprecise term and, like the term asphyxia, is best avoided when describing EFM tracings. It is far more clinically relevant to describe FHR patterns by the two currently accepted categories, reassuring and non-reassuring (Table 1).

C. Reassuring FHR Patterns

Reassuring patterns are characterized by normal baseline rate and variability and accelerations and show an absence of non-reassuring patterns. Reassuring tracings are quite reliable in predicting a baby with normal oxygen and acid-base status (high negative predictive value).

TABLE 1.   Classification of Fetal Heart Rate Tracings

Reassuring FHR Patterns	Non-reassuring FHR Patterns
Baseline	Baseline
Normal rate	Bradycardia or tachycardia
Normal variability	Minimal or absent variability
Periodic changes	Sinusoidal patterns
Accelerations	Periodic changes
	Early decelerations
	Late decelerations
	Variable decelerations
	Prolonged decelerations

D. Non-reassuring FHR Patterns

Non-reassuring patterns are characterized by any or all of the features of baseline bradycardia or tachycardia, minimal or absent variability or a sinusoidal pattern, and early, late, variable, or prolonged decelerations. Non-reassuring patterns are quite nonspecific. They cannot consistently predict whether a fetus is well oxygenated, depressed, or acidotic (i.e., many false-positives, low positive predictive value).

E. Research Guidelines

In 1997 the NIH published Research Guidelines for the Interpretation of EFM, proposing standardized and unambiguous definitions for FHR tracings upon which future research could be based.[11] In addition to the definitions of FHR variability noted above, the NIH guidelines state that a full description of any FHR tracing requires a qualitative and quantitative description of:

1. Baseline rate
2. Baseline FHR variability
3. Presence of accelerations
4. Periodic or episodic decelerations
5. Changes or trends of FHR patterns over time

The guidelines make no recommendations for treatment based on specific FHR patterns.

F. ALSO Mnemonic for EFM Interpretation

To sum up the important features of EFM interpretation, the Advanced Life Support in Obstetrics (ALSO) course has recently adopted the mnemonic, DR C BRAVADO (Table 2).[1]

V. Management of Non-reassuring FHR Patterns

A. Assess for Treatable Maternal Conditions

There are three common ways a human fetus can become hypoxic or asphyxiated.

1. Insufficiency of uterine blood flow
2. Insufficiency of umbilical blood flow
3. Decrease in maternal arterial oxygen content

B. Institute Measures to Improve Fetal Oxygenation and Placental Perfusion

1. Administer maternal oxygen by face mask, 8–10 L/min.
2. Change maternal position to improve uterine blood flow to the lateral recumbent or knee-chest position.
3. Reduce or discontinue oxytocin infusion.
4. Administer IV fluids to restore maternal intravascular volume and relieve maternal hypotension. For epidural hypotension, 2.5–10 mg ephedrine IV may be indicated.

C. Tocolytic Treatment of Fetal Intolerance of Labor[10]

Tocolytic treatment will decrease or abolish uterine activity, will remove the ischemic effect of uterine contractions and thereby improve the metabolic condition of the fetus prior to delivery.

TABLE 2. ALSO Mnemonic for EFM Interpretation[1]

DR C BRAVADO	
Define **R**isk	Low or high
Contractions	Comment on frequency
Baseline **RA**te	Bradycardia, normal, or tachycardia
Variability	At least 5–10 bpm (persistent reduced variability is a particularly ominous sign)
Accelerations	Present or absent (at least 15 bpm change from baseline lasting 15 seconds)
Decelerations	Early, variable, or late
Overall	Assessment (reassuring or non-reassuring) and plan of management

1. Indications for tocolytic treatment
   a. Significant non-reassuring FHR patterns. Tocolytic administration is indicated for treatment of significant non-reassuring FHR patterns (bradycardia, persistent late or severe variable decelerations, lack of FHR variability) or fetal acidosis (scalp pH < 7.20) for which immediate operative delivery would otherwise be indicated. Preparations should be made for cesarean delivery when the tocolytic is administered.
   b. Less severe FHR abnormalities. Tocolytic administration may be considered for less severe FHR patterns requiring operative delivery. Because of anticipated delay prior to delivery, it is thought that further fetal decompensation might occur.
2. Resumption of labor after tocolytic administration
   After administration of the tocolytic, labor may be allowed to continue/resume if:
   a. Fetal heart rate pattern resolves, with a return of normal FHR variability.
   b. Personnel are available for immediate cesarean delivery if non-reassuring FHR patterns return.
   c. A normal scalp pH is demonstrated (if available).
3. Tocolytic treatment
   a. Terbutaline, 0.25 mg subcutaneously, is the drug of choice. This may be repeated every 10–15 minutes. It can also be administered intravenously 0.25 mg in 20 ml of normal saline; this can be repeated once every 15 minutes.
      i. Contraindications. These include maternal cardiovascular disease, preexisting maternal tachycardia, fluid overload, maternal thyrotoxicosis, and possibly abruptio placentae.
      ii. Side effects. These include maternal and fetal tachycardia, cardiac arrhythmia and ischemia, increased systolic and decreased diastolic blood pressure, tremor, pulmonary edema, nausea, vomiting, and headache.
   b. Magnesium sulfate ($MgSO_4$). Two to four grams $MgSO_4$ in 10% solution (20–40 ml) IV bolus over 15–20 minutes, then infusion of 1–4 g/hr.
      i. Contraindications. A bolus is contraindicated if an $MgSO_4$ infusion is already running with a known therapeutic magnesium level.
      ii. Potential side effects include hyporeflexia and hypoventilation.
4. Outcomes
   The results of RCTs summarized in the Cochrane Library draw the following conclusions:[10]
   a. Tocolysis. Terbutaline tocolysis results in significant resolution of non-reassuring FHR patterns, improves fetal cord pH, and increases Apgar scores at birth.
   b. Adverse effects. Terbutaline is reported to have no adverse effects other than transient maternal tachycardia.
   c. Effectiveness. Terbutaline is more effective than magnesium sulfate. Terbutaline tocolysis is effective in "buying time" when fetal intolerance of labor is diagnosed.

D. Saline Amnioinfusion (see Chapter 17, section C)
Amnioinfusion is a technique of replacing amniotic fluid during labor via a transcervical intrauterine catheter. Infusion of fluid expands the amniotic cavity space, relieves cord compression, and dilutes thick meconium.
   1. Indications for saline amnioinfusion
      a. Recurrent umbilical cord compression.[6] Amnioinfusion is used for treatment of significant non-reassuring FHR patterns associated with oligohydramnios

and/or cord compression (i.e., severe or repetitive variable decelerations or bradycardia).
   b. Dilution of thick meconium (often associated with the above FHR patterns)[7]
2. Contraindications
   a. Acute fetal intolerance of labor. Amnioinfusion is not indicated for the treatment of the ominous FHR tracing for which delay in delivery could further compromise the fetus (e.g., late decelerations with absent variability, scalp pH < 7.20).
   b. Active maternal infection (chorioamnionitis, genital herpes).
   c. Known or suspected placenta previa or abruption.
   d. Malpresentations
3. Technique of amnioinfusion
   a. Insert multiple-lumen intrauterine pressure catheter (allows simultaneous measurement of contraction strength to detect uterine hypertonus).
   b. Infuse room temperature (or warmed) normal saline (or lactated Ringer's) at a rate of 10–20 ml/min to a maximum of 800 ml, then continue a maintenance infusion of 1–3 ml/min.
   c. If bedside ultrasound is available, amniotic fluid index may be monitored and maintained at 10 cm or greater.
   d. A rapid release of amniotic fluid with maternal position change may be replaced by repeat bolus of 250 ml.
4. Complications of amnioinfusion
   a. Uterine hypertonus and overdistention (polyhydramnios)
   b. Uterine perforation (especially with prior lower segment scar)
   c. Cord prolapse ("washout" by rapid infusion)
   d. Infection
5. Outcomes of amnioinfusion
   a. Treatment of umbilical cord compression.[6] RCTs of amnioinfusion for treatment of severe or repetitive variable decelerations show:
      i. Reduced variable decelerations and bradycardia
      ii. Reduced rate of cesarean sections and forceps for "fetal distress"
      iii. Less meconium-stained amniotic fluid
      iv. Improved Apgar scores and scalp pH
      v. Less postpartum endometritis
   b. Presence of thick meconium.[7] RCTs of amnioinfusion for dilution of thick meconium show similar encouraging results.
      i. Decreased rates of heavy meconium staining, meconium below the cords, and meconium aspiration syndrome.
      ii. Reduced rate of cesarean sections for "fetal distress"
      iii. Improved Apgar scores and cord pH
      iv. No significant reduction in incidence of variable decelerations was noted.
   c. Prophylactic amnioinfusion.[8] RCTs that measure the use prophylactic amnioinfusion in the setting of oligohydramnios do not demonstrate improved perinatal outcomes.

VI. Other Intrapartum Fetal Surveillance Techniques
A. Fetal Scalp pH Sampling
1. Indications
   a. Absent FHR variability without a clear cause
   b. Non-reassuring FHR patterns, unresponsive to oxygen, IV fluids, position change, amnioinfusion, and other measures
   c. Any other puzzling or worsening FHR patterns

2. Contraindications
    a. Known or suspected fetal blood dyscrasias
    b. Maternal HIV-positive status
    c. Active maternal genital infection (HSV, GBS, GC, etc.)
3. Technique of scalp pH testing
    a. Fetal scalp pH test kits are available that contain all equipment necessary for obtaining a capillary blood sample from the fetal scalp.
    b. The patient is placed in the dorsal lithotomy position or the lateral recumbent position and the fetal scalp is visualized through a cone device provided in the kit.
    c. The scalp is then prepped with betadine. Application of sterile silicone will improve beading of the capillary blood.
    d. Using a square blade device, a puncture is made in the scalp and a sample is collected in a heparinized capillary tube and sent to the lab for immediate analysis.
4. Actions based on results of scalp pH
    a. pH > 7.25—allow labor to continue and re-sample as indicated.
    b. pH 7.20–7.25—re-sample in 10–15 minutes.
    c. pH < 7.20—immediate re-sampling and delivery if confirmed.
5. Is fetal scalp pH really practical or necessary in the community hospital?
Scalp pH testing is technically difficult, time-consuming, expensive, and used relatively infrequently. However, scalp sampling yields a *diagnosis* of fetal acidemia compared to FHR monitoring which is a *screening* test that has a low positive predictive value (high rate of false-positives). A scalp sampling result that is reassuring allows the clinician to continue to carefully monitor the progress of labor when FHR tracings are non-reassuring. Continuous electronic FHR versus intermittent auscultation monitoring of high-risk pregnancies, such as the post-dates pregnancy, results in a decreased incidence of neonatal seizures *only* if scalp sampling is used as an adjunct diagnostic tool.[17] Continuous electronic FHR monitoring is associated with an increased incidence of assisted vaginal deliveries and cesarean interventions. Clinicians need to weigh the advantage of knowing the fetal pH at a given time in labor versus the technical and cost factors listed above.

B. Fetal Scalp Stimulation
Fetal scalp stimulation is a reliable clinical alternative to scalp pH testing in fetuses with non-reassuring FHR tracings. Clark has demonstrated that an FHR acceleration (15 bpm × 15 sec) in response to firm digital pressure or the pinch of an Allis clamp, correlates with a scalp pH of greater than 7.20 in all cases.[3]

C. Vibra-acoustic Stimulation
A vibrating and sound-producing stimulus (artificial larynx) is applied to the maternal abdomen. An FHR acceleration (15 bpm × 15 sec) is associated with normal fetal acid-base balance. Long-lasting (up to 2 hours) disturbances of the FHR have been reported, however, necessitating more RCTs before universal acceptance of this procedure.

D. Continuous Intrapartum Fetal Pulse Oximetry
Hardware and software are currently available, and in 2000 the FDA approved the first instrument for measurement of continuous fetal pulse oximetry.[5] A small oxygen saturation probe is used, placed next to the fetal cheek or temple.
1. Advantages
    a. Less invasive than scalp pH
    b. Continuous reading available
2. Disadvantages

a. Placement of sensor is difficult and the probe is easily dislodged.
b. Interference with hair, caput, and meconium
c. Membranes must be ruptured.
d. Higher costs of monitoring

The use of this technology in a recent RCT did *not* demonstrate a decrease in overall cesarean section rates in the presence of non-reassuring FHR tracings.[5] This technology should *not* be widely used until there are numerous RCTs demonstrating improvements in clinically important perinatal outcomes.

References

1. American Academy of Family Physicians: Advanced Life Support in Obstetrics (ALSO), 4th ed. American Academy of Family Physicians, 2000.
2. American College of Obstetricians and Gynecologists. Fetal heart rate patterns: Monitoring, interpretation and management. ACOG Technical Bulletin, No. 207, July, 1995.
3. Clark SL, Gimovsky ML, Miller FC: The scalp stimulation test: A clinical alternative to scalp pH testing. Am J Obstet Gynecol 148: 274–277, 1984.
4. Devitt N: Saline amnioinfusion for the relief of variable decelerations. Am Fam Physician 46:778–782, 1993.
5. Garite TJ, Dildy GA, McNamara YH, et al: A multicenter controlled trial of fetal pulse oximetry in the intrapartum management of nonreassuring fetal heart rate patterns. Am J Obstet Gynecol 183:1049–1058, 2000.
6. Hofmeyr GJ: Amnioinfusion for intrapartum umbilical cord compression (Cochrane Review). In The Cochrane Library, Issue 4, 2000. Oxford, Update Software.
7. Hofmeyr GJ: Amnioinfusion for meconium-stained liquor in labour (Cochrane Review). In The Cochrane Library, Issue 4, 2000. Oxford, Update Software.
8. Hofmeyr GJ: Amnioinfusion prophylactically versus therapeutically for intrapartum oligohydramnios (Cochrane Review). In The Cochrane Library, Issue 4, 2000. Oxford, Update Software.
9. Ingemarsson A: Admission test: A screening test for fetal distress in labor. Obstet Gynecol 68: 800–806, 1986.
10. Kulier R, Hofmeyr GJ: Tocolysis for suspected intrapartum fetal distress (Cochrane Review). In The Cochrane Library, Issue 4, 2000. Oxford, Update Software.
11. National Institute of Child Health and Human Development Research Planning Workshop: Electronic fetal heart rate monitoring: Research guidelines for interpretation. Am J Obstet Gynecol 177:1385–1390, 1997.
12. Parer JT: Handbook of Fetal Heart Rate Monitoring. Philadelphia, W.B. Saunders, 1997.
13. Parer JT, Livingston E: What is fetal distress? Am J Obstet Gynecol 162:1421–1427, 1990.
14. Schrimmer DB, Macri CJ, Paul RH: Prophylactic amnioinfusion as treatment for oligohydramnios in laboring patients. Am J Obstet Gynecol 165:972–976, 1991.
15. Society of Obstetricians and Gynecologists of Canada: Fetal health surveillance in labor–SOGC policy statement. J SOGC, September:859–901, 1995.
16. Sweha A, Hacker TW, Nuovo J: Interpretation of the electronic fetal heart rate during labor. Am Fam Physician 59:2487–2500, 1999.
17. Thacker SB, Stroup DF: Continuous electronic fetal heart monitoring during labour (Cochrane Review). In The Cochrane Library, Issue 4, 2000. Oxford, Update Software.

SECTION B.
SHOULDER DYSTOCIA

Osman Sanyer, M.D., and Ina May Gaskin, C.P.M., M.A.

It is 3:30 a.m. in the delivery suite. As the family physician providing obstetrical care for the primipara in the labor bed, you are relieved as the infant begins to crown after 2 hours of hard pushing. The pregnancy has been totally uncomplicated and the patient and her partner are very excited as the delivery approaches. With exhortations from you and the labor nurse, the infant's head is gradually passing through the introitus and onto the perineum. Then, unexpectedly, as you reach to check for a nuchal cord and suction the infant's nares and mouth, you discover that the infant's head is retracted firmly onto the perineum, the occiput jammed against the pubic symphysis. You can't pass a finger between the occiput and pubic arch to check for a cord. Your early morning sleepiness suddenly gives way to tension, your mind begins to race, you look to the labor nurse, your voice cracks a bit, "I think we have a shoulder dystocia!" In the next few seconds, it is as if time has slowed to a standstill. A jumble of questions race through your mind: What is going on? Should I have seen this coming? What should I do next? How much time do we have? What will happen to this infant?, to this mother?

I. Introduction

Shoulder dystocia is a potential complication of any cephalic vaginal delivery. The anterior fetal shoulder is impacted above the pubic symphysis, and attempts to deliver the fetus may result in injury to the infant and mother. The experience of managing a shoulder dystocia often proves to be memorable and emotionally traumatic to the caregivers. If efforts to reduce a shoulder dystocia are unsuccessful, fetal asphyxia will result.

Pregnancy-related characteristics that have been implicated as predictors of shoulder dystocia have later been shown to be unreliable, and the literature suggests that preventive interventions during pregnancy and labor are ineffective. Given the potentially disastrous outcomes of shoulder dystocia, it is encouraging to know that the use of specific techniques applied in rapid response to a recognized shoulder dystocia have been shown to be effective in safely delivering entrapped infants. It is most important that the birth attendant recognize the dystocia, as failure to do so is associated with increased risk of Erb's palsy.[18]

II. Background

A. Definition of Shoulder Dystocia

A shoulder dystocia is defined as the impaction of the fetal shoulder against the maternal symphysis pubis in a manner that renders it undeliverable by the usual amount of cephalic traction. This complication of delivery may occur in any vaginal birth.

B. Incidence

The incidence of dystocia is higher in infants weighing more than 4000 grams. However, it is essential that clinicians realize that more than 50% of the dystocia cases occur in infants weighing less than 4000 grams.[12] Shoulder dystocia occurs in 0.5–2% of deliveries of infants weighing less than 4000 grams, with the incidence increasing to 5–10% of infants between 4000 and 4500 grams, and 10–35% in infants weighing more than 4500 grams.[1,28]

C. Associated Risk Factors

1. Antepartum risk factors

Dystocia has been shown to occur more frequently in the presence of maternal gestational diabetes if the infant has a birth weight greater than 3000 grams.[1,28] Other antepartum characteristics inconsistently associated with increased risk of shoulder dystocia include the following: a previous LGA infant, maternal obesity, multiparity, and the use of Pitocin.[2,4] A previous delivery complicated by a shoulder dystocia is not predictive of increased risk of recurrent dystocia in subsequent deliveries.[24] Lastly, several studies show that approximately 90% of shoulder dystocias occur in the delivery of infants that are not macrosomic.[17,26]

2. Intrapartum risk factors

Labor characteristics that have been shown to be associated with an increased incidence of shoulder dystocia include a prolonged first or second stage of labor, head-bobbing in the second stage, and assisted mid-pelvic delivery of a macrosomic infant.[2,3] A large population-based study of births occurring in California in 1992 demonstrated a 35–45% increase in shoulder dystocia in vacuum- or forceps-assisted births in nondiabetic women. Similar increases of shoulder dystocia were seen in assisted deliveries in diabetic women.[27]

D. Complications Associated with Shoulder Dystocia

The outcomes from a labor complicated by shoulder dystocia include the range of possibilities from minimal injury to the mother and fetus to severe trauma or loss of life.

1. Maternal complications

Maternal complications encountered during a delivery complicated by shoulder dystocia include lacerations of the perineum, vagina, rectum, or adjacent soft tissue. Hemorrhage may result secondary to these lacerations or due to uterine atony.

2. Neonatal complications

    a. Brachial plexus injury. This injury most frequently presents as Erb's palsy. The infant's arm is flaccid, adducted at the shoulder, and internally rotated. The injury is a result of bruising and stretching of the brachial plexus nerves. The symptoms resolve spontaneously in many infants in the first few days following delivery, and recovery can continue for up to 12 months. The association between shoulder dystocia and Erb's palsy is not clearly established. Erb's palsy has been documented in infants delivered by cesarean section as well as in the posterior arm in vaginally delivered infants.[13,15] Several series evaluating outcomes of deliveries of macrosomic infants show a relatively high incidence of shoulder dystocia (5–30%), but a very low incidence of permanent neurologic sequelae (Table 3).

    b. Cervical spine injury. These injuries can occur as a result of excessive lateral stretching or rotational traction forces applied to the infant's neck.

    c. Fractures. Fractures of the clavicle and humerus are seen as the result of efforts to deliver an infant with a shoulder dystocia. Generally, these injuries heal spontaneously with minimal sequelae.

    d. Neonatal asphyxia. As a result of the entrapment of the fetal torso in the birth canal, the umbilical cord is compressed. When uteroplacental insufficiency is present prior to delivery, severe acidosis may occur in less than 7 minutes. This may result in a severely depressed infant.

III. Prevention of Shoulder Dystocia

A. Prophylactic Cesarean Section not Indicated

Efforts have been made to prevent the occurrence of shoulder dystocia through antenatal intervention. Studies have shown that early induction and prophylactic cesarean section do not reduce the incidence of dystocia.[16,32]

Efforts to identify fetal macrosomia by ultrasound have been unreliable. One study showed a predictive value of as high as 93% when fetal abdominal circumference is

TABLE 3. Incidence of Shoulder Dystocia and Permanent Neurologic Sequelae

Study	No. of Patients	Birth Weight	Shoulder Dystocia (%)	CS % (Elective/ Trial of Labor)	% Permanent Sequelae
Diani[10]	737	4000	5.3	17.6 (29/71)	0
Gregory[21]	8815	4000	11	–	–
Jayazeri[22]	254	4000	13	30	–
Blickstein[5]	236	4200	11.4%	–	–
Lipscomb[25]	227	4500	18.5%	30.8 (50/50)	0
Gonen[17]	23	4500	35%	–	–

used as the predictor of macrosomia.[22] However, other large studies show the positive predictive value of sonographic studies to be less than 50%.[17,31]

Shoulder dystocia has been to shown to occur relatively frequently in macrosomic infants. However, the same studies show the incidence of permanent sequelae from shoulder dystocia to be very low.

Studies done to evaluate the effectiveness of elective cesarean section in preventing shoulder dystocia show that large numbers of cesarean sections would need to be done to prevent permanent sequelae from shoulder dystocia. One would have to perform 150 or more cesarean sections to prevent one fetal brachial plexus injury from a shoulder dystocia.[8,23,29]

In diabetic pregnant women, there is more convincing evidence to support the use of prophylactic cesarean section to prevent brachial plexus injury. The number needed to treat has been shown to be as low as 5 cesarean sections to prevent one brachial plexus injury in fetuses estimated to be greater than 5000 g, and 48 cesarean sections to prevent one such injury in infants estimated to be greater than 4000 grams.[11] In a study that included 2000 diabetic women, there was a significant reduction in shoulder dystocia, from 2.4% to 1% (odds ratio 2.2%) with prophylactic cesarean section for infants estimated to be greater than 4250 g by ultrasound. There was a concomitant increase in cesarean section rate, from 21.7% to 25.1% (p < 0.04).[9]

B. Response to a Diagnosis of Shoulder Dystocia

Given the limited benefit of cesarean section in preventing shoulder dystocia,[3] it is worthwhile to shift the focus to the prevention of maternal and fetal injury when dystocia occurs. The development of a delivery team response incorporating specific sequential maneuvers to resolve shoulder dystocia has been shown to be effective in reducing the likelihood of injury from dystocia.[3]

IV. Management of Delivery

A. Prompt Recognition and Response

Since the fetal pH drops 0.04 every minute that the head is trapped on the perineum, it is ideal to deliver the infant within 3 or 4 minutes once the diagnosis of dystocia is made. It is essential that the birth attendants recognize and quickly identify a dystocia when it occurs. Each hospital or birthing center can set up an organized response to a birth attendant's call for help with a shoulder dystocia.

The protocol established to respond to a shoulder dystocia will vary based on the resources available to the labor and delivery unit. It may include requesting the immediate presence of additional nursing personnel, a newborn resuscitation team, and possibly calling in an additional physician. One of the roles for a delivery team member is to record the timing and sequence of the maneuvers used to relieve the dystocia, not unlike the documentation of a cardiac resuscitation. In clinical situations that raise concern that a shoulder dystocia is more likely (i.e., a suspected macrosomic fetus with a prolonged second stage of labor or requiring an instrumented delivery), the response team may be notified in advance of the delivery.

It is important to include the delivering woman and her labor room support as part of the team that is assembled to respond to a shoulder dystocia. Understanding of the maneuvers necessary to relieve the dystocia will enhance the ability of the woman to cooperate with those interventions, improving the chances for a successful and atraumatic delivery. After calling the response team, a brief explanation of the situation should be given to the mother.

B. Consider Episiotomy

If an episiotomy has not been cut, the physician should evaluate whether release of soft tissue is needed to allow more room for manipulations of the fetal shoulders and arms that may be required to relieve the dystocia.

C. McRoberts Maneuver

At this point, with the assistance of the delivery personnel and the cooperation of the laboring woman, the McRoberts maneuver is attempted. Two assistant's hyperflex the mother's thighs back onto, or alongside, her abdomen. This maneuver is easy to perform and is effective 90% of the time.[19,28]

D. Suprapubic Pressure

This maneuver may be done concurrently with or subsequent to the McRoberts maneuver. An assistant at the patient's side, often standing on a step stool, applies pressure to the maternal suprapubic region, pushing the infant's anterior shoulder forward. The assistant will need guidance from the delivering physician in regard to the baby's position to ensure that the anterior shoulder is being pushed forward and not backward. When successful, the infant's anterior shoulder will be rotated out from beneath the pubic symphysis.

E. Shoulder Rotation

If the preceding efforts are unsuccessful at reducing the dystocia, the next maneuver involves reaching the fetal shoulders through the vagina and rotating the shoulders so that they traverse the pelvis in an oblique fashion. Two fingers are applied to the anterior shoulder, usually on the scapula, and then pressure used to affect the forward rotation of that shoulder (Woods screw maneuver, Fig. 1). Alternatively, pressure may be applied to the anterior chest of the posterior shoulder, thus rotating the shoulder on that side backward (Rubin's maneuver, Fig. 2). As the anterior shoulder rotates out from under the symphysis, the dystocia is reduced.

F. Delivery of the Posterior Arm

The posterior arm may be delivered by introducing one's hand in front of the baby's face, sliding two fingers along the fetal chest into the antecubital fossa of the posterior arm. Pressure applied in this location flexes the fetal elbow, allowing the fetal forearm and hand to be grasped, drawn outward across the trunk and face, and then delivered. The posterior shoulder tends to follow the posterior arm. When delivered, this decreases the diameter of the shoulders and the forces causing impaction of the anterior shoulder against the symphysis.

G. All-Fours Position

In the event that the McRoberts maneuver is unsuccessful, assisting the mother to the "all-fours" position has been shown to quickly and atraumatically reduce most dystocias. This technique has been widely practiced by midwives and can be instituted earlier than performing the Woods screw maneuver or attempting to remove the posterior arm. Some clinicians use this maneuver as the initial one to manage a shoulder dystocia. It consists of a change in position to the hands and knees (not to

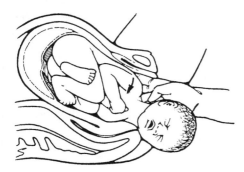 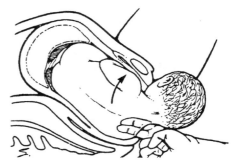

FIGURE 1. Abduction of the posterior shoulder (Woods maneuver).

FIGURE 2. Abduction of the shoulder to dislodge the shoulder girdle (Rubin's maneuver).

TABLE 4. Delivery in the "All-Fours" Position

The posterior shoulder (now uppermost) can often be delivered from this position, using a midline episiotomy if necessary. If delivery of the posterior shoulder is still not possible, posterior arm extraction may be accomplished more readily in this position by passage of the attendant's hand in front of the fetal face and splinting along the uppermost humerus with the fingers passing along the sacral curve. The attendant should attempt to flex the elbow, grasp the fetal hand or wrist, and sweep the arm across the fetal chest. If the posterior (uppermost) shoulder is still entrapped in the sacral hollow, traction on the arm may convert both shoulders to an oblique lie and relieve the anterior shoulder impaction from behind the symphysis.

This maneuver has been used effectively in a series of over 80 deliveries with shoulder dystocia.[7] The mean diagnosis-to-delivery interval in this series was 2.3 ± 1.0 (SD) minutes (range 1–6). Rotation to this position is probably enhanced by having the mother change position during labor, avoidance of internal monitoring equipment and intravenous lines, and having at least two assistants present at a birth. It may be used prophylactically as a delivery position in anticipation of the delivery of a macrosomic infant.

be confused with the knee-chest position). This position straightens the angle of the sacral promontory and may disimpact an anterior shoulder simply by the change in position. It has been reported that the maneuver increases the true diagonal conjugate by as much as 10 mm and increases the sagittal dimension of the pelvis by as much as 20 mm.[6] This maneuver is described in detail in Table 4.[7]

H. Severe Dystocia

If none of the preceding maneuvers are successful at reducing the dystocia, several other interventions may be attempted. These are regarded, to some degree, as last-resort measures. The methods result in maternal or fetal injury, although these injuries are considered acceptable when weighed against the risk of fetal asphyxia if the dystocia is not reduced.

1. Clavicular fracture

The clavicle of the anterior shoulder is deliberately fractured by applying direct pressure at its midpoint. As a result of the fracture the clavicle collapses and the anterior shoulder is able to move out from beneath the pubic symphysis.

2. Symphysiotomy

This procedure has been used infrequently in the United States, but has been used with regularity and success in developing countries. The cartilage of the symphysis pubis is sharply divided, allowing the pubis to arch upward, and the infant's anterior shoulder to slip beneath it. A Foley catheter is used to displace the urethra to one side and the incision is made under local anesthesia.[33] Patients may require 2–3 days of bedrest after the procedure, but morbidity is usually limited to a short period of discomfort with walking. Symphysiotomy may serve a role in smaller hospitals that lack the presence full-time anesthesia or easy and timely obstetrical consultation.

3. Zavanelli maneuver

This intervention involves reconstitution and flexion of the fetal head and pushing back and upwards into the vagina until the fetal head has resumed its pre-delivery position. It may require uterine relaxation, which is accomplished with terbutaline or inhaled anesthetic agents. The infant is then delivered via cesarean section.[30] In order for this maneuver to prevent fetal asphyxia, the birthing unit must have the personnel and available operating facility to perform an immediate cesarean section. The ease with which the fetal head can be returned to the vagina is unpredictable, making this intervention truly a last resort.[20]

It is now 4:00 a.m. The infant has been delivered, the mother's perineum repaired, and, as in most cases of shoulder dystocia, both are doing well. As the adrenaline ebbs from your system, you take a moment to reflect on the events of the last half-hour. You are pleased to have successfully assisted a laboring woman through one of the more frightening occurrences in obstetrical care. Before you leave the labor and delivery unit, there are a few more details that you should address.

V. Documentation

The delivery note should include documentation of the sequence and timing of the interventions used to relieve the dystocia. A description of the position of the infant, the condition of the infant at the time of delivery, and any resuscitative measures should be included.

VI. Communication

Just as communication with the laboring woman and her family prior to performing the maneuvers necessary to relieve the dystocia are important, communication with the family following delivery is equally important. The anxiety and tension experienced by the woman and her family can be tempered by a thorough explanation of this difficult obstetrical problem. A review of the efforts made to relieve the dystocia and the current status of the mother and infant may provide reassurance to a family in the face of this frightening situation.

References

1. Acker DB, Sachs BP, Friedman EA: Risk factor for shoulder dystocia. Obstet Gynecol 66:762–768, 1985.
2. Acker DB, Sachs BP, Friedman EA: Risk factor for shoulder dystocia in the average-weight infant. Obstet Gynecol 67:614–618, 1986.
3. Baskett TF, Allen AC: Perinatal implications of shoulder dystocia. Obstet Gynecol 86:14–17, 1995.
4. Benedetti TJ, Gabbe SC: Shoulder dystocia: A complication of fetal macrosomia and prolonged second stage of labor with mid-pelvic delivery. Obstet Gynecol 52:526–529, 1978.
5. Blickstein I, Ben-Arie A, Hagay ZJ: Antepartum risks of shoulder dystocia and brachial plexus injury for infants weighing 4200 g or more. Gynecol Obstet Invest 45:77–80, 1998.
6. Borell U, Fernstrom I: The mechanism of labour. Radiol Clin North Am 5:73–85, 1967.
7. Bruner JP, Drummond SB, Meenan AL, et al: All-fours maneuver for reducing shoulder dystocia during labor. J Reprod Med 43:439–443,1998.
8. Bryant DR, Leonardi MR, Landwehr JB, et al: Limited usefulness of fetal weight in predicting neonatal brachial plexus injury. Am J Obstet Gynecol 179:686–689, 1998.
9. Conway DL, Langer O: Elective delivery of infants with macrosomia in diabetic women: Reduced shoulder dystocia versus increased cesarean deliveries. Am J Obstet Gynecol 178:922–925, 1998.
10. Diani F, Venanzi S, Zanconato G, et al: Fetal macrosomia and management of delivery. Clin Exp Obstet Gynecol 24:212–214, 1997.
11. Ecker JL, Greenberg JA, Norwitz ER, et al: Birth weight as a predictor of brachial plexus injury. Obstet Gynecol 889:643–647, 1997.
12. Geary M, McParland P, Johnson H, et al: Shoulder dystocia—is it predictable? Eur J Obstet Gynecol Reprod Biol 62:15–18, 1995.
13. Gherman RB, Goodwin TM, Ouzounian JG, et al: Brachial plexus associated with cesarean section: An in utero injury? Am J Obstet Gynecol 177:1162–1164, 1997.
14. Gherman RB, Goodwin TM, Souter I, et al: The McRoberts maneuver for the alleviation of shoulder dystocia: How successful is it? Am J Obstet Gynecol 176:656–661,1997.
15. Gherman RB, Ouzounian JG, Miller DA, et al: Spontaneous vaginal delivery: A risk factor for Erb's palsy? Am J Obstet Gynecol 178:423–427, 1998.
16. Gonen O, Rosen DJ, Dolfin Z, et al: Induction of labor versus expectant management in macrosomia: a randomized study. Obstet Gynecol 89:913–917, 1997.
17. Gonen R, Spiegel D, Abend M: Is macrosomia predictable and are shoulder dystocia and birth trauma preventable? Obstet Gynecol 88:526–529, 1996.
18. Gonick B, Hoolyer BA, Allen R: Shoulder dystocia recognition: Differences in neonatal risks for injury. Am J Perinatol 8:31–44, 1991.
19. Gonick B, Stringer CA, Held B: An alternative maneuver for the management of shoulder dystocia. Am J Obstet Gynecol 145: 882–884, 1983.
20. Graham JM, Blanco JD, Wen T, et al: The Zavanelli maneuver: A different perspective. Obstet Gynecol 79:883–884, 1992.
21. Gregory KD, Henry OA, Ramicone E, et al: Maternal and infant complications in high- and normal-weight infants by method of delivery. Obstet Gynecol 92:507–513, 1998.

22. Jayazeri A, Heffron JA, Phillips R, et al: Macrosomia prediction using ultrasound fetal abdominal circumference of 35 centimeters or more. Obstet Gynecol 93:523–526, 1999.
23. Kolderup LB, Laros RK Jr, Musci TJ: Incidence of persistent birth injury in macrosomic infants: Association with mode of delivery. Am J Obstet Gynecol 177:37–41, 1997.
24. Lewis DF, Raymond RC, Perkins MB, et al: Recurrence rate of shoulder dystocia. Am J Obstet Gynecol 172:1369–1371, 1995.
25. Lipscomb KR, Gregory K, Shaw K: The outcome of macrosomic infants weighing at least 4500 grams: Los Angeles and University of Southern California experience. Obstet Gynecol 85:558–564, 1995.
26. Morrison JC, Sanders JR, Magann EF, et al: The diagnosis and management of dystocia of the shoulder. Surg Gynecol Obstet 175:515–522, 1992.
27. Nesbitt TS, Gilbert WM, Herrchen B: Shoulder dystocia and associated risk factors with macrosomic infants born in California. Am J Obstet Gynecol 179:476–480, 1998.
28. Nocon JJ, McKenzie DK, Thomas LJ, et al: Shoulder dystocia: An analysis of risks and obstetric maneuvers. Am J Obstet Gynecol 168:1732–1737, 1993.
29. Rouse DJ, Owen J, Goldenberg RL, et al: The effectiveness and costs of elective cesarean delivery for fetal macrosomia diagnosed by ultrasound. JAMA 276:1480–1486, 1996.
30. Sandberg EC: The Zavanelli maneuver: A potentially revolutionary method for the resolution of shoulder dystocia. Am J Obstet Gynecol 152:479–484, 1985.
31. Smith GC, Smith MF, McNay MB, et al: The relation between fetal abdominal circumference and birthweight: Findings in 3512 pregnancies. Br J Obstet Gynaecol 104:186–190, 1997.
32. Weeks JW, Pitman T, Spinnato JA: Fetal macrosomia: Does antenatal prediction affect delivery route and birth outcome? Am J Obstet Gynecol 173:1215–1219, 1995.
33. White S, Thorpe R, Main D: Emergency obstetric surgery performed by nurses in Zaire. Lancet 2:612–613, 1987.

SECTION C.
CHORIOAMNIONITIS

Stephen D. Ratcliffe, M.D., M.S.P.H.

Chorioamnionitis, or infection of the amniotic membrane and space, is a common intrapartum complication. Its relationship to preterm labor is discussed in Chapter 11. This section addresses the recognition and management of chorioamnionitis in preterm and term pregnancies.

I. Epidemiology
A. Preterm Labor[21]
Chorioamnionitis is commonly seen with patients experiencing preterm labor with intact membranes. Approximately 13% of such patients have a positive amniotic fluid culture, although only one of eight of patients with a positive culture have clinically apparent chorioamnionitis.[15] Very-low-birth-weight infants whose deliveries have been complicated by a clinical chorioamnionitis are at increased risk of serious neurologic compromise.[1]
B. Term Pregnancy
Chorioamnionitis occurs in 0.5–2% of all term pregnancies. Table 5 identifies factors that are associated with an increased risk of this intrapartum infection.[2] Table 6 identifies intrapartum factors that have the greatest association with chorioamnionitis.[18]

TABLE 5. Risk Factors for Acute Chorioamnionitis[2]

Presence of bacterial vaginosis	Meconium-stained fluid
Numerous vaginal exams with different providers	Previous history of spontaneous or iatrogenic abortion
Prolonged labor	Colonization with group B streptococcus or gonorrhea
Prolonged spontaneous rupture of membranes	
Premature labor	Internal fetal monitoring

TABLE 6. Predictors of Chorioamnionitis[18]

Risk Factor	Odds Ratio
> 8 digital vaginal exams (compared to 0–2 exams)	5.07
7–8 digital vaginal exams	3.80
5–6 digital vaginal exams	2.62
3–4 digital vaginal exams	2.06
Labor > 12 hours (compared < 3 hours)	4.12
Labor 9–12 hours	2.94
Labor 6–9 hours	1.97
Meconium-stained fluid	2.28
Time from ROM to active labor: > 48 hours	1.76
Time from ROM to active labor: 24–48 hours	1.77
Group B streptococcus colonization	1.71
Primipara	1.80

In the setting of premature rupture of the membranes, the risk of chorioamnionitis increases with increasing numbers of vaginal examinations.[17] There is no apparent association between water baths in labor and the development of chorioamnionitis.[14]

II. Pathophysiology
A. Microbiology
Most cases of chorioamnionitis are polymicrobial and are derived from vaginal flora.[2]

1. Aerobes
These include agents such as group B streptococcus, *Enterococcus faecalis*, *Streptococcus agalactiae* and *E. coli*.

2. Anaerobes
These include bacteria such as *Peptostreptococcus*, *Clostridium*, *Bacteroides*, *Gardnerella*, and *Fusobacterium* species. *Gardnerella* (causative agent of bacterial vaginosis) may increase the risk by a factor of 6.8 (see Chapter 8, section A).[24]

3. Other infectious agents
These include *Mycoplasma hominis*, *Ureaplasma urealyticum*, *Chlamydia*, herpes, and rarely *Candida*.[12] *Ureaplasma* and *Mycoplasma* are becoming increasingly associated with the pathogenesis of chorioamnionitis because they are isolated from infected amniotic fluid 30–45% of the time. *Ureaplasma*, unlike the other agents, is not associated with a clinically apparent infection.[3]

B. Perinatal Effects
1. Maternal
Maternal morbidity is infection-related and may result in postpartum endometritis. The risk of endometritis is increased if cesarean intervention is required. Maternal mortality, although rare, does occur.[2] There is a close association between chorioamnionitis and subsequent dystocia in labor.[11,16] This dystocia responds variably to oxytocin and may result in cesarean intervention.

2. Neonatal
Neonatal sepsis and mortality are increased when chorioamnionitis occurs in the preterm period. This is, in part, due to the increased vertical transmission of group B streptococcus in pregnancies lasting less than 35 weeks. These outcomes have become less common with preterm and term infants with the increased use of intrapartum antibiotic therapy.

III. Diagnosis
A. Clinical Presentation
As noted earlier, chorioamnionitis often occurs in the preterm pregnancy without any of the classic symptoms of infection. In the term pregnancy, the clinician should strongly suspect this diagnosis when one or more of the following signs or symptoms occurs. Of these factors, maternal fever is the most accurate predictor of infection.[2]
  1. Maternal fever (>100.5°F)
  2. Uterine tenderness
  3. Fetal tachycardia
  4. Foul-smelling amniotic fluid
  5. Maternal tachycardia, chills, or rigor

One of the potential confounding factors in making this diagnosis is the association between epidural anesthesia and low-grade intrapartum maternal fevers. Lieberman et al. demonstrated in a cohort analysis of 1500 primigravid patients that there was a fourfold increase in the diagnosis and treatment of suspected chorioamnionitis among women with epidurals compared to those without.[8] Clinicians should carefully monitor for other signs and symptoms of chorioamnionitis in patients with epidural anesthesia. If the only sign is a low-grade fever (<100.5°F), it may be prudent to withhold antibiotic therapy.

B. Laboratory Findings
Leukocytosis, total white blood count greater than 12,000, is commonly encountered with chorioamnionitis, although it may occur during normal labor as well. This degree of leukocytosis in labor has a sensitivity of 67% and a specificity of 86%.[5] A leukocytosis accompanied by a left shift or bandemia greater than 3% bands is a more sensitive marker for chorioamnionitis. When the clinical diagnosis is in question, C-reactive protein and erythrocyte sedimentation rates have been used as early markers of infection, but these tests have a low specificity (high rate of false-positive results).[13]

C. Differential Diagnosis
Other entities can mimic choriomnionitis.
  1. Genitourinary infections, including bladder and kidney infections
  2. Intra-abdominal processes, such as appendicitis and diverticulitis
  3. Upper or lower respiratory tract infections

D. Amniotic Fluid Analysis
Amniocentesis is seldom used for diagnostic purposes in the term pregnancy; however, it is a useful tool in diagnosing chorioamnionitis in the preterm pregnancy when an adequate fluid pocket can be found. Gram stains of the amniotic fluid have high positive and negative predictive values of 80–85% when the confirmation of chorioamnionitis is made based on a positive culture of the amniotic fluid.[13]

IV. Management
A. Timing of Antibiotic Therapy
  1. Preterm labor[7]

When the patient presents with preterm labor and intact membranes, an amniocentesis can be attempted to obtain fluid for Gram stain and culture if an adequate fluid pocket is available. The clinician must remain vigilant, however, for signs of clinical chorioamnionitis and allow labor to progress if they occur. Prompt introduction of antibiotic therapy is indicated if chorioamnionitis is suspected. A review of RCTs indicates that the prophylactic use of antibiotics in women with preterm premature rupture of the membranes (PPROM) results in a significant prolongation in the interval from rupture to delivery, a decrease in the incidence of neonatal sepsis, RDS, and prolonged ventilation (see Chapter

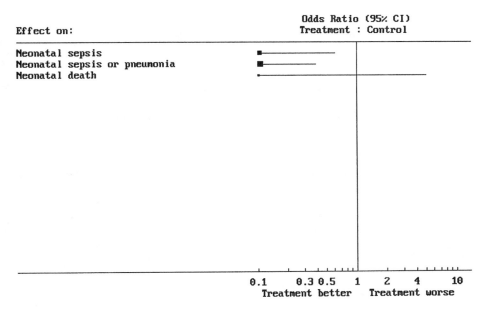

FIGURE 3. Intrapartum versus postpartum treatment of amniotic infection (one trial reviewed). (From Smaill F: Intrapartum vs. postpartum treatment of amniotic infection. In Enkin MW, Keirse MJNC, Renfrew MJ, Neilson JP [eds]: Pregnancy and Childbirth Module. Cochrane Database of Systematic Review, Review No. 07200. Cochrane Update on Disk. Oxford, Update Software, 1994, with permission.)

11, section H).[6] The use of antibiotics in the management of PPROM is not associated with an improvement in neonatal mortality.

2. Term pregnancy

Unless vaginal delivery is imminent, prompt use of antibiotic therapy is indicated when a clinical diagnosis of chorioamnionitis is made. Multiple RCTs have demonstrated decreased neonatal infection rates when antibiotics are instituted during labor as opposed to after delivery (Fig. 3).[4,20,22] Similarly, if the patient is known to be colonized with group B streptococci, neonatal infectious morbidity is decreased when intrapartum antibiotic therapy is initiated during labor.[19]

B. Choice of Antibiotic Agents[10]

Despite the presence of anaerobic bacteria in up to 50% of amniotic space infections, these infections can usually be adequately treated with antibiotics that have broad-spectrum aerobic coverage. Ampicillin, 2 g intravenously every 6 hours, or penicillin, 5 million units every 4 hours, have been shown to be effective in the treatment of women who are carriers of group B streptococcus. Ampicillin has the additional advantage of covering enterococcal infections. Expanded gram-negative coverage can be provided with the addition of an aminoglycoside, usually gentamicin. Gentamicin is given with a loading dose of 120–140 mg intravenously followed by 1–1.5 mg/kg intravenously every 8 hours. If gentamicin is used on a prolonged basis, serum peak and trough levels should be followed to avoid potential fetal ototoxicity or maternal renal toxicity. Other acceptable single-agent antibiotic regimens are listed below.[2] With the exception of penicillin-allergic patients, the authors recommend the use of ampicillin and gentamicin. In situations in which anaerobic coverage is desirable, clindamycin, 500 to 750 mg every 6 hours, can be added to the following regimens. This coverage is usually added to treat postpartum endometritis when there is a lack of response to conventional aerobic antibiotic coverage.

1. Dosing of other antibiotics
   a. Piperacillin: 3–4 g intravenously every 4 hours
   b. Mezlocillin: 3–4 g intravenously every 4 hours
   c. Ticarcillin/clavulanic acid: 3 g intravenously every 6 hours
   d. Cefoxitin: 1–2 g intravenously every 6 hours
   e. Ampicillin/sulbactam: 1.5–3 g intravenously every 6 hours
2. Chorioamnionitis, cesarean section, and use of antibiotics
   A recent RCT provides preliminary evidence that patients with chorioamnionitis who require a cesarean delivery benefit from a preoperative triple-drug regimen of ampicillin, gentamicin, and clindamycin.[23] The patients in this trial did not benefit from additional postoperative antibiotics.

C. Monitoring the Maternal Condition

The vast majority of women with chorioamnionitis remain clinically stable and can be managed in an expectant manner. Family physicians should, however, remain vigilant for the occasional patient who begins to develop symptoms of hypotension and poor peripheral perfusion, i.e., septic shock (see section H). This life-threatening complication requires an intensive-care level of treatment and monitoring.

D. Neonatal Management (see Chapter 18, section E)

There is no clear consensus as to how to manage the infant whose mother has received intrapartum antibiotics for suspected chorioamnionitis. If antibiotics are administered 4 or more hours prior to delivery, the vertical transmission of group B streptococci is only 1–2%. Newborn infants that have a normal clinical appearance and reassuring laboratory findings can be managed expectantly. Clinicians must have a low threshold to begin antibiotic coverage for infants who display any respiratory, circulatory, or neurologic compromise. This coverage consists of ampicillin (150–200 mg/kg/day intravenously or intramuscularly every 12 hours) and gentamicin (5 mg/kg/day intravenously or intramuscularly every 12 hours). Laboratory evaluation may include the following:

1. Complete blood count (CBC) with differential
   Attention must be paid to the ratio of immature (bands) to total polymorphonuclear leukocytes (bands plus neutrophils). This immature (I)/total neutrophil series (T) ratio is considered elevated if it is greater than 0.20.
2. Blood culture
3. C-reactive protein
   Serial tests for C-reactive protein (CRP), an acute-phase reactant. Two successive normal CRPs have a negative predictive value of > 98%.
4. Lumbar puncture
   Lumbar puncture should be performed when there is high index of suspicion for neonatal sepsis. Infants who have evidence of systemic infection should receive parenteral antibiotics for 7–10 days.

V. Prevention of Chorioamnionitis

Locksmith et al. have published the results of a series involving more than 20,000 women who fell into one of three management strategies designed to decrease the incidence of invasive early-onset group B streptococcus (EOGBS) infections in newborns. The strategy that incorporated GBS cultures between 35 and 37 weeks' gestation identified the maternal carriers of this infection. The treatment of these carriers in labor to prevent EOGBS resulted in a reduction in the incidence of chorioamnionitis in labor (relative risk 0.7, CI 0.6–0.8). The prevention of one case of chorioamnionitis required 23 prenatal cultures for GBS and 4 patients receiving antibiotic prophylaxis in labor.

References

1. Alexander JM, Gilstrap LC, Cox SM, et al: Clinical chorioamnionitis and the prognosis for very-low-birth-weight infants. Obstet Gynecol 91:725–729, 1998.
2. Casey B, Cox S: Chorioamnionitis and endometritis. Infect Dis Clin North Am 11:203–222, 1997.
3. Cassell F, Waites K, Watson H, et al: *Ureaplasma urealyticum* intrauterine infection: Role in prematurity and disease in newborns. Clin Microbiol Rev 6:69–73, 1993.
4. Gibbs R, Dinsmoor J, et al: A randomized trial of intrapartum versus immediate postpartum treatment of women with intra-amniotic infection. Obstet Gynecol 72:823–828, 1988.
5. Hoskins I, Johnson T, Winkel C: Leukocyte esterase activity in human amniotic fluid for the rapid detection of chorioamnionitis. Am J Obstet Gynecol 157:730–739, 1987.
6. Kenyon S, Boulvain M: Antibiotic for preterm premature rupture of membranes (Cochrane Review). In The Cochrane Library, Issue 4, 2000, Oxford, Update Software.
7. Kirschbaum T: Antibiotics in the treatment of preterm labor. Am J Obstet Gynecol 168:1239–1246, 1993.
8. Lieberman E, Lang J, Frigoletto F, et al: Epidural analgesia, intrapartum fever, and neonatal sepsis evaluation. Pediatrics 99:415–419, 1997.
9. Locksmith G, Clark P, Duff P: Maternal and neonatal infection rates with three different protocols for prevention of group B streptococcal disease. Am J Obstet Gynecol 180:416–422, 1999.
10. Maberry M, Gilstrap L: Intrapartum antibiotic therapy for suspected intraamniotic infection: Impact on the fetus and neonate. Clin Obstet Gynecol 34:345–351, 1991.
11. Mark S, Croughan-Minihane M, Kilpatrick S: Chorioamnionitis and uterine function. Obstet Gynecol 95:909–1012, 2000.
12. Mazor M, Chaim W, et al: Asymptomatic amniotic fluid invasion with *Candida albicans* in preterm premature rupture of membranes. Act Obstet Gynaecol Scand 72:52–54, 1993.
13. Ohlsson A, Wang E: An analysis of antenatal tests to detect infection in preterm premature rupture of the membranes. Am J Obstet Gynecol 162:809–818, 1990.
14. Robertson P, Huang L, Croughan-Minihane M, et al: Is there an association between water baths during labor and the development of chorioamnionitis or endometritis? Am J Obstet Gynecol 178:1215–1221, 1998.
15. Romero R, Sirtori M, et al: Infection and labor: V. Prevalence, microbiology, and clinical significance of intraamniotic infection in women with preterm labor and intact membranes. Am J Obstet Gynecol 161:817–824, 1989.
16. Satin A, Maberry M, Leveno K, et al: Chorioamnionitis: A harbinger of dystocia. Obstet Gynecol 79:913–915, 1992.
17. Schutte M, Treffers P, Kloostermen G, et al: Management of premature rupture of membranes: The risk of vaginal examination to the infant. Am J Obstet Gynecol 146:395–400, 1983.
18. Seaward P, Hannah M, Hyhr R, et al: International multicentre term prelabor rupture of membranes study: Evaluation of predictors of clinical chorioamnionitis and post partum fever in patients with prelabor rupture of membranes at term. Am J Obstet Gynecol 177:1024–1029, 1997.
19. Smaill F: Intrapartum antibiotics for group B strep colonisation (Cochrane Review). In The Cochrane Library, Issue 4, 2000, Oxford, Update Software.
20. Smaill F: Intrapartum vs. postpartum treatment of amniotic infection. In Enkin MW, Keirse MJNC, Renfrew MJ, Neilson JP (eds): Pregnancy and Childbirth Module. Cochrane Database of Systematic Review, Review No. 07200. Cochrane Update on Disk. Oxford, Update Software, 1994.
21. Sperling R, Newton E, Gibbs R: Intraamniotic infection in low-birth-weight infants. J Infect Dis 157:113–117, 1988.
22. Sperling R, Ramamurthy, Gibbs R: A comparison of intrapartum versus immediate postpartum treatment of intra-amniotic infection. Obstet Gynecol 70:861–865, 1987.
23. Turnquest M, How H, Cook C, et al: Chorioamnionitis: Is continuation of antibiotic therapy necessary after cesarean section? Am J Obstet Gynecol 179:1261–1266, 1998.
24. Watts D, Krohn M, Hillier S, et al: Bacterial vaginosis as a risk factor for postcesarean endometritis. Obstet Gynecol 75:52–56, 1990.

SECTION D.
INTRAPARTUM BLEEDING

Janis E. Byrd, M.D.

This section covers specific intrapartum diagnostic and management strategies for the following diagnoses: placenta previa, placental abruption, and vasa previa. A more general perspective is included in Chapter 6, section D.

I. Initial Management of the Bleeding Patient

A. Initial Evaluation

On arrival, the patient should be questioned whether her bleeding is spotting or "as much as a period" or "enough to soak a pad." Initial inquiries by nursing staff may also document the presence of contractions, pain, "show," or leakage of fluid. Patients may not be accurate in their description of the quantity of blood, but overestimation is preferable until medical evaluation can take place.

B. Heavy Bleeding

If bleeding is thought to be serious, a complete blood count with platelets, type and crossmatch, prothrombin time (INR), PTT, fibrinogen, and fibrin split products should be drawn. Intravenous fluids should be started and oxygen applied. Nursing protocols should specify no vaginal examinations until seen by physician. No digital examination should be performed unless the placental location is known to be distant to the cervical os. Previous ultrasounds should be obtained if available. Ultrasound for placental location should be obtained if not known from previous examinations.

C. Patient Stability

1. Immediate focus of care

This is directed at determining the stability of the maternal and fetal condition by vital signs, brief physical assessment, and fetal heart rate tracing.

2. Assessment of maternal stability

This is made more complex by the cardiovascular changes associated with pregnancy. The patient may not demonstrate any signs of shock until she has lost up to 35% of blood volume. Normal blood pressures in pregnancy tend to be lower with slight increases in maternal heart rate. Alterations in blood pressure may be most difficult to assess in the patient with pregnancy-induced hypertension, in whom a "normal" blood pressure may actually reflect substantial volume depletion.

3. Indications for immediate cesarean section

These include signs of fetal distress and severe maternal hemorrhage. Otherwise, the evaluation may proceed in a more deliberate manner.

II. Differential Diagnosis of Vaginal Bleeding

If the patient is in labor, bleeding may represent exuberant bloody "show," abruption, or possibly placenta previa. Most patients with placenta previa present before the onset of labor with bleeding. If the onset of bleeding coincided with rupture of membranes, vasa previa is more likely.

A. Vasa Previa

Bleeding from vasa previa is a fetal hemorrhage caused by the rupture of fetal vessels in a velamentous insertion. Although this condition is rare, rapid diagnosis is crucial because fetal mortality is greater than 50%. If initial fetal heart rate tracings suggest fetal distress, an immediate cesarean section should be performed with neonatal resuscitation immediately available. If fetal heart rate tracings are stable, a rapid test should be performed to determine the presence of fetal blood. Kleihauer-Betke stains are time-consuming and the following two methods are more suitable.

1. Wright's stain of smear

The presence of nucleated red blood cells is indicative of fetal blood because these are common in fetal blood and rare in adult blood.

2. Modified Apt test

Blood is collected with a syringe from the vaginal pool. The hemoglobin is lysed by the addition of tap water, and the mixture is centrifuged for several minutes. One milliliter of 1% NaOH is mixed with 5 ml of supernatant. In 2 minutes, the colorimetric reaction is read. A pink reaction indicates fetal hemoglobin; adult hemoglobin is yellow-brown.

B. Abruption

1. Painful bleeding

If bleeding is associated with pain, abruption should be considered. Pain may be mild (similar to menstrual cramping), comparable to normal labor, or excruciating. It may be accompanied with fundal tenderness or expressed solely as back pain in the patient with a posterior placenta.

2. Bleeding characteristics

Hemorrhage may be externalized, either completely or partially, or occult. The amount of bleeding is often underestimated by clinical means. Bleeding may also present as bloody amniotic fluid.

3. Ultrasound examination

This may demonstrate retroplacental or intraplacental hemorrhage, a separated placental edge, or no pathologic findings. Lack of sonographic findings should *not* be used to rule out a diagnosis of abruption.

C. Placenta Previa

1. Clinical evaluation

Patients with spotting or minor amounts of vaginal bleeding can always be evaluated by speculum examination to evaluate for cervical and vaginal causes of bleeding. Visual inspection of the cervix to ascertain a closed os is recommended by some prior to vaginal probe examination.

2. Abdominal ultrasound

This assessment can be made with a moderately full as well as an empty bladder and may avoid false-positive diagnoses.

3. Transperineal or transvaginal ultrasound

This provides the most accurate means of assessing the relationship of the cervical os to the placental edge. These scanning techniques are discussed in Chapter 17, section A and Chapter 2, section G. Transperineal scanning may be used to image a posterior placenta previa or to differentiate a marginal from a complete placenta previa. Transvaginal ultrasound may not be available in labor and delivery but may be used in the stable patient for evaluation of placenta previa. The introduction of a vaginal probe into the vagina is at right angles to the cervical canal. The vaginal probe is covered with a sterile probe cover or condom and inserted only partially into the vaginal canal to image the lower uterine segment and cervix.

III. Management of Vaginal Bleeding

Antenatal Rhogam (300 mg) should be given to all Rh-negative patients with bleeding for prophylaxis in the instance of possible fetomaternal hemorrhage. The hematocrit should be maintained greater than 30% and coagulopathy treated as outlined in Chapter 7, section D.

A. Placenta Previa

The overall strategy in managing the patient must take into account the amount of bleeding and the gestational age of the fetus.

1. Effects of prematurity

Because the greatest morbidity and mortality associated with placenta previa are due to prematurity, attempts should be made to continue a pregnancy that is less than 33 weeks' gestation. In many circumstances, the patient should be transferred as soon as stable to a perinatal center because the risk of re-bleeding is substantial in the preterm gestation with placenta previa.

2. The double set-up examination

This is a treatment modality to determine if a patient with equivocal findings of a marginal placenta previa may be permitted a trial of labor. Its utility is the prevention of unnecessary cesarean section in circumstances in which the bleeding edge of the placenta may be effectively tamponaded by the fetal head during labor. Palpation of the placental edge should not take place unless the patient is prepared and ready for immediate operative delivery, including anesthesia in attendance and blood ready. The patient may then be examined in the delivery room with palpation of the placental edge.

3. Operative delivery

This is indicated if bleeding is excessive or if the fetus is mature. There is an increased risk of placenta accreta for patients with placenta previa, especially multiparas and those with previous lower uterine incisions. The overall risk of this serious complication is 10% in patients with a low anterior placenta or placenta previa and previous cesarean section. The risk increases with each successive cesarean delivery.[4,6] Since treatment might result in a cesarean hysterectomy, it is advisable for the physician and patient to be prepared for this possibility. These issues should be kept in mind when proceeding toward operative delivery or considering transfer to a facility with more extensive blood-bank resources.

B. Placental Abruption

The management of abruption depends on the presence or absence of fetal life. In general, the risk of stillbirth in abruption is proportionate to the degree of placental separation.[1] Coagulopathy is extremely rare in acute abruption with a surviving fetus, but 30% of patients with abruptions resulting in fetal demise develop consumptive coagulopathy and disseminated intravascular coagulation from the release of thromboplastin. Although partial abruption may be stabilized such that a severely preterm gestation may continue, the following are guidelines for intrapartum management.[3]

1. Viable fetus in labor

If the fetus is alive at the time of presentation, a fetal scalp electrode should be placed. Emergency cesarean section should be performed for any signs of distress unless vaginal delivery is imminent. An individual experienced in neonatal resuscitation should be available for any delivery, vaginal or operative, when abruption is suspected.

   a. Monitoring patients with suspected abruption. The patient with abruption should be followed closely with serial complete blood counts, clotting studies, and urine output. Hematocrit should be maintained at greater than 30% and urine output at greater than 30 ml/hour. Normal pregnancy values for fibrinogen are elevated (350–650 mg/dl). A fibrinogen value less than 150 mg/dl is indicative of significant coagulopathy. The blood bank should plan to stay at least 3 units ahead in severe abruption.

   b. Bedside test for coagulopathy: the clot test. A red-top tube is drawn and taped beside the bed. Seven to 10 minutes later, the tube is checked for the presence of a clot. Absence of a clot or a fragile clot is evidence of coagulopathy.

   c. Monitoring contractions. Contractions should be monitored closely in abruption. The onset of tetanic contractions may precede fetal distress, and an intrauterine pressure catheter may be helpful. What feels like a tetanic contraction to palpation is manifested as frequent, small contractions superimposed on an elevated resting baseline.

2. The non-viable fetus and abruption

If the fetus is dead, management is directed toward the safest means of delivering the patient. Vaginal delivery is preferable, if at all possible, with no absolute time limits as long as labor is progressing. Episiotomy and other measures that increase blood loss should be avoided. Labor is often augmented to accomplish a vaginal delivery. Cesarean section is performed only for other obstetric indications or if bleeding is too excessive to replace with transfusion. These patients may be extremely ill and benefit from central venous pressure or Swan-Ganz monitoring. Fluid management in the oliguric patient may be managed more accurately by use of the pulmonary capillary wedge pressure and evaluation of the systemic vascular resistance because a subset of these patients are at risk for pulmonary edema and adult respiratory distress syndrome.[2] Other major maternal risks include the following.

     a. Coagulopathy. This is treated in preparation for cesarean section. Fresh frozen plasma and platelets are used immediately before operation because the effect of platelet transfusions is short-lived. Although evacuation of the uterus has been proposed as necessary for resolution of coagulopathy, conservative management, with stabilization of the patient before delivery, has been advocated by some due to the high risk of surgical intervention with coagulopathy. Some studies have found resolution of coagulopathy before delivery.[5]

     b. Postpartum hemorrhage. The patient with abruption is at risk for postpartum hemorrhage from uterine atony. The term Couvelaire uterus has been used to describe an enlarged uterus with hemorrhage into the myometrium. A Couvelaire uterus may contract poorly following delivery but is not an automatic indication for hysterectomy.

3. Postoperative management

This includes continued monitoring of urine output and clotting studies. The occurrence of acute tubular necrosis has decreased with more intensive monitoring of cardiovascular status.

References

1. Ananth CV, Berkowitz GS, Savitz DA, et al: Placenta abruption and adverse perinatal outcomes. JAMA 282:1646–1651, 1999.
2. Clark SL, Greenspoon JS, Aldahl D, et al: Severe preeclampsia with persistent oliguria: Management of hemodynamic subsets. Am J Obstet Gynecol 154:490–495, 1986.
3. Combs CA, Nyberg DA, Mack LA, et al: Expectant management after sonographic diagnosis of placental abruption. Am J Perinatol 9:170–174, 1992.
4. Miller DA, Chollet JA, Goodwin TM: Clinical risk factors for placenta previa-placenta accreta. Am J Obstet Gynecol 177:210–214, 1997.
5. Twaalfhoven FCM, Roosmalen JV, Briet E, et al: Conservative management of placental abruption complicated by severe clotting disorders. Eur J Obstet Gynaecol 46:25–30, 1992.
6. Zaki ZM, Bahar AM, Ali ME, et al: Risk factors and morbidity in patients with placenta previa compared to placenta previa non-accreta. Acta Obstet Gynaecol Scand 77:391–394, 1998.

SECTION E.
POSTPARTUM HEMORRHAGE

Janis E. Byrd, M.D.

Although the number of deaths by postpartum hemorrhage (PPH) has fallen in the Western world, it remains the third leading cause of maternal mortality, accounting for 25% of maternal deaths. In developed countries PPH accounts for 1 maternal death in 1000 deliveries. Women who refuse blood transfusions are at a similar risk to women in developing countries.[3]

I. Epidemiology
The incidence varies with the definition being used. Postpartum hemorrhage was previously defined as > 500 ml of blood loss in the first 24 hours after delivery with an inci-

TABLE 7.   Risk Factors for Postpartum Hemorrhage[2]

Risk Factors	Relative Relative Risk (estimate)
Prenatal	
Preeclampsia	5.0
Previous postpartum hemorrhage	3.6
Multiple gestations	3.3
Previous cesarean section	1.7
Asian or Hispanic descent	·1.7
Multiparity	1.5
Intrapartum	
Prolonged third stage (> 30 minutes)	7.5
Left mediolateral episiotomy	4.7
Midline episiotomy	1.6
Arrest of descent	3.0
Lacerations (perineal, periurethral)	2.0
Augmented labor	1.7
Forceps delivery	1.7

dence of 5%.[10] Greater than 1000-ml loss in 24 hours is now recognized as more clinically relevant and occurs in 1–2% of deliveries.

II. Diagnosis
Although numerous risk factors have been identified (Table 7), PPH occurs unpre-
dictably in low-risk women and every maternity care service must be prepared to deal
with immediate severe hemorrhage.[2,13] Likewise, providers must be vigilant for less
dramatic but steady bleeding or concealed hemorrhage. The diagnosis is often delayed
due to underestimation of blood loss and late development of the usual signs of tachycardia and hypotension due to greater blood volume in a generally young and healthy
population.[9] Patients with pre-eclampsia are at greater risk due to contracted volume
and misinterpretation of falling blood pressure readings as "normal."

III. Prevention
The most important preventive measure routinely available is prophylactic oxytocin or
so-called active management of the third stage of labor. Various protocols have been
used, usually 10 IU intramuscularly or 10-40 IU/liter of intravenous fluid given with
the anterior shoulder or immediately after delivery of the baby. This also includes immediate cord clamping and controlled traction. Cochrane data demonstrate that the
active versus expectant management of the third stage is associated with improved outcomes with respect to both moderate (> 500 ml blood loss; OR = 0.34, CI 0.28–0.41,
ARR = 10%, NNT to prevent one PPH = 10) and severe (> 1000 ml blood loss; OR =
0.40, CI 0.25–0.62, ARR = 1.5%, NNT = 65) postpartum hemorrhage.[8]

Oral and rectal misoprostol are currently under investigation because of decreased
cost, ease of administration, long shelf-life without special storage conditions, and minimal side effects. Four to six hundred micrograms are administered immediately after
birth of the infant and prior to delivery of the placenta. A randomized controlled trial of
400 μg of oral misoprostol found an incidence of PPH of 6% compared with 9% in the
placebo (RR 0.65, 95% CI 0.35–1.22).[5]

In a few women at very high risk, delivery at a center with blood banking facilities
and immediate anesthesia and surgery capabilities may be prudent. One condition was
identified by Gibb as a special risk.[4] This is the low anterior placental location in the current pregnancy with previous cesarean section. Ultrasound identification of the placental
site is recommended. If the placenta is anterior, additional cross-matched blood should
be available and the staff as well as the patient and her partner alerted to the hazard.

IV. Management

A. Uterine Atony

Uterine atony is the most frequent cause of PPH as blood loss occurs primarily from the placental site and occlusion of the spiral arteries depends on uterine contraction. The provider should begin immediate bimanual massage, with the internal hand lifting the uterus to stretch the uterine vessels. Simultaneously a large-bore IV should be started if not already in place and oxytocin given at a maximum rate of 250 ml/hour of a 40 U/L solution. If an intravenous line cannot be immediately established, 10–20 units of oxytocin can be given intramuscularly. Direct intravenous administration is not recommended because this can complicate the problem by causing transient hypotension.[14] Oxytocin acts by causing rhythmic contractions of the upper uterine segment and may also help the placenta to separate.

If bimanual massage and oxytocin are not successful, methylergonovine, 0.2 mg, may be given intramuscularly. This agent acts to cause both upper and lower uterine segments to contract in a tetanic manner. It may also cause vasoconstriction and hypertension. Caution is advisable if the patient has hypertension as a complication of the pregnancy.

If uterine atony is still suspended, prostaglandin $F_{2\alpha}$ (Hemabate) may produce dramatic effect. It can be given in a dose of 0.25 mg intramuscularly or intramyometrially through the abdominal wall by elevating the uterus with an intravaginal hand. Repeated doses can be given at 15 minutes intervals to a maximum of 2 mg. A response should be seen in 3–10 minutes, depending on route or dosage. Side effects are dose-dependent and include nausea and vomiting, diarrhea, hypertension, headache, flushing, and fever. Hemabate is supplied in 0.25-mg vials and has a shelf life of 6–12 months, allowing it to be stocked for infrequent use even in small facilities. If bleeding continues, a Foley catheter should be placed to empty the bladder and monitor urine output. Laboratory tests including CBC with platelet count, fibrinogen, fibrin split products, protime/INR, and partial thromboplastin time should be obtained. Supplemental oxygen should be administered.

B. Birth Trauma

If the uterus is not atonic and bleeding continues, the patient should be examined for vaginal or cervical lacerations or submucosal hematoma. The risk of birth trauma is increased if there has been a long or difficult labor and delivery, use of forceps or vacuum, episiotomy, or vulvar varicosities. Lacerations should be immediately repaired and hematomas larger than 3 cm incised and evacuated. Bleeding vessels may need to be identified and ligated. Adequate anesthesia/analgesia is essential for exploration and repair.

C. Uterine Inversion

Uterine inversion generally is immediately recognized as protrusion of a bluish gray mass from the vagina but may not be found until vaginal exploration is undertaken. Once it is recognized, it should be replaced immediately, either before or after removal of the placenta. Some authors believe that removing the placenta before replacement increases blood loss.[4] If the cervix is not contracted around the inverted uterus, it can usually be replaced simply by pressure on the fundus in the long axis of the vagina. The fingers of the intravaginal hand can be extended to the margins of the cervix and an abdominal hand can grasp and guide the fundus.

If the contraction ring has formed and the uterus cannot be immediately replaced, emergency management should be instituted and preparations made for surgical interventions. General anesthesia may assist in uterine relaxation, or tocolytic agents may be administered. These may produce increased bleeding, however. At laparotomy, traction may be applied to the inverted fundus simultaneously with pressure from below. In some cases, incision of the contraction ring is necessary to replace the uterus.

TABLE 8.   Clinical Conditions Associated with Uterine Rupture

Prior cesarean section	Epidural anesthesia
Previous uterine surgery	Abruptio placentae
Oxytocin hyperstimulation	Midforceps delivery
Abdominal trauma	Breech version/extraction
Parity ≥ 4	

Although there are no RCT data available, intravenous nitroglycerin 100 μg has been described as an alternative to general anesthesia.[1,6] Uterine relaxation begins in 30–90 seconds and persists for only 1 minute, thus limiting further blood loss. Sublingual application is a more convenient method that may be kept readily available in the delivery room. Hydrostatic replacement has also been described by infusing normal saline through a vacuum extractor cup used to occlude the vagina.[11]

D. Retained Fragments

If uterine atony has been treated and no birth trauma or inversion recognized, the uterus should be explored for retained placental fragments. Retained fragments may be removed manually with a gauze sponge over the fingers or by curetting with a large loop.

E. Uterine Rupture

Uterine rupture occurs in 1 in 2500 deliveries; small defects in the lower uterine segment occur more commonly but are often asymptomatic. Risk factors for uterine rupture are listed in Table 8. Signs of uterine rupture may include circulatory collapse out of proportion to the amount of blood lost externally and in the late stages, increasing abdominal girth. Management requires immediate fluid resuscitation and definitive surgery. Stop-gap measures while preparing for surgery include direct aortic compression and anteflexion, elevation, and compression of the uterus.

F. Coagulation Disorders

Coagulation disorders are rare causes of postpartum hemorrhage and are generally known antepartum. They should be suspected if lack of clotting is noted or other measures have failed to identify and control hemorrhage. Medical causes of coagulopathy include idiopathic thrombocytopenic purpura, von Willebrand's disease, and liver disease. Obstetric causes include severe hypertensive disorders, placental abruption, intrauterine fetal demise, amniotic fluid embolism, sepsis, or massive hemorrhage from any cause. If not already available, laboratory studies should be obtained. If available, an antithrombin III level should also be obtained.

Treatment guidelines include the following, but many smaller hospitals do not have platelets or fresh frozen plasma available and emergency transportation systems may need to be activated.[13]

1. Maintain fibrinogen levels at more than 100 mg/ml with fresh frozen plasma. Each unit increases the fibrinogen 10 mg/100 ml. Cryoprecipitate can be used if the fibrinogen level is less than 50 mg/ml (expected rise 2–5 mg/100 ml per bag of cryoprecipitate).
2. Maintain platelet count greater than 50,000. Each pack increases the platelet count by 5,000 to 10,000. Eight packs of random, pooled-donor platelets or one single-donor apheresis pack should be administered for every six units of packed red blood cells.
3. Maintain the hematocrit at or greater than 30% with packed red blood cells. Each unit increases the hematocrit by 3% and the hemoglobin by 1.5 g/ml.
4. Correct a prolonged prothrombin (INR) time with fresh frozen plasma. One unit is usually given for every 4–5 units of packed red blood cells or stored whole blood.

5. If at any time a patient with PPH is hemodynamically unstable, call for immediate anesthetic, surgical, and additional nursing or medical assistance.

V. Summary

Risks factors for postpartum hemorrhage should be identified antepartum when possible and appropriate precautions taken, but hemorrhage is frequent in low risk patients. The incidence of significant hemorrhage can be reduced with active management of the third stage of labor. If hemorrhage occurs, morbidity and mortality can be lessened by early recognition and a systematic approach to management. Prompt fluid resuscitation and treatment of atony with oxytocin, Methergine, and Hemabate will control the vast majority of cases and improve outcomes.

References

1. Babi DA, Sherwood DA, Campbell CE: Intravenous nitroglycerin for uterine inversion. J Clin Anesth 4:487–488, 1992.
2. Combs CA, Murphy EL, Laros RK: Factors associated with postpartum hemorrhage with vaginal birth. Obstet Gynecol 77:69–76, 1991.
3. Drife J: Management of primary postpartum hemorrhage. Br J Obstet Gynaecol 104:275–277, 1997.
4. Gibb D: Confidential inquiry into maternal death. Br J Obstet Gynaecol 97:97–101, 1990.
5. Hofmeyr GJ, Nikodem VC, de Jager M, et al: A randomized placebo-controlled trial of oral misoprostol in the third stage of labour. Br J Obstet Gynaecol 105:971–975, 1998.
6. Hood D: Anesthetic techniques in obstetric emergencies. Acta Anaesthes Scand 111:172–173, 1997.
7. Keirse MJ: What does prevent postpartum hemorrhage? Lancet 351:690–692, 1998.
8. Prendiville WJ, Elbourne D, McDonald S: Active versus expectant management in the third stage of labour (Cochrane Review). In The Cochrane Library, Issue 4, 2000. Oxford, Update Software.
9. Morey SS: ACOG releases report on risk factors, causes and management of postpartum hemorrhage. Am Fam Physician 58:1002–1004, 1998.
10. Norris TC: Management of postpartum hemorrhage. Am Fam Physician 55:635–640, 1997.
11. Ogueh O, Auoda G: Acute uterine inversion: new techniques of hydrostatic replacement. Br J Obstet Gynaecol 104:951–954, 1997.
12. Prendiville WJ, Elbourne D: Care during the third stage of labor. In Chalmers I, Enkin M, Keirse MJNC (eds): Effective care in pregnancy and childbirth. Oxford, Oxford University Press, 1989, pp 1145–1169.
13. Skye DV: Management of peripartum hemorrhage. W Med J 97:43–46, 1998.
14. Zahn CM, Yeomans ER: Postpartum hemorrhage: Placenta accreta, uterine inversion, and puerperal hematomas. Clin Obstet Gynecol 33:422–431, 1990.

SECTION F.
RETAINED PLACENTA

Janis E. Byrd, M.D.

I. Definition

The normal third stage of labor is defined as 30 minutes.

II. Classification

If the placenta is abnormally adherent, it may be either partially or completely involved. It may also be classified on the extent of invasion.

A. Placenta Accreta

The placenta is adherent to the myometrium.

B. Placenta Increta

The placenta invades the myometrium.

C. Placenta Percreta

The placenta penetrates the myometrium and the serosal surface.

TABLE 9.   Identified Risk Factors for Placenta Accreta

Placenta previa*
Prior cesarean section*
Post-pregnancy curettage
Prior retained placenta
Uterine infection

* Women with placenta previa and prior cesarean section are at much higher risk for placenta accreta; risk may be as high as 1 in 3.

III. Epidemiology
Retained placenta occurs in 2–6% of vaginal deliveries, with placenta accreta being a rare cause (1 in 2000).[4] Risk factors for placenta accreta are listed in Table 9.

IV. Pathophysiology
A. Insufficient Uterine Contractions
Sufficient uterine contractions may not occur to induce placental detachment.
B. Entrapped Placenta
The placenta may separate but become trapped by the contracted cervix.
C. Insufficient Decidual Tissue
The placenta may be abnormally adherent because of scanty or absent decidua; thus the normal line of cleavage through the decidual layer is absent. Partial separation of the placenta is more likely to cause postpartum hemorrhage because the uterus cannot contract effectively to control the bleeding.

V. Prevention
Active management of the third stage of labor with oxytocin and controlled cord traction (See section E, part III) may reduce the incidence of retained placenta. In one study the incidence of retained placenta with active management was 1.3% versus 4.5% in the expectant management group (OR 0.31, 95% CI 0.15–0.63).[3]

VI. Diagnosis and Management
A. Umbilical Cord Traction
If the cervix and uterus are contracted around the placenta, but the placenta is low in the uterine cavity, firm traction on the umbilical cord may effect delivery of the trapped placenta. The other hand should apply pressure with the tips of the fingers suprapubically to prevent uterine inversion.
B. Use of Oxytocin
If the placenta has not separated, oxytocin may induce placental detachment. It can be administered via umbilical vein injection using a dilution of 10–20 IU of oxytocin in 20 ml of saline. Three to five minutes should be allowed before deciding if the method has failed. Use of oxytocin may prevent the need for manual removal of the placenta in half or more cases.[3]
C. Uterine Relaxation for Entrapped Placenta
If the placenta has separated but remains trapped, halothane general anesthesia or tocolytics may allow delivery by relaxing the uterus. The provider needs to be prepared to reverse the uterine relaxation immediately to prevent excessive blood loss. The use of intravenous or sublingual nitroglycerin may obviate the need for general anesthesia and is short-lived, thereby reducing blood loss.[2]
D. Manual or Instrumented Placental Removal
If the placenta has not separated, attempt to identify a cleavage plane. Before attempting manual removal, make sure a large-bore intravenous line is in place, blood is available, and anesthesia and surgical backup are present. A complete placenta

accreta generally does not bleed, but once separation is attempted, blood loss can be rapid. If a cleavage plane can be identified, the provider may advance a hand between the placenta and uterus, attempting to deliver the placenta intact, if possible. When parts of the placenta are adherent, dull uterine curettage may remove fragments. Previously discussed agents may be used to induce uterine contractility. If hemorrhage still cannot be controlled, the patient may require an emergency hysterectomy. Retained placenta requiring manual removal or other procedures places the patient at higher risk for late postpartum bleeding and infection. Prophylactic antibiotics may be indicated if intervention has been extensive.

References

1. Gazvani MR, Luckas MJM, Drakeley AJ, et al: Intraumbilical oxytocin for the management of retained placenta: A randomized controlled trial. Obstet Gynecol 91:203–207, 1998.
2. Hood DD: Anesthetic techniques in obstetric emergencies. Acta Anaesth Scand 111:172–173, 1997.
3. Khan GQ, John IS, Wani S, et al: Controlled cord traction versus minimal intervention techniques in delivery of the placenta: A randomized controlled trial. Am J Obstet Gynecol 177:770–774, 1997.
4. Zahn CM, Yeomans ER: Postpartum hemorrhage: Placenta accreta, uterine inversion, and puerperal hematomas. Clin Obstet Gynecol 33:422–431, 1990.

SECTION G.
PREECLAMPSIA AND ECLAMPSIA

Janis E. Byrd, M.D.

Hypertensive disorders are the most common complication of pregnancy and the second leading cause of maternal mortality.[21,24] However, most women do not develop maternal or fetal complications[20] because current diagnostic criteria and risk factor assessment do not accurately predict outcomes (Table 10).[7] This is likely to continue until the etiologies are better understood.[19] With our current level of knowledge and medicolegal climate, however, as many as 75% of the women treated may not truly be at risk.[29] The clinical challenge is to define patients at high risk for intrapartum complications

TABLE 10. Risk Factors for Preeclampsia

Preconceptional and/or chronic risk factors	Exogenous factors
Partner-related risk factors	Smoking (risk reduction)
Nulliparity/primipaternity/adolescent pregnancy	Stress, work-related psychosocial
Limited sperm exposure, donor insemination, oocyte	strain
donation	In utero DES exposure
Oral sex (risk reduction)	Pregnancy-associated risk factors
Partner who fathered a preeclampsia pregnancy	Multiple pregnancy
in another woman	Structural congenital anomalies
Non-partner related risk factors	Hydrops fetalis
History of previous preeclampsia	Chromosomal anomalies
Age, interval between pregnancies	(trisomy 13, triploidy)
Family history	Hydatidiform mole
Presence of specific underlying disorders	Urinary tract infection
Chronic hypertension and renal disease	
Obesity, insulin resistance, low birth weight	
Gestational diabetes, type 1 diabetes mellitus	
Activated protein C resistance, protein S deficiency	
Antiphospholipid antibodies	
Hyperhomocysteinemia	
Sickle cell disease, sickle cell trait	

From Clinical Obstetrics and Gynecology, Lippincott Williams & Wilkins, 1999, p 423, with permission.

and institute the appropriate surveillance and management while avoiding unnecessary interventions that may increase morbidity in women who have only gestational hypertension or mild preeclampsia.

I. Definition
Preeclampsia is defined as new-onset hypertension > 140/90 after 20 weeks of gestation with proteinuria > 300 mg/24 hours, and significant non-dependent edema.[21] Other measures of proteinuria are > 0.1 g/L on two specimens 6 hours apart or > 2+ on a clean-catch specimen in the absence of infection.[3] Blood pressure should be obtained in the semi-reclining position and may be influenced by activity, anxiety, and pain. Preeclampsia is categorized as mild or severe. Severe preeclampsia is said to exist if the blood pressure is > 160/110 when measured two times 6 hours apart and/or proteinuria is > 500 mg/24 hours (4+ on dipstick). Severe preeclampsia also exists if there is hematologic (thrombocytopenia), renal (uric acid > 7.8), hepatic (elevated liver enzymes), central nervous system or pulmonary involvement.

II. Diagnosis
A. Laboratory Studies
The diagnosis of preeclampsia is supported by a uric acid level of greater than 5.5 to 6.0.[3,15] Many clinicians use a uric acid determination as part of the routine laboratory work-up along with hemoglobin, liver function tests, and platelet count. Unless the latter are abnormal, it is not necessary to obtain other coagulation tests such as fibrinogen, prothrombin, or partial thromboplastin times; they are often part of the initial evaluation if the diagnosis is strongly suspected.
B. History and Physical Examination
Most patients are nulliparas but older multiparas are more likely to have HELLP syndrome, as described below. Gestational age should be accurately assessed using all available data as this may affect both risk assessment and management. Major risk factors for preeclampsia/eclampsia include renal disease, diabetes mellitus, and chronic hypertension, especially if associated with early-pregnancy proteinuria.[21,25] Symptoms may include headache, visual disturbance, epigastric or right upper quadrant pain, or nausea and vomiting. Physical examination should include funduscopic, heart, lung, and abdominal exams, reflexes, and evaluation of edema in addition to routine obstetrical evaluation. Severe hypertension without proteinuria may be present in cocaine abuse.
C. Ultrasound
Ultrasound is most often used for determination of fetal size, gestational age, presentation, and fetal well-being. Uterine artery flow has not proven useful with a positive predictive value of only 27%.[6] Newer studies of cerebral perfusion may prove useful both diagnostically and therapeutically.[4] "...Eclampsia may represent the end stage of at least two very different pathophysiological pathways: one in which cerebral perfusion is low because of vasospasm and another in which cerebral perfusion is increased because of abnormal autoregulation."[5]

III. Pathophysiology
Preeclampsia is known to be a vasoconstrictive state with early abnormal placentation but the underlying cause is unknown. The three leading theories are immune maladaptation, placental ischemia, and genetic predisposition.[8] These theories have led to identification of multiple markers that may eventually prove useful in diagnosis prior to onset of clinical disease or in identifying subgroups of patients.[20] It has also led to trials of preventive and therapeutic agents such as aspirin and calcium channel blockers based on proposed mechanisms of action such as inflammation, prostacylin-thromboxane

TABLE 11. Clinical and Laboratory Characteristics of HELLP, TTP/ HUS, and AFL

	HELLP	TTP/HUS	AFL
Hypertension	++	+/-	+/-
Proteinuria	++	+/-	+/-
Thrombocytopenia	+++	+++	+/-
Lactate dehydrogenase	++	+++	++
Anemia	+	++	+/-
Bilirubin	+	++	++
AST	++	+/-	++
Fibrinogen	=	=	<
Antithrombin III	<	=	<
Ammonia	=	=	+
Glucose	=	=	<
Creatinine	+	++	++

+/-, equivocal; +, possible; ++, likely; +++, definitive; =, normal; <, decreased.
From Clinical Obstetrics and Gynecology, Lippincott Williams & Wilkins, 1999, p 558, with permission.

imbalance, and other thrombophilic states.[2,9,10,16,22] To date no theory or treatment alone has been sufficient to predict or prevent preeclampsia. Most likely the pathophysiology involves interaction of immune maladaptation with multiple underlying genetic factors such as hypertension, obesity, carbohydrate intolerance, and thrombophilic disorders. Placental ischemia is probably an end-stage phenomenon.

IV. Differential Diagnosis for Preeclampsia
Several rare disorders may mimic certain clinical and laboratory aspects of preeclampsia/eclampsia, although hypertension is less prominent (Table 11).[11]

A. Intrahepatic Cholestasis
Intrahepatic cholestasis generally presents only with pruritus and/or jaundice. The bilirubin is < 5 and there is no significant elevation of transaminases (Fig. 4).[13]

B. Acute Fatty Liver
Acute fatty liver (AFL) can be very confusing as patients often present with headache, nausea, vomiting, or abdominal pain. Platelets and fibrinogen may be decreased with prolongation of the PT and PTT. The bilirubin is often markedly elevated with only modest elevations of the transaminases at < 1000 IU.

C. Thrombotic Thrombocytopenic Purpura/Hemolytic Uremic Syndrome
Thrombotic thrombocytopenic purpura or hemolytic uremic syndrome (TTP/HUS) may also present with decreased platelets, hemolysis, headache, confusion, abdominal pain, and renal abnormalities. Fever may be present and the white blood cell count may be elevated. Fibrinogen, PT, and PTT are normal, but transaminases may be > 1000 IU. Haptoglobin is decreased and the Coombs' test is negative.

D. Maternal Sepsis
Finally, sepsis should be considered when the differential diagnosis is in doubt. Management of these disorders is beyond the scope of this text and the interested reader is referred to additional sources.[11,13]

V. Management
A. Initial Treatment
The fetus should be continuously monitored with the mother at bed rest in the left lateral decubitus position. She should be kept NPO with an eclamptic tray nearby. An intravenous line should be started and fluids (D5/0.45NS) kept at < 150 ml/hour. This should be reduced if oliguria (< 100 ml/4 hours) is present. Accurate intake and output should be recorded hourly and may require placement of a Foley catheter.

Alanine Aminotransferase Elevation During Pregnancy

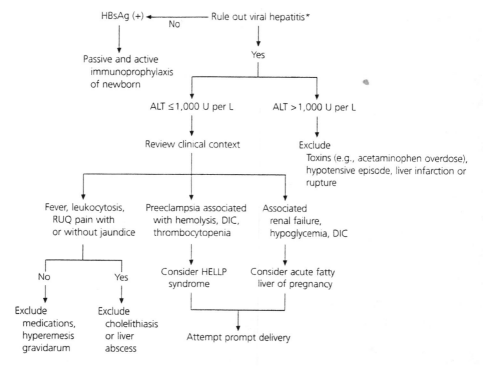

Recommended serologic tests: Hepatitis A IgM, hepatitis B surface antigen and hepatitis B core antibody, hepatitis C antibodies, cytomegalovirus IgM, herpes simplex virus IgM, and Epstein-Barr virus IgM.

FIGURE 4. Algorithm for the evaluation of alanine aminotransferase elevation during pregnancy. HBsAg, hepatitis B surface antigen; ALT, alanine aminotransferase; RUQ, right upper quadrant; DIC, disseminated intravascular coagulopathy; HELLP, hemolysis, elevated liver enzymes, low platelets. (From Hunt CM, Sharara AI: Liver disease in pregnancy. Am Fam Physician 59:829–836, 1999, with permission.)

B. Seizure Prophylaxis

The effectiveness of magnesium sulfate has been well validated, although the exact mechanism of action has not been fully elucidated and therapeutic levels have never been established.[14,23] Higher levels are needed to stop seizures than to prevent them.[29] A loading dose of 4–6 grams is generally given over 10–20 minutes followed by a continuous infusion at 2 g/hour. An initial level is checked at 1 hour after loading. Levels of 6–8 are generally considered therapeutic. Loss of reflexes may occur at a level of 10 with respiratory depression and/or arrest at levels of 12–15. Calcium gluconate, 10 ml of a 10% solution is given intravenously over 3 minutes as an antidote to magnesium sulfate toxicity. Magnesium sulfate does not have a significant tocolytic effect when used for treatment of preeclampsia in women at term in active labor. Although a theoretical risk of neuromuscular blockade and hypotension exists with concurrent use with nifedipine, in practice this appears to be relatively uncommon.[14]

C. Continuing Surveillance

Vital signs should be recorded every 15–30 minutes with hourly reflexes and lung auscultation. Magnesium levels, platelets, hemoglobin, liver functions, uric acid,

TABLE 12. Parenteral and Oral Drugs for Treatment of Severe Hypertension in Pregnancy

Drug	Dose	Onset of Action	Duration	Adverse Effect
Parenteral drugs				
Hydralazine	5–10 mg IV q 20 min	10–20 min	3–6 hr	Tachycardia, headache, flushing, aggravation of angina
Labetalol	20–80 mg IV q 10 min	5–10 min	3–6 hr	Scalp tingling, vomiting, heart block
Sodium	0.25–10 µg/ kg/min IV	Immediate	1–2 min	Nausea, vomiting, muscle twitching, thiocyanate and cyanide intoxication
Nitroglycerin	5–100 µg/min IV	2–5 min	3–5 min	Headache, methemoglobinemia, tachyphylaxis
Nicardipine	5–15 mg/hr IV	5–10 min	1–4 hr	Tachycardia, headache, phlebitis
Oral drugs				
Nifedipine	10 mg PO q 30 min	10–15 min	4–5 hr	Headache, tachycardia, synergistic interaction with magnesium sulfate
Clonidine	0.2 mg PO then 0.1 mg PO q 1 hr	30 min	6–8 hr	Drowsiness, bradycardia, ortho- static hypotension, rebound hypertension with abrupt withdrawal

From Clinical Obstetrics and Gynecology, Lippincott Williams & Wilkins, 1999, p 558, with permission.

renal function, and clotting studies should be obtained every 4–6 hours in labor depending on severity of disease.

D. Antihypertensive Therapy

Blood pressures > 160/110 mmHg should be treated to prevent cerebral hemorrhage, infarction, edema, and other cardiovascular complications, but will not prevent abruption. Table 12 lists oral and parenteral agents.[17] Hydralazine is still considered the drug of choice because of its safety and efficacy. Labetalol is a common second-line agent and nifedipine is frequently used "off-label" due to availability in an oral form. Epidural anesthesia alone lowers the blood pressure by 15%. Spinal anesthesia, although controversial, has shown similar declines.[12]

E. Management of Complications

1. HELLP syndrome

HELLP syndrome, defined as hemolysis (H), elevated liver enzymes (EL), and low platelets (LP) may first be diagnosed intrapartum and deteriorate rapidly, necessitating careful decisions regarding timing, route, and place of delivery.[18] Maternal and perinatal morbidity and mortality are significant. Management and transfer to a perinatal center is advisable if patient stability and time allow, especially if prematurity is present. One small RCT of expectant management of severe preeclampsia at 28–32 weeks' gestation showed a significantly higher gestational age at delivery (32.9 ± 1.5 vs. 30.8 ± 1.7 weeks, p = 0.0001).[26] Hematologic complications often require blood bank resources not available at smaller hospitals.

2. Route of delivery

Vaginal delivery is ideal when possible, but in numerous situations cesarean delivery will be necessary. Epidural anesthesia can be used if the platelet count is > 100,000. Additional risks of hypertension, intracranial hemorrhage, pulmonary edema, and laryngeal edema remain regardless of route.[27] A vertical incision may result in fewer wound complications.[18] Platelet transfusion should be given preoperatively for counts < 40,000 and prior to vaginal delivery for counts < 20,000 (see Chapter 7, section D for treatment of coagulopathy).

3. Corticosteroids

Dexamethasone, 10 mg IV every 12 hours for two doses, enhances fetal lung maturity, keeps maternal platelet counts above 100,000, and results in more rapid postpartum recovery.[18]

4. Liver rupture and hemodynamic monitoring

Sudden onset of hypotension in the setting of HELLP syndrome is often the first signal of liver rupture and generally requires immediate surgical intervention, although support exists for initial conservative management.[27] A pulmonary artery catheter is not necessary in all patients with severe preeclampsia but may be indicated if oliguria, pulmonary edema, and/or other multisystem organ involvement is present.

5. Encephalopathy and cerebrovascular accident (CVA)

Confusion, stupor, and coma without focal or lateralizing neurologic signs suggests hypertensive encephalopathy. The diastolic pressure is usually but not always > 130. Associated signs and symptoms include headache, visual disturbance, nausea, vomiting, and seizures. Differentiation from eclampsia may be difficult, but seizures unresponsive to magnesium dictate CT scanning, as do focal neurologic signs.

6. Eclampsia

Forty percent of eclamptic seizures occur antepartum prior to hospitalization. If a seizure occurs after magnesium loading, an additional 2-gram bolus should be given intravenously over 3–5 minutes. Recurrent convulsions on adequate magnesium may be treated with a short-acting barbiturate such as amobarbital 250 mg IV over 3–5 minutes. Most eclamptic seizures resolve in 60–90 seconds.

7. Abruption

The incidence of placental abruption is increased in hypertensive disorders (see Chapter 6, section B) and the odds ratio is stronger in smokers with severe preeclampsia (OR 5.9, CI 3.4–10.3).[1]

8. Fetal growth

Preeclampsia increases the risk of intrauterine growth restriction and low birthweight (OR 2.65, CI 1.73–4.39) as well as increases the risk of severe preeclampsia (OR 2.53, CI 1.19–4.93).[30]

F. Postpartum Management

Delivery is the definitive treatment for preeclampsia and eclampsia but HELLP syndrome and eclampsia may both manifest themselves in the postpartum period. Mild preeclampsia usually resolves in 24 hours but intensive monitoring should continue until (1) the platelet count shows an upward trend, (2) liver enzymes show a downward trend, (3) hypertension is well-controlled, and (4) diuresis of at least 100 ml per hour occurs without fluid bolus or diuretics.[18] Daily monitoring of laboratory values is sufficient for mild disease but should be obtained every 4–6 hours with severe disease until improvement is seen. Corticosteroids should be continued until HELLP syndrome is resolved. Neonates should be observed for hypermagnesemia, hypocalcemia, respiratory depression, hyporeflexia, excessive drowsiness, or ileus.

VI. Patient Counseling

Our limited knowledge of the cause(s) of preeclampsia prevents us from predicting in most cases which women are at risk. We do know that women with severe chronic hypertension are at increased risk but cannot predict those who will be at even greater risk if they develop superimposed preeclampsia.[28] Conversely, we can advise those with mild chronic hypertension or gestational hypertension that risks are minimal. All women can be counseled regarding good nutrition, smoking cessation, warning signs, and the importance of prenatal visits.

VII. Summary

Despite much research, the cause of hypertensive disorders in pregnancy remains unknown and the intrapartum management of preeclampsia/eclampsia continues to be a problem for obstetric providers. Family physicians and midwives must be prepared to diagnose preeclampsia, recognize the degree of severity, and institute emergency management.

References

1. Ananth CV, Smulian JC, Vintzileos AM: Incidence of placental abruption in relation to cigarette smoking and hypertensive disorders during pregnancy: A meta-analysis of observational studies. Obstet Gynecol 93:622–628, 1999.
2. Arias F, Romero R, Joist H, et al: Thrombophilia: A mechanism of disease in women with adverse pregnancy outcome and thrombotic lesions in the placenta. J Matern Fet Med 7:277–286, 1998.
3. Barton JR, Witlin AG, Sibai BM: Management of mild preeclampsia. Clin Obstet Gynecol 42:455–469, 1999.
4. Belfort MA, Anthony J, Saade GR: Prevention of eclampsia. Semin Perinatol 23:65–78, 1999.
5. Belfort MA, Giannina G, Herd JA: Transcranial and orbital doppler ultrasound in normal pregnancy and preeclampsia. Clin Obstet Gynecol 42:479–506, 1999.
6. Benedetto C, Valensise H, Marozio L, et al: A two-stage screening test for pregnancy-induced hypertension and preeclampsia. Obstet Gynecol 92:1005–1011, 1998.
7. Dekker GA: Risk factors for preeclampsia. Clin Obstet Gynecol 42:422–435, 1999.
8. Dekker GA, Sibai BM: The immunology of preeclampsia. Semin Perinatol 23:24–33, 1999.
9. Duley L: Aspirin for preventing and treating pre-eclampsia. BMJ 318:751–752, 1999.
10. Dumont A, Flahault A, Beaufils M, et al: Effect of aspirin in pregnant women is dependent on increase in bleeding time. Am J Obstet Gynecol 180:135–140, 1999.
11. Egerman RS, Sibai BM: Imitators of preeclampsia and eclampsia. Clin Obstet Gynecol 42:551–562, 1999.
12. Hood DD, Durry R: Spinal versus epidural anesthesia for cesarean section in severely preeclamptic patients: A retrospective survey. Anesthesiology 90:1252–1254, 1999.
13. Hunt CM, Sharara AI: Liver disease in pregnancy. Am Fam Physician 59:829–836, 1999.
14. Idama TO, Lindow SW: Magnesium sulphate: A review of clinical pharmacology applied to obstetrics. Br J Obstet Gynaecol 105:1040–1041, 1998.
15. Lim KH, Friedman SA, Ecker JL, et al: The clinical utility of serum uric acid measurements in hypertensive diseases of pregnancy. Am J Obstet Gynecol 178:1067–1071, 1998.
16. Liu HS, Chu TY, Chang YK, et al: Thromboxane and prostacyclin in maternal and fetal circulation in pre-eclampsia. Inter J Gynaecol Obstet 63:1–6, 1998.
17. Mabie WC: Management of acute severe hypertension and encephalopathy. Clin Obstet Gynecol 42:519–531, 1999.
18. Magann EF, Martin JN Jr: Twelve steps to optimal management of HELLP syndrome. Clin Obstet Gynecol 42:532–550, 1999.
19. Mattar F, Sibai BM: Prevention of preeclampsia. Semin Perinatol 23:58–64, 1999.
20. Myatt L, Miodovnik M: Prediction of preeclampsia. Semin Perinatol 23:45–57, 1999.
21. Norwitz ER, Robinson JN, Repke JT: Prevention of preeclampsia: Is it possible? Clin Obstet Gynecol 42:436–454, 1999.
22. Redman CW, Sacks GP, Sargent IL: Preeclampsia: An excessive maternal inflammatory response to pregnancy. Am J Obstet Gynecol 180:499–506, 1999.
23. Sander R, Konijeneberg A, Huijgen HJ, et al: Intracellular and extracellular, ionized and total magnesium in pre-eclampsia and uncomplicated pregnancy. Clin Chem Lab Med 37:55–59, 1999.
24. Sibai BM: Hypertension in pregnancy. Clin Obstet Gynecol 42:421, 1999.
25. Sibai BM, Lindheimer M, Hauth J, et al: Risk factors for preeclampsia, abruptio placentae, and adverse neonatal outcomes among women with chronic hypertension. National Institute of Child Health and Human Development Network of Maternal-Fetal Medicine Units. N Engl J Med 339:667–671, 1998.
26. Sibai BM, Mercer BM, Schiff E, Friedman SA: Aggressive versus expectant management of severe preeclampsia at 28 to 32 weeks' gestation: A randomized controlled trial. Am J Obstet Gynecol 171:818–822, 1994.
27. Van Hook JW: Management of complicated preeclampsia. Semin Perinatol 23:79–90, 1999.
28. Witlin AG: Counseling for women with preeclampsia or eclampsia. Semin Perinatol 23:91–98, 1999.
29. Witlin AG: Prevention and treatment of eclamptic convulsions. Clin Obstet Gynecol 42:507–518, 1999.
30. Xiong X, Mayes D, Demianczuk N, et al: Impact of pregnancy-induced hypertension on fetal growth. Am J Obstet Gynecol 180:207–213, 1999.

SECTION H.
MEDICAL EMERGENCIES IN PREGNANCY

Carol Osborn, M.D.

Pulmonary embolism and septic shock are uncommon but potentially lethal complications of pregnancy. Usually unanticipated, these disease processes require an astute evaluation and rapid decision making to decrease perinatal morbidity and mortality. While the evaluation occurs, ongoing resuscitation directed at basic life support prevents further deterioration of the mother and fetus.

The lack of prospective clinical trials as to the optimal treatment makes management of these emergencies controversial and stressful. Given that these events are rare, clinical trials in the future are unlikely. Instead, large existing databases and national registries provide retrospective case reviews to help define disease incidence and risk factors. These reviews also help to understand clinical presentations and therapeutic efficacy.

I. Pulmonary Embolism

Pulmonary embolism (PE) is the leading maternal cause of death in the developed world.[9,10] These deaths are often preventable. Assessing and intervening for risk factors, obtaining objective diagnoses, and starting timely treatment will reduce both the mortality and morbidity associated with PE.

A. Incidence

Maternal death from pulmonary embolism is still rare at 1 per 100,000.[9] These deaths occur throughout the antenatal and postnatal period with the greatest risk in the postpartum period. Although 75% of the deep vein thromboses occurred before delivery, 66% of the PE developed after delivery, especially following cesarean sections.[20]

B. Natural History

Since PEs arise from the pelvic and lower extremity venous system, recognizing deep venous thrombosis (DVT) is essential in preventing further illness from embolization. The Glasgow database of 72,000 deliveries revealed an incidence of 0.6 per 1,000 for women under 35 and 1.2 for women over 35 years.[14] Failure to recognize and diagnosis DVTs results in a 15–24% increased risk of a PE. Maternal death occurs in 15% of this underdiagnosed group.[23]

C. Risk Factors

1. Pregnancy

Pregnant women are 5–6 times more likely to develop a PE than nonpregnant women.[18] Furthermore, pregnant women over 35 years have a double risk of pulmonary embolism.[14]

2. Cesarean section

The highest risk period for a PE occurs immediately following an operative delivery.[20] The risk of PE increases 8 times from an emergency cesarean section under general anesthesia.[6]

3. Parity and obesity

These are risk factors independent of age. Although restricted movement such as long automobile and air travel is associated with increased risk, bed rest has not clearly shown to increase the risk of an embolism.[3]

4. Factor V Leiden and antithrombin III deficiency

Patients with these disorders are three times more likely to experience thromboembolic disease in pregnancy. With each pregnancy those with antithrombin III deficiency increase their risk for a DVT between 12–60%.[7]

D. Pathophysiology

Three factors increase the risk of pulmonary thromboembolism in the pregnant state.

1. Hypercoagulable state

There are changes in coagulation factors that promote clotting.

2. Reduction in the venous blood flow

The reduction in venous flow in early pregnancy occurs from an increase in venous capacity. Compression of the inferior vena cava from the gravid uterus causes the reduced venous flow during the later stages of pregnancy. Because this obstruction occurs especially on the left side, 85% of DVTs are on the left side.[8]

3. Tissue injury

Tissue injury is common during instrumented vaginal deliveries or cesarean sections.

E. Diagnosis

Many symptoms are associated with pulmonary embolism, including dyspnea, tachycardia, pleuritic chest pain, and hypotension, but patients tend to present with the following signs and symptoms.[22]

1. Hypotension
2. Change in mental status, often with loss of consciousness
3. Chest tightness
4. Pleuritic chest pain with or without hemoptysis
5. Dyspnea

Physical findings associated with embolisms include a transient friction rub. If the embolism is massive, cyanosis, hypotension, and an elevated jugular venous pressure are obvious findings.

Symptoms and signs are often subtle and may be confused with typical findings in pregnancy, such as lower extremity edema and dyspnea. Therefore, diagnostic testing is essential. Avoidance of a diagnostic test due to potential x-ray exposure of the fetus is a common error. Given the seriousness of this diagnosis, a complete work-up is essential if clinically suspicious findings are present. Table 13 includes diagnostic tools that assist in this evaluation. Usually the combination of a clinical assessment, V/Q scanning, and duplex ultrasound will lead to a diagnosis. However, with an indeterminate V/Q scan and negative duplex scans, additional imaging is often necessary.[22]

F. Medical Decision-Making

1. Initial management

Initial management of a potential PE focuses on the patient's hemodynamic stability. The hypoxic, hypotensive patient requires immediate resuscitation. High-flow oxygen and IV access are necessary measures. Central venous pressure monitoring helps in following right heart filling pressure.[2]

2. Rapid assessment for other diagnoses

Although pulmonary embolism remains the most common etiology of acute pulmonary distress in pregnancy, other diagnostic possibilities to consider include pneumonitis, spontaneous pneumothorax, air or amniotic fluid embolism, and septic shock. The clinical presentation and a chest x-ray may help differentiate these possibilities.

3. Initial treatment of suspected PE

If the clinical probability of an embolism remains high, begin unfractionated heparin IV with a 5000-unit bolus (75 U/kg) followed by a continuous infusion.[1] As the patient stabilizes, begin a complete diagnostic work-up, including CBC, coagulation screening, thrombophilia screen, chest x-ray, EKG, V/Q scan, and lower extremities Doppler scans.

TABLE 13.   Diagnostic Tests in Suspected Pulmonary Embolus

Test	Finding	Usefulness of Test
D-dimer	Levels increased in pregnancy[6]	Little value
Chest radiograph	Atelectasis, pleural effusion, raised diaphragm, wedge-shaped infiltrate	Nonspecific
EKG	Sinus tachycardia, RAD, S-wave in lead I, Q waves in leads II and III, and nonspecific changes	Nonspecific
ABG	PaO_2 decreased, PaO_2 normal or low (PaO_2 in normal pregnancy may vary as much as 15 mmHg from the supine to the sitting position)[23]	Nonspecific
Ventilation/perfusion	Perfusion defects	Primary test, useful if normal or high probability
Doppler US	Visualize clot in the lower extremities	Useful if V/Q shows low or intermediate probability
Pulmonary angiography	Constant luminal filling defect or an abrupt cut-off of a pulmonary artery	Gold standard, useful if V/Q probability is intermediate and US negative
Helical CT	Image clot directly	Helpful in life-threatening presentations[22]
MRI	Image clot directly without radiation	Not well studied in pregnancy

4. Management of the unstable patient

If the patient remains seriously unstable, aggressive interventions such as thrombolysis (streptokinase or TPA) or thrombectomy should be considered. Both interventions require angiography or a helical CT, not only to confirm the diagnosis, but also to guide the procedure. These interventions require experienced staff in a tertiary care center. Thrombolysis with TPA and streptokinase, both intravenous and catheter-directed, has been used in gravely ill patients during pregnancy with some success, although bleeding complications have occurred.[11,17]

5. Indications for immediate delivery

Immediate delivery is required if the resuscitation does not resolve the hypoxia and hypotension, and fetal distress is prolonged.[19]

6. Management of the stable patient

In the clinically stable patient, more methodical diagnostic testing is done before treatment is initiated. The primary diagnostic test for PE is the ventilation/perfusion scan (Table 14). The diagnosis is further supported with a DVT demonstrated on Doppler ultrasound of the legs. More definitive or repeat testing is necessary if the diagnosis remains unclear; this includes pulmonary angiography, helical CT scans, or MRI testing. Once a diagnosis is made, one of two anticoagulation regimens is recommended.

   a. Unfractionated heparin IV 5000 units bolus, followed by a continuous IV infusion for 5–10 days. Twice-daily subcutaneous dosing is then initiated after the IV heparin is discontinued in antepartum patients. The dose

TABLE 14.   Probability of Pulmonary Thromboembolism Based on V/Q Scans Report[22]

Scan Category	Probability (%)
High probability	87
Intermediate probability	30
Low probability	14

needs to be adjusted based on activated partial prothrombin time (APTT) with the therapeutic range 1.5–2.5 times normal. Commonly, this will result in total daily doses of 10,000 units in the first trimester up to 20,000 units in the third trimester. Postpartum patients may be anticoagulated with Coumadin in the usual manner with the goal of achieving an INR of 2–2.5.

  b. Low-molecular-weight heparin (LMWH) dosed at 1 mg/kg (based on early pregnancy weight) every 12 hours. The advantage of LMWH includes fewer side effects than unfractionated heparin and minimal monitoring. Recommendations on monitoring LMWH are not established in pregnancy; however, some experts suggest measuring anti-Xa activity 3 hours post-injection (therapeutic range 0.4–1.0 U/ml).[6]

7. Duration of anticoagulation

Anticoagulation is recommended for 3–6 months after diagnosis. Although lacking evidence, most experts also advise anti-coagulation until 6 weeks postpartum due to a persistent hypercoaguable state. Postpartum therapies include the following:

  a. Switch from unfractionated heparin to Coumadin 24 hours after delivery.
  b. Continue LMWH at 40 mg twice daily.[22]

II. Amniotic Fluid Embolism

This is a rare, unexpected, and often catastrophic event in pregnancy. The incidence varies from 1/8000 to 1/80,000 pregnancies with a mortality rate as high as 80%.[5] Due to the low incidence all data originate from retrospective case analyses. The original description of this event by Steiner and Luschbaugh has been revised especially as national databases and registries are developed and analyzed.[5,21]

A. Risk Factors

This condition was originally described in association with precipitous deliveries and hypertonic contractions. Meconium was also implicated as a risk factor. Further review and study of cases have revealed no specific risk factors. In 12% of the cases artificial rupture of membranes occurs within minutes of this catastrophic event.[5] At least two cases of amniotic fluid embolism occurred during a saline amnioinfusion.[15]

B. Pathophysiology

Steiner and Luschbaugh theorized that a bolus of amniotic fluid forced into the intravascular system by tetanic contractions caused hemodynamic instability and cardiopulmonary failure.[21] Recent case analysis suggests an anaphylactoid syndrome develops when a small amount of amniotic fluid sensitizes the maternal system. This results in platelet-fibrin thrombi formation and deposition in the pulmonary vasculature. Clotting factors depletion and disseminated intravascular coagulation (DIC) also develop.[4]

C. Clinical Features

Sudden onset of dyspnea followed by hypotension and rapid decomposition to cardiopulmonary arrest characterizes the clinical presentation of amniotic fluid embolism. If the woman survives the initial resuscitation, secondary pulmonary edema, adult respiratory distress syndrome, and DIC soon follow.

D. Diagnostic Work-up

An amniotic fluid embolism is sudden and often catastrophic. Although the clinical presentation suggests the diagnosis, post-mortem aspiration of central venous blood is usually needed to confirm the presence of amniotic fluid debris. The following tests are nonspecific but support an amniotic fluid embolism and help differentiate other conditions such as a pulmonary embolism or MI.

1. EKG: right ventricular strain pattern
2. Chest x-ray: perihilar infiltrate
3. Arterial blood gases: deceased PaO_2
4. Coagulation studies: DIC features

E. Medical Management

Initial attention with this unexpected event includes securing the airway, and using endotrachial intubation and 100% oxygen. IV access is crucial. Placement of a central venous or pulmonary artery catheter to administer and monitor effects of pressor agents such as dopamine and dobutamine is recommended. Blood work should include CBC, type cross, coagulation panel, electrolytes, renal function, and ABG. Other tests to consider include chest x-ray, V/Q scan, and cardiac enzymes. Clotting studies need to be repeated every 2 hours and blood products administered as indicated.[12]

III. Septic Shock

Septic shock in pregnancy is rare with the estimated incidence of 1 in 8,000 pregnancies. The associated mortality varies widely from 20–60%.[13]

A. Clinical Features

Predisposing factors to the development of sepsis includes prolonged rupture of membranes (resulting in chorioamnionitis and postpartum endometritis), surgical delivery, uterine evaluation for retained products, and infections of the urinary tract. Patients presenting with fevers, especially with hypotension, require an immediate investigation of the source of an infection, which is essential for treatment.[22]

B. Management

1. Hemodynamic stabilization
Volume replacement (crystalloid with wedge pressure monitoring)
Inotropic therapy (dopamine or dobutamine)
Peripheral vasoconstrictors (phenylephrine)
Extreme caution is advised if inotropic or peripheral vasocontrictors are administered antenatally.
2. Identify the infectious source
   a. Blood, urine and/or cervical cultures
   b. Abdominal CT, uterine ultrasound scans, consider amniocentesis
   c. Chest x-ray
   d. Exploratory laparotomy for suspected peritonitis or intra-abdominal abscess
3. Other laboratory tests
   a. DIC panel
   b. CBC
   c. Liver function tests
4. Broad-spectrum antibiotics, such as:
   a. Ampicillin, gentamicin, or clindamycin
   b. Imipenem

IV. Cardiovascular Resuscitation in Late Pregnancy

A. Advanced Cardiac Life Support (ACLS) Recommendations

ACLS recommends that CPR is most effective if the patient is in a supine position on a firm surface. In advanced pregnancy, however, this position compresses the vena cava and reduces venous return to the heart. Because of this anatomic condition, CPR performed in late pregnancy is most effective with the patient in a lateral position at 30° or manually deviating the uterus to the left and slightly cephalad with the leg raised in the supine position.[16]

B. Timing of Cesarean Intervention

Case reviews of cardiac arrest in late pregnancy found improved outcome if a crash cesarean section was performed within 10 minutes of initiating CPR. In cases where CPR was performed for more than 10 minutes much poorer fetal outcomes were noted.[19]

References

1. British Society for Haematology: Guidelines on the prevention and management of thrombosis associated with pregnancy. J Clin Path 46:489–496, 1993.
2. British Thoracic Society: Suspected acute pulmonary embolism: A practical approach. Thorax 52:511–524, 1997.
3. Carr MH, Towers CV, Eastenson AR, et al: Prolonged bed rest during pregnancy. J Matern Fet Med 6:264–267, 1997.
4. Clark SL: Amniotic fluid embolism. Clin Perinatol 13:801–815, 1986.
5. Clark SL, Hankins GD, Dudley DA, et al: Amniotic fluid embolism: Analysis of the national registry. Am J Obstet Gynecol 172:1158–1169, 1995.
6. De Sweit M: Management of pulmonary embolus in pregnancy. Eur Heart J 20:1378–1385, 1997.
7. Friderich PW, Sanson BJ, Simioni P, et al: Frequency of pregnancy related venous thromboembolism in anticoagulant factor-deficient women: Implications for prophylaxis. Ann Intern Med 125:955–960, 1996.
8. Gherman RB, Goodwin TM, Leung B, et al: Incidence, clinical characteristics, and timing of objective diagnosed venous thromboembolism during pregnancy. Obstet Gynecol 94:730–734, 1999.
9. HMSO. Report on Confidential Inquires into Maternal Deaths in the United Kingdom 1994–1996, 1998.
10. Koonin LM, Atrash HK, Lawson HW, et al: Maternal morbidity surveillance, U.S., 1979–86. MMWR CDC Surveillance Summary 40:1–13, 1991.
11. Krishnamurthy P, Martin CB, Kay HH, et al: Catheter directed thrombolysis for thromboembolic disease during pregnancy. J Matern Fetal Med 8:24–27, 1999.
12. Locksmith GJ: Amniotic fluid embolism. Ob Gyn Clin North Am 26:435–444, 1999.
13. Mabie WC, Barton JR, Sibai B: Septic shock in pregnancy. Obstet Gynecol 90:553–561, 1997.
14. Macklon NS, Greer IA: Venous thromboembolic disease in obstetrics and gynaecology: The Scottish experience. Scot Med J 41:83–186, 1996.
15. Maher JE, Wenstrom KD, Hauth JC: Amniotic fluid embolism after saline amnioinfusion: Two cases and review of the literature. Obstet Gynecol 83:851–853, 1994.
16. Marx GF: Cardiopulmonary resuscitation of late pregnant women. Anesthesiology 56:156, 1982.
17. Mazeika PK, Oakley DM: Massive pulmonary embolism in pregnancy treated with streptokinase and percutaneous catheter fragmentation. Eur Heart J 15:1281–1283, 1994.
18. National Institutes of Health: Prevention of venous thrombosis and pulmonary embolism: NIH Consensus Development. JAMA 256:744–749, 1986.
19. Oates S, Williams GH, Rees GA: Cardiopulmonary resuscitation in late pregnancy. BMJ 297:404–405, 1988.
20. Rutherford S, Montoro M, McGhee W, et al: Thrombembolic disease associated with pregnancy: An eleven-year review. Am J Obstet Gynecol 164:286–290, 1991.
21. Steiner PE, Luschbaugh CC: Maternal pulmonary embolism by amniotic fluid. JAMA 117:1245–1254, 1941.
22. Thomson AJ, Greer IA: Non-haemorrhage obstetric shock. Baillieres Clin Obstet Gynecol 14:19–41, 2000.
23. Toglia MR, Weg JG: Venous thromboembolism during pregnancy. N Engl J Med 335:108–114, 1996.

CHAPTER 16

Malpresentations and Malpositions

This chapter discusses the management of face, brow, transverse lie, transverse arrest, twin delivery, and breech presentations. It also discusses the recognition and treatment of the persistent occiput posterior malposition. Section H addresses the procedure of external cephalic version.

SECTION A.
DIAGNOSIS

Elizabeth G. Baxley, M.D.

I. Introduction

The lie is the relation of the long axis of the fetus to the mother; longitudinal lies are present in over 99% of pregnancies. The presenting part is the portion of the body of the fetus that is closest to the birth canal; it is the presenting part that determines the presentation. In the longitudinal lie, the presenting part is either breech or vertex. When the long axis is transverse, the shoulder is most often the presenting part.

In 95% of pregnancies near term the fetus assumes a longitudinal lie with the vertex directed at the maternal pelvis, the back convex, and the head sharply flexed on the neck such that the chin is nearly in contact with the chest. In the remaining 5% of cases, a deviation occurs from this normal lie, constituting a malpresentation. Common factors associated with malpresentations include grand multiparity with lax maternal abdominal support, high fundal or lower uterine segment implantation of the placenta, prematurity, macrosomia, hydramnios, uterine malformations, fetal anomalies, and a contracted maternal pelvis. The literature also suggests that malpositions are more often seen with the use of epidural anesthesia.[5,8,9] It is not clear, however, if the relationship is causal. It may be that by excessive relaxation of the pelvic musculature epidural anesthesia prevents appropriate rotation of the vertex, leading to occiput posterior, persistent transverse, or asynclitic presentations.

Careful attention to prenatal diagnosis of a fetal malpresentation is essential to maximize fetal outcomes. Higher rates of maternal and perinatal mortality have been reported with fetal malpresentation. In unstable or transverse lie, perinatal mortality rates from 3.9% to 24% have been reported, with up to 10% maternal mortality in some series.[6] Cord prolapse occurs twenty times as often in cases of transverse lie as compared to vertex presentations.

II. Incidence

At or near term the incidence of various malpresentations is as follows:

A. Face Presentation

The reported incidence of face presentation varies widely, from 0.1% to 2.0%; the majority of reports place the average incidence of this particular malpresentation at 0.2–0.3%, or 1 in 500–600 deliveries.[1,2,4,6,7]

B. Brow Presentation

Brow presentation is less common than face, with a reported incidence ranging from 1/468 to 1/3543 deliveries; most reports give an average incidence of 0.007% or 1 in 1400 deliveries.[1,3,4,6,7]

C. Transverse Lie

This malpresentation complicates 0.3% to 0.4% of all births, or 1/300 births.[1,4,6,7]

D. Breech Presentation

The incidence of breech presentation is highly dependent on gestational age, decreasing in frequency as the pregnancy progresses:

1. Incidence at 28 weeks: 22–25%
2. Incidence at 32 weeks: 7–13%
3. Incidence at 36 weeks: 5–7%
4. Incidence at 40 weeks: 2.5–6%

III. Diagnosis

Several diagnostic measures can be used to determine the lie and presentation of a fetus, including abdominal palpation, vaginal examination, auscultation, and radiography or ultrasonography.

A. Abdominal Palpation

Abdominal palpation can be performed throughout the latter weeks of gestation, and between contractions in early labor, to gain information about the presentation and position of the fetus. A systematic set of four maneuvers, called Leopold maneuvers, are used to examine the gravid abdomen (Fig. 1).[4]

1. First maneuver

After outlining the contour of the uterus, the examiner gently palpates the fundus to determine which fetal pole is present.

2. Second maneuver

This portion of the maneuver involves placing the palms of the examiner's hands on either side of the abdomen with gentle but deep pressure. This indicates the side on which the fetal back is located (hard, resistant structure) versus where the fetal limbs are located (numerous nodulations).

3. Third maneuver

Using the thumb and fingers of one hand and grasping the lower portion of the maternal abdomen above the pubic symphysis, the examiner can differentiate between the head and breech.

4. Fourth maneuver

Facing the mother's feet and using the fingertips of each hand, the examiner palpates above and to the sides of the symphysis pubis to determine the degree of head flexion in a cephalic presentation.

B. Vaginal Examination

Vaginal examination may be helpful in palpating the presenting part, although it can be inconclusive if the presenting part is very high or when palpating through a closed cervix and thick lower uterine segment. If the cervix is dilated enough to admit the examiner's gloved finger, the head versus breech usually can be readily distinguished from one another by differentiation of the sutures and fontanels from the sacrum and ischial tuberosities.

C. Auscultation

Auscultation by itself does not determine the fetal position, but may reinforce what the examiner suspects from palpation. In the vertex and breech positions, fetal heart tones are best heard through the fetal back, whereas in a face presentation they are heard through the fetal thorax. In vertex presentations, heart tones are heard with maximal intensity between the umbilicus and the anterior superior iliac spine of the

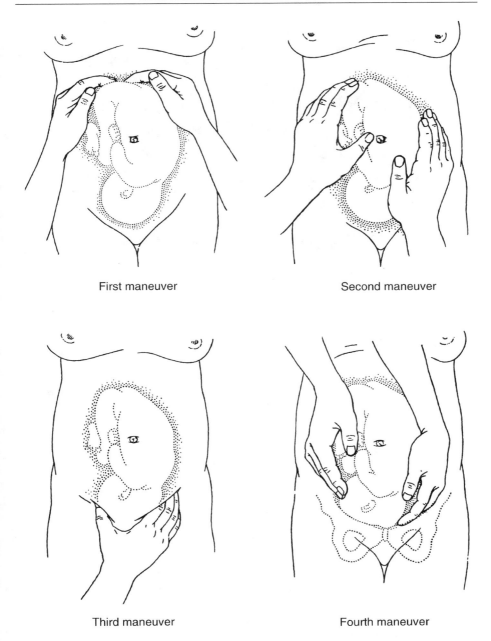

First maneuver   Second maneuver

Third maneuver   Fourth maneuver

FIGURE 1. Illustration of Leopold maneuvers. (From Pritchard JA, Mac Donald PC, Gant NF: Williams Obstetrics, 17th ed. Norwalk, CT, Appleton-Century-Crofts, 1985, with permission.)

mother. In breech presentations, this point of maximal intensity is closer to the level of the umbilicus. In the more common occipito-anterior position, fetal heart tones are heard best near the midline, whereas in transverse presentations they are more lateral and in posterior presentations the point of maximal intensity is back toward the mother's flank.

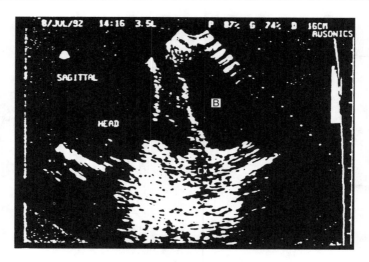

FIGURE 2. Sagittal ultrasound scan of cephalic presentation. The infant's head is seen adjacent to the cervix (CX) and maternal bladder (B).

D. Diagnostic Ultrasonography
Bedside ultrasound in labor and delivery can be used to determine fetal presentation when abdominal and vaginal examinations are not confirmatory. Visualization of the fetal head versus breech in the lower uterine segment is definitive (Fig. 2). When the presenting part is high, cord presentation may be discovered, although the absence of cord preceding the head does not guarantee safety of artificial rupture of membranes. Ultrasound also allows identification of placental location and may indicate fetal malformations associated with an abnormal lie. Visualization with real-time ultrasound is an important adjunct to external cephalic version.

E. X-Ray Examination
A single x-ray film may be used to aid in the diagnosis of fetal presentation. Information received in these cases far exceeds the minimal risk from plain film exposure. This type of examination may be more helpful in obtaining specific types of information, including type of breech presentation, extent of fetal neck extension, and gross maternal pelvic deformity.

References

1. Cruickshank DP: Malpresentations and umbilical cord complications. In Scott JR, DiSaia PJ, Hammond CB, Spellacy WN (eds): Danforth's Obstetrics and Gynecology, 6th ed. Philadelphia, J.B. Lippincott, 1990.
2. Duff P: Diagnosis and management of face presentation. Obstet Gynecol 57:105–112, 1981.
3. Levy DL: Persistent brow presentation: A new approach to management. South Med J 69:191–192, 1976.
4. Pritchard JA, MacDonald PC, Gant NF: Dystocia caused by abnormalities in presentation, position, or development of the fetus and presentation, position, attitude and lie of the fetus. In Pritchard JA, MacDonald PC, Gant NF (eds): Williams Obstetrics, 17th ed. Norwalk, CT, Appleton, 1985, pp 659–666.
5. Saunders NJ Sr, Spiby H, Gilbert L, et al: Oxytocin infusion during second stage of labour in primiparous women using epidural analgesia: A randomized double-blind placebo-controlled trial. BMJ 299:1423–1426, 1989.
6. Seeds JW: Malpresentations. In Gabbe SG, Niebyl JR, Simpson JL (eds): Obstetrics: Normal and Problem Pregnancies, 2nd ed. New York, Churchill Livingstone, 1991, pp 539–549.
7. Shields JR, Medearis AL: Fetal malformations. In Hacker NF, Moore JG (eds): Essentials of Obstetrics and Gynecology, 2nd ed. Philadelphia, W.B. Saunders, 1992.
8. Thorp JA, Hu DH, Albin RM, et al: The effect of intrapartum epidural analgesia on nulliparous labor: A randomized, controlled prospective trial. Am J Obstet Gynecol 169:851–858, 1993.
9. Wittels B: Does epidural anesthesia affect the course of labor and delivery? Semin Perinatol 15:358–367, 1991.

SECTION B.
FACE PRESENTATION

Elizabeth G. Baxley, M.D.

I. Introduction

Face presentation occurs when the fetal head hyperextends such that the fetal face, between the chin and the orbits, is the presenting part. High maternal parity and a pendulous abdomen predispose to this presentation, as do a contracted pelvis and fetal macrosomia.[4] Anencephalic fetuses almost always present by the face, due to lack of cranium development; this malformation has been reported to be seen in one-third of cases of face presentation.[6]

II. Diagnosis

The diagnosis of face presentation is usually not made until late in labor.[4] Only 3% of face presentations are diagnosed antepartum, with 35% being diagnosed in the first stage, 27% in the second stage, and 35% at the time of delivery.

A. Abdominal Palpation

On Leopold maneuvers, face presentation is suspected when the cephalic prominence is on the same side as the fetal spine, occasionally with a palpable groove between them. Fetal heart tones are usually heard on the side of the small parts, below the umbilicus.[4]

B. Vaginal Examination

Face presentation is more often diagnosed by palpation of fetal mouth, nose, malar bones, and orbital ridges during vaginal examination. It is possible to confuse a face presentation with a breech presentation. In face presentations, the fetal mouth and malar prominences form the corners of a triangle, whereas in the breech the fetal anus is always on a line with the ischial tuberosities.

C. Radiologic Examination

Bedside ultrasound quickly reveals if the breech or head is presenting, and may demonstrate that the fetal neck is hyperextended. If ultrasound is not available or the diagnosis is uncertain, a conventional x-ray film of the abdomen also may demonstrate hyperextension of the fetal head.[4]

III. Management

The delivery position of the face is categorized according to the position of the fetal chin, or mentum. The majority (60–80%) of face presentations are in the mentum anterior position, whereas 10–12% are mentum transverse and 20–25% are mentum posterior.[2,6,7] This is an important clinical distinction, as the mentum anterior position delivers by spontaneous vaginal delivery 75% of the time, with the delivery of the head occurring by flexion rather than extension. The chin and mouth appear at the vulva initially followed by the nose, mouth, and brow. This is represented in an old obstetrical adage "if a face is progressing, leave it alone."[2]

Protracted labor is not uncommon in face presentations and can be an ominous sign, as it has been associated with an increased number of intrapartum deaths.[6] An increased incidence of fetal heart rate abnormalities also has been reported in labors with face presentations (predominantly variable decelerations), and continuous electronic fetal monitoring is recommended in these cases.[1,5] Internal fetal monitors must be applied very carefully, avoiding ocular and cosmetic damage and preferentially placing the electrode over the fetal chin.

Almost all mentum transverse and one-half to one-third of mentum posterior presentations spontaneously rotate to a mentum anterior position. However, a persistent mentum posterior position cannot deliver vaginally, since the additional extension required to negotiate the pelvic curvature during descent is not possible. Cesarean section is indicated for persistent mentum posterior or when there is an arrest of dilatation or descent in any face presentation.[3] Maneuvers to convert a face presentation to a vertex result in increased perinatal morbidity and mortality, and should not be attempted. Face presentation is not a contraindication to use of oxytocin or forceps, although vacuum extraction should not be applied to the fetal face.

Close observation of the neonate must occur after delivery of a face presentation, as laryngeal and tracheal edema are possible sequelae of the birth process and may require nasotracheal intubation if severe.[6] There is almost always severe facial edema in the newborn, causing transient distortion, about which parents need reassurance.

References

1. Benedetti TJ, Lowensohn RI, Truscott AM: Face presentation at term. Obstet Gynecol 55:199–202, 1980.
2. Cruickshank DP: Malpresentations and umbilical cord complications. In Scott JR, DiSaia PJ, Hammond CB, and Spellacy WN (eds): Danforth's Obstetrics and Gynecology, 6th ed. Philadelphia, J.B. Lippincott, 1990.
3. Danforth DN: Dystocia due to abnormal fetopelvic relations. In Danforth DN, Scott JR (eds): Obstetrics and Gynecology, 5th ed. Philadelphia, J.B. Lippincott, 1986.
4. Duff P: Diagnosis and management of face presentation. Obstet Gynecol 57:105–112, 1981.
5. Schwartz Z, Dgani R, Lancet M, et al: Face presentation. Aust N Z J Obstet Gynaecol 26:172–176, 1986.
6. Seeds JW: Malpresentations. In Gabbe SG, Niebyl JR, Simpson JL (eds): Obstetrics: Normal and Problem Pregnancies, 2nd ed. New York, Churchill Livingstone, 1991, pp 539–549.
7. Shields JR, Medearis AL: Fetal malformations. In Hacker NF, Moore JG (eds): Essentials of Obstetrics and Gynecology, 2nd ed. Philadelphia, W.B. Saunders, 1992.

SECTION C.
BROW PRESENTATION

Elizabeth G. Baxley, M.D.

I. Introduction

A brow presentation occurs as a result of extension of the fetal head midway between the vertex (flexion) and the face (hyperextension). The presenting part of the fetus visualized is that between the orbits and the anterior fontanelle. The frontal bones form the point of designation (e.g., right frontal transverse), with frontum anterior as the most common position. Brow presentations are usually unstable, occurring when the head is in the process of converting from a vertex to a face or vice versa.

The etiology of brow presentation is similar to that of a face presentation. Any condition that causes abnormal neck extension and prevents descent of the fetal head can predispose to brow presentation. Fetal neck masses should be considered (e.g., cystic hygroma or teratoma) and ruled out by ultrasonography.

II. Diagnosis
A. Abdominal Palpation
Rarely, by Leopold maneuvers, a brow presentation may be diagnosed when the examiner is able to palpate both the fetal chin and occiput.
B. Vaginal Examination
Brow presentation is more commonly diagnosed by palpating orbital ridges, eyes, frontal sutures, or the anterior fontanelle during vaginal examination. Like with a face presentation, this diagnosis is made before the second stage of labor in fewer than half of cases.[1,3]

C. Ultrasound versus X-Ray Diagnosis

Plain-film abdominal x-rays can demonstrate the degree of neck flexion better than ultrasonography, and should not be avoided due to concerns about ionizing radiation, particularly in cases where labor is prolonged or has a secondary arrest.

III. Management

The prognosis of a brow presentation depends on the final presentation of the fetal vertex. It is an unstable lie, converting to a face or an occiput presentation two-thirds of the time. As with face presentations, management is expectant as long as labor is progressing normally. However, prolonged labors have been observed in 33–50% of brow presentations and secondary arrest is common.[3,4] Persistent brow presentations are unable to deliver vaginally unless the fetus is very small or the pelvis very large, because of the large presenting diameter. Methods to convert the brow presentation are contraindicated. Cesarean section is the safest delivery method for a persistent brow presentation.[2]

References

1. Cruickshank DP: Malpresentations and umbilical cord complications. In Scott JR, DiSaia PJ, Hammond CB, Spellacy WN (eds): Danforth's Obstetrics and Gynecology, 6th ed. Philadelphia, J.B. Lippincott, 1990.
2. Danforth DN: Dystocia due to abnormal fetopelvic relations. In Danforth DN, Scott JR (eds): Obstetrics and Gynecology, 5th ed. Philadelphia, J.B. Lippincott, 1986.
3. Seeds JW: Malpresentations. In Gabbe SG, Niebyl JR, Simpson JL (eds): Obstetrics: Normal and Problem Pregnancies, 2nd ed. New York, Churchill Livingstone, 1991, pp 539–549.
4. Shields JR, Medearis AL: Fetal malformations. In Hacker NF, Moore JG (eds): Essentials of Obstetrics and Gynecology, 2nd ed. Philadelphia, W.B. Saunders, 1992.

SECTION D.
TRANSVERSE LIE

Elizabeth G. Baxley, M.D.

I. Introduction

In a transverse lie, the long axis of the fetus is perpendicular to that of the mother. Persistence of a transverse lie beyond 36–38 weeks' gestation is a significant clinical problem that must be managed carefully and systematically. In a transverse lie, the fetal head is in one iliac fossa of the mother, while the breech lies in the other iliac fossa. The fetal shoulder is typically the presenting part, and this condition is called a shoulder presentation.

The incidence of transverse lie is ten times higher in grand multiparous patients (parity of four or more) than in nulliparous women. Additionally, any condition that obstructs the lower uterine segment predisposes to transverse lie, including placenta previa or low-lying placenta, lower uterine segment uterine myomas, uterine anomalies, and fetal masses.

II. Diagnosis
A. Abdominal Palpation

Even before abdominal palpation, a transverse lie is often recognizable by inspection alone, when the maternal abdomen is observed to be wider from side to side and the fundus does not extend very far beyond the umbilicus. In the case of a transverse lie, the fetal spine is either positioned up toward the maternal head or down toward the maternal cervix. With the first Leopold maneuver neither the head nor the breech is found in the fundus, and on the second maneuver the fetal head and buttocks are palpable in opposite iliac fossas. With abdominal palpation, the location of the fetal back (up or down) is readily identified.

B. Vaginal Examination
Neither the fetal head nor breech is found to be presenting on vaginal examination.
C. Radiologic Examination
Ultrasonography can rapidly confirm the diagnosis of transverse lie, as well as indicate the position of the fetal spine, the placental implantation site, and any fetal abnormalities that predispose to the transverse lie.

III. Management
A. External Version
Before the onset of labor, attempts at external cephalic version are worthwhile if membranes are intact, and if placenta previa and pelvic masses have been excluded as a cause. Emergency cesarean section and neonatal resuscitation capabilities must be immediately available if external version is attempted. Internal cephalic version is contraindicated because of the high rate of fetal and maternal complications. If the attempted version fails, or if rupture of membranes has occurred, vaginal delivery is impossible and cesarean section should be performed.[3]
B. Labor and Delivery Management
Spontaneous delivery of a term infant in impossible in cases of a persistent transverse lie. All of these women should be managed with elective cesarean section, often with a vertical uterine incision necessitated by the difficulty encountered in extraction of the fetus.

Unexpected spontaneous rupture of membranes (SROM) or artificial rupture of membranes (AROM) without a fetal part filling the pelvic inlet results in cord prolapse twenty times more often than in a vertex presentation, particularly for a "back up" transverse lie. AROM should be avoided when a shoulder presentation is present. Even with appropriate care, rates of maternal and fetal morbidity and death are higher with transverse lie due to the frequent association of this malpresentation with placenta previa, the higher risk of cord accidents, and the inevitability of abdominal delivery.

In cases of neglected transverse lie, the fetal shoulder is forced into the pelvis by the strength of the uterine contractions. After rupture of membranes, the corresponding arm often prolapses into the vagina. The shoulder arrests in the margins of the pelvic inlet after some descent, but becomes impacted here as labor continues. This is an obstetric emergency. If not recognized and managed promptly, the uterus eventually ruptures as it contracts and tries to overcome the obstruction. The mother and fetus usually die without treatment.

References
1. Danforth DN: Dystocia due to abnormal fetopelvic relations. In Danforth DN, Scott JR (eds): Obstetrics and Gynecology, 5th ed. Philadelphia, J.B. Lippincott, 1986.

SECTION E.
TRANSVERSE ARREST

Stephen D. Ratcliffe, M.D., M.S.P.H.

I. Definitions and Causes
The classic definition of this condition is arrest of descent of the fetal head with the sagittal suture in a transverse position at the level of the mid-pelvis without the normal rotation of the head into the anteroposterior plane for 30 minutes.[1] This condition is caused by the shape of the maternal pelvis (flattened in the anteroposterior plane) or by ineffective uterine contractions.

II. Management
A. Change in Maternal Position
A change in maternal position may encourage the fetus to rotate spontaneously.
B. Attempted Manual Rotation from Occiput Transverse to Occiput Anterior
Once complete dilatation has occurred, the clinician can attempt a manual rotation from the occiput transverse (OT) position to occiput anterior (OA) position using the maneuver described in section F. Maintaining flexion of the fetal head and using an abdominal hand to gently sweep the fetal shoulder out of the anterior-posterior plane are important aids to successfully complete this maneuver.
C. Ineffective Uterine Contractions (see Chapter 13, section A)
If the cause is believed to be ineffective uterine contractions, oxytocin augmentation is indicated. It is difficult to make a diagnosis of cephalopelvic disproportion until this step has been carried out.
D. Cephalopelvic Disproportion (CPD)
If the above maneuvers have not been successful and the cause of the transverse arrest is believed to be an abnormally flattened maternal pelvis, cesarean section is indicated unless the operator is skilled in mid-forceps rotation with Kielland or Barton forceps. Mid-forceps rotations or applications at a station of 0 to + 2 carry greater maternal and infant morbidity than cesarean section.[1,2] Mid-forceps application or rotation should not be attempted by family physicians if cesarean intervention is readily available.

References
1. Danforth DN: Dystocia due to abnormal fetopelvic relations. In Danforth DN, Scott JR (eds): Obstetrics and Gynecology, 7th ed. Philadelphia, J.B. Lippincott, 1998.
2. Plauche WC: Operative vaginal delivery and abnormal vertex presentation. In Plauche WE, Morrison JC, O'Sullivan MJ (eds): Surgical Obstetrics. Philadelphia, W.B. Saunders, 1992.

SECTION F.
OCCIPUT POSTERIOR POSITION

Stephen D. Ratcliffe, M.D., M.S.P.H.

I. Definition, Causes, and Effects
The occiput posterior (OP) position occurs when the occipital portion of the fetal head presents in the posterior portion of the birth canal. The baby is often said to be looking upward. This malposition is a common challenge for the clinician to recognize and manage.
A. Epidemiology
At the onset of labor 10–20% of fetuses are in the OP position. Ultimately about 5% of vaginal deliveries occur in a persistent OP position. There is an increase in the incidence of the persistent OP position in women receiving epidural anesthesia (OR 4.5, CI 1.5–13.5, NNH = 10).[3]
B. Natural History
Gardberg et al. conducted a prospective study of 408 women in labor to track fetal positions throughout labor using bedside ultrasounds.[1] Sixty-eight percent of the persistent OP positions began labor in the occiput anterior (OA) position. Eighty seven percent of the fetuses that began labor in the OP position rotated spontaneously to OA prior to delivery. Women in labor whose fetuses are in the OP position tend to have "back labor" and may experience slower cervical dilatation and fetal descent. The duration of stage two is increased with persistent OP positions.[4]

C. Effect on Perinatal Outcome[4]
1. Maternal morbidity

Laboring women with persistent OP position experience an increase in the following complications.
   a. Number of episiotomies
   b. Third- and fourth-degree extensions
   c. Operative deliveries
   d. Cesarean deliveries
   e. Maternal blood loss
   f. Length of stay
2. Neonatal morbidity

Most, if not all, of the neonatal morbidity is associated with the use of forceps or vacuum-assisted deliveries. Pearl et al. reported an increased incidence of Erb's and facial nerve palsies with the use of forceps-assisted deliveries of babies in the persistent OP position.[4]

II. Diagnosis
The practitioner should be alerted to the possibility of an OP position when labor pains are primarily felt in the back. The clinician can make a diagnosis of OP position when the anterior fontanel (diamond-shaped, with four sutures emanating from the fontanel) is palpated in the anterior portion of the vagina and the posterior fontanel is palpated in the posterior portion of the birth canal. Occasionally the fetal ears can be felt to assist in making the diagnosis. Use of a bedside ultrasound scanner can confirm a diagnosis that is in doubt.

III. Management
A. Maneuvers to Correct an OP Position
1. Change of maternal position

There is no RCT evidence upon which to make recommendations. There is much "experience-based" opinion that encourages women to change positions frequently, particularly to the "hands and knees" position. It is thought that this may be helpful to rotate the fetus to the preferred OA position.
2. Manual rotation

Rotation of the persistent OP to an OA position can avoid prolongation of stage two and the entire list of maternal/infant complications listed above. The following steps to rotate a fetus from the OP position to OA are the methods used by the author.
   a. Inform your patient that effective pushing on her part is essential to help guide the rotation of her baby's head.
   b. If the fetus is in a left occiput posterior position (LOP), the clinician should rotate the head in a counterclockwise direction about 90° to a left occiput anterior (LOA) position. Likewise, if the fetal head is in an ROP position, the clinician should rotate the head in a clockwise direction (also about 90°) to the ROA position.
   c. Use of an assistant's hand to assist the rotation of the fetal shoulder can be a valuable addition to this procedure. The assistant's hand is applied in a "kneeding" fashion to the patient's left lower abdomen when making a LOP to LOA rotation to help rotate the right fetal shoulder in a counterclockwise direction (from the vantage point of the clinician). This allows the fetus to make a rotation of its entire body and not merely its head. Likewise, the assistant's hand should apply gentle pressure to the right lower abdomen to move the left fetal shoulder in a clockwise direction when making a ROP to ROA rotation.

d. It is important that the clinician's first maneuver when entering the vagina is to place the middle finger in the fetal posterior fontanel and then flex the fetal head by putting the middle finger on the posterior fontanelle and gently flexing the finger. *Do not elevate the fetal head.* During the ensuing manual rotation, every attempt should be made to maintain the fetal head in a flexed position.

e. During a contraction the mother is asked to push and the assistant is asked to begin a "kneading" motion over the appropriate side of the lower maternal abdomen. The clinician will have already flexed the fetal head and now places the middle finger along the upper lambdoidal suture and uses the torque of the hand to move the head in a rotary motion from LOP to LOA or from ROP to ROA. Remember to try to maintain flexion of the fetal head.

It is helpful to perform a number of manual rotations under the supervision of a practitioner skilled in this procedure to improve one's skills.

B. Delivery from an OP Position

1. Spontaneous vaginal delivery (SVD)

Women are often able to have an uneventful spontaneous vaginal delivery of an infant who was in a persistent OP position. During the final moments of pushing the fetus may undergo a spontaneous rotation to OA. There is, however, an increased risk of third- and fourth-degree extensions with an SVD.[4] This is thought to be due to the larger biparietal diameter that the persistent OP position presents with delivery of the infant's head.

2. Vacuum-assisted vaginal delivery (see Chapter 17, section D)

The vacuum device should be applied over the apex of the head 2–3 cm from the posterior fontanel. This may be difficult to do with the persistent OP position. Paramedian placement of the vacuum cup is associated with an increased risk of neonatal cephalhematomas.[5] There is RCT evidence that the use of softer vacuum cups versus rigid ones is associated with a decreased number of successful vaginal deliveries, particularly with delivery of the fetus in the OP position (OR = 1.64 , CI 1.11–2.41, NNH = 20), but the use of the soft cups is associated with a decrease in significant scalp trauma (OR = 0.55, CI 0.38–0.79, NNT = 14).[3]

3. Forceps-assisted vaginal delivery

Forceps may be applied to deliver an infant in the OP position. All of the prerequisites discussed in Chapter 17, section C should be met. The handles of the forceps should not be elevated in order to deliver the baby's face in the OP position. As a result, third- and fourth-degree extensions are common. In Pearl's series, the percentage of infants experiencing Erb's palsy was 1% and facial nerve palsy was 3% when forceps was used to deliver babies in the OP position.[4] Family physicians must be prepared to abandon this procedure and proceed to cesarean section if excessive traction is required to effect a vaginal delivery.

4. Cesarean section

When managing the woman with a persistent OP position, the clinician should make plans for the possibility of the diagnosis of cephalopelvic disproportion (CPD) that will necessitate a cesarean intervention. This is especially true for the nulliparous patient. The diagnosis of CPD is usually made with failure to descend with adequate uterine contractions with complete cervical dilatation or when there is an unsuccessful attempt at a vacuum- or forceps-assisted delivery.

References

1. Gardberg M, Laakkonen E, Salevaara M: Intrapartum sonography and persistent occiput posterior position: A study of 408 deliveries. Obstet Gynecol 91:746–749, 1998.
2. Howell CJ: Epidural versus non-epidural analgesia in labour (Cochrane Review). In The Cochrane Library, Issue 1, 2000, Oxford, Update Software.

3. Johanson R, Menon V: Soft versus rigid vacuum extractor cups (Cochrane Review). In The Cochrane Library, Issue 1, 2000. Oxford, Update Software.
4. Pearl M, Roberts J, Laros R, et al: Vaginal delivery from the persistent occiput posterior position: Influence on maternal and neonatal morbidity. J Reprod Med 38:955–961, 1993.
5. Teng FY, Sayre JW: Vacuum extraction: Does duration predict scalp injury? Obstet Gynecol 89:281–285, 1997.

SECTION G.
BREECH PRESENTATION

Stephen D. Ratcliffe, M.D., M.S.P.H.

I. Epidemiology[17]

A. Incidence
Breech deliveries occur in 4% of all deliveries, but occur in 15% of infants weighing less than 2500 grams.

B. Predisposing Factors[7]
1. Fetal anomalies
These include major structural abnormalities such as hydrocephaly and anencephaly as well as the major chromosomal anomalies.
2. Uterine overdistention
Major causes of overdistention include polyhydramnios and multiple gestation.
3. Uterine abnormalities/pelvic obstruction
Conditions include septate and bicornuate uterus. Pelvic obstructions include uterine fibroids, placenta previa, and low-lying placenta.

II. Natural History[7]

A. Spontaneous Conversion from Breech to Vertex
Of all fetuses that are breech at 32 weeks' gestation, about 60% spontaneously convert to vertex. Factors that reduce the conversion to vertex include nulliparity, previous breech, and extended fetal legs.[18]

B. Associated Fetal/Neonatal Conditions[12]
Central nervous system malformations occur in 1.5–2.0% of infants with a breech presentation. The incidence of trisomy 21 is 0.5%. Overall, 9% of all infants with breech presentations have some type of congenital malformation.

C. Effect on Perinatal Morbidity/Mortality
There is a fourfold increase in perinatal mortality among term infants and a threefold increase among preterm infants.[6,13,15] Two-thirds of these deaths are a result of congenital malformations or infections. Thus, only one-third of the increased risk of perinatal mortality is attributed to preventable factors, such as trauma and asphyxia.[4] The newborn may sustain trauma either via a vaginal or cesarean delivery. Asphyxia occurs most commonly as a result of umbilical cord compression.

III. Diagnosis[7]
When the clinician performs the Leopold maneuvers during an antenatal exam, the fetal head is palpated in the fundus and the softer breech is felt over the lower abdomen. A vaginal examination may be done to reveal soft fetal buttocks, genitalia, an anus or small parts. When the exam is in doubt, an ultrasound examination will resolve any questions as to the presenting fetal part. The types of breech presentations at term are shown in Figure 3.

A. Frank Breech
This occurs when the fetal hips are flexed and the knees are extended; this accounts for about 60% of breeches.

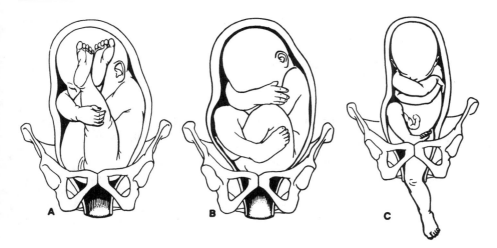

FIGURE 3. Variations of breech presentation. *A*, frank breech; *B*, complete breech; *C*, footling breech. (From Danforth DN, Scott JR: Obstetrics and Gynecology, 5th ed. Philadelphia, J.B. Lippincott, 1986, with permission.)

B. Incomplete Breech
The fetus has one or both of its hips incompletely flexed so that some part of the lower extremity is the presenting part. This presentation occurs about 25–35% of the time and is more common among premature fetuses.

C. Complete Breech
The fetus has its hips and knees flexed. This accounts for 5% of breech presentations.

IV. Management
The family physician should have a strategy to recognize and manage the breech presentation during the third trimester and in labor.

A. Antenatal Management
1. Recognition

   It is important to begin to assess the fetal lie beginning at 32 to 34 weeks' gestation using the techniques as described above.

2. Maneuvers to convert the breech to the vertex position

   a. External version. This maneuver can be carried out safely by a qualified operator beginning at 36 weeks' gestation for the nullipara and 38 weeks' gestation for the multipara. See section H in this chapter for a complete description of the procedure.

   b. Use of moxibustion. This is a type of traditional Chinese medicine that uses moxibustion (burning herbs to stimulate acupuncture points) of acupoint BL 67 (located beside the outer corner of the fifth toenail). A recent RCT in JAMA reported that the application of moxibustion for nullipara breech presentations beginning at 33 weeks' gestation resulted in increased fetal activity during the treatment period and an increased spontaneous conversion to the vertex presentation (relative risk 1.58, CI 1.29–1.94).[2]

   c. Postural management. The Cochrane meta-analysis of three RCTs involving a total number of 192 women showed that the use of postural management (elevation of the maternal pelvis) was associated with a nonsignificant trend towards fewer noncephalic births. The author of this review states "there is not enough evidence to evaluate the use of postural management for breech presentation."[11,14]

B. Intrapartum Management

After breech presentation is diagnosed and the patient is in active labor, one must decide whether to perform a cesarean section or attempt vaginal delivery. If the patient is not in active labor, external version can be considered (see section H). There are only two RCTs that assess the effect of a routine policy for performing cesarean versus attempted vaginal deliveries of a breech presentation at term. The preliminary evidence from these studies indicates an improved short-term neonatal morbidity and increased maternal morbidity with the practice of elective cesarean intervention. No difference in perinatal mortality was noted.[5,10] Long-term outcomes are not improved when comparing school-age children who were delivered with elective cesarean compared to vaginal breech deliveries.[8] There is a need for a large multicenter RCT to provide additional evidence to support the safety of elective vaginal breech delivery or to support the common practice of elective cesarean delivery.[9]

C. Factors Favorable for Vaginal Breech Delivery[7]

1. Frank breech
2. Gestational age between 36 and 38 weeks
3. Multiparous patient with previous vaginal breech delivery of infant over 3200 g or cephalic delivery of infant over 3600 g
4. Estimated fetal weight between 2700 and 3200 g (6 and 7 pounds)
5. Favorable (soft, effaced) cervix dilated 3 cm or more
6. Presenting part at or below 0 station at labor's onset
7. Adequate pelvimetry (particularly in the anteroposterior diameter): anteroposterior dimension of the inlet, 11 cm or greater transverse diameter of the inlet and anteroposterior diameter of the mid-pelvis, 12 cm or greater interspinous distance of the mid-pelvis, 9.5 cm or greater
8. Flexed fetal neck
9. Experienced operator

D. Factors Unfavorable for Vaginal Breech Delivery

1. Footling or complete breech presentation
2. Gestational age less than 36 or more than 38 weeks
3. Estimated fetal weight of less than 2700 g or more than 3800 g
4. No previous vaginal deliveries or difficult previous vaginal delivery
5. Unfavorable cervix
6. High presenting part at onset of labor
7. Maternal pelvis flattened in the anteroposterior diameter
8. Hyperextended fetal neck
9. Inexperienced operator

E. Special Precautions for Estimating Fetal Weight in Labor

A sonographic estimate of fetal weight can be helpful in deciding whether or not to attempt a vaginal breech delivery. It is important to note, however, that even skilled sonographers can estimate plus or minus 15% of the actual fetal weight. See section A for a more detailed discussion of this matter.

F. Techniques to Assess Maternal Pelvimetry

Once a determination of estimated fetal weight has occurred, a number of methods are available to assess maternal pelvimetry. The initial test of choice is a radiograph or bedside ultrasound of the maternal abdomen to assure that the fetal head is not extended and to look for other congenital anomalies. X-ray pelvimetry can produce the pelvic measurements as detailed above. CT pelvimetry has the advantage of using radiation that is 80% lower than conventional x-rays. A recent RCT that compared the use of MRI versus clinical pelvimetry showed that the use of this technology did not significantly reduce the overall cesarean rate. MRI pelvimetry was associated with a lower emergency cesarean rate.[16]

G. Technique of Vaginal Breech Delivery[7,19]

The following is the procedure for expediting vaginal delivery of the breech fetus. This procedure is commonly advocated with the assumption that progressive fetal acidosis occurs between delivery of the umbilical cord and the head. No trials of expedited breech delivery exist, however, on which to base clinical practice.

1. Expect spontaneous dilatation and descent at a normal rate

If the progress of labor is abnormal, consider abandoning vaginal delivery in favor of cesarean section. Avoid early amniotomy as it may increase the risk of cord prolapse.

2. Use of anesthesia

If used, anesthesia that permits full maternal cooperation is best (i.e., local, pudendal, low spinal, or epidural rather than general). Epidural anesthesia is associated with a prolonged stage two but not with an increase in breech extraction or cesarean sections.[1,3] Anesthesia personnel should be available on standby for the second stage of labor in case general anesthesia is required.

3. Delivery of the breech

The operator needs to have patience during this process and should monitor for fetal well-being throughout the delivery. Await descent of the breech until the perineum is distended. Delivery of the infant up to the umbilicus should occur by spontaneous contractions and maternal pushing. Once the fetal umbilicus has passed the perineum, the fetal head will have entered the maternal pelvis and vaginal breech delivery becomes the only available route of delivery.

4. Ensure that the fetal back is anterior

Grasp the hips to assure that the fetal back is anterior (Fig. 4). If the back rotates posteriorly, the head will be occiput posterior and the chin is likely to extend against the symphysis pubis with potentially disastrous results.

5. Freeing the umbilical cord

After the umbilicus is delivered, pull out a few inches of the umbilical cord if it appears to have excessive traction on it; otherwise, do not manipulate the umbilical cord.

6. Delivery of the body

Maternal pushing should be the major force to help deliver the fetal body. The operator can use a towel placed around the fetal pelvis with thumbs applied over the sacroiliac joints and fingers over the anterior thigh to apply very gentle downward traction. *The operator must not apply pressure to the fetal abdomen that could result in significant visceral injuries.*

7. Delivery of the shoulders and arms

If the shoulders and arms do not deliver spontaneously, sweep the posterior arm across the chest and out. If this is not effective, rotate the trunk to place the other shoulder posterior and sweep that arm out if it does not deliver spontaneously (Figs. 5 and 6). It is often helpful to have an assistant elevate the fetal trunk and legs by cradling it in a towel sling.

8. Delivery of the fetal head

An assistant maintains suprapubic pressure to keep the head flexed. An episiotomy may be necessary to provide the exposure to accomplish the following maneuvers.

    a. Digital pressure on the malar eminence with the same hand supporting the chest and the opposite hand pulling downward on the shoulders (Mauriceau-Smellie-Veit maneuver) (Fig. 7)

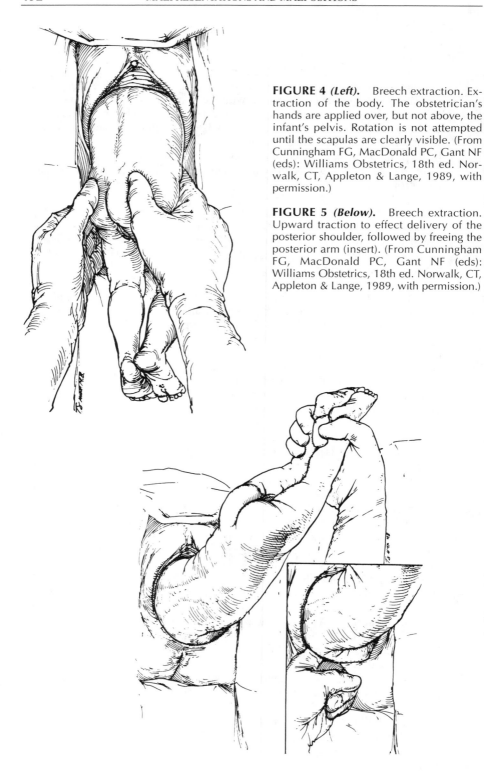

FIGURE 4 *(Left)*. Breech extraction. Extraction of the body. The obstetrician's hands are applied over, but not above, the infant's pelvis. Rotation is not attempted until the scapulas are clearly visible. (From Cunningham FG, MacDonald PC, Gant NF (eds): Williams Obstetrics, 18th ed. Norwalk, CT, Appleton & Lange, 1989, with permission.)

FIGURE 5 *(Below)*. Breech extraction. Upward traction to effect delivery of the posterior shoulder, followed by freeing the posterior arm (insert). (From Cunningham FG, MacDonald PC, Gant NF (eds): Williams Obstetrics, 18th ed. Norwalk, CT, Appleton & Lange, 1989, with permission.)

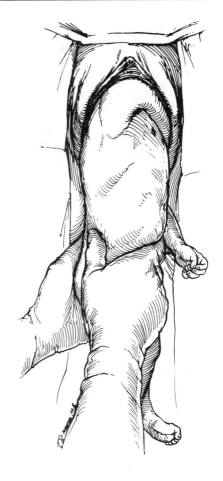

FIGURE 6 (*Right*).   Breech extraction. Delivery of the anterior shoulder by downward traction. The anterior arm may then be freed the same way as the posterior arm in Figure 5. (From Cunningham FG, MacDonald PC, Gant NF (eds): Williams Obstetrics, 18th ed. Norwalk CT, Appleton & Lange, 1989, with permission.)

FIGURE 7 (*Below*).   Delivery of aftercoming head. Note that as the fetal head is being delivered, flexion of the head is maintained by suprapubic pressure provided by an assistant and simultaneously by pressure on the maxilla (insert) by the operator as traction is applied. (From Cunningham FG, MacDonald PC, Gant NF (eds): Williams Obstetrics, 18th ed. Norwalk, CT, Appleton & Lange, 1989, with permission.)

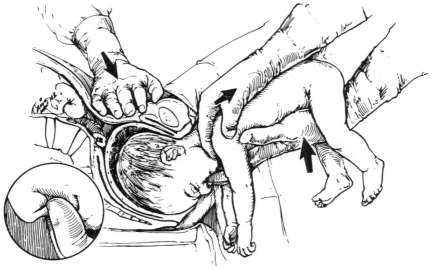

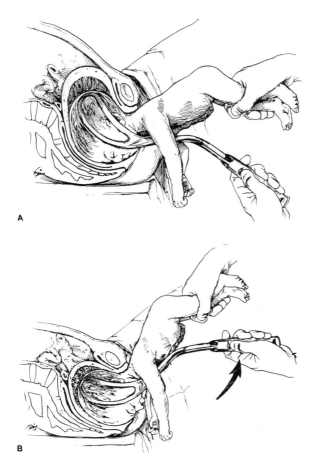

FIGURE 8. *A,* Forceps applied to the aftercoming head. The head has entered the pelvis and forceps have been applied. *B,* Forceps delivery of aftercoming head. Note the direction of movement (arrow). (From Cunningham FG, MacDonald PC, Gant NF (eds): Williams Obstetrics, 18th ed, Norwalk, CT, Appleton & Lange, 1989, with permission.)

   b. Digital pressure on the malar eminence as above with the opposite hand applying suprapubic pressure to maintain head flexion (Wigand-Martin maneuver)

   c. Piper forceps application (Fig. 8)

   The fetal body should not be elevated any more than being parallel to the floor to avoid hyperextension injuries. The operator may need to kneel on the floor to deliver the fetal head, particularly if forceps are applied.

References

1. Bingham P, Hird V, Lilford R: Management of the mature selected breech presentation: An analysis based on the intended method of delivery. Br J Obstet Gynaecol 94:746–749, 1987.
2. Cardini F, Weixin H: Moxibustion for correction of breech presentation. JAMA 280:1580–1584, 1998.
3. Chadha YG, Mahmoud TA, Dick MJ, et al: Breech delivery and epidural analgesia. Br J Obstet Gynaecol 99:96–100, 1992.
4. Cheng M, Hannah M: Breech delivery at term: A critical review of the literature. Obstet Gynecol 82:605–610, 1993.
5. Collea JV, Chein C, Quilligan EJ: The randomized management of term frank breech presentation: A study of 208 cases. Am J Obstet Gynecol 137:235, 1980.
6. Croughan-Minihane MS, Petitti DB, et al: Morbidity among breech infants according to method of delivery. Obstet Gynecol 75:821–825, 1990.

7. Cruickshank DP: Malpresentations and umbilical cord complications. In Danforth DN, Scott JR (eds): Obstetrics and Gynecology, 7th ed. Philadelphia, J.B. Lippincott, 1998.
8. Danielian PJ, Wang J, Hall M: Long-term outcome of term breech presentation by method of delivery. BMJ 312:1452–1453, 1996.
9. Hannah, M, Hannah W: Caesarean section or vaginal birth for breech presentation at term. BMJ 312:1433–1434, 1996.
10. Hofmeyr GJ, Hannah MC: Planned elective cesarean section for term breech presentation (Cochrane Review). In The Cochrane Library, Issue 1, 2000, Oxford: Update Software.
11. Hofmeyr GJ: Cephalic version by postural management (Cochrane Review). In The Cochrane Library, Issue 1, 2000, Oxford, Update Software.
12. Kaupilla O: The perinatal mortality in breech deliveries and observations on affecting factors: A retrospective study of 2227 cases. Acta Obstet Gynaecol Scand 39:1–10, 1975.
13. Kiely JL: Mode of delivery and neonatal death in 17,587 infants presenting by the breech. Br J Obstet Gynaecol 98:898–904, 1991.
14. Smith C, Crowther C, Wilkinson C, et al: Knee-chest postural management for breech at term: A randomized controlled trial. Birth 26:71–75, 1999.
15. Thorpe-Beeston JG, Banfield PJ, Saunders NJ Sr: Outcomes of breech delivery at term. BMJ 305:746–747, 1992.
16. Van Loon AJ, Mantingh A, Serlier D, et al: Randomised controlled trial of magnetic-resonance pelvimetry in breech presentation at term. Lancet 350:1799–1804, 1997.
17. Weiner CP: Vaginal breech delivery in the 1990s. Clin Obstet Gynecol 35:559–569, 1992.
18. Westgren M, Edvall H, Nordstrom L, et al: Spontaneous cephalic version of breech presentation in the last trimester. Br J Obstet Gynaecol 92:19–24, 1985.
19. Yasin S, O'Sullivan MJ: Assisted breech extraction. In Plauche WC, Morrison JC, O'Sullivan MJ (eds): Surgical Obstetrics. Philadelphia, W.B. Saunders, 1992, pp 325–346.

SECTION H.
EXTERNAL CEPHALIC VERSION

Kent Petrie, M.D.

External cephalic version is a procedure to manually guide a fetus from the breech to a vertex presentation performed to reduce the incidence of breech presentation at delivery. Fetuses found to be in the breech presentation at 36 weeks' gestation or later are candidates for external cephalic version.

I. Incidence of Breech[1,4]
There is a natural tendency toward spontaneous version from breech to cephalic presentation as pregnancy progresses. Twenty-five percent of fetuses are breech at 28 weeks' gestation. This number drops to 13% by 32 weeks. Nine percent of fetuses are breech at 36 weeks' gestation and half of these will revert spontaneously to cephalic presentation in the last month of pregnancy.[12]

Smaller fetuses are more likely to be breech at 40 weeks. Eight percent of 2000-gram fetuses are breech while only 3% of 3000-gram fetuses are breech.

II. Natural History
A. Conditions Associated with Breech Presentation
Multiple gestation, multiparity and uterine relaxation, polyhydramnios and oligohydramnios, pelvic tumors, uterine fibroids and septa, and a prior history of breech are factors increasing the incidence of breech presentation.
B. Congenital Anomalies
Congenital anomalies are seen more frequently in breech fetuses. These include hydrocephaly and anencephaly, and disorders of the gastrointestinal, genitourinary, cardiovascular, and musculoskeletal systems. Fetuses with Down syndrome also are more commonly found in the breech presentation.

III. Effect on Perinatal Outcome
A. Morbidity Associated with Breech Presentation
Breech presentation is a common problem that can cause hazards to both mother and fetus. Perinatal morbidity and mortality for vaginal breech delivery at term are significantly higher than for vertex delivery.
B. Maternal Morbidity and Mortality with Cesarean Section
Twelve percent of cesarean sections in the U.S. are now performed for breech presentation, ranking third most frequent indication, following repeat cesarean and labor dystocia.[4] This modern trend toward cesarean section for breech presentation at term has been accompanied by increased postsurgical maternal morbidity and mortality compared to vaginal delivery. Potential injury to the infant in breech, however, still exists at cesarean section.

IV. Diagnosis
Ultrasound is useful for confirmation of breech presentation and for ruling out certain birth defects and uterine anomalies that predispose to breech presentation.

V. Alternative Treatments for Version of the Breech Presentation
A. Prenatal Exercises
A small study[3] in which the patient assumed the knee-chest position with chest and head against the floor or bed and hips elevated, accompanied by gentle pelvic rocking for 20 minutes three times a day, demonstrated version rates significantly higher than controls. This posture allows the fetus to "fall forward" out of the pelvis and promotes turning. If the knee-chest position is uncomfortable, the patient may achieve the same effect by lying supine with her hips supported on several firm pillows. As stated in section G, the Cochrane meta-analysis shows an overall nonsignificant trend towards a reduction in a persistent breech presentation with these exercises.
B. Hypnosis
Mehl[8] studied 100 volunteer patients whose fetuses were found to be breech at 37–40 weeks' gestation. The patients received weekly office hypnosis sessions with suggestions for general relaxation and release of fear and anxiety. Relaxation audiotapes were provided for each subject to use daily at home. Mehl reported 81% of the fetuses in the intervention group turned compared to 48% in a matched control group.
C. Traditional Chinese Medicine
Moxibustion has been studied when applied at acupuncture point UB 67 on the lateral aspect of the fifth toe. When performed bilaterally for 15 minutes each day beginning at 33 weeks' gestation, Cardini[2] demonstrated a 75% version rate by 35 weeks compared to 47% in matched controls. It is postulated that this stimulation causes increased maternal adrenocortical activity, increasing uterine tone and fetal activity that stimulates spontaneous version.

VI. Predicting Success of External Cephalic Version
A. Success Rates
The overall success rate of external cephalic version (ECV) has been reported in the literature as 60–70%.[13] Favorable prognostic factors for external cephalic version success include multiparity, placental location lateral or fundal, normal, or increased amniotic fluid volume, fetuses whose abdominal circumference is over the 5th percentile, and a non-frank breech presentation with the fetal spine crossing the maternal midline.
B. Scoring System for External Cephalic Version
A scoring system (Table 1) has been proposed that can help predict success of ECV. One study using this system showed no successful versions with a score of 2 or less and 100% success with scores of 9 or 10.[9]

TABLE 1. Scoring System to Predict Success of External Cephalic Version

	0	1	2
Parity	0	1	≥ 2
Dilation	≥ 3 cm	1–2 cm	0 cm
Estimated fetal weight	< 2500 g	2500–3500	> 3500 g
Placenta	Anterior	Posterior	Lateral/fundal
Station	≥ –1	–2	< –3

C. Tocolysis

Although the benefit from tocolysis during ECV remains unproven, most protocols recommend administration of a tocolytic in all but the most relaxed multiparas.

VI. Contraindications to External Cephalic Version
A. **Multiple pregnancy (except version of the second twin after delivering first)**
B. **Oligohydramnios**
C. **Uterine malformation**
D. **Placenta previa**
E. **Any fetal anomaly**
F. **Previous placental abruption during this pregnancy**
G. **Suspected fetal distress or IUGR**
H. **Ruptured membranes (because of the risk of cord prolapse)**
I. **Non-reassuring fetal heart rate tracings**
J. **Preeclampsia (relative contraindication due to increased risk of abruption)**
K. **Previous uterine surgery**
This is considered by some to be a relative contraindication. Other authors feel an ECV is not contraindicated after prior cesarean section, and can be performed prior to attempted vaginal birth after cesarean (VBAC).[6]

VIII. Performing an External Cephalic Version[1,4,5]
A. Informed Consent
Written informed consent should be signed after careful discussion of the procedure, alternatives, and risks.
B. Preparation
1. The procedure should be performed in a labor room with the operating room notified in the event of complications requiring emergency cesarean section. A non-stress test may be performed while an IV is started and blood sent for possible type and crossmatch.
2. The patient should empty her bladder, be placed in a hospital gown, and assume a supine position in bed with a slight left lateral tilt, mild Trendelenburg, with knees slightly bent.
3. If tocolysis is chosen, it may be administered as terbutaline 5–10 mg orally 30 minutes before the procedure or 0.25 mg subcutaneously 10 minutes before the procedure.
4. Two operators are recommended as the procedure can be strenuous.
5. Operators should have well-trimmed fingernails.
6. Ultrasound gel or mineral oil applied to the abdomen will reduce friction on the skin as the baby is moved.
C. Procedure
1. Elevate the breech with a hand placed in the suprapubic area below the breech.
2. With slow, steady pressure, push the breech into the iliac fossa with the lower hand in the direction to begin a forward roll movement of the fetus.

3. Keeping the head flexed, manipulate the fetus into the oblique and then transverse diameter. Avoid rapid, sharp movements. Firm pressure will allow the progress to occur in stages. Pause occasionally to allow the infant to "squirm" a bit. Typically, about two thirds of the force needs to be applied to the breech, while one third is applied to the head, mainly to keep the head flexed.

4. When the technique is applied using two operators, the second may monitor the progress with frequent ultrasound observations of fetal position and heart rate as well as assist the first operator with manual pressure on one of the fetal poles.

5. When the baby is just past transverse, it will usually rotate the rest of the way with little effort on the part of the operators.

6. Set the head into the pelvis by manual manipulation and fundal pressure. Move the patient out of the Trendelenburg position.

7. If a forward roll fails, try a backward flip, particularly if the head and breech lie on the same side of the midline.

8. If the procedure is unsuccessful in 15–20 minutes, discontinue the procedure.

9. If bradycardia occurs during the procedure, stop. If it persists, revert to the original breech position and apply oxygen. If bradycardia persists despite oxygen administration and maternal position change, prepare for emergency cesarean section.

10. Perform a non-stress test when the version is completed, whether or not the procedure is successful.

11. Administer Rhogam to Rh-negative women.

IX. Complications of External Cephalic Version
A. Fetal and Maternal Complications
The overall incidence of complications is 1–2%. They include fetal bradycardia and fetal distress due to knotted or entangled cords, placental abruption, fetal hemorrhage, maternal hemorrhage, preterm labor, and premature rupture of the membranes. Fetal heart rate changes are the most common complications, but are usually transient. One series found a 39% incidence of FHR changes, but they had no relation to the final outcome of the pregnancy.[10]

    1. Fetal and maternal mortality

Fetal mortality has been reported, but only in cases of attempted ECV under general anesthesia or in settings without electronic monitoring and ultrasound. Maternal mortality due to amniotic fluid embolus also has been reported.

    2. Vaginal birth after successful version

After successful version, the intrapartum cesarean section rate has been reported to be twice that of a control group.[7]

    3. Feto-maternal transfusion

This has been reported to occur in up to 6% of patients undergoing external version, but effects are minimized by Rhogam administration.

B. Reversion to Breech
Reversion rates of up to 40% occur when version is attempted before 36 weeks' gestation, emphasizing that fetal lie is generally unstable until the last month of pregnancy. Most reports of ECV after 36 weeks show a stable vertex presentation at labor in 90–100% of cases. ECV prior to term is not recommended because of this higher rate of reversion, the risk of premature birth, and the potential need to perform an emergency cesarean section of a premature infant due to fetal distress.

X. Management After Attempted External Cephalic Version
A. If ECV Is Unsuccessful
Version may be attempted again in several days to one week, cesarean section may be scheduled, or cesarean section may be performed when patient presents in labor.

B. If ECV Is Successful

Patient may resume routine prenatal care until onset of labor with close surveillance by exam and/or ultrasound to assure maintenance of vertex presentation. If the cervix is favorable and the patient is term, induction of labor may be considered.

XI. Multiple Pregnancy
A. Version of the Second Twin

Although multiple pregnancy is listed as a contraindication to external cephalic version, version of the second twin after the first twin has been delivered vaginally is acceptable. After delivery of the first twin and before rupture of the membranes surrounding the second twin, the head of the second twin generally can be guided into the pelvis for vertex delivery. The procedure is made easier if real-time ultrasound is available at the bedside in the delivery room.

References

1. American College of Obstetricians and Gynecologists: External cephalic version. ACOG Practice Patterns, no. 4. Washington, DC, ACOG, 1997.
2. Cardini F, Weixin H: Moxibustion for correction of breech presentation: A randomized controlled trial. JAMA 280:1580–1584, 1998.
3. Chenia F, Crowther CA: Does advice to assume the knee-chest position reduce the incidence of breech presentation at delivery? A randomized clinical trial. Birth 14:75–78, 1987.
4. Coco AS, Silverman SD: External cephalic version. Am Fam Phys 58:731–748, 1998.
5. Eisinger SH, Koller WS: Malpresentations, malpositions and multiple gestations. In Advanced Life Support in Obstetrics (ALSO) Course Syllabus, 3rd ed. Kansas City, MO, American Academy of Family Physicians, 1996.
6. Flamm BL, Fried MW, Lonky NM, et al: External cephalic version after previous cesarean section. AJOG 165:370–372, 1991.
7. Lau TK, Lo KW, Robers M: Pregnancy outcomes after successful external cephalic version for breech presentation at term. Am J Obstet Gynecol 176: 218–223, 1997.
8. Mehl LE: Hypnosis and conversion of the breech to vertex presentation. Arch Fam Med 3:883–887, 1994.
9. Newman RB, Peacock BS, VanDorsten JP, Hunt HH: Predicting success of external cephalic version. Am J Obstet Gynecol 169:245–250, 1993.
10. Phelan JP, Stine LE, Mueller E, et al: Observations of fetal heart rate characteristics related to external cephalic version and tocolysis. Am J Obstet Gynecol 149:658–661, 1984.
11. Tiran D, Mack S: Complementary Therapies for Pregnancy and Childbirth. London, Bailliere Tindall, 1995.
12. Westgren W, Edvall H, Nordstrom L, et al: Spontaneous cephalic version of breech presentation in the last trimester. Br J Obstet Gynaecol 92:19–22, 1985.
13. Zhang MJ, Bowes WA, Fortney JA: Efficacy of external cephalic version: A review. Obstet Gynecol 82:306–313, 1993.

SECTION I.
TWIN GESTATION

Ellen L. Sakornbut, M.D.

I. Distribution of Twin Gestation[1,25]
A. Twin A vertex, twin B vertex: 43% of twins
B. Twin A vertex, twin B nonvertex: 38% of twins
C. Twin A nonvertex, twin B any presentation: 19% of twins

II. Management of Twin Labor
A. Intrapartum Ultrasound

It is helpful to have ultrasound available for use both at presentation to the labor unit and during vaginal delivery for assessment of position, presentation, and heart rate of the fetuses. With practice, the clinician can determine degree of fetal head flexion and position of extremities in the non-vertex second twin (frank, complete, footling breech).

B. Use of Oxytocin

One study comparing oxytocin augmentation and induction of labor in twin and singleton pregnancies found use of oxytocin to be safe and effective.[11] In this study, patients with twin pregnancy were not more likely to encounter hyperstimulation or less likely to respond to oxytocin therapy than patients with singleton pregnancies.

C. Timing of Delivery

A 7-year study of uncomplicated twin gestations in one center found a 13-fold increased risk of neonatal complications in pregnancies delivered before 38 weeks compared to pregnancies delivered at or after 38 weeks.[23]

D. Fetal Heart Rate Monitoring

In twin pregnancies it may be technically more difficult to obtain adequate documentation of fetal heart rates. A combination of methods may be needed to monitor the status of each twin.

III. Choice of Route of Delivery[21]

A. Vertex Presentations

Vaginal delivery can be attempted. Both twins should be monitored. If the second twin shows signs of distress after delivery of the first twin, either assisted vaginal delivery or cesarean section can be performed, depending on which is more expedient.

B. Vertex, Nonvertex Presentations

Choice of delivery in this situation is subject to judgment. The vertex twin may be delivered vaginally followed by external version of the second twin under sonographic guidance in the delivery room. Alternatively a breech delivery can be performed for the second twin, or cesarean section can be performed for both. The twin presentation ideally should be diagnosed before the onset of labor, enabling delivery plans to be made beforehand with a consultant if necessary. Cesarean section for the second twin has not been shown to improve neonatal outcome near term, even for low-birth-weight infants.[8,9] It is associated with increased maternal morbidity.[8]

C. First Twin Nonvertex

Cesarean section is usually chosen in this situation.

D. Decision-Making and Outcome Expectations

1. Literature summary

The issue of whether all breech fetuses must be delivered by cesarean section is a controversial one. In some large retrospective studies, vaginal breech delivery appears to be associated with increased morbidity and mortality.[13,15,16,20,22] Other studies have not shown these associations.[6,7,14,15] Prospective studies using strict criteria for vaginal breech delivery have shown that such deliveries can be safe.[25] These studies have shown no differences in neonatal outcomes except that umbilical cord arterial pH is lower in breech infants delivered vaginally than in those delivered by cesarean section.[5] The Zatuchni-Andros scoring system for vaginal delivery of breech fetuses (Table 1)[27] is the only such system said to have been tested prospectively.[25] Breech fetuses have been shown to be at risk for lower Apgar scores regardless of route of delivery; this leads to the suggestion that such fetuses have some inherent abnormality leading to both the breech presentation and neonatal compromise.[3] Despite the increasing trend of delivering breech infants operatively (reaching nearly 100% in some centers), a corresponding decrease in birth asphyxia, trauma, and neonatal death has not been demonstrated.[12]

2. Informed consent

Considerations in choosing the method of delivery should include any special issues about either or both fetuses, such as structural anomalies, operator experience, and maternal characteristics.

    a. External version of the second twin. This may be complicated by cord entanglement, cord prolapse, or premature separation of the placenta. Uterine rupture is an unlikely, but possible complication.

    b. Risk of breech extraction. Many clinicians consider breech extraction of the second twin to be less risky than other vaginal breech deliveries. Nonetheless, issues relative to vaginal breech delivery should be covered in counseling and obtaining informed consent. Patients under consideration for vaginal breech delivery should otherwise meet the criteria discussed earlier in this section. The risk of vaginal breech delivery is mainly that of fetal injury, including death in the event of head entrapment. However, when patients are carefully selected for vaginal breech delivery and the operator is experienced, a vaginal delivery can be as safe as a cesarean section.[26]

    c. Risks associated with cesarean section. These risks include bleeding, infection, rare damage to internal organs (bladder, bowel), increased risk of blood loss requiring transfusion, longer recovery time, and anesthesia complications. These should be discussed with the patient.

    d. Cost-effectiveness. A prospective study in three groups of twin pregnancies found the lowest costs for maternal and neonatal care in the group managed by vaginal delivery with breech extraction of the second twin. Intermediate costs for newborn care were encountered in the group managed by vaginal delivery and external version of the second twin. The highest costs for newborns were encountered in the group managed by cesarean delivery. These groups did not differ in maternal complications, gestational age, birth weights, or other clinical parameters.[17] This would appear to suggest that neonatal morbidity is not decreased by cesarean delivery and may be increased.

3. Anesthesia

The use of epidural anesthesia in vaginal breech delivery also is controversial. Some argue that epidural anesthesia increases labor time, use of oxytocin, and rate of cesarean section.[4] Others believe that epidural anesthesia facilitates vaginal delivery.[25]

4. Resuscitation

Additional personnel for pediatric resuscitation should be provided at all twin deliveries, vaginal or operative. If at all possible, two setups with warmers and two sets of equipment with assigned personnel should be ready. Although it has been proposed that the after-coming twin is at greater risk than the presenting twin, the most experienced pediatric resuscitator should initiate activity with the presenting twin if that infant appears unstable at birth.

5. Twin vaginal birth after previous cesarean

Three separate studies of twin vaginal births after cesarean, each including approximately 10 years' experience at a single institution, appear to indicate that vaginal birth after cesarean is safe and effective. Although the smallest study found a slightly longer NICU length of stay for the second twin, this was not a consistent finding in the other studies.[18,19,24]

6. Monoamniotic twin gestation

Limited information is available about this infrequently encountered clinical problem. Overall information about prognosis has been poor, with frequent intrauterine mortality from cord entanglement and other cord problems. At the current time, the most prudent course of action appears to be weekly ultrasound observation from the late second trimester and delivery by cesarean at approximately 32–34 weeks. Even with such close monitoring, sudden intrauterine demise may occur due to cord compression.[2,10]

IV. Summary

Intrapartum twin management should be individualized using patient, operator, and institutional factors. At present, evidence from the literature does not support routine delivery of vertex/vertex or vertex/nonvertex twins by cesarean section.

References

1. Adams PM, Chervenak FA: Intrapartum management of twin gestation. Clin Obstet Gynecol 33:52–60, 1990.
2. Beasley E, Megerian G, Gerson A, Roberts NS: Monoamniotic twins: Case series and proposal for antenatal management. Obstet Gynecol 93:130–134, 1999.
3. Calvert JP: Intrinsic hazard of breech presentation. BMJ 281:1319–1320, 1980.
4. Chadha YG, Mahmoud TA, Dick MJ, et al: Breech delivery and epidural analgesia. Br J Obstet Gynaecol 99:96–100, 1992.
5. Christian SS, Brady K: Cord blood acid-base values in breech-presenting infants born vaginally. Obstet Gynecol 78:778–781, 1991.
6. Collea JV, Chein C, Quilligan EJ: The randomized management of term frank breech presentation: A study of 208 cases. Am J Obstet Gynecol 137:235–244, 1980.
7. Croughan-Minihane MS, Petitti DB, et al: Morbidity among breech infants according to method of delivery. Obstet Gynecol 75:821–825, 1990.
8. Crowther CA: Effect of cesarean delivery on the second twin. In Enkin MW, Keirse MJNC, Renfrew MJ, Neilson JP (eds): Pregnancy and Childbirth Module. Cochrane Database of Systematic Reviews, Review No. 06467. Oxford, Update Software, 1994.
9. Davidson L, Easterling TR, Jackson C, Beredette TJ: Breech extraction of low-birth weight second twins: Can cesarean section be justified? Am J Obstet Gynecol 166:497–502, 1992.
10. Dubecq F, Dufour P, Vinatier D, et al: Monoamniotic twin pregnancies: Review of the literature, and a case report of vaginal delivery. Eur J Obstet Gynecol Reprod Biol 66:183–186, 1996.
11. Fausett MB, Barth WH Jr, Yoder BA, Satin AJ: Oxytocin labor stimulation of twin gestations: Effective and efficient. Obstet Gynecol 90:202–204, 1997.
12. Green JE, McLean F, Smith LP, Usher R: Has an increased cesarean rate for term breech delivery reduced the incidence of birth asphyxia, trauma, and death? Am J Obstet Gynecol 142:643–648, 1982.
13. Hellstrom AC, Nilsson B, Stange L, Nylund L: When does external cephalic version succeed? Acta Obstet Gynaecol Scand 69:281–285, 1990.
14. Hofmeyr GJ: Planned elective cesarean section for term breech presentation. In Enkin MW, Keirse MJNC, Renfrew MJ, Neilson JP (eds): Pregnancy and Childbirth Module. Cochrane Database of Systematic Reviews, Review No. 05287. Cochrane Updates on Disk. Oxford, Update Software, 1994.
15. Kiely JL: Mode of delivery and neonatal death in 17,587 infants presenting by the breech. Br J Obstet Gynaecol 98:898–904, 1991.
16. Mahomed K, Seeras R, Coulson R: A randomized controlled trial using tocolysis. Br J Obstet Gynaecol 98:8–13, 1991.
17. Mauldin JG, Newman RB, Mauldin PD. Cost-effective delivery managment of the vertex and nonvertex twin gestation. Am J Obstet Gynecol 179:864–869, 1998.
18. Miller DA, Mullin P, Hou D, Paul RH. Vaginal birth after cesarean section in twin gestation. Am J Obstet Gynecol 175:194–198, 1996.
19. Myles TD, Miranda R: Vaginal birth after cesarean delivery in twin gestation. Obstet Gynecol 95(4 Suppl 1):S65, 2000.
20. Ranney B: The gentle art of external cephalic version. Am J Obstet Gynecol 116:239–251, 1973.
21. Tchabo J, Tomai T: Selected intrapartum external cephalic version of the second twin. Obstet Gynecol 79:421–423, 1992.
22. Thorpe-Beeston JG, Banfield PJ, Saunders NJ Sr: Outcomes of breech delivery at term. BMJ 305:746–747, 1992.
23. Udom-Rice I, Singlis SR, Skupski D, et al: Optimal gestation age for twin delivery. J Perinatol 20:231–234, 2000.
24. Wax JR, Philput C, Mather J, et al: Twin vaginal birth after cesarean. Conn Med 64:205–208, 2000.
25. Weiner CP: Vaginal breech delivery in the 1990s. Clin Obstet Gynecol 35:559–569, 1992.
26. Yasin S, O'Sullivan MJ: Assisted breech extraction. In Plauche WC, Morrison JC, O'Sullivan MJ (eds): Surgical Obstetrics. Philadelphia, W.B. Saunders, 1992, pp 325–346.
27. Zatuchni GI, Andros GJ: Prognostic index for vaginal delivery in breech presentation at term. Am J Obstet Gynecol 98:854–857, 1967.

CHAPTER 17

Intrapartum Procedures

SECTION A.
USE OF ULTRASOUND IN LABOR AND DELIVERY

Ellen L. Sakornbut, M.D.

Many patients presenting to labor and delivery are in need of sonographic evaluation. Common indications for diagnostic use of ultrasound in labor and delivery include the evaluation of patients with unknown dates or size-dates discrepancy, determination of fetal position, evaluation of preterm labor or preterm premature rupture of membranes, evaluation of patients with vaginal bleeding, and investigation of possible fetal demise. This section addresses the use of ultrasound as it is used in urgent or emergent intrapartum problems. Physicians who provide intrapartum care can become familiar with basic intrapartum use in this context. Some intrapartum applications require more advanced skills and extended amounts of training. The practitioner must recognize that intrapartum sonographic examinations are often difficult to perform due to fetal crowding, low station of the presenting part, oligohydramnios, and patient discomfort. Sonographic examinations in labor and delivery may be limited to specific information that is quickly sought owing to clinical necessity. The use of ultrasound in this context is not intended to supplant standard or basic obstetric examination as defined by the American Institute of Ultrasound in Medicine and the American College of Obstetricians and Gynecologists (ACOG).[24]

I. Applications
Initially, the clinician should perform a general uterine survey with longitudinal and transverse sweeps of the maternal abdomen. This should reveal the following basic information:
A. Fetal Presentation
1. Breech
If breech, it may be difficult to ascertain whether it is complete, frank, or footling. It is possible to identify extremity position, but a single plain film (fetogram) more completely defines position of extremities if one is considering vaginal delivery and sonographic findings are inconclusive.
2. Transverse lie
If transverse lie is confirmed, the position of the spine (back up or down) is important to determine. Cord prolapse is much more likely with the back up, and the uterine incision may be modified for operative delivery.
B. Multiple Gestation
Multiple gestation is usually suspected when fetal size is greater than dates would indicate or if more than two fetal poles are palpated. Confirmation of twins is achieved by visualizing two separate fetal heads and heartbeats. Diagnosis of twin gestation should always be followed by a careful check to detect a greater than twin gestation.

If twin gestation is diagnosed, the examiner should attempt to locate a separating membrane. The membrane may be difficult to visualize owing to crowding, but a gentle tap on the side of the maternal abdomen may demonstrate the membrane fluttering in the fluid wave. Monoamniotic twins are rare; owing to the danger of cord entanglement, delivery is usually operative. Position and presentation of each fetus should be determined for intrapartum management. Difficulties in the diagnosis of a twin gestation include the following:

    1. Diagnosis of a "stuck" twin

    The "stuck" twin, either demised or living, may be contained within an oligohydramniotic sac. This fetus may be difficult to visualize depending on its position in the uterus.

    2. Diagnosis of conjoined twins

    Although rare, this diagnosis may be suspected because of persistent face-to-face or chest-to-chest presentation.

C. Fetal Life

Locating fetal heart tones may be difficult in some patients on presentation to labor and delivery. Sonographic location of fetal cardiac activity is usually easy to determine. Diagnosis of fetal demise can be confirmed by the following findings.

    1. No cardiac activity

    2. Hydropic changes (pleural effusions, skin edema, and ascites)

    3. Overriding of cranial bones, as with x-ray

D. Amniotic Fluid Assessment

    1. Technique

    Using the midline and the umbilicus, the maternal abdomen is divided into four quadrants. Keeping the transducer perpendicular to the floor, the deepest pocket of amniotic fluid is located in each quadrant. A vertical measurement of this pocket is performed, avoiding any areas of the pocket that contain extremity or cord. The sum of these measurements (in centimeters) is the amniotic fluid index. Less than 5 cm is considered oligohydramnios, 5–8 borderline, 8–20 normal and greater than 20–25 is considered polyhydramnios.[5]

E. Placental Evaluation

The placenta is generally easy to identify by its characteristic homogeneous appearance; some lobulation often appears in late pregnancy. Certain challenges and pitfalls can be encountered.

    1. Placental grading

    Ultrasound is not reliable as a means of assessing fetal lung maturity. Less than 50% of patients will demonstrate a grade 3 placenta at term, so lack of a "mature" placenta does not indicate inadequate lung maturation. By the same token, the presence of a grade 3 placenta is usually associated with fetal lung maturity.[11]

    2. Placenta previa

        a. Anterior placenta previa. When this is suspected in a patient with a full bladder, the patient should empty her bladder with repeat scanning to eliminate the possibility of a false-positive in a low-lying anterior placenta.

        b. Posterior placenta previa. When this is suspected, place the patient in the Trendelenburg position and attempt to displace the fetal presenting part gently so that the lower uterine segment and cervical os may be visualized.

        c. Transvaginal or transperineal scanning (Table 1). This can be used to define more completely the relationship of the placenta to the cervical os when transabdominal scanning is inconclusive. Transvaginal ultrasound results in lower rates of false-positives and false-negatives than transabdominal ultrasound,[6] with a positive predictive value of 71% and a

TABLE 1. Performance of Transperineal Scanning

The patient is placed in a supine position with legs abducted and flexed (frog-legged) or in stirrups.
A sector or small curvilinear transducer is prepared by covering it with ultrasound gel, then a condom, transducer cover, or similar plastic covering is placed to prevent transmission of infection.
More gel is then placed on the transducer, and gel is also placed between the labia.
The transducer is placed at the introitus or on the perineum.
Orientation is similar to transvaginal ultrasound with longitudinal or sagittal images and coronal images.
A transducer frequency of 3 or 3.5 mHz produces a depth of field in which the lower segment is well-imaged.

negative predictive value of 100%. Many labor and delivery units do not have transvaginal transducers, and transperineal scanning may be substituted. This technique produces a similar field of view, demonstrating the internal cervical os and placental relationships. Transvaginal scanning of placenta previa can be performed safely because the probe is only partially inserted into the vagina for optimal visualization of the cervix; the endocervical canal is approximately perpendicular to the vagina, making intracervical insertion unlikely.

3. Succenturiate lobes

These lobes may be missed with ultrasound scanning.

4. False-positive diagnosis

Other structures that may be mistaken for placental tissue are as follows:
   a. Segmental myometrial contractions. These may be seen throughout pregnancy and last 20 to 30 minutes. Usually there is a slight difference in echogenicity and a characteristic contour to the segmental contraction. There is no echogenic reflection from the subsegmental contraction, unlike the chorionic plate of the placenta.
   b. Blood clots. Blood clots may have a similar echodensity and consistency as does placental tissue.

II. Assessment of Preterm Labor and Preterm Rupture of Membranes (see Chapter 11)

A. Gestational Age/Estimated Fetal Weight Assessment

Patients presenting in labor may have scanty or no documentation of gestational age. Even when there is some estimate of gestational age from menstrual dating and antenatal visits, accuracy of dating may be limited. Because ultrasound dating in the third trimester is no more accurate than ±3 weeks, estimates made in labor and delivery may be erroneous. Nonetheless, an estimate of fetal size is of some management and prognostic value.

1. Fetal biometry

Fetal biometry is a more advanced skill and beyond the scope of this chapter. Fetal weight estimates in the third trimester commonly vary from actual weights by 10–15%.[17,22]

2. Estimation of fetal weight

This is most accurate when based on measurement of multiple parameters, preferably fetal head, abdomen, and femur measurements.

B. Assessment of the Lower Uterine Segment and Cervix

This can be facilitated by use of transperineal or transvaginal scanning (see Table 1), avoiding the acoustic shadows created by the symphysis pubis and avoiding the risks of digital examination for patients with ruptured membranes or placenta previa.[12,15,26]

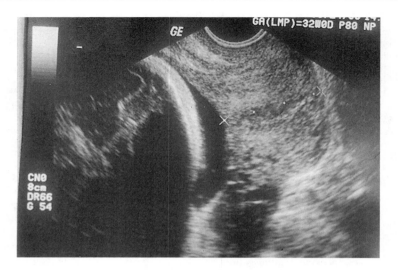

FIGURE 1. A transvaginal image of the cervix demonstrates the echogenic mucus of the endocervix and the internal cervical os. The fetal head is presenting. The calipers are placed to measure the cervical length.

1. Technique for visualization of the cervix and lower uterine segment
The curvilinear probe is placed on the perineum or the vaginal probe is partially inserted into the vagina. The image is oriented so that a symmetric image of the external cervical os is obtained with the internal os visualized as a "T" or an isosceles triangle or funnel.[2] Transperineal and transvaginal scanning demonstrate comparable results.[14] The use of transvaginal ultrasound does not increase the risk of infection in women with preterm premature rupture of membranes (Fig. 1).[3]
2. Accuracy of the technique
Cervical dilatation has been demonstrated with some accuracy up to 4 cm. Cervical effacement and lower uterine segment changes may antedate cervical dilatation.
    a. "Funneling" of the lower uterine segment or development of a V-shaped or U-shaped segment. This can be seen in early preterm labor.
    b. Cervical effacement. This has been determined with more accuracy than dilatation. The uneffaced cervix in the third trimester usually measures between 3.5 and 4.8 cm. Fifty percent effacement corresponds to a cervical length of 1.5 cm, and 75% effacement corresponds to 1.0 cm. A cervical length ≤ 2.0 cm has been associated with a short time interval between ruptured membranes and delivery.[18] In addition, a cervical length ≤ 2.0 cm has been strongly associated with premature delivery at < 27 weeks in women who were being evaluated for cervical incompetence.[10]

III. Assessment for Abruption
Abruption is a clinical diagnosis. It may be supported by sonographic findings, but lack of sonographic evidence does not rule out an abruption. The size of a bleed is often underestimated by ultrasound examination. Possible sonographic findings of abruption include the following.
A. Abnormal Thickening of the Placenta
This may be caused by the presence of a recent retroplacental hemorrhage. Fresh hemorrhage is usually echogenic.

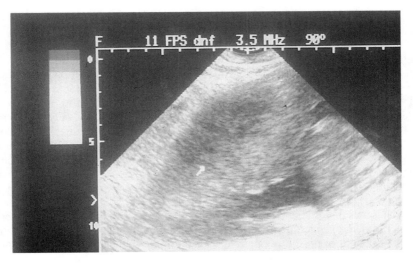

FIGURE 2. The arrow indicates a small abruption which is demonstrated as an echolucent retroplacental clot. The patient presented following a motor vehicle accident and was tender to palpation over this aspect of the uterine fundus.

B. "Torn up" or Abnormally Rounded Edge of the Placenta
C. Increased Area of Sonolucency
This may occur between the myometrium and the placenta and represent a retroplacental clot (Fig. 2). Areas of sonolucency may occur within the substance of the placenta. These may be mimicked by placental lakes, which are normal in mature placentas.

IV. Assessment of Fetal Well-Being
A. Amniotic Fluid Index (AFI)
The use of the AFI to assess fetal well-being is discussed in Chapter 10, section B.
B. Biophysical Profile
The use of the biophysical profile is discussed in Chapter 10, section B. The technique as described by Manning[16] is as follows:
1. Amniotic fluid pocket measuring 1×2 cm: 2 points
2. Fetal breathing movements, three periods of 30 seconds each in 30 minutes: 2 points
3. Fetal extremity movements, three in 30 minutes: 2 points
4. Fetal tone, three episodes of extension with return to flexion in 30 minutes: 2 points
5. Reactive NST: 2 points

A perfect score on a biophysical profile is described as 10/10 with an NST or 8/8 without NST.

V. Use of Ultrasound to Determine Excess Fetal Weight
A. Abdominal Circumference
This measurement appears to be the critical measurement[19,23] and is more predictive than transverse abdominal diameter[9] or other formulas for fetal weight estimation when predicting macrosomia. Other measurements reflective of nutritional status of the fetus have been evaluated and they have not been shown to demonstrate reproducible results in multiple studies.

B. Study Protocols

Studies to determine macrosomia by ultrasound show low sensitivity and low positive predictive value (17% and 36%, respectively) with improved sensitivity (43%) and positive predictive value (53%) from clinical estimation alone.[8] Ultrasound prediction of macrosomia appears to influence clinical behavior with increased rates of labor induction (and failed induction) without reduction in shoulder dystocia or birth trauma.[25] One large series that used protocols for detection of macrosomia found that shoulder dystocia occurred 93% of the time in infants weighing less than 4500 g. Conversely, a trial of labor was evaluated for outcomes in almost 200 pregnancies resulting in infants weighing 4500 g or more. Eight two percent delivered vaginally, with 18.5% experiencing shoulder dystocia with no permanent sequelae. Increased infectious morbidity was found in both women who underwent cesarean following trial of labor (OR 7.1, 95% CI 3.9–13.1) and women undergoing elective repeat cesarean section (OR 5.4, 95% CI 3.1–9.4).[13] Other studies demonstrate similar outcomes in non-diabetic women.[5] Thus, although rates of shoulder dystocia are higher in macrosomic infants, ultrasound determination has not been demonstrated to be of benefit in preventing permanent neurologic sequelae in infants of non-diabetic women who are suspected of macrosomia.

C. Clinical Management Based Upon Ultrasound Findings

Three policies of management for the ultrasound diagnosis of macrosomia in non-diabetic women were compared in a decision analysis model. Elective cesarean section at 4000 g or 4500 g estimated fetal weight resulted in decreased rates of shoulder dystocia and permanent brachial plexus injury, but the cost for each preventable brachial plexus injury ranged between 4.9 and 8.7 million and approximately 2300 to 3700 additional cesarean sections. The same decision-analysis, when applied to diabetic women, was more favorable, with 443 to 489 additional cesarean sections performed to prevent one permanent brachial plexus injury.[20]

A large study of 2600 diabetic women found a threshold of 4250 g for elective cesarean delivery and induction for estimated fetal weights greater than or equal to the 90th percentile, but < 4250 g reduced the rate of shoulder dystocia to 7.4%. This resulted in 10.6% of all diabetic pregnancies at term requiring intervention (induction or elective cesarean section).[4] Both of these studies may provide improved evidence that diabetic women should be managed differently with respect to the diagnosis of macrosomia, and that ultrasound may be of benefit in making a decision regarding management.

VI. Use of Ultrasound for Intrapartum Procedures

A. **Amniocentesis** (see section F)

B. **External Version** (see Chapter 16, section I)

C. **Twin Delivery** (see Chapter 16, section H)

Monitoring of position and cardiac activity of the second twin may be helpful while manually guiding the twin into cephalic position.

VII. Summary

Ultrasound is frequently useful in the intrapartum setting. Although some skills are easily learned, other skills, such as biometry and assessment of preterm labor, may take greater amounts of training and experience. The use of ultrasound in labor and delivery for limited examinations has been recognized as a valid and valuable adjunct in patient management.[24] Use of ultrasound for limited examinations is in no way intended to supplant diagnostic use of ultrasound for basic and targeted exams as defined by the American College of Obstetricians and Gynecologists and the American Institute of Ultrasound in Medicine (which includes full biometry and organ survey). The physician performing the sonographic examination must be aware of the pitfalls in diagnosis and the limitations associated with the intrapartum setting.

References

1. Antepartum Obstetrical Ultrasound Examination Guidelines: Official Guidelines and Statements on Obstetrical Ultrasound. The American Institute of Ultrasound in Medicine, October 1985.
2. Burger M, Weber-Rossler T, Willmann M, et al: Measurement of the pregnant cervix by transvaginal sonography: An interobserver study and new standards to improve interobserver variability. Ultrasound Obstet Gynecol 9:188–193, 1997.
3. Carlan SJ, Richmond LB, O'Brien WF: Randomized trial of endovaginal ultrasound in preterm premature rupture of membranes. Obstet Gynecol 89:458–461, 1997.
4. Conway DL, Langer O: Elective delivery of infants with macrosomia in diabetic women: Reduced shoulder dystocia versus increased cesarean deliveries. Am J Obstet Gynecol 178:922–925, 1998.
5. Diani F, Venanzi S, Zanconato G, et al: A fetal macrosomia and management of delivery. Clin Exp Obstet Gynecol 24:212–214, 1997.
6. Farine D, Peisner DB, Timor-Trisch IE: Placenta previa—is the traditional approach satisfactory? J Clin Ultrasound 18:328–330, 1990.
7. Finberg HJ, Kurtz AB, Johnson RL, et al: The biophysical profile: A literature review and reassessment of its usefulness in the evaluation of fetal well-being. J Ultrasound Med 9:583–587, 1990.
8. Gonen R, Spiegel D, Abend M: Is macrosomia predictable, and are shoulder dystocia and birth trauma preventable? Obstet Gynecol 88:526–529, 1996.
9. Grange G, Favre F, Goffinet F, et al: Comparative value of transverse abdominal diameter and fetal abdominal perimeter, 3844 biometric examinations. J Gynecol Obstet Biol Reprod (Paris) 24:843–849,1995.
10. Guzman ER, Mellon R, Vintzileos AM, et al: Relationship between endocervical canal length between 15–24 weeks and obstetric history. J Matern Fet Med 7:269–272, 1998.
11. Hopper KD, Komppa GH, Williams BP, et al: A reevaluation of placental grading and its clinical significance. J Ultrasound Med 3:261–265, 1984.
12. Jeanty P, d'Alton M, Romero R, et al: Perineal scanning. Am J Perinatol 3:289–295, 1986.
13. Kurtzman JT, Goldsmith LJ, Gall SA, et al: Transvaginal versus transperineal ultrasonography: A blinded comparison in the assessment of cervical measurement at midgestation. Am J Obstet Gynecol 179:852–857, 1998.
14. Lipscomb DR, Gregory D, Shaw K: The outcome of macrosomic infants weighing at least 4500 g: Los Angeles County and the University of Southern California experience. Obstet Gynecol 85:558–564, 1995.
15. Mahony BS, Nyberg DA, Luthy DA, et al: Translabial ultrasound of the third trimester cervix. J Ultrasound Med 9:717–723, 1990.
16. Manning FA, Baskett TF, Millison I, et al: Fetal biophysical profile scoring: A prospective study in 1,184 high-risk patients. Am J Obstet Gynecol 140:289–293, 1981.
17. Ott WJ, Doyle S, Falmm S: Accurate ultrasonic estimation of weight. Am J Perinatol 2:178–182, 1985.
18. Rizzo G, Capponi A, Angelini E, et al: The value of transvaginal ultrasonographic examination of the uterine cervix in predicting preterm delivery in patients with preterm rupture of membranes. Ultrasound Obstet Gynecol 11:23–29, 1998.
19. Rotmensch S, Celentano C, Liberati M, et al: Screening efficacy of the subcutaneous tissue width/femur length ratio for fetal macrosomia in the non-diabetic pregnancy. Ultrasound Obstet Gynecol 13:340–344, 1999.
20. Rouse DJ, Owen J, Goldenberg RL, et al: The effectiveness and costs of elective cesarean delivery for fetal macrosomia diagnosed by ultrasound. JAMA 276:1480–1486, 1996.
21. Rutherford SE, Phelan JP, Smith CV, et al: The four-quadrant assessment of amniotic fluid volume: An adjunct to antepartum fetal heart rate testing. Obstet Gynecol 70:353–356, 1987.
22. Sabbagha RE, Minogue J, Tamura RK: Estimation of birth weight by use of formulas targeted to large-, appropriate-, and small-for-gestational-age fetuses. Am J Obstet Gynecol 160:854–862, 1989.
23. Smith GC, Smith MF, McNay MB, et al: The relation between fetal abdominal circumference and birth weight: Findings in 3512 pregnancies. Br J Obstet Gynaecol 104:186–190, 1997.
24. Ultrasound imaging in pregnancy. American College of Obstetricians and Gynecologists Committee Opinion, Number 96, August 1991.
25. Weeks JW, Pitman, T, Spinnato JA: Fetal macrosomia: Does antenatal prediction affect delivery route and birth outcome? Am J Obstet Gynecol 173:1215–1219, 1995.
26. Zilianti M, Azuaga A, Calderon F, et al: Transperineal sonography in second trimester to term pregnancy and early labor. J Ultrasound Med 10:481–485, 1991.

SECTION B.
PUDENDAL AND PARACERVICAL BLOCKS

Janis E. Byrd, M.D.

Emphasis on nonpharmacologic methods of pain relief and increased use of epidural anesthesia have largely replaced the relatively simple and readily available techniques of pudendal and paracervical blocks.

I. Paracervical Block
A. Indications
The paracervical block provides relief of pain from cervical dilatation and pressure on the bony pelvis during the first stage of labor.[1,5] A paracervical block may also alleviate an uncontrolled urge to push that some patients experience prior to complete dilatation, thus decreasing the risk of cervical laceration. Paracervical anesthesia blocks the ganglion containing visceral sensory fibers from the uterus, cervix, and upper vagina but does not affect the perineum. A successful block lasts from 30 to 90 minutes.
B. Contraindications
Contraindications include:
1. Allergy to local anesthetic agent
2. Fetal distress
3. Pelvic infection
4. Coagulopathy

Informed consent should be obtained prior to performing the procedure.
C. Complications
1. Transient fetal bradycardia

These episodes of bradycardia may last up from 3 to 6 minutes, occur commonly, but are not associated with adverse fetal outcome (unless delivery occurs during the event). The resultant patient and provider anxiety, however, has led to infrequent use of this technique for obstetric anesthesia since the advent of electronic fetal monitoring.

2. Intravascular or intrafetal injection

This may occur with improper technique.

3. Inhibition of labor

If given before 4 cm of dilatation, labor may be inhibited.
D. Technique
The patient is placed in a modified lithotomy position with a pillow under the side to avoid inferior vena cava and aortic compression, which can cause decreased maternal cardiac output, hypotension, and uteroplacental insufficiency manifesting in fetal bradycardia.[3]

1. Place fetal monitor.
2. Check cervical dilatation.
3. Perform perineal preparation
4. Using a 10 ml syringe with a 20- or 22-gauge 6-inch needle and trumpet guide, draw up 10 ml of 1% lidocaine, 1% mepivacaine or 1.5% chloroprocaine.
5. Using the index and middle fingers, guide the trumpet to the cervicovaginal junction (Fig. 3) at the 3–4 o'clock position, depending on the cervical dilatation. Earlier in labor, the nerves are located at 4 and 8 o'clock; later they migrate to 3 and 9 o'clock.
6. Allowing no more than 3 mm of the needle tip to protrude, aspirate for blood and, if negative, inject 5–10 ml of anesthetic.

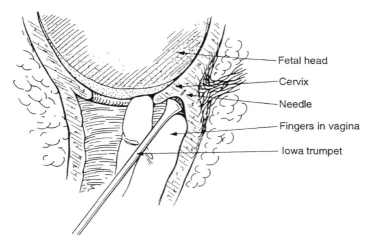

Fetal head

Cervix

Needle

Fingers in vagina

Iowa trumpet

FIGURE 3. Technique of administering a paracervical block during labor using an Iowa trumpet. (From Pfenninger JL, Fowler GC (eds): Procedures for Primary Care Physicians. St. Louis, Mosby, 1994, p 800, with permission.)

7. If no bradycardia occurs after 5 minutes, repeat at the 8–9 o'clock position.
8. Continue fetal monitoring for 30 minutes after the procedure.

II. Pudendal Block
A. Indications
Pudendal blocks provide pain relief during the second stage of labor and for episiotomy and repair. It is most often used for vacuum or low forceps deliveries. A successful procedure blocks all three branches of the pudendal nerve, which supplies sensory and motor innervation to the perineum.[5]
B. Contraindications
Contraindications are the same as for paracervical block with the exception of fetal distress, which is not a risk with pudendal block unless amounts are injected intravascularly or intrafetally causing systemic reactions.
C. Complications
1. Intravascular injection
2. Hematoma
3. Failure of bilateral block, which occurs 50% of the time despite good technique. This is probably due to aberrant pathways of the three branches.[4]
D. Technique[2]
Place the patient in the modified dorsal lithotomy position as for a pudendal.
1. Institute electronic fetal monitoring
2. Perform a vaginal exam for dilatation and descent to avoid injection of the fetal scalp.
3. Perform a perineal prep.
4. Using a 10 ml 20-gauge 6-inch needle, draw up 10 ml of 1% lidocaine.
5. Using the index and middle fingers, guide the tip to the ischial spine (Fig. 4).
6. Allowing 7–10 mm of the tip to protrude, aspirate for blood. The vessels are lateral to the nerve, so if blood is aspirated, move the needle tip medially. If negative, inject 2–4 ml of 1% lidocaine at 2–3 sites—inferior to the tip of the ischial spine, medial to the tip of the spine, and into the ligament. Limit the total amount injected to 10 ml per site to avoid systemic reactions.

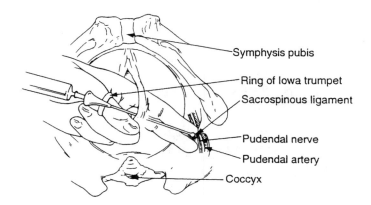

FIGURE 4. Left hand is directing guide and needle toward the pudendal nerve. This illustration shows the hand directed more laterally to better show the anatomy. (From Pfenninger JL, Fowler GC (eds): Procedures for Primary Care Physicians. St. Louis, Mosby, 1994, p 797, with permission.)

    7. Repeat on the opposite side.

    8. After 5 minutes, check anesthesia by gently drawing an Allis forceps over each side of the perineum and observing for the anal "wink" response. Additional local anesthesia may be required prior to performing other procedures.

References

1. Fields SA, Wall EM: Obstetrics analgesia and anesthesia. Prim Care 20:705–712, 1993.
2. Henderson S: Paracervical block. In Pfenninger JL, Fowler GC (eds): Procedures for Primary Care Physicians. St. Louis, Mosby, pp 799–802, 1994.
3. Jayasinghe C, Blass NH: Pain management in the critically ill obstetric patient. Crit Care Clin 15:201–228, 1999.
4. Marquardt DN: Paracervical block. In Procedures for Primary Care Physicians. St. Louis, Mosby, pp 794–798, 1994.
5. Stephens MB, Ford RE: Intrathecal narcotics for labor analgesia. Am Fam Physician 56: 463–470, 1997.

SECTION C.
AMNIOINFUSION AND USE OF
INTRAUTERINE PRESSURE CATHETER

Stephen D. Ratcliffe, M.D., M.S.P.H.

The clinical significance of oligohydramnios and its relationship to placental insufficiency and umbilical cord compression is discussed in Chapter 6, section H and Chapter 10, section B. The scientific basis for the use of amnioinfusion is described in Chapter 15, section A. This section describes the related procedures of placement of an intrauterine pressure catheter (IUPC) and administration of an amnioinfusion.

I. Intrauterine Pressure Catheter
A. Indications
Intrauterine pressure catheters (IUPCs) are often used for administering high doses of oxytocin (greater than 20 mU/minute). In the setting of dystocia and suspected inadequate uterine contractions, placement of an IUPC yields objective measurements of intrauterine pressure.

B. Contraindications
The following are relative contraindications:
1. Chorioamnionitis
2. Malpresentation
3. Known or suspected placenta previa
4. Known or suspected placental abruption

C. Complications
Clinically significant complications are rare, but there are case reports of uterine perforation, umbilical cord trauma, and placental abruption.

D. Equipment
Single- and double-lumen catheters are available. Double-lumen catheters allow for simultaneous monitoring of intrauterine pressure and amnioinfusion.

E. Placement Technique
1. The fetal presenting part is known; the cervix is usually dilated more than 1 cm.
2. Using sterile technique, the clinician introduces the tip of the plastic guide posteriorly into the endocervical os.
3. The IUPC is then gently inserted to a depth of 30 cm. The clinician should encounter only mild resistance in placing the IUPC. Marked resistance should be an indication to abort the procedure.
4. The fetal monitor is then calibrated so that intrauterine pressures can be readily measured. Resting tone should be less than 15 mm Hg.

II. Amnioinfusion
A. Indications
1. Evidence of umbilical cord compression

A major indication for amnioinfusion is to provide a protective fluid cushion when there is evidence of umbilical cord compression during labor. Repetitive variable decelerations, particularly if they are severe or prolonged, are thought to be a result of umbilical cord compression. Amnioinfusion is more effective in relieving variable decelerations in the presence of oligohydramnios (AFI < 5 cm).[8] A summary of published RCTs indicates that there is strong evidence that use of amnioinfusion for the treatment of suspected cord compression results in a decreased rate of variable decelerations (NNT = 3), cesarean section (NNT = 8), cord pH less than 7.20 (NNT = 8), and postpartum endometritis (NNT = 17) (Fig. 5).[3] Prophylactic amnioinfusion in the presence of oligohydramnios is not associated with an improvement in the outcomes noted above.[5]

2. Presence of thick meconium-stained fluid

Another indication for amnioinfusion is the presence of moderate to thick meconium-stained fluid. Ten RCTs have demonstrated a number of significantly improved outcomes with the use of procedure (Table 2).[5] It is not known whether this beneficial effect is due to the dilution of the meconium or the primary alleviation of umbilical cord compression.[1,10]

B. Contraindications
These are the same contraindications noted previously with regard to placement of an IUPC. A large retrospective study has demonstrated that amnioinfusions can be safely used with patients undergoing an attempt at vaginal birth after a previous cesarean section.[6]

C. Complications
1. Polyhydramnios

In addition to the rare complications associated with placement of an IUPC, polyhydramnios may occur if the rate and duration of the amnioinfusion are not carefully monitored.

Review: Amnioinfusion for umbilical cord compression in

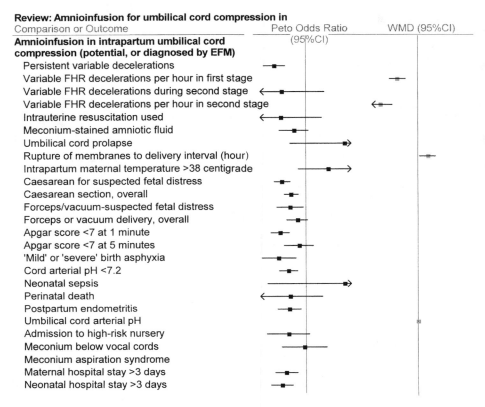

FIGURE 5. Review: Amnioinfusion for umbilical cord compression in comparison of outcome. (From Hofmeyr GJ: Amnioinfusion in intrapartum umbilical cord compression. In The Cochrane Library, Issue 4, 2000. Oxford, Update Software.)

 2. Uterine hypertonus
A possible effect of polyhydramnios is uterine hypertonus.[2] The incidence of cord prolapse is not increased with the use of amnioinfusion.
   D. Equipment
      1. Intrauterine pressure catheter
      2. Intravenous tubing
      3. Normal saline or lactated Ringer's solution
      4. Fetal monitor
   E. Procedure
      1. Indications are met for amnioinfusion.
      2. Informed consent is obtained.
      3. The IUPC is placed.

TABLE 2. Use of Amnioinfusion for Meconium-Stained Amniotic Fluid[5]

Improved Perinatal Outcomes	Number Needed to Treat (NNT)
Decrease in heavily stained meconium fluid	1.4
Prevention of one infant with cord pH < 7.20	11
Prevention of one case of meconium aspiration syndrome	10
Prevention of one neonatal ventilation/admission to newborn ICU	12

4. Performing the amnioinfusion

An initial bolus of 250–600 ml of normal saline (NS) or lactated Ringer's (LR) solution is administered. The infusion may be administered using gravity drainage or a pump. The case reports of complications due to uterine overdistention have occurred with the use of an infusion pump; hence some centers have opted to use the gravity drainage method. There is no evidence to support the original recommendation that the NS or LR be warmed prior to starting the amnioinfusion.[2]

5. Post-amnioinfusion maintenance

After the initial bolus, a maintenance infusion of 1–3 ml/minute is used. If intrapartum ultrasound is used, the amnioinfusion can be adjusted to keep the AFI between 8 and 12 cm. An infusion of 250 ml of fluid results in an average increase of the AFI of 4 cm and often results in a small increase in the basal uterine tone.[7,9] Clinicians who can obtain an AFI during labor can easily determine when an adequate fluid cushion has been achieved (an AFI between 8 and 12 cm). When an AFI is not available, it is recommended that the total quantity infused not exceed 800 ml.

References

1. Dye Taubry R, Gross S, et al: Amnioinfusion and the intrauterine prevention of meconium aspiration. Am J Obstet Gynecol 171:931–935, 1994.
2. Glantz J, Letteney D: Pumps and warmers during amnioinfusion: Is either necessary? Obstet Gynecol 87:150–155, 1996.
3. Hofmeyr GJ: Amnioinfusion in intrapartum umbilical cord compression (Cochrane Review). In The Cochrane Library, Issue 4, 2000. Oxford, Update Software.
4. Hofmeyr GJ: Amnioinfusion for meconium stained liquor in labour (Cochrane Review). In The Cochrane Library, Issue 4, 2000. Oxford, Update Software.
5. Hofmeyr GJ: Amnioinfusion prophylactically versus therapeutically for intrapartum oligohydramnios (Cochrane Review). In The Cochrane Library, Issue 4, 2000. Oxford, Update Software.
6. Ouzounian J, Miller D, Paul R: Amnioinfusion in women with previous cesarean births: A preliminary report. Am J Obstet Gynecol 174:783–786, 1996.
7. Posner MD, Ballagh SA, Paul RH: The effect of amnioinfusion on uterine pressure and activity: A preliminary report. Am J Obstet Gynecol 163: 813–818, 1990.
8. Spong C, McKindsey F, Ross M: Amniotic fluid index predicts the relief of variable decelerations after amnioinfusion bolus. Am J Obstet Gynecol 175:1066–1070, 1996.
9. Strong TH, Hetzler G, Paul RH: Amniotic fluid volume increase after amnioinfusion of a fixed volume. Am J Obstet Gynecol 162: 746–748, 1990.
10. Weismiller D: Transcervical amnioinfusion. Am Fam Physician 57:504–510, 1998.

SECTION D.
ASSISTED DELIVERIES

James R. Damos, M.D.

This section discusses the indications and prerequisites for an assisted vaginal delivery using forceps and vacuum extraction. The prerequisites that should be met prior to attempting an assisted vaginal delivery are presented. The evidence comparing forceps with vacuum extraction is examined.

I. Rationale for Family Physicians Doing Assisted Deliveries
The assisted vaginal delivery, either with forceps or vacuum extraction, is an important skill to acquire when managing the second stage of labor.
A. The Clinician's Role in Small Hospitals
Twenty-three percent of the nation's population lives in rural America. Two-thirds of the obstetric providers in rural areas are family physicians or general practitioners.[11]

Obstetricians tend to be concentrated in larger cities and teaching centers. Thus, the care of low-risk obstetric patients in smaller hospitals is often the primary responsibility of family physicians and nurse midwives. Emergencies that require the use of instruments in vaginal delivery may occur at times when an obstetrician may not be readily available even for clinicians who practice in more urban areas.

B. Effects of Losing Local Perinatal Services

Women who leave their rural communities to obtain maternity care elsewhere experience an increase in adverse perinatal outcomes.[16] There is an increased incidence of complicated deliveries, prematurity, and low birth weight. As a result, higher costs of maternal and neonatal care occur. Nesbitt has replicated this study that demonstrates that poor local access to providers of maternity care is associated with the following conditions.[17]

1. Neonatal risk

There is a greater risk of having a non-normal neonate for both Medicaid- and privately insured patients.

2. Hospital costs

There are higher charges and increased hospital length of stay for the privately insured.

II. History of Assisted Deliveries

A. Forceps—Pre-Twentieth Century

In the year 1600, Peter Chamberlen invented forceps for delivery of a live-born infant. The secret, however, was kept in the family for more than 100 years. In the 1740s, the Chamberlen forceps became public medical knowledge. Between the 1740s and 1900s, the Chamberlen forceps were modified by practitioners such as Smellie, Kielland, Barton, and Piper (over 600 modifications have been developed).

B. Forceps—Twentieth Century

In the early 1920s, DeLee promoted the principle of prophylactic forceps. By 1950, forceps were used in more than 50% of deliveries. Since then, the rate of forceps deliveries has declined owing to the introduction of oxytocin, increased use of cesarean section, and changes in maternal anesthesia practices.

C. Vacuum

In 1849, Simpson described a trumpet-shaped cup with a pump handle. Its use in the next 100 years was quite limited. In the early 1950s, the Swedish obstetrician Malmstrom was among the first to advocate applying a vacuum device through a partially dilated cervix to facilitate the first stage of labor. This, however, was quickly abandoned owing to maternal trauma that developed.

In the 1960s, the vacuum was further developed as a replacement for forceps in Europe. With the subsequent introduction of plastic cups, vacuum extraction has become more popular in the United States.

III. Indications for Assisted Vaginal Delivery

A. Maternal Indications

1. Maternal exhaustion

This occurs commonly if stage 1 or stage 2 labor is prolonged. Other factors associated with maternal fatigue include timing of the onset of pushing and the presence or absence of a labor support companion (see Chapter 13, sections D and F).[18]

2. Anesthesia and analgesia

The use of epidural anesthesia is strongly associated with an increased use of an assisted vaginal delivery (Fig. 6).[12] For every ten patients receiving epidural

Review: Epidural versus non-epidural analgesia for pain

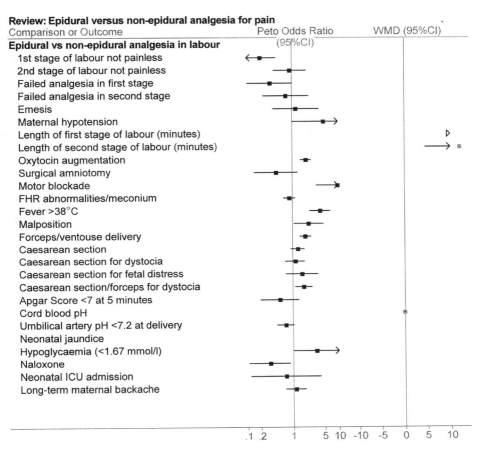

FIGURE 6.   Review: Epidural versus nonepidural analgesia for pain comparison or outcome. (From Howell CJ: Epidural vs. non-epidural analgesic for pain relief. In The Cochrane Library, Issue 4, 2000. Oxford, Update Software, with permission.)

anesthesia an additional forceps- or vacuum-assisted delivery occurs. This can be partially mitigated with discontinuance of the epidural at 8 cm of dilatation or with the use of oxytocin during stage 2 labor.[9] Drug-induced analgesia that interferes with the woman's voluntary expulsive efforts may also occur.

3. Soft-tissue dystocia

Some practitioners cite inflexible perineal and vaginal musculature as factors associated with an assisted vaginal delivery, although evidence to support this belief is lacking.

4. Patients with chronic medical conditions

Women with chronic conditions whose health will be adversely affected with repeated Valsalva maneuvers are clearly candidates for an assisted delivery.

B. Prolonged Second Stage of Labor

The American College of Obstetricians and Gynecologists (ACOG) previously defined prolonged stage 2 labor as greater than 1 hour for the multiparous patient and greater than 2 hours for the primigravid patient.[1] In recognizing that regional anesthesia has the effect of prolonging stage 2 labor, ACOG amended these definitions for women with epidural anesthesia as follows.

    1. Prolonged stage 2 labor for the multigravid patient lasting greater than 2 hours
    2. Prolonged stage 2 labor for the primigravid patient lasting more than 3 hours

C. Maternal-Fetal Reasons for Assisted Vaginal Delivery
    1. Relative cephalopelvic disproportion (CPD)
The diagnosis of CPD is often made retrospectively after an unsuccessful attempt of an assisted vaginal delivery. The clinician should also anticipate the possibility of an impending shoulder dystocia.
    2. Malposition and malpresentation
Examples of this include persistent occipitoposterior or transverse presentation and mild degrees of deflexion or asynclitism (see discussion in Chapter 16).

D. Fetal Reasons for Assisted Vaginal Delivery
    1. Non-reassuring fetal heart tones
Non-reassuring fetal heart tones should be superimposed on an overall reassuring preceding fetal tracing. If the family physician does not believe that an assisted vaginal delivery can be effected expeditiously, then preparations should be made to have immediate access to a cesarean section.
    2. Premature separation of the placenta with hemorrhage
When a clinical abruption occurs, an assisted vaginal delivery can be undertaken if the criteria are met regarding fetal descent and presentation.

IV. Prerequisites for Assisted Vaginal Delivery[6]
A. Membranes Must Be Ruptured
Knowledge of the presence or absence of meconium-stained fluid can affect neonatal management.

B. Cervix Must Be Completely Dilated
In order to avoid maternal trauma, the clinician must be certain that there is no remaining cervical lip or rim before applying the forceps or vacuum. The clinician should also do a vigorous exam to rule out the presence of a cervical rim before proceeding with the assisted delivery.

C. Vertex Presentation Exists
D. Position of the Head Must Be Known
Throughout stage 1 labor, it is important to determine the fetal head position. It becomes increasingly difficult to make this determination during stage 2 as the fetal caput develops.
    1. The anterior fontanelle is larger and forms a cross or a diamond with *four* sutures emanating from it.
    2. The posterior fontanelle is smaller and forms a Y with *three* sutures extending from it.
    3. The clinician can feel for an ear and see which way it bends. When in doubt, the clinician may use the bedside ultrasound to determine the position.

E. Head Must Be Deeply Engaged
    1. If the cephalic prominence can still be palpated above the pubic symphysis on abdominal exam, the fetal head is probably not sufficiently engaged.
    2. The vertex presentation with considerable molding may appear to be at a lower station of descent than it actually is. Practitioners should assess to what degree the vertex occupies the sacral hollow. If much of the sacral hollow is empty, fetal descent is likely to be higher than a +2 station. This would involve a mid-forceps or vacuum application and should be avoided if at all possible.

F. Knowledge of Delivering Instruments
Family physicians and other clinicians performing assisted vaginal deliveries must know what types of forceps and suction devices are available at their institution.

G. Maternal-Fetal Size Relationship Should Be Assessed
Large fundal measurement or estimated fetal weight greater than 4000 to 4500 g increase the possibility of a shoulder dystocia. This clearly affects management of stage 2, including the timing of an attempted assisted delivery versus cesarean intervention.

H. Adequate Anesthesia
Regional anesthesia usually provides adequate anesthesia. An effective pudendal block provides some relief that may be augmented with local infiltration of 1% lidocaine (see section B). The application of 1% lidocaine topical gel may provide additional relief.

I. Abandoning the Procedure
The clinician must have a willingness to abandon the procedure if forceps or vacuum does not proceed easily, and be prepared for emergency cesarean section if the fetal condition deteriorates. During the transition time to cesarean section, if the fetal condition is in jeopardy, an intrauterine fetal resuscitation can be done by administering subcutaneous terbutaline (0.25 to 0.5 mg) and oxygen to the patient (see Chapter 15, section A).[1]

V. Classification of Forceps Application
A. Engagement (Fig. 7)
Engagement occurs when the biparietal diameter of the fetal head has passed the plane of the pelvic inlet. Clinically, one can determine engagement when on vaginal exam the presenting part is at the level of the ischial spine (station 0).

B. Problems Defining Engagement
After vigorous labor, the fetal skull may be elongated and molded with caput formation. There may be asynclitism in which the sagittal suture is not in the midline of

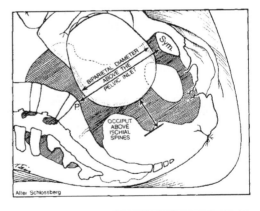

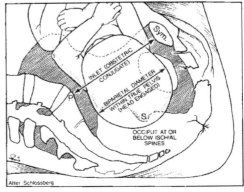

FIGURE 7. *Top,* When the lowermost portion of the fetal head is above the ischial spines, the biparietal diameter of the head is not likely to have passed through the pelvic inlet and therefore is not engaged. (P = sacral promontory; Sym = symphysis pubis.) *Bottom,* When the lowermost portion of the fetal head is at or below the ischial spines, it is usually engaged. Exceptions occur when there is considerable molding, caput formation, or both. (P = sacral promontory; S = ischial spine; Sym = symphysis pubis.) (Reprinted with permission from Cunningham FG, MacDonald P, Gant N, et al (eds): Williams Obstetrics, 19th ed. East Norwalk, CT, Appleton and Lange, 1993, pp 283–296.)

the pelvis. These factors may create the erroneous impression that engagement has occurred when, in fact, the biparietal diameter has not passed through the inlet.

C. Forceps Definitions

Because of problems defining engagement and guidelines for mid-forceps application, the Maternal-Fetal Medicine Committee of the ACOG in 1988 reclassified forceps applications.[1]

    1. Outlet forceps

The fetal skull has reached the pelvic floor. The scalp is visible between contractions. The sagittal suture is in the anteroposterior diameter or in the right or left occiput anterior or posterior position, but not more than 45° from the midline.

    2. Low forceps

The leading edge of the fetal skull is at +2 station or lower. The head is not on the pelvic floor but fills the hollow of the sacral space. Rotations are divided into 45° or less and more than 45°.

    3. Mid-forceps

The head is engaged, but the leading edge of skull is above +2 station.

VI. Procedure for Forceps[6]

A. Choice of Instrument (Fig. 8)

    1. The Simpson forceps and its modifications have long, shallow, tapered blades and are most suitable to large and extensively molded fetal heads (Simpson, Luikart-Simpson, and DeLee).

    2. The Elliot forceps and its modifications have shorter blades and an accentuated cephalic curve that is more suitable to the rounded fetal head that has not undergone extensive molding (Elliot, Tucker-McLane, Tucker-Luikart). In addition, Elliot instruments, because of their overlapping shanks, do not distend the perineum as do the separated shanks of the Simpson-type forceps.

B. Application

    1. Insertion of the forceps

After the clinician is assured that the indications and prerequisites for forceps procedures exist, many physicians coat the forceps blades with soapy lubricant for ease of application. There is preliminary evidence from RCTs that the application of foam pads to the forceps blades may decrease neonatal facial trauma.[13] The left (with regards to maternal position) forceps handle is held in the left hand during insertion with a pencil grip and the cephalic curve inward toward

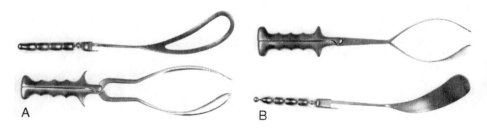

FIGURE 8. *A*, Simpson forceps. Note the ample pelvic curve in the single blade above and cephalic curve evident in the articulated blades below. The fenestrated blade and the wide shank in front of the English-style lock characterize the Simpson forceps. *B*, Tucker-McLane forceps. The blade is solid the the shank is overlapping. (From Cunningham FG, MacDonald P, Gant N, et al (eds): Williams Obstetrics, 19th ed. East Norwalk, CT, Appleton and Lange, 1993, pp 283–296, with permission.)

the vulva and the shank perpendicular to the floor. The blade is applied to the left side of the fetal head (in occiput anterior positions) normally with the right hand protecting the maternal left pelvis and guiding the blade into position. The thumb is placed on the heel, and this is the inserting force, not the handle. The right forceps handle is then held in the right hand during insertion and is applied to the right side of the fetal head on the mother's right with the left hand protecting the maternal right pelvis and guiding the blade into position. The handles should fit together and lock if the blades are correctly applied.

2. Position for safety

The posterior fontanel should be midway between the shanks and 1 cm anterior or above the plane of the shanks. This ensures proper flexion of the head to present the narrowest diameter to the pelvis. If the posterior fontanelle is higher than 1 centimeter above the plane of the shanks, traction will cause extension of the head, present greater fetal diameters to the pelvis, and make the delivery more difficult. If there is a fenestration in the forceps being used, it should be just barely palpable. Not more than a fingertip should be able to be inserted. If more is felt, then the blades are not inserted far enough to be below the malar eminence. Finally, one should check fetal sutures. The sagittal suture should be midway between the shanks. Some also check the lambdoidal sutures that should be above and equidistant from the upper or superior surface of each blade. The sagittal suture should be in the midline between the blades to assure proper forceps application. In summary, to make sure the forceps are applied correctly, check **P**osition **F**or **S**afety—**P**osterior fontanel, **F**enestration, **S**utures.

C. Delivery (Fig. 9)

Traction is made with a gentle pulling motion that gradually increases and decreases to mimic the uterine contraction unless circumstances dictate a more expedient approach. Using Pajot's maneuver, the pelvic curve will be followed. As the fetal head begins to descend under the pubic symphysis, the handle of the forceps should be elevated to lessen the pressure and distention of the perineum. It is at this junction that the clinician may need to perform an episiotomy that should be modest and extended into the vaginal mucosa and away from the anal sphincter. It is quite feasible to avoid making an episiotomy for the multiparous patient. Once the fetal head has "crowned," the forceps should be removed carefully to avoid causing a sulcus or vaginal sidewall laceration. A modified Ritgen maneuver may be necessary to help deliver the head at this point.

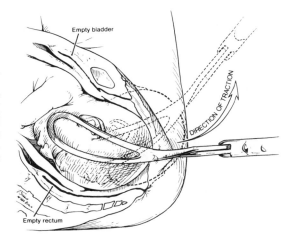

FIGURE 9. Occiput anterior. Delivery by outlet forceps (Simpson). The direction of gentle traction for delivery of the head is indicated. (From Cunningham FG, MacDonald P, Gant N, et al (eds): Williams Obstetrics, 19th ed. East Norwalk, CT, Appleton and Lange, 1993, pp 555–576, with permission.)

D. Follow-up Care

1. A thorough maternal cervical, vaginal, and rectal examination is conducted to rule out lacerations.

2. The infant should be examined for evidence of birth trauma (fractured clavicle, cephalhematoma, lacerations or abrasions, facial nerve palsy).

3. Write or dictate an operative note that includes a detailed account of the indications for the procedure and all pertinent details of the operation.

4. On first postpartum day, mother and any other significant family members should be questioned on their perceptions of the need for operative intervention and how delivery went. Clarification of any misperceptions can be carried out with support and empathy.

5. The clinician should provide stool softeners, particularly when 3rd- or 4th-degree extensions have occurred. Patients should be given the anticipatory guidance to expect that the first bowel movement or two may be painful.

VII. Vacuum Extraction[8]

Vacuum rivals forceps in safety and efficacy depending on the experience of the operator. Plastic cup extractors are safer and easier to assemble. Metal cups, no longer available in the United States, are more capable of solving rotational problems and can provide more traction.

A. Indications and Prerequisites

The same indications and prerequisites outlined for forceps application apply for use of the vacuum device.

B. Advantages of Vacuum Application

1. The vacuum is easy to apply.

2. The vacuum-assisted delivery teaches the clinician to follow the pelvic curve.

3. Vacuum applies less force to the fetal head.

4. The vacuum requires less anesthesia (local often suffices) and results in fewer vaginal and cervical lacerations.

5. Some studies show a lower incidence of anal sphincter tears with vacuum application compared with forceps.[8,22,23]

C. Disadvantages

1. Traction can only be applied during contractions.

2. Proper traction is necessary to avoid losing vacuum.

3. Delivery may take longer than with forceps (not ideal when rapid delivery is necessary).

4. There may be difficulty in holding the vacuum if molding is present.

5. There is an increase in the incidence of cephalhematomas and retinal hemorrhages compared to spontaneous vaginal delivery or the use of forceps.[14] Pre-delivery factors found to predispose to neonatal cephalhematoma formation include increasing asynclitism, paramedian placement of the vacuum, and time from application to delivery exceeding 5–10 minutes.[3,24]

6. Potentially fatal subgaleal hemorrhages have been reported in recent years resulting in an FDA Advisory described in section G.[1]

D. Contraindications

1. Caution with prematurity (less than 37 weeks of gestation)*

2. Breech, face, brow, or transverse presentation

---

* Although indicated use of the silicone-rubber vacuum to assist vaginal delivery of neonates weighing ≤ 2000 g does not appear to be associated with an increased risk of periventricular or intraventricular hemorrhage or other neonatal complications, it would be prudent for family physicians to avoid vacuum in these situations if possible.[25]

3. Incomplete cervical dilatation
4. Cephalopelvic disproportion
5. Head not engaged
6. Caution if greater than 45 degrees rotation is necessary

E. When to Stop

1. Failure to achieve extraction after 10 minutes at maximal pressure.
2. Failure to achieve extraction within 30 minutes of initiation of procedure.
3. Disengagement of extractor cup three times.
4. No significant progress in three consecutive pulls.
5. Fetal scalp trauma inflicted by extractor cup.
6. An unsuccessful trial of forceps and/or vacuum in a setting where a cesarean section can promptly occur is not associated with increased morbidity of either mother or baby.[20]

F. Procedure (Figs. 10 and 11)

The cup is inserted and positioned over the apex of the fetal head (approximately 2 cm anterior to the posterior fontanelle). A finger is swept around the cup to make sure no maternal tissue is trapped beneath the cup. The cup can be rotated several times to ensure that no maternal soft tissue has been caught. Negative pressure is then raised to the yellow area on the dial (10 or 100 depending on the instrument used). The cup is re-examined for position and maternal tissue. With the next contraction, the negative pressure is rapidly raised to the green area on the dial. Traction is applied while trying to avoid a rotary force that may break the seal. The J-shaped pelvic curve can be appreciated when using the vacuum as the head descends through the pelvis.

G. Complications

On May 21, 1998, an FDA public advisory was published cautioning health care providers when using vacuum assisted delivery devices. This advisory stated: "Over the past four years, the FDA has received reports of twelve deaths and nine serious injuries among newborns on whom vacuum assisted delivery devices were used, an average of five events per year. In contrast, during the preceding 11 years, there were four deaths and five serious injuries reported, fewer than one event per year.

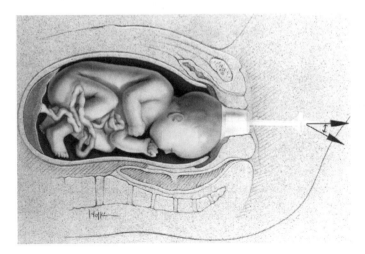

FIGURE 10. Correct position of the vacuum cup and the correct direction of traction before the vertex clears the symphysis pubis. (From Epperly T, Breitinger R: Vacuum extraction. Am Fam Physician, Sept 205–210, 1988, with permission.)

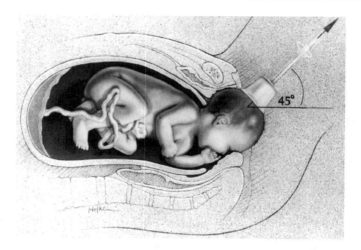

FIGURE 11. Change in the direction of traction as the vertex crowns. (From Epperly T, Breitinger R: Vacuum extraction. Am Fam Physician, Sept 205–210, 1988, with permission.)

Part, but probably not all, of this five-fold increase can be explained by an increase in usage—based upon data from 1989–1995, it is estimated that use of vacuum-assisted delivery devices increased from 3.5 percent of all deliveries to 5.9 percent." One type of life-threatening complication noted was subgaleal hematoma. This occurs when emissary veins are damaged and blood accumulates in the potential space between the galea aponeurotica and the periosteum of the skull. Signs of subgaleal hematoma include diffuse swelling of the head that may shift dependently when the infant's head is repositioned. This swelling indents easily on palpation and may be significant enough to result in hypovolemic shock. Intracranial hemorrhage (subdural, subarachnoid, intraventricular, and/or intraparenchymal hemorrhage) may also be life-threatening. Signs of intracranial hemorrhage include convulsions, lethargy, obtundation, apnea, bulging fontanelle, poor feeding, increased irritability, bradycardia, and/or shock.[5]

H. Follow-up Care Following Vacuum

1. Documentation

If possible, dictate an operative report that describes the indication, procedure, and complications (if any) of the procedure.

2. Patient communication

Attempt to understand the perceptions of the patient and her family as to why the assisted delivery occurred and to address any possible misunderstanding. Misunderstandings are common and may persist indefinitely.

3. Fetal scalp trauma

If fetal scalp emphysema or erythema has occurred after the vacuum was applied, it will resolve within 1 week without complications. Examine for cephalhematomas, subgaleal hemorrhages, and subsequent jaundice. Parental reassurance plays an important role.

VIII. How to Deliver an Occipitoposterior (OP) Presentation by Forceps/Vacuum[6]

The fetus in the OP position rotates spontaneously to an OA presentation in more than 90% of cases. If the OP presentation is persistent, delivery can occur in this position. Vacuum or forceps delivery with the fetus in an OP position or a cesarean section is safer and in most cases preferable to forceps rotation. Also, the persistent OP presentation is a cause of relative cephalopelvic disproportion and is associated with an increased incidence of a failed assisted delivery. Therefore, preparations should be made for emergent cesarean section if the procedure fails or the fetal condition deteriorates.

A. Vacuum

The vacuum may be particularly good for this because auto-rotation may occur without trauma to maternal sidewalls. A built-in safety factor is disengagement of the cup three times.

B. Forceps

Forceps rotation should be done only by skilled and experienced operators. For less experienced clinicians, a vacuum or forceps delivery with the fetus in an OP position or a cesarean intervention is safer. Forceps delivery when the fetus is in an OP position occurs as follows:

1. Forceps is applied in the same manner.
2. Traction initially is straight out because flexion of the head is limited and extension of the head presents greater diameters to the pelvis and will not occur.
3. Traction is applied until the nose is visible beneath the symphysis, then upward motion brings the occiput into view, which is followed by downward pressure to deliver the rest of the face.

IX. Forceps versus Vacuum: Which Is Better?[2,10,21,26]

The vacuum extractor rivals forceps in safety and efficacy depending on the experience of the operator. Use of the vacuum extractor is associated with an increased risk of cephalhematoma (absolute risk increase of 5.5%, number needed to harm = 18) and retinal hemorrhage (absolute risk increase of 15.4%, number needed to harm = 6.5).[14] However, use of vacuum prevents significant maternal injury (absolute risk reduction = 11%, number needed to treat = 9). Forceps is often preferred in emergent situations when time is a factor.

References

1. American College of Obstetricians and Gynecologists Practice Bulletin: Operative Vaginal Delivery. Number 17, June, 2000.
2. Berkus MD, Ramamurthy RS, O'Connor PS: Cohort study of silastic obstetric vacuum cup deliveries: I. Safety of the instrument. J Obstet Gynecol 66:503–509, 1985.
3. Bofill JA, Rust OA, Devidas M, et al: Neonatal cephalohematoma from vacuum extraction. J Reprod Med 42:565–569, 1997.
4. Broekhuizen FF, Washington JM, Johnson F, et al: Vacuum extraction versus forceps delivery: Indications and complications, 1979 to 1984. Obstet Gynecol 69:338–342, 1987.
5. Burlington, DB: FDA Public Health Advisory: Need for CAUTION When Using Vacuum-Assisted Delivery Devices, May 21, 1998.
6. Cunningham FG, MacDonald P, Gant N, et al: Forceps delivery and related techniques. In Cunningham FG, MacDonald P, Grant N (eds): Williams Obstetrics, 19th ed. East Norwalk, CT, Appleton & Lange, 1993, pp 555–576.
7. Damos JR, Koller WS: Forceps and vacuum extraction: Advanced life support in obstetrics. American Academy of Family Physicians Course Syllabus, 1996, pp 119–130.
8. Epperly T, Breitinger R: Vacuum extraction. Am Fam Physician, September 205–210, 1988.
9. Fraser WD: Oxytocin during 2nd stage with epidural. In Enkin MW, Keirse MHNC, Renfrew MJ, Neilson JP (eds): Pregnancy and Childbirth Module. Cochrane Database of Systematic Reviews, Review No. 06448. Cochrane Updates on Disk. Oxford, Update Software, 1994.
10. Gray DL, Nelson, DM: Cord blood acid-base status in neonates delivered by silastic vacuum cup extraction: Comparison with forceps and spontaneous deliveries. J Obstet Gynecol 71:76–80, 1988.
11. Hogg W, Lemelin J: The case for small hospital obstetrics. Can Fam Physician 32:2135–2139, 1986.
12. Howell CJ: Epidural vs. non-epidural analgesic for pain relief (Cochrane Review). In The Cochrane Library, Issue 4, 2000. Oxford, Update Software.
13. Johanson RB: Obstetric forcep pad designed to reduce trauma. In Enkin MW, Keirse MHNC, Renfrew MH, Neilson JP (eds): Pregnancy and Childbirth Module. Cochrane Database of Systematic Reviews, Review No. 07086. Cochrane Updates on Disk. Oxford, Update Software, 1994.

14. Johanson RB, Menon VJ: Vacuum extraction versus forceps delivery (Cochrane Review). In The Cochrane Library, Issue 4, 2000. Oxford, Update Software.
15. Johanson RB, Menon VJ: Soft versus hard vacuum extraction cups for assisted vaginal delivery (Cochrane Review). In The Cochrane Library, Issue 4, 2000. Oxford, Update Software.
16. Nesbitt TS, Connell FA, Hart LG, et al: Access to obstetric care in rural areas: Effect on birth outcomes. Am J Public Health 80:814–818, 1990.
17. Nesbitt TS, Larson EH, Rosenblatt RA, et al: Access to maternity care in rural Washington: Its effect on neonatal outcomes and resource use. Am J Public Health. 87:85–90, 1997.
18. Nikoderm VC: Early vs. late pushing with epidural anesthesia in 2nd stage of labor. In Enkin MW, Keirse MHNC, Renfrew MJ, Neilson JP (eds): Pregnancy and Childbirth Module. Cochrane Database of Systematic Reviews, Review No. 03403, Cochrane Updates on Disk. Oxford, Update Software, 1994.
19. Pelosi MA: A randomized comparison of assisted vaginal delivery by obstetric forceps and polyethylene vacuum cup. Obstet Gynecol 79:638–639, 1992.
20. Revah A. Ezra Y, Farine D, et al: Failed trial of vacuum or forceps—maternal and fetal outcome. Am J Obstet Gynecol 176:200–204, 1997.
21. Seidman DS, Laor A, Gale R, et al: Long-term effects of vacuum and forceps deliveries. Lancet 337: 1583–1585, 1991.
22. Sultan AH, Johanson RB, Carter JE: Occult anal sphincter trauma following randomized forceps and vacuum delivery. Inter J Gynaecol Obstet 61:113–119, 1998.
23. Sultan AH, Kamm MA, Hudson CN, et al: Anal sphincter disruption during vaginal delivery. N Engl J Med 329:1905–1911, 1993.
24. Teng FY, Sayre JW: Vacuum extraction: Does duration predict scalp injury? Obstet Gynecol 89:281–285, 1997.
25. Thomas SJ, Morgan MA, Asrat T, et al: The risk of periventricular-intraventricular hemorrhage with vacuum extraction of neonates weighing 2000 grams or less. J Perinatol 17:37–41, 1997.
26. Williams WC, Knupper RA, O'Brien WS, et al: A randomized comparison of assisted vaginal delivery by obstetrical forceps and polyethylene vacuum cup. J Obstet Gynecol 78:789–794, 1991.

SECTION E.
EPISIOTOMY AND REPAIR OF LACERATIONS

Elizabeth G. Baxley, M.D., and Robert Gobbo, M.D.

I. Definitions and Classification

A full discussion of the evidence for the selective use of episiotomy is found in Chapter 13, section G. All clinicians will have the occasion to perform elective episiotomies and will also encounter third- and fourth-degree extensions. This section describes the classification of these wounds and how to repair them.

A. Midline Episiotomy

The incision is performed in the median or midline raphe of the perineal body.

B. Mediolateral

This is performed with the incision directed from the posterior fourchette either to the right or left at a 30° to 45° angle from the vertical. This type of incision is not commonly used in the United States because of increased postpartum maternal discomfort. This approach is associated with a decreased incidence of third- and fourth-degree extensions.

C. Episiotomy Classification

For purposes of classification, perineal lacerations, episiotomies, and extensions of episiotomies are considered in the same manner. However, it is usually unnecessary and unwise to deliberately cut a third- or fourth-degree episiotomy. The latter incision is referred to as an episioproctotomy.

1. First-degree episiotomy

These incisions or extensions are confined to the mucosal and skin layer and usually do not need repair unless they are actively bleeding. They generally do not extend behind the hymenal ring.

2. Second-degree episiotomy

These involve the mucosa and deeper muscular and fascial tissues of the vagina and perineum, but spare the sphincter.

3. Third-degree episiotomy or extension

This involves the anal sphincter. A third-degree extension completely transects the anal sphincter; a partial third-degree partially extends through the fascia into the muscular tissue of the anal sphincter.

4. Fourth-degree episiotomy or extension

This extension dissects into the rectal mucosa, usually transecting the anal sphincter in the process. In cases in which the sphincter is preserved, a "button-hole" fourth-degree extension may be noted. It commonly occurs about 3–4 cm above the anorectal verge, where the vagina and the rectum are separated by a very thin layer of areolar or connective tissue.

II. Indications for Episiotomy

Indications for episiotomy are listed below, and include circumstances in which additional room may be needed to facilitate the performance of a maneuver or procedure.

A. Shoulder Dystocia

Shoulder dystocia is a soft tissue dystocia, and episiotomy does not relieve the dystocia. However, it may help provide room for the birth attendant's hands if internal rotational maneuvers are needed.

B. Breech Delivery

This is a relative indication depending on gestational age and fetal size.

C. Forceps Delivery

This is also a relative indication depending on gestational age, fetal size, and room available at the introitus for applying forceps. The decision to do an episiotomy is operator-dependent.

III. Relative Contraindications to Episiotomy

These include maternal conditions in which the performance of an episiotomy could lead to excessive maternal bleeding, such as coagulopathies or the presence of large perivulvar varicosities. Episiotomies should not be performed when the avoidance of maternal blood exposure to the newborn, such as with the delivery of an HIV-infected mother, is important.

IV. Performance of Episiotomy and Repair

A. When to Perform an Episiotomy

An episiotomy is performed when the fetal head is crowning 3–4 cm. Performing an episiotomy earlier than this usually does not hasten delivery and may lead to increased blood loss. The perineum is distended between two fingers and divided with Mayo scissors, taking care not to incise the anal sphincter. Midline episiotomies increase the risk of a third- or fourth-degree extension.[6,8] The incision should be extended approximately 5–6 cm into the vagina.

B. Anesthesia

Local anesthesia, when needed, can be administered prior to cutting an episiotomy or before the repair. Anesthetic choice is at the discretion of the provider, but commonly used anesthetic agents include lidocaine, chloroprocaine, or bupivacaine. In addition to local anesthesia, options for anesthesia include pudendal nerve block, intravenous analgesia, or "topping-off" an existing epidural.

C. Repair Techniques

Perineal lacerations can be repaired in the same manner in which an episiotomy is repaired. First-degree lacerations need not be repaired unless there is active bleeding.

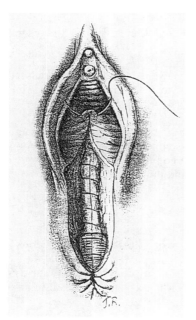

FIGURE 12. Repair of the midline episiotomy. Similar to the principal with the mediolateral episiotomy, an anchor stitch is placed approximately 1 cm beyond the most superior extent of the episiotomy. This is an important stitch to ensure that cut or bleeding vessels are not missed at the apex of the wound. (From Hankins GDV, Clark SL, Cunningham FG, Gilstrap III LC (eds): Operative Obstetrics. East Norwalk, Appleton & Lange, 1995, p 104, with permission.)

1. The vaginal mucosa (Fig. 12)
This is repaired by placing a stitch above the apex of the incision or tear in order to incorporate any retracted blood vessels and prevent bleeding. If the apex is deep in the vagina, it may be difficult to visualize. The clinician can place a single interrupted suture as high in the defect as possible and then pace a hemostat on the free end of the suture. The wound can then be retracted inferiorly, exposing the apex for repair.

Once the apex suture is secured, the vaginal mucosa is approximated by passing the needle through one side of the vagina deep into the muscular layer and back out to the opposing side through the vaginal mucosa. Locking each stitch provides better hemostasis, but is not necessary if the tissue is not bleeding. Care should be taken not to place the sutures too lateral to the midline incision. This may result in excessive imbrication of the vaginal epithelium that can lead to epidermal inclusion cysts as the wound heals. The suture is then brought under the hymenal ring and held for repair of superficial layers of the perineum. Appropriate sutures for this repair include 3–0 chromic catgut and polyglycolic acid. Absorbable synthetic suture (e.g., polyglycolic acid and polyglactin sutures) versus chromic material appears to decrease the women's experience of short-term pain (OR 0.53, 95% CI 0.43–0.64, ARR 13%, NNT 7.5), less need for analgesia (OR 0.63, 95% CI 0.49–0.80, ARR 11%, NNT 9), and less suture dehiscence (OR 0.41, 95% CI 0.25–0.67, ARR 10%, NNT 10).[4,5]

2. Repair of the perineum (Fig. 13)
Some patients may have too deep of a defect to repair the perineum with single bites of the remaining suture. In this situation, the deep layers of the perineum can be closed with interrupted stitches. In most situations, this portion of the wound can be repaired with the suture material used to close the vaginal mucosa. With the suture that has been passed under the hymenal ring, the needle is held horizontally to take a deep lateral bite of the fascia and bulbocavernous muscle that borders the posterior fourchette of the vagina. This stitch is called

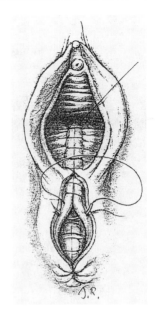

FIGURE 13. Repair of the midline episiotomy. The technique of using one suture for closure of the midline episiotomy is demonstrated. Once the vaginal mucosa has been reapproximated to the hymenal ring, the needle is passed from the midline of the vagina out onto the perineal body. The same suture can now be used for placement of the crown stitch. (From Hankins GDV, Clark SL, Cunningham FG, Gilstrap LC III (eds): Operative Obstetrics. East Norwalk, CT, Appleton & Lange, 1995, p 105, with permission.)

the "crown" or "bulbocavernosus" stitch. It is then completed by taking a similar bite on the opposite side. The remainder of the wound may then be closed in a running fashion extending to the inferior apex of the perineum apex.

From this point, the clinician may tie the suture or continue the repair in a subcuticular fashion approximating the wound edges. At the top of this closure, the needle is passed into the vagina behind the hymenal ring and tied to itself. Alternatively, the superficial perineal layer may be closed with interrupted sutures. The continuous subcuticular versus interrupted approach is associated with less pain for up to 10 days postpartum (OR 0.68, 95% CI 0.53–0.86, ARR 7%, NNT 14).[4,5]

3. Repair of third- and fourth-degree lacerations

Extensions of episiotomies or lacerations into deeper tissues are associated with routine episiotomy, delivery with stirrups, instrumented delivery (forceps > vacuum), prolonged second stage of labor, nulliparity, occiput transverse or occiput posterior positions, anesthesia (local and epidural), patient age ≤ 21 years, use of oxytocin, and experience of the birth attendant.[1]

    a. Rectal mucosa repair. A thorough inspection of the full extent of the wound is necessary. Identifying the apex of the rectal mucosal tear and the often-retracted ends of the external rectal sphincter and its fascia is essential to re-approximate the anatomy for proper healing and function. Irrigating the area with warm saline, re-draping and re-gloving may aid in reducing the potential complications of tissue breakdown and secondary infection.

        The rectal mucosa is repaired first. A Gelpie retractor may be helpful in providing exposure or additional assistance should be obtained to provide necessary exposure. A continuous suture of 4-0 plain, chromic or polyglycolic acid on a tapered needle is started at the apex of the mucosal incision to approximate the mucosa, muscularis, and serosa. The suture is placed in a manner that imbricates or inverts the rectal mucosa. The sutures should be placed so as to avoid passing the needle into the bowel lumen and should be directed to pass through the serosa and muscularis layers of the rectal wall. Some operators find it helpful to place a double-gloved little finger of the nondominant hand into the rectum to assist in providing optimal exposure while performing this phase of the repair.

At this point, the operator should re-irrigate the wound and change gloves again. A second layer of 3-0 chromic or polyglycolic acid sutures is placed next to provide additional support and strength. The first stitch of this second layer is placed at the apex of the wound approximately 0.5 cm above the repaired rectal mucosa. It is placed to gather adjacent smooth muscle of internal anal sphincter in a running or interrupted fashion down to the anopectineal line to help provide a bridge of connective tissue support.

Once this layer is complete, some find it helpful to approximate a few centimeters length of skin from the anopectineal line up to the perineum before closing the rectal sphincter. This may help in preventing a button-hole defect and make it easier to close the skin in this area rather than waiting until later in the repair.

b. Anal sphincter repair. The ends of the sphincter must be clearly identified. They often retract into the capsule laterally. The muscle and its capsule can be grasped and brought anteriorly and medially using Allis clamps. The severed ends of the sphincter muscle and its capsule should be oriented to identify the posterior, inferior, superior, and anterior poles (PISA, Fig. 14). The sphincter is re-approximated using four carefully placed 2-0 or 3-0 polyglycolic acid or chromic interrupted sutures on a tapered needle. The first suture should be placed at the bottom, which is the most

"PISA"

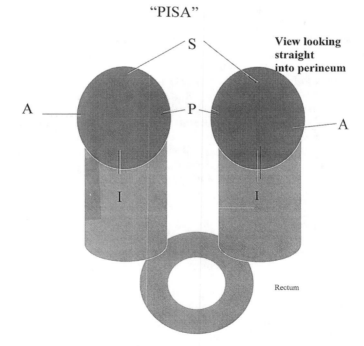

FIGURE 14. Four simple interrupted or "figure of eight" sutures are placed to carefully approximate each side of the external sphincter (posterior, inferior, superior and anterior) together.)

posterior portion of the sphincter using a simple mattress placement. Sutures are then placed in the inferior, superior, and anterior poles to complete the PISA repair. Avoiding figure-of-eight sutures has been recommended because of the theoretical risk of tissue strangulation with resultant devascularization and poor healing.[3] Stitches should incorporate a minimum of muscle to prevent necrosis of muscle tissue.

4. Lacerations of the vulva and anterior vaginal wall

Anterior vaginal wall lacerations are more common with restrictive use of episiotomies.[2] The urethra, bladder, and clitoris can all be involved with resulting hemorrhage and/or fistula formation. The placement of a Foley catheter can aid in distinguishing the urethra from the surrounding structures. Careful attention to repair of these lacerations with correct anatomic re-approximation should be done if the wounds are deep or if hemostasis is required.

V. Postpartum Care
A. Comfort Measures
Ice packs are used initially, followed by local heat and anesthetic sprays.
B. Third- or Fourth-Degree Lacerations
No medications are administered rectally, including enemas, suppositories, and stool softeners.

VI. Follow-Up Care for Complications
A. Infection
Infection of episiotomy sites is an uncommon complication. Superficial infection is characterized by local erythema, edema, exudate, and tenderness. Management includes opening the perineal wound and debridement of the infected tissue. It should be left to heal by secondary intention. Simple, noninfected hematomas should be drained and hemostasis secured, unless they are very small and not expanding.
B. Third- and Fourth-Degree Extension
Patients with a third- or fourth-degree laceration repair initially may experience a sensation of tearing or pulling with bowel movements. Rectovaginal fistulas are uncommon, but some degree of decreased rectal tone may still occur with an appropriate repair of the sphincter. Patients with concerns of fecal incontinence should be examined with digital examination during postpartum follow-up. Fecal incontinence or flatal incontinence may present as late concerns and can be related to direct damage to the sphincter or damage to its innervation.[7]

References

1. Canavan T: Third- and fourth-degree perineal lacerations.In Damos J, Eisinger S (eds): ALSO Manual, 4th ed. Kansas City, MO, American Academy of Family Physicians, 2000.
2. Carroli G, Belizan J, Stamp G: Episiotomy policies in vaginal births (Cochrane Review). In The Cochrane Library, Issue 4, 2000. Oxford, Update Software.
3. Delancey JOL, Hankins GDV: Episiotomy. In Hankins GDV, Clark SL, Cunningham EG, Gilstrap LC (eds): Operative Obstetrics. East Norwalk, CT, Appleton & Lange, 1995, pp 93–127.
4. Kettle C, Johanson RB: Absorbable synthetic versus catgut suture material for perineal repair. In The Cochrane Library, Issue 4, 2000. Oxford, Update Software.
5. Kettle C, Johanson RB: Continuous versus interrupted sutures for perineal repair. In The Cochrane Library, Issue 2, 2000. Oxford, Update Software.
6. Klein M, Gauthier R, Jorgensen S, et al: Does episiotomy prevent perineal trauma and pelvic floor relaxation? Online J Curr Clin Trials, 1992; Doc. 10.
7. Snooks SJ, Henry MM, Swash M: Faecal incontinence due to external anal division in childbirth is associated with damage to the innervation of the pelvic floor musculature: A double pathology. Br J Obstet Gynaecol 92:824–828, 1985.
8. Thorp JM, Bowes WA, Brame RF, et al: Selected use of midline episiotomies. Obstet Gynecol 70:260–262, 1987.

SECTION F.
AMNIOCENTESIS DURING THE THIRD TRIMESTER
OF PREGNANCY

Mark Deutchman, M.D.

I. Indications
A. Assessing Fetal Lung Maturity
Amniocentesis is done to obtain amniotic fluid for lung maturity testing in any of the following situations.

1. Prior to repeat cesarean delivery if questions persist about fetal lung maturity
2. Premature labor
3. For patients in labor with very questionable dates and unresolved gestational age by history, physical examination, and ultrasound fetal biometry
4. As an aid to deciding when to stop tocolysis in prematurely laboring patients

B. Suspected Chorioamnionitis
Amniocentesis may be performed to obtain amniotic fluid for white blood cell count, Gram stain and culture, or other tests. The clinical settings in which this testing is most commonly done are preterm labor, preterm premature rupture of the membranes, and maternal fever and fetal tachycardia.

C. Rh Isoimmunization
In Rh-isoimmunized pregnancies, serial amniocentesis procedures may be performed to diagnose and follow the degree of fetal hemolysis as represented by increasing amniotic fluid bilirubin levels.

II. Parameters and Interpretation
A. Lung Maturity Testing
1. Lecithin: sphingomyelin (L:S) ratio
The L:S ratio is the traditional standard for fetal lung maturity testing. A ratio of greater than 2:1 is 98% predictive of fetal lung maturity. Falsely mature values can be obtained in diabetic mothers (classes A through C), asphyxiated infants, or in cases of Rh isoimmunization.[8] Because this test is cumbersome and time-consuming, it is commonly replaced by one of the following tests.
2. Phosphatidyl glycerol
The presence of phosphatidyl glycerol (PG) in excess of 3% (positive test) indicates functional lung maturity and is a more reliable predictor of mature lungs than the L:S ratio in clinical situations in which the L:S may be falsely mature, such as maternal diabetes. The appearance of PG is also accelerated in clinical situations associated with fetal stress, such as maternal hypertension and premature rupture of the membranes.[8] Testing for PG is performed by thin-layer chromatography or by a slide agglutination test using antisera.
3. Fetal Lung Maturity (Abbott Laboratories, Irving, TX)
This is a test for total surfactant relative to albumin in amniotic fluid using fluorescent polarization technology. A value of 70 or greater is considered mature.
4. Foam Stability Index (Beckman Instruments, Fullerton, CA)
This is a kit test that measures total surfactant activity. It is a modern quantitative variant of the older shake test. Amniotic fluid is added to wells in a cassette that contains varying preloaded volumes and concentrations of ethanol. The entire cassette is shaken vigorously for 30 seconds and observed after an additional 60 seconds. The endpoint is the observation of stable bubbles in the wells of varying ethanol:amniotic fluid concentrations. Stable bubbles in the well labeled "47" or greater indicate lung maturity.

5. The tap test

This is a bedside test in which 1 ml of amniotic fluid is mixed with one drop of 6 N hydrochloric acid and 1.5 ml of diethyl ether. The tube containing this mixture is tapped three or four times, creating 200 to 300 bubbles in the ether layer. Fluid from a mature fetus causes the bubbles to break down rapidly. If no more than five bubbles persist in the ether layer after 10 minutes, the result is considered mature.[14] Faster disappearance of bubbles provides more assurance of lung maturity.[5]

6. Turbidity of amniotic fluid

This is a potent indicator of fetal lung maturity. If a tube of amniotic fluid is turbid enough to prevent the reading of newsprint through it, fetal lung maturity is predicted with 97% certainty.[5] This test is fast, simple, and inexpensive, and should be considered the primary rapid screening test.

7. Optical density

The optical density of amniotic fluid at 650 nm is a useful test of fluid contaminated by blood but not by meconium. OD values ≥ 0.15 predict maturity and agree well with L:S ratio testing.[5]

8. Causes of false-positive results

Meconium and blood can affect lung maturity test results. Both blood and meconium can cause falsely mature results for the Fetal Lung Maturity test, Foam Stability Index, and shake and tap tests.[9] An assay for phosphatidyl glycerol should be reliable even in the face of meconium[15] and bloody fluid.[1,12]

9. Testing from vaginal pool specimens

Testing on amniotic fluid sample obtained from the vaginal pool following spontaneous rupture of membranes must be interpreted with caution. Some studies have found testing for phosphatidyl glycerol testing to be more reliable than L:S testing, but others have found that certain vaginal bacteria can create false-positive results.[5] Because they are surfactants, soaps and detergents should be carefully excluded from any amniotic fluid sample being tested for fetal lung maturity.

Commonly available tests are so strongly predictive of lung maturity that testing by multiple methods is not recommended if the result of a first test is "positive."[1] Efficacy of common tests as published in a recent study is shown in Table 3.[10]

B. Diagnosis of Chorioamnionitis

1. Gram stain

Any organisms seen on a Gram stain of unspun amniotic fluid obtained by amniocentesis are abnormal.[6] If fluid is obtained by aspiration through an intrauterine pressure catheter, the first 10 ml of this fluid should be discarded to avoid contamination.[11]

2. Amniotic fluid white cell count (AFWBC)

The use of this technique to diagnose chorioamnionitis is controversial. Some reports consider AFWBC not to be predictive of chorioamnionitis[11] or of positive fetal and amniotic fluid bacterial cultures.[3] Other investigators have found AFWBC greater than 50/mm^3 to be predictive of positive bacterial cultures,

TABLE 3

	Phosphatidyl glycerol test	Tap test
Sensitivity	83%	80%
Specificity	92%	91%
Predictive value for lung maturity	96%	95%
Predictive value for immaturity	73%	68%

clinical chorioamnionitis, and neonatal morbidity in patients with preterm premature rupture of membranes.[17] In patients with preterm labor and intact membranes. AFWBC was found to be the best predictor of positive bacterial cultures, clinical chorioamnionitis, early delivery, neonatal sepsis, and neonatal complications.[16]

3. Rapid test for leukocyte esterase
This has been tested to diagnose chorioamnionitis and has been said to be helpful by some authors[7] and not by others.[4]

4. Amniotic fluid culture
Fluid obtained by amniocentesis or through an intrauterine pressure catheter can be cultured and may help guide later therapy of mother or infant.

5. Amniotic fluid glucose
Levels less than 10 mg/dl help predict chorioamnionitis.[4]

A rapid, convenient laboratory test for chorioamnionitis that is both highly sensitive and specific does not exist. The diagnosis of chorioamnionitis remains primarily clinical and is indicated by maternal fever, maternal or fetal tachycardia, uterine tenderness, and malodorous amniotic fluid.

C. Amniotic Fluid Bilirubin Levels
Bilirubin levels are indirectly assessed by measuring the optical density of amniotic fluid at 450 nm. The value obtained is plotted against gestational age on a Liley graph, which is available in standard textbooks. The absolute value and trend over time determines management, which may include continued surveillance, intrauterine transfusion, or delivery.

III. Ultrasound Examination Before the Procedure
Before a patient undergoes an amniocentesis, she should have an ultrasound evaluation with particular attention paid to assessment of fluid volume, location of fluid pockets, fetal presentation, and placental location. It is desirable but not absolutely essential to avoid the placenta. The main contraindication to amniocentesis is severe oligohydramnios. Unless a prior ultrasound evaluation has been performed to rule out fetal anomalies and establish accurate dating, an ultrasound should be obtained before amniocentesis because the finding of anomalies or readjustment of dating may alter the clinical diagnosis and management plan.

IV. The Procedure[2,13]
A. Written Informed Consent
This should be obtained, making sure that the patient understands the reason for the procedure, alternatives, and risks.

B. Identifying a Fluid Pocket
Ultrasound is used to locate an accessible pocket of fluid. Ideally, a pocket not close to the fetal face and free of umbilical cord should be chosen. In cases of oligohydramnios or a large anterior placenta, examiner may lift the fetal head, creating a pocket of fluid in the lower uterine segment appropriate for amniocentesis. The maternal bladder should be empty. This suprapubic technique carries an increased risk of rupture of the membrane. The transplacental route for amniocentesis is less desirable, but not absolutely contraindicated if no other appropriate site is available.

C. Use of Anesthesia/Local Preparation
Local anesthesia (1% lidocaine) may be used. Some operators think that since this is a "one-stick" procedure, local anesthesia is not necessary. This option should be discussed with the patient. After an appropriate site is selected, the skin is prepped in a sterile fashion. Making a "dent" in the skin with the hub of a needle or other round object can help keep the operator from losing the operative site during the prep.

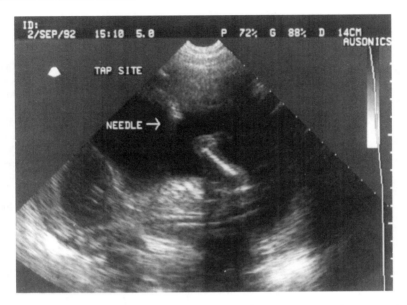

FIGURE 15. The needle tip is observed as a bright echo as it traverses the maternal tissues and enters the amniotic fluid.

D. Preparation for the Amniocentesis
Prior to doing the tap, the anticipated depth of insertion of the needle is measured sonographically. A 3.5-inch, 21-gauge spinal needle is commonly used, but a 1.5-inch needle may be sufficient in thin patients.

E. The Procedure
1. Technique

The operator holds the needle in one hand and the ultrasound transducer in the other hand, continuously observing the progress of the needle through the maternal tissues into the target pocket of amniotic fluid (Fig. 15). The transducer is held a few centimeters away from the tap site, often under the sterile drape. Alternatively, an experienced assistant may hold the ultrasound transducer. The transducer is not sterile and should not contact the needle; it may be covered with a sterile glove. Antiseptic soaps such as povidone iodine and chlorhexidine work well as ultrasound conductive media during the procedure.

2. Aspiration of amniotic fluid

The stylet is removed from the needle and if amniotic fluid is seen to appear in the hub, a short piece of flexible tubing is attached and a 20–30-ml syringe is used to aspirate fluid. If the operator is holding both the needle and the transducer, an assistant can connect the tubing and aspirate the fluid. If no fluid comes back, the needle is repositioned, usually slightly deeper. If the needle tip is seen to be within fluid but there is no fluid return, the membranes may be tented over the tip. This can be alleviated either by rotating the needle, which causes the bevel of the needle to tear through the membranes, or by further advancing the needle under sonographic guidance. If blood-tinged fluid is obtained, the first few milliliters are discarded until clear fluid is obtained.

3. Post-amniocentesis

After a sample is obtained, usually 10–30 ml, the needle is withdrawn. It is not unusual for the baby to "bump" the needle during the procedure, usually resulting in a withdrawal response by the fetus.[12] If a large amount of fetal movement is noted while the preparation is being done, the patient should be rescanned to confirm the presence of the target pocket. Another site should be chosen if the pocket has disappeared. The fluid is placed in a sterile container and taken directly to the laboratory for analysis. It is strongly recommended that the laboratory be warned prior to the procedure that a sample is on the way. If a kit test is being used, the results can be available in a few minutes.

Following the amniocentesis, the tap site is inspected sonographically. "Streaming" of blood into the amniotic fluid is sometimes seen and usually stops promptly. If this continues, the pregnancy should be monitored closely. A period of maternal observation for contractions is necessary, and nonstress testing should be considered.

4. Special considerations

If optical density testing is to be performed in case of Rh isoimmunization (bilirubin testing), the fluid should be shielded from light. Mothers who are Rh-negative should receive Rh_o (D) immune globulin.

V. Risks of Amniocentesis

Amniocentesis risks can be minimized by using simultaneous real-time sonographic guidance to avoid injury to maternal and fetal structures. Most studies of amniocentesis risks deal with early second-trimester procedures performed for genetic testing, not the third-trimester applications discussed here.[13] Many reports of fetal injury were made before sonographic monitoring was available.

A. Maternal Risks

The following risks occur rarely.
1. Perforation of intra-abdominal organs with infection or bleeding
2. Amniotic fluid embolism
3. Rh isoimmunization

B. Fetal Risks

1. Initiation of labor
2. Amnionitis
3. Rupture of the membranes
4. Puncture of fetus or umbilical cord
5. Placental abruption

References

1. American College of Obstetricians and Gynecologists: Assessment of Fetal Lung Maturity. ACOG Educational Bulletin No. 230, November, 1996. Washington, DC, American College of Obstetricians and Gynecologists.
2. Bowman J: Technique of amniocentesis. In Creasy R, Resnik R (eds): Maternal-Fetal Medicine: Principles and Practice. Philadelphia, W.B. Saunders, 1989, p 628.
3. Carroll SG, Philpott-Howard J, Nicolaides KH: Amniotic fluid Gram stain and leukocyte count in the prediction of intrauterine infection in preterm prelabour amniorrhexis. Fetal Diag Ther 11:1-5, 1996.
4. Coultrip LL, Grossman JH: Evaluation of rapid diagnostic tests in the detection of microbial invasion of the amniotic cavity. Am J Obstet Gynecol 167:1231–1242, 1992.
5. Field NT, Gilbert WM: Current status of amniotic fluid tests of fetal maturity. Clin Obstet Gynecol 40:366–386, 1997.
6. Gibbs RS, Blanco JD, St Clair PJ, et al: Quantitative bacteriology of amniotic fluid from patients with clinic intra-amniotic infection at term. J Infect Dis 145:1–8, 1982.
7. Hoskins IA, Johnson TRB, Winkel CA: Leukocyte esterase activity in human amniotic fluid for the rapid detection of chorioamnionitis. Am J Obstet Gynecol 157:730–732, 1987.
8. Jobe A: Evaluation of fetal lung maturity. In Creasy R, Resnik R (eds): Maternal-Fetal Medicine: Principles and Practice. Philadelphia, W.B. Saunders, 1989.
9. Keniston RC, Noland GL, Pernoll ML: The effect of blood, meconium and temperature on the rapid surfactant test. Obstet Gynecol 48:442–445, 1976.

10. Kucuk M: Tap test, shake test and phosphatidylglycerol in the assessment of fetal pulmonary maturity. Int J Gynaecol Obstet 60:9–14, 1998.
11. Listwa HM, Sobel AS, et al: The predictability of intrauterine infection by analysis of amniotic fluid. Obstet Gynecol 48:31–33, 1976.
12. Petrikovsky MB, Kaplan GP: Fetal responses to inadvertent contact with the needle during amniocentesis. Fetal Diagn Ther 10:83–85, 1995.
13. Romero R, Pupkin M, Oyarzun E, et al: Amniocentesis. In Fleischer AC, et al (eds): The Principles and Practice of Ultrasonography in Obstetrics and Gynecology, 4th ed. East Norwalk, CT, Appleton & Lange, 1991.
14. Socol M: The tap test: Confirmation of a simple, rapid, inexpensive, and reliable indicator of fetal pulmonary maturity. Am J Obstet Gynecol 162:218–222, 1990.
15. Strassner HT Jr, Golde SH, Mosley GH, Platt LD: Effect of blood in amniotic fluid on the detection of phosphatidylglycerol. Am J Obstet Gynecol 138:697–701, 1980.
16. Yoon BH, Yang SH, Jun JK, et al: Maternal blood C-reactive protein, white blood cell count, and temperature in preterm labor: A comparison with amniotic fluid white blood cell count. Obstet Gynecol 87:231–237, 1996.
17. Yoon BH, Jun JK, Park KH, et al: Serum C-reactive protein, white blood cell count and amniotic fluid white blood cell count in women with preterm premature rupture of membranes. Obstet Gynecol 88:1034–1040, 1996.

SECTION G.
CESAREAN DELIVERY

Mark Deutchman, M.D., and Neil Murphy, M.D.

I. Introduction

This section covers indications for cesarean delivery, perioperative patient care, and an overview of surgical technique. The actual techniques of cesarean delivery must be learned by practical, supervised experience. The ability to perform cesarean delivery as primary surgeon is part of the surgical skills of many family physicians, particularly those in rural areas. Every family physician should be able to function as a good first assistant at surgery and should be prepared to perform perimortem cesarean delivery.

A. Overview and Incidence

The use of operative delivery has been increasing and now accounts for nearly 25% of births in many locations in the United States. Cesarean delivery had become the most common operation in the United States by 1984. However, the rise in cesarean delivery has not been accompanied by an improvement in perinatal outcome, and hospitals and individual physicians vary widely in their cesarean delivery rate with no direct relationship to perinatal outcome. The economic cost differential of cesarean delivery versus vaginal birth is significant, with average charges for cesarean delivery exceeding vaginal birth by about $3000 per case, including a combination of hospital and physician fees. The Centers for Disease Control and Prevention has set a national health objective for the year 2000 to reduce the overall cesarean delivery rate to 15% and the cesarean delivery rate for primigravidas to 12%.[8,28]

B. Role of the Family Physician

Family physicians and midwives have established a positive record of lower than average cesarean delivery rates in several published outcome studies.[3,15,25] Family physicians who perform their own cesarean deliveries have reported excellent patient outcomes.[13,14] Clinicians can help assure their patients a reasonable chance of vaginal delivery by using these approaches.[3,26,27,30]

1. Encourage a trial of vaginal birth after previous cesarean section (VBAC).
2. Adhere to the definition of active labor before admitting low-risk mothers to the hospital (see Chapter 13, section A).
3. Interpret fetal heart rate patterns properly to avoid overdiagnosis of fetal distress (see Chapter 15, section A).
4. Use intrapartum amnioinfusion in appropriate situations (see section C).
5. Use epidural anesthesia judiciously.

6. Use oxytocin to judiciously augment labor but avoid hyperstimulation and resultant fetal distress (see Chapter 14, sections A and B).

7. Encourage patients to be informed about and prepared for their childbirth experience.

8. Establish "second opinion" or preoperative consultation guidelines within the hospital.

II. Indications for Cesarean Delivery
A. Maternal Indications
1. Hemorrhage due to placenta previa or placental abruption
2. Inability of mother to tolerate labor due to cardiac, pulmonary, or other medical disease
3. Contracted pelvis due to congenital deformity or old fracture
4. Previous reconstructive vaginal surgery, particularly vesicovaginal fistula
5. Pelvic tumors
6. Previous placement of a cerclage by the abdominal route
7. When trial of labor is contraindicated due to history of uterine surgery involving the active segment of the uterus (myomectomy or cesarean delivery)
8. Repeat when mother refuses trial of labor
9. Perimortem, as a possible aid to maternal resuscitation when cardiopulmonary resuscitation has been in progress for more than 4 or 5 minutes.[2]

B. Fetal Indications
1. Transverse lie (including shoulder presentation)
2. Transverse arrest
3. Brow presentation
4. Face presentation with mentum posterior
5. Failed forceps delivery
6. Failed vacuum extraction if head too high for forceps
7. Truly arrested labor after trial of augmentation
8. Breech presentation not meeting criteria for vaginal delivery (Chapter 16, section F)
9. Failed external cephalic version of breech infant
10. Non-reassuring fetal heart rate pattern, usually after intrauterine resuscitation efforts
11. Umbilical cord prolapse
12. Infant with very low birth weight (< 1500 g)
13. Macrosomic infant (be aware of the inaccuracy of sonographic estimation of fetal weight; see section A)
14. Conjoined twins
15. Active maternal genital herpes simplex virus infection
16. Maternal thrombocytopenia
17. Uterine rupture including abdominal trauma or rupture of previous cesarean delivery scar
18. For delivery of infant of an HIV-positive mother to decrease likelihood of transmission to the infant (see Chapter 8, section A).[5,29,34]
19. Perimortem for fetal salvage in case of mother undergoing cardiopulmonary resuscitation for more than 4 or 5 minutes.[2]

III. Technique and Other Surgical Issues and Choices
A. Preoperative Preparation
1. Make sure patient's prenatal record, including laboratory data, is available. Review preoperative hematocrit levels. Assess the patient's risk for

complications and consider whether appropriate facilities and personnel are available.

2. If time permits, it is desirable to check mother's blood type and check for antibodies in case blood is required for transfusion. It is usually not necessary to crossmatch blood unless the likelihood of transfusion is high.

3. Normotensive patients who will receive epidural or spinal anesthesia should be volume-loaded with 1000 ml of lactated Ringer's solution or normal saline.

4. Consider administration of nonparticulate antacid and/or H_2 blocker/metoclopramide in case of vomiting to minimize risk of pulmonary damage if aspiration occurs.

5. Establish whether or not father or other support person will be present.

6. Identify family members and, if possible, have them designate a spokesperson for communications.

7. Document in the chart the indications for the procedure and the discussion with the patient providing the basis for her informed consent. Risks to document include bleeding, infection, damage to maternal organs, hysterectomy, and death.

8. Note that for mothers with low to moderate risk for bacterial endocarditis, the American Heart Association no longer recommends the administration of antibiotics for prophylaxis of subacute bacterial endocarditis.[11]

B. Choice of Anesthesia[33]

1. General anesthesia

General anesthesia is usually used in life-threatening emergency cases such as cord prolapse, severe hemorrhage, or severe fetal distress.

2. Spinal or epidural anesthesia

This is used if time is not critical. This permits the mother to be awake and avoids passage of anesthetic agents to the infant across the placenta.

3. Spinal anesthesia

Spinal anesthesia is easier to perform and has faster onset than epidural anesthesia but carries increased risk of hypotension due to peripheral vasodilatation. In either case, the patient should receive a fluid bolus (500 to 1000 ml of normal saline or lactated Ringer's solution) before anesthesia, and ephedrine should be available in case hypotension occurs (25–50 mg intramuscularly or 10 mg intravenously).

4. Technique of spinal anesthesia

    a. Perform a lumbar puncture at L4–5 or L3–4 interspace with mother in sitting or lateral decubitus position. A 21-gauge or smaller needle should be used to avoid a spinal headache due to presumed leak from tap site. Insert the needle with the bevel parallel to the long axis of the spine to make smaller hole in dura (along its fibers) rather than create a flap in dura. A smaller needle (25-gauge) can be used through a larger, shorter needle inserted through the skin.

    b. Mix 0.8 mg of tetracaine, 0.2 ml of 1:1000 epinephrine, and 1.0 ml of 10% dextrose in a syringe. When cerebrospinal fluid flows from the needle hub, attach the syringe containing anesthetic mixture and draw a few drops of cerebrospinal fluid into it to demonstrate free flow, then inject over a period of a few seconds and immediately withdraw needle and place mother supine with uterus displaced to one side. While testing abdominal skin sensation, roll operating table to right, left, head up or down to control level of block.

    c. A small dose of narcotic may be added to provide long-lasting postoperative analgesia.

5. Local anesthesia may be used as a primary technique or to augment an incomplete spinal or epidural block. After the infant has been delivered, general anesthesia can be induced or sedation can be added.

C. Instruments Used During the Cesarean Section

1. Scalpel to open skin and deeper layers
2. Electrocautery pencil set to "coagulation" current to control bleeding
3. Electrocautery pencil set to "cutting" current to open subcutaneous tissue and fascia
4. Scissors (curved Mayo or Metzenbaum) to open fascia and peritoneum
5. Hemostats to clamp bleeding vessels prior to electrocoagulation or ligature
6. Kocher or Ochsner clamps to hold fascia
7. Bladder retractor
8. Richardson retractors for abdominal wall
9. Thumb forceps (Russian or Bonney) to elevate peritoneum and bladder reflection as these tissues are handled
10. Smooth thumb forceps to handle peritoneum upon entering the abdomen
11. Ring forceps to help remove membranes and placental fragments
12. Allis or Pennington clamps to hold the cut edges of the uterus and limit blood loss
13. Suction tips: pool or Yankauer depending on stage of operation
14. The choice of suture is entirely optional. Absorbable suture is appropriate for all layers. A long-lasting suture should be chosen for the fascia if absorbable suture is used.

D. Essential Steps in the Operation

1. Prepare the patient as described above.
2. Anesthesia administration
3. Skin scrub and patient positioning
   a. A variety of skin scrub regimens are suitable, including but not limited to povidone iodine and chlorhexidine, as for any other abdominal surgery.
   b. Consider clipping pubic hair that interferes with the incision area.
   c. The patient should be positioned with a lateral tilt to decrease hypotension due to vena cava compression by the uterus. Lateral tilting has been shown to result in higher infant Apgar scores and higher umbilical cord pH.[17]
4. Decompress the urinary bladder with an indwelling Foley bladder catheter.
5. Perform the skin incision.
   a. A Pfannenstiel incision is cosmetically preferable but may take longer depending on experience of the surgeon. Its repair is stronger because there is 30 times less strain on the underlying transversely incised fascia than when fascia is incised vertically.[31] This incision is made transversely about two finger breadths above the symphysis pubis. Incisions at least 15-cm long provide greater ease of infant delivery than shorter incisions.[4]
   b. A midline vertical incision from the symphysis to the umbilicus can offer more room, particularly if difficulty is expected delivering the infant owing to abnormal lie, hydrocephalus, or other unusual conditions.
   c. In either case, the rectal muscles may also be divided to obtain more room.
   d. If a previous skin scar is present, it may be excised as the incision is made or closed, although this is not usually necessary in cases of Pfannenstiel incision.
6. Divide subcutaneous tissues and secure hemostasis. The assistant should be ready with sponges, a hemostat, and electrocautery or ligation material depending on operator's preference.

7. Divide the fascia in the same direction as the skin incision. When making a low transverse abdominal entry, the assistant should be ready with Kocher clamps to grasp the fascia upper and lower edges.

8. Free the fascia from underlying rectus muscles in the case of Pfannenstiel incision. This is usually done bluntly with fingers; if adhesions are present, sharp dissection may be necessary. This is a critical step in obtaining good exposure and must be done both above and below the incision. Be prepared to identify and clamp the inferior epigastric arteries, which are exposed during this step.

9. Separate the rectus muscles by placing fingers between the rectus muscles and pulling laterally.

10. Open the peritoneum: Using a hemostat or smooth thumb forceps, grasp the peritoneum high in the incision to avoid injury to the bladder. Regrasp the peritoneum close to the original spot and drop the original site to allow bowel to fall away, then carefully open the peritoneum with Metzenbaum scissors.

11. Palpate the uterus and presenting part.

12. Develop the bladder flap: Grasp the peritoneum where it reflects off the bladder onto the uterus and open the plane with scissors. Extend the flap to both sides as the assistant rotates the bladder and abdominal wall retractors to the side the operator is working on.

13. Open the uterus[1]
   a. The low transverse incision is most commonly used. The initial uterine incision is made with a knife. Lateral extension is made with blunt pressure or with bandage scissors. The assistant should maintain exposure using suction and retractors.
      i. In most cases, the lower uterine segment is thin and therefore less vascular.
      ii. This incision heals well, reducing the risk of dehiscence in later pregnancies, thus permitting subsequent trial of labor.
      iii. The main risk of transverse incision is lateral extension into the uterine vessels.
   b. The classical incision reaches into the "active" upper uterine segment or the fundus. Vertical extension is made with a knife or bandage scissors. It is associated with increased blood loss and rupture during subsequent pregnancies but is appropriate in these situations:
      i. The lower uterine segment is very thick, underdeveloped, or occupied by fibroids or an anterior placenta previa.
      ii. When delivering a very-low-birth-weight infant
      iii. The infant is in a transverse lie with back down.
      iv. Fetal anomalies are present requiring a large incision (e.g., hydrocephalus).
   c. The low vertical incision may also be used but often extends upward into the active uterine segment making it similar to the classical incision.

14. Deliver the infant
   a. If the infant is in a cephalic presentation, scoop the head out of the pelvis and deliver the body in the usual fashion.
   b. If the infant is in a breech presentation, grasp the pelvis or feet and then follow the same steps described for assisted vaginal delivery (see Chapter 16, section F). Be prepared with a larger incision and maneuvers to maintain neck flexion including availability of Piper forceps.
   c. During this time, the assistant should be prepared to perform these functions at the operator's request:

    i. Suction amniotic fluid and blood from the surgical field.
    ii. Remove the bladder retractor to give the operator room to grasp the presenting part
    iii. Suction the infant's nose and mouth.
    iv. Apply fundal pressure.
    v. Reinsert retractors after infant is delivered.

15. Deliver the placenta and membranes

Allowing the placenta to expel spontaneously through the incision results in decreased maternal blood loss and decreased incidence in postpartum endometritis compared to manual removal.[20] Ring forceps are used to retrieve fragments.

16. Request oxytocin and antibiotic administration at this time.
    a. Prophylactic antibiotics: Cesarean deliveries are by definition "contaminated cases," particularly if the membranes were ruptured prior to surgery. Prophylactic antibiotic use has been shown to reduce postpartum morbidity, wound infection, and serious infections.[2,7,29]
    b. There appears to be no advantage to multiple doses over a single perioperative dose.[24]
    c. Ampicillin or a first-generation cephalosporin (such as cefazolin, 1 g intravenously, after delivery of the infant) is inexpensive and effective.[24]
    d. Irrigation with antibiotic is less effective than systemic antibiotic administration.[24]

17. Place ring, Allis, or Pennington clamps on the cut edges of the uterus to aid closure and limit blood loss.

18. Evacuate the uterus of remaining fluids and tissues using a laparotomy sponge.

19. Close the uterus.
    a. The assistant should maintain exposure and be ready to remove clamps before sutures are placed to avoid sutures being placed through the opening in the clamps.
    b. Some operators bring the uterus out of the abdomen while it is being closed. This may make the uterine incision more accessible if exposure is difficult, but often causes an awake patient to become nauseated due to vagal stimulation when traction is applied to the peritoneum.[21]
    c. The uterus may be closed in one layer.[19] Additional or imbricating layers can be added if required for hemostasis.

20. Evacuate blood and amniotic fluid from the pelvis using a pool suction tip or gauze wrapped over a Yankauer suction tip. Many clinicians choose to irrigate the peritoneal cavity with normal saline to assist in the evacuation of blood clots. Laparotomy sponges may be used.

21. Bladder flap and peritoneal closure is not necessary.[18]

22. Close the fascia. Grasp the fascia in the midline with Kocher clamps. The assistant should demonstrate the corner of the fascial incision with a small Richardson retractor at the start of the repair.

23. Irrigate the subcutaneous tissues. Closure of the subcutaneous tissue (Camper fascia closure) has been shown to decrease the incidence of wound infection, separation, seromas, and hematomas, independent of all factors except obesity and four or more vaginal examinations.[12] Drains are normally not necessary in a cesarean delivery, but may be indicated if there is concern about incomplete hemostasis, a hematoma, or possible infection.[16]

24. Close the skin with suture or staples. Subcuticular closure of Pfannenstiel incisions results in less pain and better cosmetic appearance.[22]

25. Apply a sterile dressing.

26. To ensure uterine drainage, compress the uterus with the palm of a hand on the abdomen to squeeze out blood and clots. If necessary, palpate the cervical os from below to make sure it is open for drainage, particularly for patients whose membranes were not ruptured prior to surgery.

E. The Simplified "Misgav Ladach" Cesarean Section Technique
This modification of the Joel-Cohen method of cesarean delivery is faster and produces less blood loss. This technique involves these main features:[9]
1. The skin incision is made just through the skin and not the subcutaneous tissue. Incision placement is higher than a Pfannenstiel incision, about 1 inch below a line connecting the anterior superior iliac spines.
2. The subcutaneous fat is opened sharply only in the midline to expose the fascia which is opened in the midline with a knife.
3. The fascia is "zipped" open with slightly opened scissors tips beneath the fat.
4. The fascia is pulled off the midline cranially and caudally.
5. The muscles, fascia, and subcutaneous fat are slowly pulled laterally seeking to open the incision bloodlessly.
6. The peritoneum is opened bluntly by stretching with fingers.
7. The uterus is closed in a single layer.
8. The bladder flap and peritoneum are not closed.
9. The fascia is closed with one running layer of 1-0 Vicryl with the operator working away from himself or herself.
10. Skin is closed loosely with widely spaced mattress sutures.

F. The "Bloodless" Cesarean Section
This cesarean delivery technique has been described for use on mothers infected with human immunodeficiency virus. The main features of this technique are:[35]
1. The wound is irrigated and re-draped before the uterus is opened.
2. The surgeon cleans or changes gloves before the uterus is opened.
3. The uterus is opened without rupturing membranes and a surgical stapling device is used to enlarge the uterine incision
4. The infant is delivered leaving membranes intact over the presenting part if possible.
5. The infant is initially bathed on the operating table before being handed off.

G. Writing an Operative Note
1. For cesarean delivery, specify type of skin and uterine incision and note if tubal ligation has been done. When the uterine incision is vertical, note whether or not it extended into the active segment.
2. Indication, preoperative and postoperative diagnoses
3. Age of mother, G__P__ at ____ weeks
4. Gender, cord vessel number, weight, Apgar scores, cord pH of baby (if obtained)
5. Anesthesia type
6. Estimated blood loss. The average blood loss at cesarean delivery is 1000 ml.[37]
7. Tubes/drains
8. Complications
9. Surgeons

IV. Complications
A. The Difficult Cesarean Delivery (Abdominal Dystocia)
1. If the abdominal incision is too tight, it may be extended (both skin and fascia) or the rectus muscles may be divided.
2. If the head is deeply engaged, it can be lifted from below (vaginally) by an assistant or grasped with forceps or a vacuum extractor. A vacuum extractor should not be applied over the infant's face.

3. Low transverse or low vertical incisions may be extended vertically to get extra room. Low transverse incisions may be extended in either a "T" (central) or "L" (lateral) fashion. If the vertical extension reaches into the active segment of the uterus, the patient should not try labor in a subsequent pregnancy because of the risk of uterine rupture.

B. Cesarean Delivery Complicated by Chorioamnionitis

1. Chorioamnionitis affects up to 10% of pregnancies.

2. Infectious complications are increased when patients with chorioamnionitis undergo cesarean delivery.

3. A randomized controlled trial of chorioamnionitis patients undergoing cesarean delivery found that continuing antibiotics postoperatively did not show any benefit in reducing endometritis over treatment with ampicillin during labor and a single dose of clindamycin and gentamycin preoperatively.[36]

C. Uterine Hemorrhage

Uterine hemorrhage may be treated with a variety of techniques. Significant intraoperative blood loss should be treated in a timely fashion with blood products and/or autotransfusion (by cell saver) if available.

1. Administer oxytocin, 5 to 20 units intravenously, intramuscularly, or directly into the uterus for atony.

2. Administer Methergine, 0.2 mg intramuscularly for atony.

3. Prostaglandin $F_{2\alpha}$ (Hemabate) may be given intramuscularly or into the myometrium in doses of 0.25 mg every 30–60 minutes to a maximum dose of 2.0 mg for atony.

4. The lower uterine segment may be tourniquetted by tying a latex or rubber urinary-type catheter around it. This can buy time for uterine artery ligation or hysterectomy or while help is being summoned.

5. Directly suture bleeding points.

6. Ligate the uterine artery by placing sutures in the lateral aspect of the uterus.

7. Ligate the uterine arteries medial to the ovaries.

8. Place interrupted circular sutures parallel to the uterine incision anteriorly and completely through the wall of the uterus posteriorly.[10]

9. Proceed with hypogastric artery ligation.

10. Inflate a Foley catheter balloon (30 ml) in the lower uterine segment with the rest of the catheter protruding out the vagina and apply moderate traction.

11. Selective arterial embolization may be used but is often not timely or feasible.

12. Hysterectomy is often the procedure of last resort.

D. Bladder Injury

Bladder injury usually occurs during repeat cesarean delivery and is due to adhesions.[38]

1. Superficial or partial thickness injuries can be repaired with a single layer of 3-0 absorbable suture.

2. Larger injuries should be repaired in two layers with 2-0 or 3-0 absorbable suture.

3. Bladder repair integrity can be tested by inflating the bladder with sterile milk (infant formula), which, unlike methylene blue or indigo carmine, does not stain tissues.

4. Bladder drainage with a Foley catheter for 1–5 days is indicated for larger injuries.

E. Bowel Injury

Bowel injury is rare. Previous surgery or pelvic infection with adhesion formation are predisposing factors.[38]

1. Simple serosal tears can be oversewn with 3-0 or 4-0 absorbable suture.

2. Enterotomy should be repaired in two layers.

3. The suture line should be placed at a right angle to the bowel long axis to avoid narrowing the bowel lumen and creating stenosis.

4. Extensive bowel injury should be repaired by end-to-end anastomosis.

5. Any defects in the mesentery should be closed to avoid internal hernias.

6. After bowel repair, patients must be observed for return of bowel motility and for infection.

F. Criteria for Postoperative Blood Replacement

Young, stable, otherwise healthy patients can tolerate a very low hematocrit level if blood volume is maintained with crystalloid. Blood replacement should be based on symptoms rather than laboratory data.

G. Postoperative Fever[23]

1. The differential diagnosis includes the following:
   a. Endomyometritis
   b. Urinary tract infection
   c. Respiratory infection
   d. Pulmonary atelectasis
   e. Wound infection
   f. Septic pelvic thrombophlebitis

2. The work-up includes the following:
   a. Perform a general physical examination with particular attention to the wound, the uterus and lochia, and the lungs, particularly in smokers.
   b. Obtain a complete blood count, urinalysis and urine culture, culture of uterine cavity obtained during a sterile speculum examination, and culture of wound drainage.
   c. Order a chest x-ray if there are abnormal lung findings on physical examination.
   d. Open the wound if signs of wound infection are present.
   e. Consider blood cultures.

3. Treatment

This includes broad-spectrum antibiotic therapy to cover both aerobic and anaerobic organisms while cultures are pending. A synthetic penicillin and an aminoglycoside, or a second- or third-generation cephalosporin are acceptable initial choices. Lack of defervescence after initiation of antibiotics should prompt suspicion of septic pelvic thrombophlebitis. Treatment consists of a trial of anticoagulation with heparin, which usually produces defervescence in 48–72 hours. Anticoagulation is not usually necessary beyond 7–10 days.

H. Pulmonary Embolus

This diagnosis should be considered as in any other postoperative patient with chest pain, respiratory distress, or other suggestive symptoms.

I. Spinal Headaches

Headaches following spinal anesthesia or a "wet" epidural anesthetic (in which the dura was punctured) can usually be dramatically alleviated by injecting 10 ml of the patient's own blood into the epidural space close to the original puncture site (epidural blood patch).

V. Postoperative Care and Patient Counseling

A. General Principles of Postoperative Care and Order-Writing

1. As with all orders, strive for clarity and simplicity.

2. Avoid nonstandard abbreviations.

3. When possible, specify start and stop times for medications, particularly antibiotics.

4. Each patient's postoperative course is unique; avoid automatic changes in care items that must be individualized, such as diet.

5. Remember that anyone whose abdomen has been opened is likely to have a period of ileus and therefore will not tolerate solid foods or oral medications for a variable period of time.

6. There is no substitute for frequent hands-on patient reevaluation by a consistent observer.

B. Typical Initial Postoperative Orders

Always record date and time of postoperative orders.

1. Vital signs are obtained every 15 minutes until stable, every 30 minutes until anesthesia wears off, and then every 4 hours after the patient is returned to her room.

2. Nothing by mouth (NPO) is ordered until anesthesia has worn off and the patient is not nauseated; then offer clear liquids. Do not advance diet except with specific orders.

3. The patient should sit up at bedside and dangle legs as soon as anesthesia has worn off.

4. Intravenous fluids: D5/0.45 normal saline at 125 ml per hour continuously

5. Add 10 units of oxytocin to first 1000 ml of intravenous fluids and reassess need for continuation.

6. Hematocrit on the morning of (specify date, usually first postoperative day)

7. Foley catheter to closed drainage

8. Reinforce dressing with dry gauze as needed. Call physician if dressing becomes saturated or wound becomes swollen.

9. Antibiotics (if used other than perioperative dose)

10. If patient is a smoker, consider incentive inspirometer and nicotine patch.

11. Call physician if patient develops a fever over 100.4°F, increasing uterine tenderness, or foul-smelling lochia.

12. Record number and degree of saturation of perineal pads.

13. If vaginal flow is excessive, give 5 units of oxytocin by intravenous push and call physician.

14. Pain medication options include:
   a. If patient had intraspinal narcotics administered at the time of surgery, there may be no need for additional pain medication during the first 24 hours postoperatively.
   b. Patient-controlled analgesia pump (usually specified by additional institutional protocol)
   c. Meperidine, 50–75 mg, with hydroxyzine, 50 mg intramuscularly, every 3 to 4 hours as needed
   d. Avoid writing orders for oral medications immediately after surgery because the patient may get them and get nauseated. Write oral pain medication orders when the patient can tolerate them on subsequent postoperative days.

15. Antiemetic options include:
   a. Promethazine, 50 mg intramuscularly, every 4 hours as needed
   b. Prochlorperazine, 10 mg intramuscularly, every 4 hours as needed
   c. Trimethobenzamide, 250 mg intramuscularly, every 4 hours as needed
   d. Ondansetron, 4 mg intravenously or intramuscularly

16. Indicate if work-up for Rh_o (D) immune globulin is to be done or not.

17. Review prenatal laboratory data to see if hepatitis prophylaxis is needed for baby.

18. Specify that this is a family practice patient and indicate the phone number to be called if there are questions or problems.

C. Immediate Postoperative Patient Counseling
1. Offer a simple statement of condition of her baby and herself.
2. Inform her of where her baby and family are and when she will be able to see them.
3. Explain that the usual postoperative length of hospital stay is about 3 days barring any complications.
4. Tell her how to get pain medication (call button or use patient-controlled analgesia).
5. Tell her that her uterus will cramp and that nurses will be massaging her uterine fundus.
6. Offer to try to answer any additional questions, particularly a review of the circumstances leading to the cesarean delivery if it was not planned.

D. Considerations on First Postoperative Day
1. Review nurse's notes and graphic chart.
2. Ask patient how she feels; acknowledge her incisional pain and uterine cramps.
3. Ask if her pain medication is adequate.
4. Review the items listed previously as "immediate postoperative counseling."
5. Listen to patient's chest and abdomen and remove dressing to inspect incision. If necessary, reapply only a light dressing.
6. Review results of postpartum hematocrit if available and compare to preoperative value.
7. Encourage patient to ambulate and warn her of postural hypotension.
8. Typical orders include the following:
   a. Discontinue Foley catheter.
   b. Ambulate at least once during each day and evening shift.
   c. May shower and wash hair with help.
   d. Advance diet by specific order if bowel sounds were heard and patient is hungry. *Avoid writing: "Diet as tolerated."*
   e. If GI motility has returned, stop parenteral medications and change to oral.
   f. Consider a decrease in intravenous fluids or convert to a heparin lock if the patient has been taking oral fluids well.
   g. Follow up on work-up of need for Rho (D) immune globulin if it was ordered.
9. If patient is nursing, ask how nursing is progressing and order lactation consultant if needed.
10. Consider ordering rooming-in if mother desires and is capable.
11. Consider performing a newborn examination in the presence of parents; if necessary, arrange to return to do that when father can be present.
12. Assess the progress of maternal-infant bonding.
13. Assess if social services will be needed, particularly for single mothers or if the patient seems vague about where she will live, lacks support people, or does not have baby clothes and accessories already assembled.
14. Remind her that an infant car seat is needed prior to discharge.
15. Instruct patient in how to hug a pillow to splint abdomen during coughing.

E. Considerations on Second Postoperative Day
1. Repeat items 1 through 6 as on the first day.
2. Advance diet by specific order based on physical findings and return of GI motility.
3. Change to oral pain medication if not done the previous day. Reserve intramuscular medication as an option for bedtime, if needed.

4. Make sure that if prophylactic antibiotics were ordered, they are being stopped on schedule.

5. For constipation, consider 30 ml of milk of magnesia.

6. For "gas pains," consider ambulation or a return flow enema.

7. Repeat items 9 through 15 as on the first day.

F. **Considerations on Subsequent Postoperative Days**

1. Repeat items 1 through 6 and 9 through 13 as on the first day.

2. Arrange feeding, bathing, cord care, circumcision care, and breast care demonstrations.

3. For non-nursing mothers, discuss breast binding and ice packs.

4. Discuss birth control.

5. Restart prenatal vitamins for nursing mothers.

6. Start iron if needed.

7. Administer rubella vaccine if indicated

G. **Considerations Prior to Discharge**

1. The mother should be able to eat, ambulate, urinate, and have her pain controlled by oral medications prior to discharge.

2. Baby care and self-care teaching should have been completed.

3. Birth control and resumption of intercourse should be discussed.

4. Discuss expectations for vaginal bleeding.

5. Write instructions or prescriptions for pain medication, iron, and vitamins if applicable.

6. If patient has a stapled transverse wound, consider removing staples by the third or fourth day and applying tape reinforcing strips. If the wound was closed using subcuticular sutures, consider applying fresh tape. In either case, tell her what bathing is permitted, that powder can help itching and ingrown hairs, that a light dressing is helpful to prevent rubbing on clothes, and that a thick scar will normally develop as healing progresses, then smooth out over subsequent months.

7. Answer questions about lifting and exercise. Patients with Pfannenstiel incisions should have their exercise dictated by their comfort. For vertical skin incisions, avoid lifting anything heavier than the baby until the 6-week follow-up. Kegel exercises, single leg lifts, and "cat and cow" pelvic tilt back exercise can start as soon as comfort permits.

8. Consider a dietary consult for overweight or underweight patients and those who are nursing for the first time.

9. Make specific appointments in writing for mother and baby at 1–2 weeks postpartum and 6–8 weeks postpartum. Mothers who go home very soon (second or third postoperative day) should be seen sooner (at 5–7 days postoperatively for wound checks or removal of staples from vertical incisions and to answer questions about self- and infant care). Telephone follow-up may suffice in some systems.

10. Discuss the importance of well-child visits and immunizations.

11. Direct mother to community services, including Women, Infants, and Children (WIC), for assistance with nutritional services if indicated.

12. Baby car seat is needed.

H. **Considerations at the First Outpatient Visit**

1. Review reasons for the cesarean delivery and how mother feels about having had the surgery rather than a vaginal delivery.

2. Answer specific questions.

3. Discuss the possibility of a future trial of labor.

4. Examine incision. Confirm that the thickening under the incision is a normal process that indicates healing and that it will smooth out over a few months.

5. Discuss normal postpartum vaginal bleeding.
6. Discuss resumption of intercourse and need for extra lubrication owing to the relative estrogen deficiency normally present postpartum and particularly during lactation.
7. Discuss birth control.
8. Discuss physical activity.
9. Discuss diet.
10. Always allow time for questions about the baby and an examination of the baby.
11. Discuss medications (pain, vitamins, iron, bowel care).
12. Set specific date for next visit.

References

1. Abuhamad A, O'Sullivan MJ: Operative techniques for cesarean section. In Plauche WC, Morrison JC, Sullivan MJ (eds): Surgical Obstetrics. Philadelphia, W.B. Saunders, 1992, pp 417–429.
2. American Heart Association: Advanced Cardiac Life Support 1997–99: Cardiac arrest associated with pregnancy. Dallas, TX, American Heart Association, 1999.
3. Applegate JA, Walhout MF: Cesarean section rate: A comparison between family physicians and obstetricians. Fam Pract Res J 12:255–262, 1992.
4. Ayers JWT, Morley GW: Surgical incision for cesarean section. Obstet Gynecol 70:706-710, 1987.
5. Brocklehurst P: Interventions aimed at decreasing the risk of mother-to-child transmission of HIV infection (Cochrane Review). In The Cochrane Library, Issue 4, 2000. Oxford, Update Software.
6. Byrd JE: Diagnostic criteria and the management of dystocia. J Fam Pract 27:595–599, 1988.
7. Cartwright PS, Pittaway DE, Jones HW, Entman SS: The use of prophylactic antibiotics in obstetrics and gynecology: A review. Obstet Gynecol Surv 39:537–544, 1984.
8. Centers for Disease Control and Prevention. MMWR 42:285–289, 1993.
9. Chez RA: The Misgav Ladach Method of Cesarean Section. Contemp Ob/Gyn June 81–88, 1998.
10. Cho JY, Kim SJ, Cha KY, et al: Interrupted circular suture: Bleeding control during cesarean delivery in placenta previa accreta. Obstet Gynecol 78:876–879, 1991.
11. Dajani A, Bolger A, Taubert K, et al: Prevention of bacterial endocarditis: American Heart Association recommendations. JAMA 277:1794–1801, 1997.
12. Del Valle GO, Combs P, Qualls C, et al: Does closure of camper fascia reduce the incidence of post-cesarean superficial wound disruption? Obstet Gynecol 80:1013–1016, 1992.
13. Deutchman ME, Connor PD: Cesarean Section by Family Physicians: A National Multisite Study of Surgical Outcomes and Training. Presented at the 25th Annual Meeting of the North American Primary Care Research Group Orlando, FL, 1997.
14. Deutchman M, Connor P, Gobbo R, et al: Outcomes of cesarean sections performed by family physicians and the training they received: A 15-year retrospective study. J Am Board Fam Pract 8:81–90, 1995.
15. Deutchman ME, Sills D, Connor PD: Perinatal outcomes: A comparison between family physicians and obstetricians. J Am Board Fam Pract 8:440–447, 1995.
16. Enkin MW: Closed suction wound drainage at cesarean section. In Chalmers I (ed): Oxford Database of Perinatal Trials, Version 1.3. Oxford, Update Software, 1992.
17. Enkin MW, Wilkinson C: Lateral tilt during cesarean section (Cochrane Review). In The Cochrane Library, Issue 4, 2000. Oxford, Update Software.
18. Enkin MW, Wilkinson CS: Peritoneal non-closure cesarean section (Cochrane Review). In The Cochrane Library, Issue 4, 2000. Oxford, Update Software.
19. Enkin MW, Wilkinson C. Single versus two-layer closure of uterine incision at cesarean section (Cochrane Review). In The Cochrane Library, Issue 4, 2000. Oxford, Update Software.
20. Enkin MW, Wilkinson C: Manual removal of placenta at Caesarean section (Cochrane Review). In The Cochrane Library, Issue 4, 2000. Oxford, Update Software.
21. Enkin MW, Wilkinson C. Uterine exteriorization vs. intraperitoneal repair at cesarean section (Cochrane Review). In The Cochrane library, Issue 4, 2000. Oxford: Update Software.
22. Frishman GN, Schwartz T, Hogan JW: Closure of Pfannenstiel skin incisions, staples vs. subcuticular suture. J Reprod Med 42:627–630, 1997.
23. Gabert HA: Complications common to obstetric operative procedures. In Plauche WC, Morrison JC, Sullivan MJ (eds): Surgical Obstetrics. Philadelphia, W.B. Saunders, 1992, pp 65–76.
24. Hopkins L, Smaill F: Antibiotic prophylaxis regimens and drugs for cesarean section. (Cochrane Review). In The Cochrane Library, Issue 4, 2000. Oxford, Update Software.
25. Hueston WJ: Specialty differences in primary cesarean section rates in a rural hospital. Fam Pract Res J 12:245–253, 1992.

26. Iglesias S, Burn R, Saunders LD: Reducing the cesarean section rate in a rural hospital. Can Med Assoc J 145:1459–1463, 1991.
27. Meyers SA, Gliecher N: A successful program to lower cesarean section rate. N Engl J Med 319:1511–1516, 1988.
28. Public Health Service. Healthy People 2000: National Health Promotion and Disease Prevention Objectives. DHHS publication No. (PHS) 91–50212. Washington, DC, U.S. Department of Health and Human Services, Public Health Service, 1991.
29. Riley LE, Greene MF: Elective cesarean delivery to reduce the transmission of HIV (editorial). N Engl J Med 340:1032–1033, 1999.
30. Sanchez-Ramos L, Peterson HB, Martinex-Schnell B, et al: Reducing cesarean sections at a teaching hospital. Am J Obstet Gynecol 163:1081–1088, 1990.
31. Sloan GA: A new upper abdominal incision. Surg Gynecol Obstet 45:678–682, 1927.
32. Smaill F, Hofmeyr GJ: Antibiotic prophylaxis for cesarean section. (Cochrane Review). In The Cochrane Library, Issue 4, 2000. Oxford, Update Software.
33. Spielman FJ, Cefalo RC: Anesthesia for obstetrics. In Plauche WC, Morrison JC, Sullivan MJ (eds): Surgical Obstetrics. Philadelphia, W.B. Saunders, 1992, pp 77–99.
34. The International Perinatal HIV Group: The mode of delivery and the risk of vertical transmission of human immunodeficiency virus type 1. N Engl J Med 340:977–987, 1999.
35. Towers CV, Deveikis AA, Asrat T, et al: A "bloodless cesarean section" and perinatal transmission of the human immunodeficiency virus. Am J Obstet Gynecol 179:708–714, 1998.
36. Turnquest MA, How HY, Cook CR, et al: Chorioamnionitis: Is continuation of antibiotic therapy necessary after cesarean section? Am J Obstet Gynecol 179:1261–1266, 1998.
37. Wilcox CF, Hunt AB, Owen CA: The measurement of blood loss during cesarean section. Am J Obstet Gynecol 77:772–776, 1959.
38. Yasin SY, Walton DL, O'Sullivan MJ: Problems encountered during cesarean delivery. In Plauche WC, Morrison JC, Sullivan MJ (eds): Surgical Obstetrics. Philadelphia, W.B. Saunders, 1992, pp 431–445.

CHAPTER 18

The First Month of Life

Patricia Fontaine, M.D.

SECTION A.
INITIAL MANAGEMENT OF THE
NORMAL NEWBORN

Family physicians have a unique advantage in providing care for infants they deliver. Having already established a relationship with one or both parents, and being well acquainted with maternal prenatal factors that can have significant impact on the newborn's condition, family physicians can provide high-quality medical care for infants while promoting bonding and family adjustment.

I. Care of the Infant at Birth
A. Initial Steps
The infant is delivered into a warm environment and quickly dried. The nose and mouth are suctioned with a bulb syringe. When necessary, further stimulation may be provided by vigorously rubbing the infant's back with a dry towel, or slapping or flicking the infant's feet. Every attempt should be made to respect parents' expressed preferences for their involvement in the delivery, such as having the father cut the umbilical cord or having the baby placed immediately in skin-to-skin contact with the mother. Early breastfeeding is also an option. As long as the infant appears stable and hypothermia is avoided, these activities may be encouraged due to their value in family bonding.
B. Apgar Scoring
1. General use
The Apgar score provides a systematic appraisal of the infant's adaptation to extrauterine life. Five characteristics (heart rate, respiratory effort, tone, reflex response, and color) are scored at 1 minute and 5 minutes of life (Table 1).
2. Apgar scores
Infants with Apgar scores of 7 to 10 are considered normal; a score of 4 to 6 indicates mild to moderate depression; and a score of 0 to 3 indicates severe depression. If the 5-minute score is less than 7, additional scores are noted every 5 minutes, up to 20 minutes. Although the Apgar score has little value in predicting long-term outcomes, a low 1-minute score generally reflects the need for resuscitation and the 5-minute score reflects the effectiveness of resuscitation[19] (see section B, Neonatal Resuscitation).
C. Physical Examination in the Delivery Room
The physician's initial examination in the delivery room should be brief in order to minimize stress on the infant and unnecessary disruption of the family. It should include an ongoing assessment of heart rate, breathing, and color, auscultation of the heart and lungs, and a visual survey for obvious physical abnormalities.

TABLE 1.   Determination of Infant Apgar Score

Sign	0	1	2
Color (Appearance)	Blue, pale	Body pink, extremities blue	Completely pink
Heart rate (Pulse)	Absent	Under 100	Over 100
Reflex response (Grimace)	No response	Grimace	Cough, sneeze, cry
Muscle tone (Activity)	Limp	Slow flexion of extremities	Well flexed
Respiratory Effort	Absent	Weak cry, hypoventilation	Strong cry

1. Assessment of heart rate, breathing, and color
   a. The heart rate should always be over 100 beats per minute and generally stabilizes in the 120–160 range. Irregularities in cardiac rhythm are occasionally present, most often due to premature atrial contractions that are benign and self-limited.[19]
   b. The normal respiratory rate is 30–60 breaths per minute. Moist rales are often present during the first several minutes of life. Rales are not a concern as long as the infant is well suctioned, is not cyanotic, and is not showing signs of respiratory distress such as grunting or retractions.[19]
   c. Acrocyanosis—a blue coloration of the hands and feet—is common in normal newborns, especially in response to a cool environment. Generalized cyanosis and pallor are two signs reflecting inadequate oxygenation or poor peripheral circulation. Generalized cyanosis requires immediate evaluation for significant cardiac or lung abnormalities.[19]
2. Inspection for physical anomalies and evidence of birth injury.
   a. Major anomalies. These are ideally detected during prenatal care, by ultrasound or other studies, so that an appropriate management plan is in place for the delivery.
   b. Common minor deviations. These deviations from normal may be noted for the first time after birth. Features, significance and management of selected abnormalities are described in Table 3.
   c. Birth injury. Injuries may result from unavoidable pressure as the infant passes through the birth canal, or from medical interventions such as the vacuum extractor. Scalp edema (caput succedaneum) and bruising occur commonly over the presenting part. Subperiosteal hemorrhage (cephalhematoma) tends to occur over the fetal parietal bones after passage through a tight maternal pelvis, and may be seen following a prolonged second-stage labor.[21]
   d. Shoulder dystocia. When shoulder dystocia occurs, the infant should be examined for a fractured clavicle or brachial plexus palsy.[21]

D. Disposition

The infant may either room in with the mother or be transferred to a normal newborn nursery, according to parental request and hospital practices. The optimal family-centered program is the rooming-in situation, where mother and infant spend time together with attention from an understanding and helpful nurse and with essentially unrestricted visits from the father, siblings, and other key support persons.[1] Rooming in offers advantages for breastfeeding instruction, as well as potential protective effects against hospital-acquired infections as the infant becomes colonized with maternal microorganisms.

II. Care in the Normal Newborn Nursery
A. Physical Examination

When the initial delivery room assessment is normal, the first complete newborn examination takes place sometime during the first 24 hours of life, after admission routines have been accomplished and the infant's general condition and temperature have stabilized.

1. Estimation of gestational age

The maternal due date often provides a reliable estimate of the infant's gestation, and is used to plot the infant's weight, length, and head circumference against standard growth curves. When maternal dates are uncertain, the infant's physical and neurologic maturity can be assessed using the instrument shown in Figure 1. Infants are classified as small for gestational age (SGA) when weight is less than the 10th percentile for gestational age and large for gestational age (LGA) when weight is greater than the 90th percentile. Associated conditions are listed in Table 2.[19]

2. Physical examination by organ system

The physician reviews the infant's measurements and vital signs (temperature, pulse, respiratory rate) and then examines in the following order:

NEUROMUSCULAR ACTIVITY

	0	1	2	3	4	5
POSTURE						
SQUARE WINDOW	90°	60°	45°	30°	0°	
ARM RECOIL	180°		100°-180°	90°-100°	< 90°	
POPLITEAL ANGLE	180°	160°	130°	110°	90°	< 90°
SCARF SIGN						
HEEL-TO-EAR MANEUVER						

PHYSICAL MATURITY

	0	1	2	3	4	5
SKIN	gelatinous red, transparent	smooth, pink, visible veins	superficial peeling and/or rash, few veins	cracking pale areas, rare veins	parchment, deep cracking no vessels	leathery, cracked, wrinkled
LANUGO	none	abundant	thinning	bald areas	mostly bald	
PLANTAR CREASES	no crease	faint red marks	anterior transverse crease only	creases ant. 2/3	creases cover entire sole	
BREAST	barely percept.	flat areola, no bud	stippled areola, 1–2 mm bud	raised areola, 3–4 mm bud	full areola, 5–10 mm bud	
EAR	pinna flat, stays folded	sl. curved pinna, soft w/slow recoil	well curv. pinna, soft but ready recoil	formed and firm with instant recoil	thick cartilage, ear stiff	
GENITALS	scrotum empty, no rugae		testes descending, few rugae	testes down, good rugae	testes pendulous, deep rugae	
GENITALS	prominent clitoris, and labia minora		majora and minora equally prominent	majora large, minora small	clitoris and minora completely covered	

TOTAL MATURITY RATING	SCORE	5	10	15	20	25	30	35	40	45	50
	WEEKS	26	28	30	32	34	36	38	40	42	44

FIGURE 1. To assess gestational age, rate the neuromuscular activity and physical maturity of the infant. Then combine these ratings to derive the total maturity rating at the bottom of the form. (From Klaus MH, Fanaroff AA: Care of the High-Risk Infant. Philadelphia, W.B. Saunders, 1977, p 47, with permission.)

TABLE 2.   Conditions Associated with SGA and LGA Infants

SGA Infants	LGA Infants
Uteroplacental insufficiency	Genetic
Intrauterine infection (e.g., TORCH)	Maternal diabetes
Maternal hypertension	
Maternal alcohol consumption, smoking, drugs	
Congenital anomalies, trisomies	

    a. Heart and lungs auscultation. These are the initial maneuvers, because they are best accomplished while the infant is quiet.

    b. Examination. Examine the head, eyes, ears, nose, throat, neck, chest, abdomen, genitalia, back, and extremities in head-to-toe order.

    c. Neurologic assessment. Perform neurologic examination including assessment of resting posture, muscle tone, and reflexes. Check for the rooting, suck, and grasp reflexes. Evaluate the traction response (head lag) as the infant is pulled to sitting position, and observe the Moro reflex.

Table 3 summarizes the typical physical findings and minor deviations from normal that can be observed on newborn physical examinations.[14,21]

B. Preventive Health Care Measures for Newborns

Screening tests and treatments routinely administered in the newborn nursery are designed to prevent short- and long-term morbidity. The American Academy of Pediatrics and the American College of Obstetricians and Gynecologists have developed clinical guidelines describing the recommended measures.[1]

    1. Vitamin K prophylaxis against hemorrhagic disease of the newborn (HDN)

        a. Background. Hemorrhagic disease of the newborn is due to deficiency of the vitamin K-dependent clotting factors II, VII, IX, and X. It classically develops in the first week of life, although it may occur early (within the first 24 hours) or late (beyond the first week).[18] Common sites of bleeding include the skin, nose, circumcision site, umbilical cord, and gastrointestinal tract. Cerebral hemorrhage may cause significant morbidity and death.[17] A prolonged protime (or INR) coupled with a normal fibrinogen level and platelet count are typical laboratory findings in the infant with vitamin K deficiency.

        b. High-risk infants

            i. Breastfed infants are at increased risk for HDN compared to those who are formula-fed. Vitamin K is not present in appreciable amounts in breast milk, and the newborn is unable to synthesize the vitamin.[9,19]

           ii. Infants whose mothers take anticonvulsants or warfarin while pregnant or nursing are also at higher risk for vitamin K deficiency and may require supplementation (see Chapter 7, section G).[19]

        c. Dosage for prophylaxis

           i. In the United States, the standard is to administer 0.5–1 mg of vitamin K by the intramuscular route within 1 hour of birth.[1] This has been shown to be an effective strategy for preventing HDN. The risk of an infant developing significant hemorrhage despite one-time IM prophylaxis is extremely low, an estimated 0.25 bleeding incidents for every 100,000 infants treated.[15]

           ii. In other countries, concerns over high vitamin K levels after intramuscular injection and a controversial association with childhood leukemia (subsequently substantially refuted) have prompted investigation into more physiologic oral dosage schedules.[4] One milligram of vitamin K

TABLE 3. Common and Uncommon Deviations from Normal
on Newborn Physical Examinations

Condition	Description	Causes	Evaluation/Treatment
HEENT			
Cephalhematoma	Subperiosteal hemorrhage causing localized swelling, usually over parietal bones	Pressure against fetal skull as it passes through birth canal	Observation; if severe, rule out underlying fracture
Subconjunctival hemorrhage	Red patch in sclera, adjacent to iris	Rupture of small conjunctival capillaries during birth process	Observation; resolves in 7–10 days
Abnormal red reflex; "white pupil"	Ophthalmoscope exam— lack of typical red-yellow reflection from retina	Cataract; neuroblastoma (rare)	Ophthalmologic referral for complete evaluation
Congenital glaucoma	Cornea cloudy, large (> 11 mm)	Congenital	Early recognition and referral for treatment
Nasolacrimal duct obstruction	Eye watering; conjunctivitis may develop secondarily	Developmental; may manifest during first few days to weeks of life	Warm pack, massage; treat conjunctivitis with topical antibiotic; refer for probing if not resolved by 9–12 months
Low-set external ear	Upper attachment of ear (not pinna) falls below a horizontal line determined by the inner and outer canthus of the eye	Renal anomalies (Potter's syndrome); trisomies; other congenital anomalies	Investigate for trisomy, renal anomalies as indicated
Preauricular skin tags	Uni- or bilateral; broad vs. pedunculated base; mainly cosmetic concern	Familial/embryogenic anomaly	Pedunculated tag: ligate tightly at base; sloughs in 1–2 weeks. Broad-based tag, or one containing cartilage; refer to surgeon, consider Goldenhar's syndrome
Cleft lip or palate	Incomplete closure of lip's vermilion border; may also involve nasolabial fold, palate	Multifactorial: genetic, chromosomal, and nongenetic. Cleft lip-palate occurs in 1/1000 births. Cleft palate alone occurs in 1:2500 births.	Multidisciplinary team approach; surgical correction (lip) as early as 1–3 months; feeding assessment important
Gingival retention cysts (epithelial pearls)	"Rice-like" white nodules on gingiva (may be mistaken for teeth)	Keratin-containing cysts lined with squamous epithelium	Observation; anticipate spontaneous resolution
Neck mass	Brachial cleft cyst/sinus; thyroglossal duct cyst; cystic hygroma	Developmental/ embryogenic anomalies	Surgical referral
Chest			
Heart murmur	Characterize quality, intensity, and timing in cardiac cycle.	1. Transitional—change over from fetal to infant circulatory system 2. Functional 3. Pathologic—congenital anomalies	Evaluate infant's overall status. Cyanosis or respiratory distress in the presence of murmur needs urgent evaluation.
Abdomen			
Mass	Palpable mass	50% are of genitourinary origin	Ultrasound exam of urinary tract
Two umbilical vessels (check freshly cut cord section at birth)	Only one umbilical artery present in cord stump	More common in twins; other congenital defects possible (cerebrovascular, gastrointestinal, genitourinary), but low incidence	Perform additional diagnostic tests if other findings also suggest abnormality

(Table continued on next page.)

TABLE 3. Common and Uncommon Deviations from Normal on Newborn Physical Examinations *(Continued)*

Condition	Description	Causes	Evaluation/Treatment
Genitalia			
Vaginal tags/ discharge	Mucosal skin tags protrude from vagina; mucus or blood-tinged discharge in first days of life	Tags: common variant Discharge: probably normal response to maternal hormone withdrawal	Tags: observe; surgical removal rarely needed
Undescended testes	Location of testes: intra-abdominal, in inguinal canal, high scrotal, or ectopic	Etiology unclear Incidence: 3–5% term births, higher for preterm If bilateral cryptor-chidism, consider ambiguous genitalia	Observe for spontaneous descent between 3–6 months; refer for surgical exploration/ orchiopexy at 6–12 months; long-term risk for testicular malignancy, infertility
Hypospadias	Urethral meatus located proximal to tip of glans (base of glans, penile shaft, scrotum)	Developmental anomaly Incidence: 1/500 male births	Avoid circumcision; surgical referral, repair at 6–9 months
Hernia, inguinal	Inguinal swelling or mass; may extend into scrotum; does not transilluminate; may be reducible	Less common in newborn than hydrocoele	Prompt surgical referral due to risk of incarceration
Hydrocoele	Scrotal swelling that transilluminates	Patent processus vaginalis allows fluid accumulation around testes	Observe for resolution over 4–6 months; refer for surgical repair if persists beyond 6–12 months
Extremities, Back			
Clavicle fracture	Infant cries when affected side is examined; de-creased movement of arm on that side	LGA infant, shoulder dystocia. Break often occurs as anterior shoulder is delivered from under maternal pubic symphysis.	Heals spontaneously
Hip dislocation	Head of femur lies outside or is easily displaced from acetabulum. Leg lengths may be unequal, and hip abduction may be limited, with palpable "click"	Multifactorial: genetic pre-disposition to acetabular dysplasia and joint laxity; environmental (breech position). Incidence: 1/1000 births	Early detection important; orthopedic referral
Pilonidal dimple/tract	Pinpoint invagination of skin over caudal portion of spinal column	May be associated with spina bifida occulta, nonfusion of posterior arches of spine. Patch of abnormal hair, lipoma or hemangioma may also mark spina bifida occulta	Perform neurologic examination; neurosur-gical referral if deficits present
Skin			
Salmon patch or "Stork's beak mark"	Light red, irregularly shaped macule found on the upper eyelids, glabella, or occiput	Superficial capillary malformation, extremely common among light-skinned newborns	Facial lesions fade over months, occipital lesions may persist into adulthood
Port wine stain or "nevus flammeus"	Dark red or purplish macule that does not blanch to pressure	Capillary malformation. On the face, suggests Sturge-Weber syndrome; on extremity, Klippel-Trenaunay syndrome	Refer to dermatologist for pulsed dye laser treat-ment. Evaluate for underlying syndromes as appropriate.

(Table continued on next page.)

TABLE 3. Common and Uncommon Deviations from Normal
on Newborn Physical Examinations *(Continued)*

Condition	Description	Causes	Evaluation/Treatment
Skin *(cont.)*			
Hemangioma	Red, rough-surfaced nodule	Benign tumor of capillary endothelial cells	Expect lesion to enlarge initially, then involute; 50% are gone by age 5, 70% by age 7, 90% by age 9.
Milia	Pinpoint-sized white papules scattered over the nose, cheeks, and forehead	Sebaceous retention cysts; present in up to 40% of newborns	Expect spontaneous rupture and disappearance within a few weeks
Erythema toxicum	Blotchy erythematous macules; may develop urticarial centers. Size varies from a few mm to 2–3 cm. Appears on trunk or extremities during the first days of life.	Etiology not known. Smears of lesions show eosinophils. More common in term infants; in preterm, seek other etiologies for rash.	Expect spontaneous resolution within 7–10 days.

administered as a single oral dose on the first day of life prevents clotting deficiencies in the first week. However, the single dose is not effective against late-onset hemorrhagic disease.[22] Repeated doses may confer additional benefit, and additional studies are needed to determine the optimal dosing schedule.[10] There is currently no oral preparation of vitamin K licensed for use in newborns in the United States.[1]

2. Prophylaxis against ophthalmia neonatorum
   a. Background. *Ophthalmia neonatorum*, or conjunctivitis of the newborn, refers to the presence of conjunctival inflammation and discharge in an infant less than 1 month old.[11,16] In the United States, the most common cause of newborn conjunctivitis is *Chlamydia trachomatis*, with an incidence of 8 per 1000 live births. Gonococcal ophthalmia neonatorum is less common (0.3 cases per 1000 live births) but is significant because of its potential to result in corneal scarring and blindness if left untreated.[11,16] Without prophylaxis, ophthalmia will develop in approximately one-third of infants exposed to chlamydia and 30–50% exposed to gonococci.[12]
   b. Routine prophylaxis. In the United States, federal law mandates prophylaxis against ophthalmia neonatorum. The most common agents used for prophylaxis are 1% silver nitrate solution (single-dose wax ampules), 0.5% erythromycin ointment, and 1% tetracycline ointment (single-dose tubes).[16] All three treatments are effective in preventing gonococcal ophthalmia,[11,16] but none reliably reduce the incidence of conjunctivitis due to chlamydia.[8]
   c. Timing. Topical prophylaxis is most effective when the solution or ointment is instilled into the infant's inferior conjunctival sacs as soon as possible after birth. However, a delay of 1 hour may be acceptable to facilitate maternal/infant bonding.[1,3]
   d. Prophylaxis for infants exposed to active maternal infections. In addition to receiving ocular prophylaxis with the topical agents listed above, infants born to mothers with active gonococcal disease should receive a single intramuscular or intravenous dose of ceftriaxone (25–50 mg/kg, maximum dose 125 mg). Because no topical agent has been shown to prevent exposed infants from developing nasopharyngeal colonization with chlamydia, infants born to mothers with untreated chlamydial infections

should be treated with oral erythromycin (30 mg/kg/d in divided doses every 8–12 hours for 14 days).[19]

3. Immunization against hepatitis B virus

    a. Background. Reducing perinatal hepatitis B virus (HBV) transmission by immunizing newborns is part of a comprehensive strategy to prevent HBV infection in the United States.[2,5] The risk of perinatal HBV transmission when the mother is hepatitis B surface antigen (HbsAg)-positive ranges from 10–85%. Ninety percent of infants thus infected go on to become chronic carriers of HBV, and up to 25% die in adulthood of HBV-associated liver disease, including cirrhosis and hepatocellular carcinoma. Appropriate immunization has been shown to decrease perinatal transmission and to reduce the number of chronic carriers by 90%. Because the acute and chronic consequences of HBV infections are major health concerns, and because strategies that rely on vaccinating only high-risk groups have not been successful, universal HBV immunization is recommended for all infants born in the United States.[1,2,5]

    b. Hepatitis B immune globulin (HBIG). HBIG is administered to infants of HBsAg-positive mothers to provide passive immunity until the hepatitis B vaccine series is completed. It is prepared from human plasma known to contain a high titer of antibody against HbsAg. The plasma is screened for antibodies to HIV and prepared by a process that would inactivate the HIV virus if present.[5]

    c. Hepatitis B vaccine (Hep B). Hepatitis B vaccines are produced by recombinant DNA technology. A series of three immunizations are required to induce immunity. Until 1999, all hepatitis B vaccines contained mercury, as a component of the preservative thimerosal. Because of the potential for mercury toxicity with repeated doses of childhood vaccines, preservative-free preparations are now preferred (Recombivax HB, Merck & Co., Inc., West Point, PA or Engerix-B, SmithKline Beecham Biologicals, Philadelphia, PA).[6]

    d. Administration and dosage schedule[7]

        i. Infants born to HBsAg-positive mothers should receive HBIG and Hep B injected simultaneously but at different sites within 12 hours of birth.

        ii. If the mother's hepatitis B status is unknown at the time of delivery, the infant should receive Hep B within 12 hours of birth. Maternal blood should be drawn to check her HbsAg status. If the mother tests HbsAg-positive, the infant should receive HBIG as soon as possible, within the first week of life.

        iii. For infants whose mothers are HBsAg-negative, only the hepatitis B vaccine is required. It is acceptable to use thimerosal-free Hep B within 12 hours of birth; however, the first dose of Hep B may be given any time until age 2 months. The second dose is given at least 1 month after the first dose, generally at 1–2 months of age. The third dose is given at least 4 months after the second dose, often at age 6 months, but it may be as late as age 18 months.

        iv. Table 4 summarizes specific dosage recommendations for hepatitis B vaccination in newborns.

        v. Adverse effects of hepatitis B vaccine in infants appear to be minimal.

C. Screening Tests

    1. Newborn screening tests

Hospitals may be governed by state laws requiring newborn screening for inborn errors of metabolism and other medical conditions.[13] Examples include

TABLE 4.   Hepatitis B Vaccination Recommendations for Newborns

Maternal HBsAg status	Initial Vaccine Doses and Timing			
	Hepatitis B immune globulin*	Recombivax HB[†] vaccine mg (ml)	Engerix-B[†] vaccine mg (ml)	Timing
HBsAg-negative	Not given	2.5 (0.25) or	10 (0.5)	Vaccine[†] Two alternatives: • At birth • Age 1–2 months
HBsAg-positive	0.5 ml	5.0 (0.5) or	10 (0.5)	HBIG and vaccine[†] within 12 hours of birth
HBsAg unknown (draw mother's blood for HBsAg when admitted in labor)	0.5 ml (if HBsAg-positive)	5.0 (0.5) or	10 (0.5)	HBIG: as soon as mother is found to be HBsAg-positive; not later than 1 week after birth Vaccine[†] within 12 hours of birth

* Hepatitis B immune globulin (HBIG) is prepared from human plasma known to contain a high titer of antibody against HBsAg. Both screening and processing ensure elimination of human immunodeficiency virus (HIV) from HBIG.
† Recombivax HB (Merck, Sharp & Dohme) and Engerix-B (SmithKline Beecham Biologicals) are the two vaccine preparations licensed for use in the United States. Both are produced by recombinant DNA techniques.
‡ Two additional doses of hepatitis B vaccine are necessary to complete the series.

phenylketonuria, galactosemia, hypothyroidism, and hemoglobinopathies. The family physician should make sure that results of tests performed in the newborn nursery are documented on the infant's outpatient medical record after discharge, and that appropriate follow-up is arranged for any abnormal results.

2. Hearing screening
   a. Prevalence. The prevalence of congenital hearing loss is 2 to 3 per 1000 live births.[20] Infants at risk for hearing loss include those with a family history of hereditary sensorineural hearing loss; a history of cytomegalovirus, rubella, syphilis, herpes, or toxoplasmosis infection in utero; craniofacial anomalies, including morphologic abnormalities of the pinnae and ear canals; ototoxic medications, including aminoglycosides used in multiple courses or in combination with loop diuretics; birth weight less than 1500 g; mechanical ventilation lasting 5 days or longer; and bacterial meningitis.[1]
   b. Early identification. The rationale for early identification of hearing loss is to allow interventions that will optimize the infant's development and acquisition of language skills.[1,20] A national public health goal outlined in *Healthy People 2010* is to "increase the proportion of newborns who are screened for hearing loss by age 1 month, have audiologic evaluation by age 3 months, and are enrolled in appropriate intervention by age 6 months."[20] As of 1999, twenty U.S. states require hearing screening for all newborns before hospital discharge.[20]

References

1. American Academy of Pediatrics and American College of Obstetricians and Gynecologists: Guidelines for Perinatal Care, 4th ed. 1997, pp 152–162.
2. American Academy of Pediatrics, Committee on Infectious Diseases: Universal hepatitis B immunization. Pediatrics 89:795–800,1992.
3. Bausch LC: Newborn eye prophylaxis—where are we now? Nebr Med J 78:383–384,1993.

4. Brousson MA, Klein MC: Controversies surrounding the administration of vitamin K to newborns: A review. CMAJ 154:307–315, 1996.
5. CDC: Hepatitis B virus: A comprehensive strategy for eliminating transmission in the United States through universal childhood vaccination. Recommendations of the Immunization Practices Advisory Committee (ACIP). MMWR 40:1–25, 1991.
6. CDC: Recommendations regarding the use of vaccines that contain thimerosal as a preservative. MMWR 48:996–998, 1999.
7. CDC: Recommended childhood immunization schedule—United States, 2000. MMWR 49:35–38, 2000.
8. Chen JY: Prophylaxis of ophthalmia neonatorum: Comparison of silver nitrate, tetracycline, erythromycin and no prophylaxis. Pediatr Infect Dis J 11:1026–1030, 1992.
9. Cornelissen EM, Kollee LA, De Abreu RA, et al: Prevention of vitamin K deficiency in infancy by weekly administration of vitamin K. Acta Paediatr 82:656–659, 1993.
10. Cornelissen M, von Kries R, Loughnan P, et al: Prevention of vitamin K deficiency bleeding: efficacy of different multiple oral dose schedules of vitamin K. Eur J Pediatr 156:126–130, 1997.
11. De Toledo AR, Chandler JW: Conjunctivitis of the newborn. Infect Dis Clin North Am 6:807–813, 1992.
12. Foster A, Klauss V: Ophthalmia neonatorum in developing countries. N Engl J Med 332:600–601,1995.
13. Laws of Minnesota for 1994. Chapter 636, Article 2, Section 2.
14. Lewan RB, Sander RW, Ambuel B, et al: Problems of the newborn and infant. In Taylor RB (ed): Family Medicine Principles and Practice, 5th ed. New York, Springer-Verlag, 1998, pp 146–162.
15. McMillan DD: Administration of vitamin K to newborns: Implications and recommendations. CMAJ 154:347–349, 1996.
16. O'Hara MA: Ophthalmia neonatorum. Pediatr Rev 40:715–725, 1993.
17. Rutty GN, Smith CM, Malia RG: Late-form hemorrhagic disease of the newborn: A fatal case report with illustration of investigations that may assist in avoiding the mistaken diagnosis of child abuse. Am J Forensic Med Pathol 20:48–51, 1999.
18. Sutor AH, von Kries R, Cornelissen EA, et al: Vitamin K deficiency bleeding (VKDB) in infancy. ISTH Pediatric/Perinatal Subcommittee. International Society on Thrombosis and Haemostasis. Thromb Haemost 81:456–461, 1999.
19. Thilo EH, Rosenberg AA: The newborn infant. In Hay WW, Hayward AR, Levin MJ, Sondheimer JM (eds): Current Pediatric Diagnosis and Treatment, 14th ed. New York, NY, Appleton & Lange, 1999, pp 19–28.
20. U.S. Department of Health and Human Services. Healthy People 2010: Understanding and improving health. January 2000. http://www.health.gov/healthypeople/default.htm.
21. Variations and Minor Departures in Infants. Evansville, IN, Mead Johnson, 1978, pp 1–48.
22. Zipursky A: Prevention of vitamin K deficiency bleeding in newborns. Br J Haematol 104:430–437, 1999.

SECTION B.
NEONATAL RESUSCITATION

Patricia Adam, M.D., M.S.P.H., and Patricia Fontaine, M.D.

I. Preparation for Resuscitation

Even under the best of circumstances, instruments for scoring ante- and intrapartum risk will not identify all infants at risk for adverse outcomes.[14] Family physicians who practice obstetrics should acquire and maintain skills in neonatal resuscitation so they can respond with confidence when called upon to attend to an infant in unanticipated distress.

A. Anticipation

Anticipate the need for resuscitation in high-risk situations. See Table 5 for obstetric events associated with adverse newborn outcomes.

B. Assemble Team

Have one to two additional people present whose sole responsibility is the newborn. These individuals should be skilled or certified in neonatal resuscitation. The first person should be trained in all aspects of resuscitation, including endotracheal intubation and administration of medications. The second person is needed if the resuscitation becomes complicated; he or she should be able to assist with tactile stimulation, suctioning, bag and mask ventilation, or chest compressions.[1,18]

C. Equipment

Assemble and check necessary equipment (see Table 6).

TABLE 5.   Anticipating a Depressed Infant: High-Risk Conditions[3]

Maternal disease (e.g., diabetes, hypertension, preeclampsia, substance abuse)	Abnormal presentation
	Fetal distress
Prematurity (< 36 weeks)	Persistent bradycardia (< 120 beats/minute)
Premature or prolonged rupture of membranes	Persistent tachycardia (> 160 beats/minute)
Prolonged second stage of labor	Severe variable or late decelerations
Meconium in amniotic fluid	Loss of beat-to-beat variability

II. Resuscitation of the Depressed Infant
A. Pathophysiology of Neonatal Asphyxia

It is essential that the physician resuscitating the neonate be familiar with the pathophysiology of neonatal asphyxia and the concepts of primary and secondary apnea. Primary apnea develops in response to hypoxemic stress, which can occur in utero or peripartum. The neonate experiencing primary apnea demonstrates gasping or absent breathing and a mild decrease in heart rate and tone. Primary apnea can be reversed simply with tactile stimulation and oxygen. Secondary apnea occurs if hypoxia continues, or if there is no resuscitative effort. It is characterized by absent or gasping respirations, along with a more profound decrease in PaO_2, blood pressure and heart rate. Only aggressive ventilatory resuscitation will reverse this more severe neonatal depression.

Because it is impossible to determine by clinical appearance whether the depressed newborn is in primary or secondary apnea, all infants with absent or gasping respirations should be assumed to be in secondary apnea and in need of aggressive resuscitation.[1]

TABLE 6.   Preparation of Delivery Room Equipment

Procedure	Equipment	Preparation
Thermal protection	Radiant warmer Towel/blanket	Preheat warmer Warm towel/blanket

Clearing airway	Bulb syringe
	Mechanical suction
	Suction catheters:
	  5 or 6, 8, and 10 French
	For meconium infants:
	  Laryngoscope
	    (#0 and 1 straight blade)
	  Endotracheal tubes
	    (2.5, 3.0, 3.5, 4.0 mm)
	  Stylet
	  Endotracheal tube suction adapter
		Set pressure to 100 mm Hg
		
		Attach appropriate-size blade
		  and check light

Positive-pressure ventilation	Oxygen tubing/flowmeter Resuscitation bag Mask Feeding tube, 8 French 20-ml syringe Endotracheal tube Stethoscope	Attach to bag; set at 5 L flow Check for function Select appropriate size On hand for gastric suction
Medications	Epinephrine 1:10,000 Sodium bicarbonate 0.5 mEq/ml Naloxone Volume expander Syringes and needles	Keep dosage card with medications
Universal precautions	Gloves	

B. Neonatal Resuscitation

This consists of a disciplined series of well-ordered steps in which evaluation of the infant's respiratory effort, heart rate, and peripheral perfusion leads to decisions regarding appropriate actions. The guidelines reviewed here have been established by the American Heart Association and endorsed by the American Academy of Pediatrics.[1] Many of these guidelines are only now being tested in rigorous controlled trials.[18]

1. Initial steps
   a. Warm, dry, suction, and stimulate the infant during the first 30 seconds after delivery. For normal newborns, this can be accomplished at the foot of the bed.
   b. If necessary, place the infant, head toward you, under a preheated radiant warmer.
   c. Position the infant's head so the airway is open. Suction the mouth and then the nose with a bulb syringe, removing mucus and amniotic fluid. A suction catheter attached to mechanical suction set at 100 mm Hg may also be used.
   d. Dry the infant with a warm towel, stimulating with vigorous strokes over the back. Remove the wet towel. Newborns lose body heat rapidly from wet skin, particularly given their large surface area to body mass ratio. Cold stress must be avoided because it causes peripheral vasoconstriction and exacerbates metabolic acidosis.[1]
2. Rapid assessment
   a. Simultaneously assess, with the initial steps described above, the infant's breathing, heart rate, and color to guide further management. A useful protocol is given in Figure 2.
   b. Positive-pressure ventilation should be instituted immediately for an infant with heart rate below 100 beats per minute or with gasping or absent respiratory effort. The longer it takes to restore spontaneous heart rate and breathing, the greater the likelihood of anoxic cerebral insult.[1]

C. Bag and Mask Ventilation

This simple and effective means of delivering positive-pressure ventilation with 100% oxygen restores respiration in most moderately depressed newborns (Apgar score of 4–6).[1]

1. Indications
   a. Heart rate less than 100 beats per minute
   b. Absent or gasping respirations
2. Equipment
   a. Self-inflating bags. Bags such as Hope II or neonatal Laerdal are most commonly used. Check for connection to oxygen supply, oxygen reservoir (needed in order to deliver 100% oxygen to patient), and pressure relief or pop-off valve. The pop-off valve prevents pressures over 30–40 cm H_2O from being delivered to the infant, a precaution against pneumothorax.
   b. Masks. These should have cushioned rims for adapting to the contours of the face. Sizes are available for infants from 500 to 4500 g. Proper fit is achieved when the infant's nose and mouth, but not eyes, are covered by the mask.
3. Technique
   a. Position the infant with the neck slightly extended to open the airway in the "sniffing" position.
   b. Place the mask on the face to obtain a seal while avoiding pressure over the eyes or larynx.

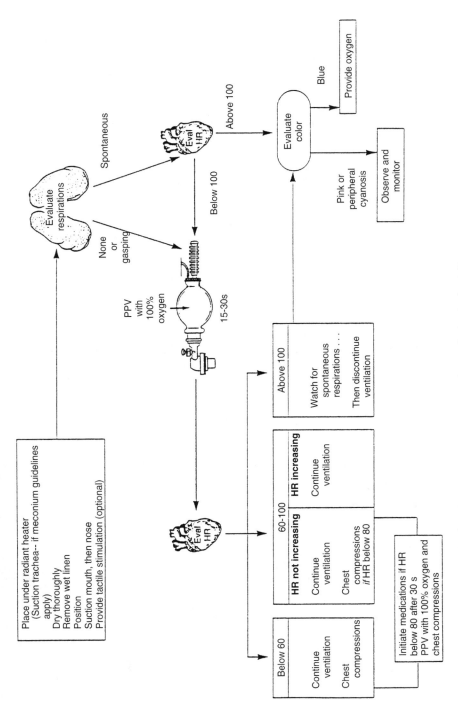

FIGURE 2. Overview of resuscitation in the delivery room.

  c. Ventilate by compressing the bag enough to achieve visible, easy rise of the infant's chest. Remember that the first breath requires more pressure than subsequent breaths. If there is difficulty getting the infant's chest to rise, check for air leak around the mask from improper size or positioning, airway blocked by excessive secretions, or equipment malfunction, such as a pop-off valve stuck in the open position.

  d. Continue to ventilate 40–60 times per minute. (The addition of chest compressions decreases the amount of time available for ventilations, so the rate drops to 30 times per minute.)

  e. If bag and mask ventilation is needed for more than a few minutes, insert an orogastric tube to evacuate air that accumulates in the stomach, which could potentially compromise diaphragmatic excursion.

  f. Discontinue ventilation when central cyanosis has resolved, the heart rate is greater than 100 beats per minute, and spontaneous respirations have returned.

D. Chest Compressions

Chest compressions are required for severe depression, equivalent to an Apgar score of 0–3. This step should be instituted only after ventilation has been established, because chest compression in the absence of ventilation is of little if any value.[1]

 1. Indications

  a. Heart rate less than 60 beats per minute

  b. Heart rate of 60–80 beats per minute and not increasing.

 2. Technique

  a. Hand position. Both hands encircle the infant's chest, with the two thumbs placed over the sternum below the nipple line and above the xiphoid process. Alternatively, the index and middle fingers of one hand can perform compressions in the same location.

  b. Technique. The sternum should be depressed one half to three quarters of an inch at a rate of 90 compressions per minute.

  c. Use of bag and mask. Bag and mask ventilation at 30 breaths per minute should accompany the compressions in a 3-to-1 ratio.

  d. Chest compressions. Chest compressions may be discontinued when the heart rate is over 80 beats per minute and increasing. There should be evidence of improved circulation, such as good femoral pulses, improved capillary filling, and return to normal pink color.

E. Endotracheal Intubation

Endotracheal intubation requires more skill than bag and mask ventilation, but it does offer more control over ventilation and eliminates the concern that air will enter the infant's stomach.[1]

 1. Indications

  a. Ineffective or prolonged bag and mask ventilation

  b. Tracheal suctioning for the infant born through amniotic fluid with meconium

  c. Anticipated need for longer-term ventilation (e.g., birth weight 1250–1500 g, gestational age below 30–31 weeks)

  d. An infant with a known diaphragmatic hernia.

 2. Personnel and equipment

  a. Two people are needed—one to intubate and ventilate, and one to assist in managing equipment and confirming proper tube placement by listening to the infant's lungs.

  b. A laryngoscope with a straight blade, size 0 or 1, should be tested and in good working order. A spare light bulb should always be available.

    c. Endotracheal tubes (2.0 mm to 4.0 mm in internal diameter) should be available. A 3.5- or 4.0-mm tube works well for most infants over 38 weeks or 3000 g. Stylets are often used to stiffen the tube. The stylet must be secured so that its tip does not extend beyond the tube itself.

    d. A suction catheter of appropriate caliber for the endotracheal tube should be available. The catheter is connected to mechanical suction set at a maximum of 100 mmHg.

3. Technique

    a. Position the infant with the head slightly extended to open the airway. A small towel roll behind the infant's shoulders may be helpful. Hyperextension moves the trachea forward and makes landmarks difficult to visualize.

    b. With the laryngoscope in the left hand (for both left- and right-handed individuals), advance the blade carefully over the infant's tongue until the glottis is visualized. Use a lifting motion in the direction of the scope handle rather than a lever-like motion, which places undue pressure on the infant's maxilla. Have an assistant put gentle pressure over the larynx, which may help bring the glottis into view in difficult circumstances.

    c. When properly positioned, the tip of the blade will be either in the vallecula behind the epiglottis, or over the epiglottis, with the vocal cords clearly in view.

    d. Insert the endotracheal tube by advancing it gently from the right side of the infant's mouth. A common mistake is to advance the tube through the center of the laryngoscope blade, preventing direct visualization of the intubation. The clinician should be able to see the endotracheal tube pass directly through the vocal cords.

    e. The depth of insertion should be 1–1.5 cm below the vocal cords, placing the tip of the endotracheal tube just above the carina.

    f. Shorten the endotracheal tube so that less than 4 cm extends from the lips and tape it into place.

    g. Attach a ventilation bag to the endotracheal tube and deliver positive-pressure ventilations (not if meconium is present). If the assistant hears bilateral breath sounds, the endotracheal tube is most likely in proper position.

F. Drugs and Volume Expansion

Drugs for neonatal resuscitation are given for the following indications. The dosages and routes of administration are summarized in Table 7.[1,2]

1. Acidosis

    a. Indications for treatment include fetal asphyxia with progressive hypercarbia and prolonged resuscitation, and a cord pH of less than 7.0 to 7.1.

    b. Treatment begins with providing adequate ventilation to correct respiratory acidosis. Volume expansion (10 ml/kg of normal saline over 5–10 minutes) may be additionally helpful in restoring tissue perfusion and correcting a moderate metabolic acidosis. Sodium bicarbonate, 4.2% solution, is not routinely recommended but may be used (2 mEq/kg IV over 2 minutes) to correct a severe, persistent acidosis.[2]

2. Hypovolemia

    a. Hypovolemia in the neonate occurs in conjunction with maternal shock, sepsis, or hemorrhage.

    b. Treatment consists of volume expansion with 5% albumin or normal saline, given through an umbilical catheter or peripheral intravenous line. The initial bolus of 10 ml/kg over 5–10 minutes can be repeated if necessary. Whole blood may be used for volume replacement in situations where fetal blood loss is suspected.

TABLE 7. Medications for Neonatal Resuscitation

Medication	Concentration to Administer	Preparation	Dosage/Route*	Weight	Total Dose/Infant	Rate/Precautions
Epinephrine	1:10,000	1 ml	0.1–0.3 ml/kg IV or ET	**Weight** 1 kg / 2 kg / 3 kg / 4 kg	**Total ml** 0.1–0.3 ml / 0.2–0.6 ml / 0.3–0.9 ml / 0.4–1.2 ml	Give rapidly. May dilute with normal saline to 1–2 ml if giving ET
Volume expanders	Whole blood, 5% Albumin, Ringer's lactate, Normal saline	40 ml	10 ml/kg IV	**Weight** 1 kg / 2 kg / 3 kg / 4 kg	**Total ml** 10 ml / 20 ml / 30 ml / 40 ml	Give over 5–10 minutes
Sodium bicarbonate	0.5 mEq/ml (4.2% solution)	20 ml or two 10-ml prefilled syringes	2 mEq/kg IV	**Weight** 1 kg / 2 kg / 3 kg / 4 kg	**Total Dose** 2 mEq / 4 mEq / 6 mEq / 8 mEq **Total ml** 4 ml / 8 ml / 12 ml / 16 ml	Give *slowly*, over at least 2 minutes. Give only if infant is being effectively ventilated
Naloxone hydrochloride	0.4 mg/ml	1 ml	0.1 mg/kg (0.25 ml/kg) IV, ET, IM, SQ	**Weight** 1 kg / 2 kg / 3 kg / 4 kg	**Total Dose** 0.1 mg / 0.2 mg / 0.3 mg / 0.4 mg **Total ml** 0.25 ml / 0.50 ml / 0.75 ml / 1.00 ml	Give rapidly. IV, ET; ET preferred. IM, SQ acceptable
	1.0 mg/ml	1 ml	0.1 mg/kg (0.1 ml/kg) IV, ET, IM, SQ	**Weight** 1 kg / 2 kg / 3 kg / 4 kg	**Total Dose** 0.1 mg / 0.2 mg / 0.3 mg / 0.4 mg **Total ml** 0.1 ml / 0.2 ml / 0.3 ml / 0.4 ml	
Dopamine	$\dfrac{6 \times \text{Weight (kg)} \times \text{Desired dose } \mu g/kg/min}{\text{Desired fluid (ml/h)}} = \text{mg of dopamine per 100 ml of solution}$		Begin at 5 µg/kg/min (may increase to 20 ug/kg/min if necessary) IV	**Weight** 1 kg / 2 kg / 3 kg / 4 kg	**Total mg/min** 5–20 µg/min / 10–40 µg/min / 15–60 µg/min / 20–80 µg/min	Give as a continuous infusion using an infusion pump. Monitor heart rate and blood pressure closely. Seek consultation

From Bloom RS, Cropley C: Textbook of Neonatal Resuscitation. American Heart Association, 1996, with permission.

* IM, intramuscular; ET, endotracheal; IV, intravenous; SQ, subcutaneous.

3. Bradycardia or cardiac arrest
    a. Bradycardia is defined as a neonatal heart rate less than 80 beats per minute that does not respond to oxygen and positive-pressure ventilation.
    b. Treatment consists of epinephrine, 1:10,000 solution, given either intravenously or via endotracheal tube.
4. Narcotic-induced respiratory depression
    a. Narcotic analgesics administered to the mother prior to delivery can result in poor respiratory effort and decreased tone in the newborn.
    b. Treatment consists of naloxone hydrochloride (1 mg/ml solution) given intravenously, intramuscularly, or via endotracheal tube.

III. Management of Meconium-Stained Amniotic Fluid
A. Background
Meconium in amniotic fluid has traditionally been regarded as a sign of fetal distress because the passage of meconium can result from hypoxia and subsequent parasympathetic stimulation of the fetal gut and anal sphincter.[8] It was reported in the 1950s that the fetus passes meconium in utero when the oxygen saturation in the umbilical vein declines to 30% or less, approximately half the normal level.[15] The combination of thick meconium and a fetal heart rate under 100 beats per minute was associated with a perinatal mortality rate of approximately 22% in one early study.[7]

B. Pathophysiology
It is now known that meconium alone is not always a sign of fetal distress. In mature fetuses, physiologic activation of the vagal system may be responsible for meconium passage in the absence of distress. Meconium-stained amniotic fluid (MSAF) is present in 25–30% of post-term pregnancies, a rate roughly twice that found at term.[8]

It is estimated that 13% of infants are born through MSAF and that 5–12% of these go on to develop meconium aspiration syndrome (MAS), a significant cause of perinatal morbidity and mortality.[17] Fortunately, the incidence of meconium aspiration syndrome has declined since the mid-1970s with the initiation of combined suctioning of the infant's oropharynx before delivery of the shoulders and the trachea once delivery is complete.[17]

C. Recognition and Characterization of Meconium in Amniotic Fluid
Identifying the presence and type of meconium in amniotic fluid is the critical first step in planning management.
1. At-risk pregnancies
Pregnancies at risk for meconium are those in which intrauterine hypoxia has led to some degree of fetal stress. Intrauterine growth restriction or postdates pregnancies are examples. Antenatal testing (such as an abnormal biophysical profile) may alert the physician to potential fetal distress. In pregnancies with these risk factors, amniotomy should be considered if spontaneous rupture of membranes has not occurred prior to the second stage of labor. This provides adequate time to make the necessary preparations for delivery when meconium is present.
2. Consistency of the meconium-stained fluid
Thin meconium results when relatively small amounts of meconium are well dispersed throughout the amniotic fluid. The fluid is slightly discolored, but no solid particles are visible. Moderately thick meconium is opaque fluid without particles. Thick meconium is both opaque and particulate, often likened to "pea soup." The thicker the meconium, the greater the risk for developing MAS. In a study of over 2000 infants born through MSAF, the odds of developing MAS

with thick meconium were nearly ten times that with thin meconium. (Odds ratio 9.85; 95% CI 4.4–22.1).[17]

D. Management

1. Endotracheal intubation

During the last quarter of the 20th century, the standard management of infants born through thick meconium involved oropharyngeal suction prior to delivery of the shoulders, followed immediately by endotracheal intubation and suction.[3] The goal was to prevent the baby from aspirating particulate meconium into its lungs. However, a small number of neonates continued to develop MAS despite appropriate suctioning, while others suffered tracheal and pulmonary complications from the intubation itself.[5,17]

Recently, a meta-analysis by the Cochrane Library[9] and a large international randomized trial[17] concluded that vigorous infants do not require routine intubation, regardless of the consistency of the MSAF. In the trial of 2094 vigorous infants—defined as having a heart rate over 100 beats per minute, spontaneous respiration and some movement, extremity flexion at birth—all received oropharyngeal suction. There was no difference in the incidence of MAS between those who were additionally assigned to routine intubation (3.2%) and those treated expectantly (2.7%).[17] The study also confirmed the important role of oropharyngeal suction prior to delivery of the shoulders. When that step was omitted the odds of MAS were significantly increased.

2. Amnioinfusion

Intrapartum amnioinfusion is another management option for decreasing the likelihood of MAS.[4,11,16] The Cochrane Library, in a meta-analysis combining the results of 10 trials, found that amnioinfusion decreased the occurrence of MAS by at least 50%. (RR 0.24, 95% CI 0.12–0.48, absolute risk reduction 6%, number needed to treat to prevent one case of MAS = 17).[10] The improved outcomes were most likely in the presence of thick meconium and oligohydramnios. The largest trial (325 subjects undergoing amnioinfusion) found no complications from this procedure.[13]

3. Intrapartum management

   a. Continuous intrapartum monitoring is recommended to evaluate for fetal distress.

   b. Consider starting an amnioinfusion for thick meconium, oligohydramnios, or significant variable decelerations (see Chapter 17, section C).[16]

4. Neonatal management

   a. As soon as the baby's head is delivered, prior to delivery of the shoulders, suction the mouth, oropharynx, and hypopharynx thoroughly. A DeLee suction device connected to wall suction is commonly used (e.g., the Argyle DeLee Mucus Trap with a 10 French diameter catheter, Sherwood Medical, St. Louis). However, a hand-held bulb suction is equally effective.[17]

   b. If the baby is vigorous (by criteria listed above), the 1-minute Apgar score will be 8 or greater and routine assessment and care are the only steps needed. Intubation and endotracheal suction are not necessary unless subsequent respiratory distress develops.[17]

   c. If there are any signs of distress, either intrapartum or at delivery, the newborn should be intubated and endotracheal suction performed.[1]

   d. The procedure is repeated with reintubation and suctioning until the returns from the trachea are free of meconium. If at any point the infant develops profound bradycardia and central cyanosis, the resuscitator may need to give positive-pressure ventilation, despite the fact that not all the meconium has been cleared.[1]

References

1. Bloom RS, Cropley C: Textbook of Neonatal Resuscitation. Dallas, TX, American Heart Association/American Academy of Pediatrics, 1996.
2. Burchfield DJ: Medication use in neonatal resuscitation. Clin Perinatol 26:683–691, 1999.
3. Carson BS, Losey RW, Bowes WA, et al: Combined obstetric and pediatric approach to prevent meconium aspiration syndrome. Am J Obstet Gynecol 126:712–717, 1976.
4. Cleary GM, Wiswell TE: Meconium-stained amniotic fluid and the meconium aspiration syndrome: an update. Pediatr Clin North Am 45:511–529, 1998.
5. Davis RO, Phillips JB, Harris BA, et al: Fatal meconium aspiration syndrome occurring despite airway management considered appropriate. Am J Obstet Gynecol:151:731–736, 1985.
6. Dye T, Aubry R, Gross S, et al: Amnioinfusion and the intrauterine prevention of meconium aspiration. Am J Obstet Gynecol 171:1601–1605, 1994.
7. Fenton AN, Steer CM: Fetal distress. Am J Obstet Gynecol 83:354, 1962.
8. Freeman RK, LaGrew DC Jr: Postdate pregnancy. In Gabbe SG, Niebyl JR, Simpson JL (eds): Obstetrics: Normal and Problem Pregnancies, 3rd ed. NY, Churchill Livingstone, 1996.
9. Halliday HL: Endotracheal intubation at birth for preventing morbidity and mortality in vigorous, meconium-stained infants born at term (Cochrane Review). In The Cochrane Library, Issue 1. Oxford, Update Software, 2000.
10. Hofmeyr GJ: Amnioinfusion for meconium-stained liquor in labour (Cochrane Review). In The Cochrane Library, Issue 3. Oxford, Update Software, 2000.
11. Hofmeyr GJ, et al: The collaborative randomised amnioinfusion for meconium project (CRAMP): 1 . South Africa. Br J Obstet Gynaecol 105:304–308, 1998.
12. Linder N, Aranda JV, Tsur M, et al: Need for endotracheal intubation and suction in meconium stained neonates. J Pediatr 112:613–615, 1988.
13. Mahomed K, Mulambo T, Woelk G, et al: The collaborative randomised amnioinfusion for meconium project (CRAMP): 2 . Zimbabwe. Br J Obstet Gynaecol 105:309–313, 1998.
14. Smith M, Stratton WC, Roi L: Labor risk assessment in a rural community hospital. Am J Obstet Gynecol 151:569–574, 1985.
15. Walker J: J Obstet Gynaecol Br Emp 61:162, 1954.
16. Weismiller DG: Transcervical amnioinfusion. Am Fam Physician 57:504–510, 1998.
17. Wiswell TE, Gannon CM, Jacob J, et al: Delivery room management of the apparently vigorous meconium-stained neonate: Results of the multicenter, international collaborative trial. Pediatrics 105:1–7, 2000.
18. Wolkoff LI, Davis JM: Delivery room resuscitation of the newborn. Clin Perinatol 26:641–658, 1999.

SECTION C.
NEONATAL CIRCUMCISION

I. Background

Newborn circumcision is a common procedure in the United States, performed largely for cultural reasons. At the peak of its acceptance between the late 1940s and the early 1970s, up to 1.5 million newborn circumcisions were performed annually, and in some U.S. hospitals 85–90% of male infants were circumcised.[19] Today, the number of circumcisions is estimated at 1.2 million, and the rate varies according to ethnic, religious, and socioeconomic affiliation. White Americans are more likely to be circumcised (81%) than African Americans (65%) or Hispanics (54%).[15] Jewish and Moslem religious teachings stipulate newborn circumcision.

The question whether circumcision conveys medical benefit sufficient to outweigh its risks and costs has sparked ongoing debate. In 1999, the American Academy of Pediatrics issued a policy statement concluding that existing scientific evidence is not sufficient to recommend routine neonatal circumcision, that the procedure is not essential to an infant's well-being, and that parents should be the ones to decide what is in their son's best interest.[1] In this context, the family physician's roles are the following: (1) to provide accurate and unbiased information for parents' decisions; (2) to support the decision once made; and (3) when circumcision is elected, to perform it with skill, using appropriate analgesia.

II. Risks, Benefits, and Informed Consent

Ideally, the family physician should discuss the potential risks and benefits of circumcision with one or both parents during prenatal visits. Table 8 can serve as a guide for obtaining informed consent; it outlines indications, contraindications, risks and benefits, and supporting evidence.

TABLE 8. Newborn Circumcision: Risks and Benefits

	Comments
Indications for Circumcision	
Religious belief	Jewish and Moslem religions have stipulations regarding circumcision.
Strong parental preference	
Contraindications to Circumcision	
Medically unstable infant	Delay circumcision until the infant is stable or, for preterm, until
Preterm infant	ready for discharge.
Genital anomalies— hypospadias, webbed penis, congenital megalourethra	Do not circumcise. Obtain surgical consultation. With hypospadias, the foreskin may be needed for later surgical correction.
Abnormal bleeding or family history of bleeding disorder	Check appropriate coagulation studies prior to circumcision.
Potential Risks	Most complications are minor. The overall incidence of complications is approximately 0.2–0.6%[1]
Pain and behavioral changes	CNS pain pathways are well developed in newborns. Heart rate, blood pressure, cortisol levels, and crying all increase during circumcision; use of local anesthesia can blunt these effects.
Hemorrhage	Bleeding requiring treatment occurs in approximately 0.1% of circumcisions.[1] Typical management includes direct pressure and use of hemostatic agents (silver nitrate, absorbable gelatin or cellulose products). If bleeding skin edges are widely separated, circumferential sutures may be needed.
Infection	The true incidence of infection is unknown. Minor erythema or yellowish crusting not uncommon during healing.
Removal of too much or too little skin	A poor cosmetic result can be avoided with careful attention to technique. Identify the coronal sulcus and aim to remove skin 1–2 mm distal to that landmark. Avoid excessive traction on the foreskin which can pull skin from the penile shaft into the cone or bell.
Foreskin adhesions, skin bridges	Make sure the tissue plane between foreskin and glans is completely developed before removing the foreskin.
Retained plastic bell apparatus	The plastic bell should be removed after 7 days if it has not dropped off spontaneously. Rarely, prolonged attachment may result in urosepsis or formation of a permanent sulcus.
Potential Benefits	
Reduced risk of penile cancer	Penile cancer is rare, 9–10 cases per year per million U.S. men. Invasive penile cancer is associated with being uncircumcised (relative risk > 3), with phimosis, and with human papillomavirus infection.[1]
Reduced incidence of urinary tract infection	The risk for uncircumcised infants is 4–10 times higher than circumcised.[1,22] Most of the excess risk occurs in infants < 12 months old. The absolute risk of UTI in an uncircumcised infant is 1%.
Reduced risk of STDs/ HIV infection	Behavioral factors are more important than circumcision status in acquiring STDs. Conclusions from studies are conflicting and vary by disease; however, noncircumcised status appears to be a risk factor for syphilis and HIV.[5]
Avoiding circumcision later in life	Conditions requiring circumcision later in life are uncommon: Phimosis (non-retractable foreskin)—90% of uncircumcised males have a fully retractable foreskin by age 5 years Paraphimosis (retracted foreskin trapped behind the glans)—may occur in elderly men requiring bladder catheterization. Balanitis (infection of the glans and foreskin) is more common in uncircumcised boys and men.[6]

III. Analgesia

A. Rationale

Newborns demonstrate physiologic stress responses to circumcision including increased crying, changes in heart rate and blood pressure, decreased oxygen saturation, and increased serum cortisol levels. These responses are attenuated or eliminated by local anesthesia. The importance of pain control for newborn circumcision is highlighted by the AAP's 1999 Circumcision Policy Statement that "analgesia is safe and effective in reducing the procedural pain . . . and should be provided if neonatal circumcision is performed."[1]

B. Options for Pain Management

1. Dorsal penile nerve block (DPNB)

DPNB achieves anesthesia of the foreskin, glans, and distal penile shaft by blocking the dorsal penile nerves as they exit from beneath the symphysis pubis. To date, DPNB is the most thoroughly studied method for managing the pain of neonatal circumcision. Several small randomized controlled trials (RCTs) have confirmed DPNB's effectiveness in achieving decreased crying, smaller increases in heart rate, smaller decreases in oxygen saturation, and lower serum cortisol levels than placebo injections or no analgesia.[2,10,17,20,23] DPNB carries a low risk of minor side effects, the most common being ecchymosis or brief bleeding at the injection site.[7] Detailed technique is presented in the next section. Risks and benefits of DPNB are presented in Table 9.

2. "Ring block"

Local infiltration of 1% xylocaine in a circumferential ring at the base of the penis or at mid-shaft ("ring block"). One RCT (52 infants total) found ring block to be equivalent to DPNB and EMLA cream in reducing infant crying, and more effective than either in minimizing heart rate changes during lysis of foreskin adhesions.[14]

3. "Distal branch block"

Injecting lidocaine at the base of the glans ("distal branch block" or "local anesthesia") has been tested against DPNB in one randomized trial (30 infants total)

TABLE 9. Risks and Benefits of Anesthesia for Newborn Circumcision

Risks	Comments
Bleeding from injection site: ecchymosis or hematoma at injection site	Bleeding and ecchymosis are usually of minor degree. Incidence of small ecchymoses is 10% in a series of DPNB
Methemoglobinemia	Rare; may be induced by a variety of local anesthetics; presents with cyanosis and decreased oxygen saturation
Transient penile ischemia	Theoretical; not reported in newborn circumcision with local anesthesia
Lidocaine toxicity: cardiac arrhythmias, seizures	Theoretical; should not occur if dosage is kept within guidelines and intravascular injection is avoided
Benefits	
During circumcision procedure: 1. Less crying 2. Better transcutaneous oxygen levels 3. Smaller increases in heart rate, BP	Overall, local anesthesia has been shown to reduce pain and stress of newborn circumcision (most studies have involved the dorsal penile nerve block)
Postoperatively: 1. Cortisol levels less indicative of stress 2. Less interference in infant's behavioral state and sleep patterns 3. Less interference in maternal-infant interaction	Behavioral changes are transient; have not been documented beyond 24 hours after the procedure.

and found to be associated with significantly smaller increases in heart rate, less time crying, and lower serum cortisol levels.[18] However, distal injections can distort anatomic landmarks, making the circumcision procedure more difficult and leading in some cases to unsatisfactory cosmetic results.[16]

4. Topical anesthesia

Topical application of a lidocaine/prilocaine mixture, also known as eutectic mixture of local anesthetics (EMLA) has been shown to be effective in reducing overall infant crying and heart rate changes when compared to placebo.[3,21] 1–2 grams of EMLA cream are applied to the distal half of the penis and secured with an occlusive dressing 60–90 minutes prior to the procedure.

5. Adjuvant measures

A sucrose-flavored pacifier has been shown to reduce crying during the procedure,[4] and acetaminophen can be used postoperatively.[11]

C. Technique of Dorsal Penile Nerve Block[8]

1. Assemble the necessary equipment: a 1-ml tuberculin syringe, a 31–33-gauge needle, and 1% lidocaine without epinephrine.
2. Prepare the penis and the prepubic skin with a topical surgical scrub.
3. Draw 0.8 ml of 1% lidocaine into the tuberculin syringe; 3–4 mg/kg may be used for more precise dosing.
4. Stabilize the penis by gentle traction with one hand.
5. Identify the two injection sites at the base of the penis. They will be at the 10 o'clock and 2 o'clock positions, 0.5 to 1.0 cm distal to the point where the penile root passes under the pubic symphysis.
6. Pierce the skin with the needle at an acute angle, directed slightly downward. A depth of 1–3 mm is required to reach the appropriate fascial layer superficial to the corpora cavernosa.
7. Check that the tip of the needle is freely mobile, i.e., not embedded in the corpus cavernosum.
8. Aspirate to ensure against intravascular injection.
9. Inject 0.4 ml, or half the total calculated dose of lidocaine.
10. Repeat the injection at the second site.
11. Allow 3–5 minutes for the block to take effect.

D. Circumcision Technique

Clamp techniques (e.g., Gomco or Mogen) and the Plastibell all achieve good results with appropriate patient selection, attention to asepsis, and careful surgical technique.[9] Steps and diagrams for Gomco and Plastibell circumcision follow (Fig. 3):[12]

1. Steps for circumcision with the Gomco method
    a. Set up the sterile circumcision tray; check all equipment.
    b. Identify anatomic landmarks; consider marking the coronal sulcus with sterile pen.
    c. Grasp the rim of the foreskin at 10 o'clock and 2 o'clock with curved mosquito hemostats.
    d. Insert a blunt-tipped probe or straight hemostat under the foreskin to the coronal sulcus. Sweep the probe or hemostat over the glans penis, freeing the foreskin from the glans.
    e. Make the crush line for the dorsal slit by inserting one blade of a straight hemostat under the foreskin at 12 o'clock, to within a few millimeters of the corona. One technique is to slide the hemostat blade all the way to the corona and then withdraw it by one third of the total distance. Close the hemostat and hold for a few seconds, then remove it.
    f. Cut the dorsal slit along the crush line with scissors.

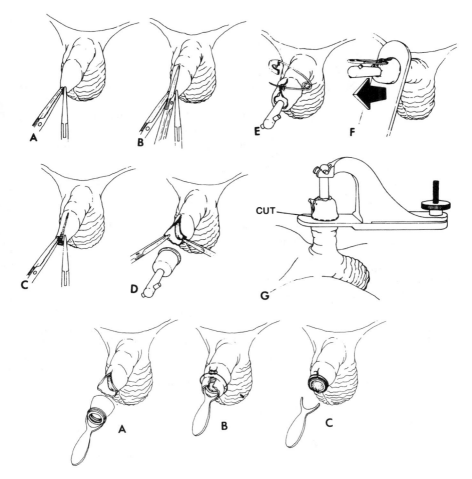

FIGURE 3. Two common techniques for newborn circumcision. Top, using the Gomco clamp; bottom, using the plastic bell.

g. Retract the foreskin to expose the entire glans and coronal sulcus. Break down any remaining adhesions with the probe or a gauze 4 × 4.

h. Insert a properly sized cone over the glans. Cones of 1.1 or 1.3 cm are usually appropriate for term infants.

i. Draw the foreskin back over the cone, bring the two edges of the dorsal slit together, and secure with a sterile safety pin.

j. Bring the safety pin up parallel with the shaft of the cone. Use the pin to draw the foreskin through the hole in the Gomco base plate. (An alternative technique is to use a curved mosquito hemostat to approximate the edges of the dorsal slit and guide the foreskin through the base plate.)

k. Hook the Gomco top plate under the arms of the cone and position it properly over the base plate.

l. Check landmarks
    i. Is there a symmetric cuff of foreskin above the base plate?
    ii. Is the entire length of the dorsal slit visible above the base plate?

    m. Attach the nut to the bolt on the base plate and fasten firmly. Many authorities recommend waiting 5 minutes to assure hemostasis.

    n. Excise the foreskin just above the base plate, holding the scalpel nearly parallel to the plate.

    o. Unfasten the nut and remove the upper and lower plates.

    p. Gently brush the crushed skin line off the cone with gauze and remove the cone.

    q. Cover the glans with petroleum jelly or precut petrolatum gauze.

2. Steps for circumcision with the Plastibell technique

    a. Free adhesions and make a dorsal slit as in preceding steps 1 through 6.

    b. Place the plastic cone inside the foreskin. It should fit snugly, but without pressure on the glans. The groove in the cone should lie beyond the apex of the dorsal slit.

    c. If the cone catches on the frenulum, use scissors to shape the lower edge of the cone to fit.

    d. Hold the foreskin firmly over the cone and tie a suture around the cone to compress the foreskin into the groove.

    e. Trim off the foreskin distal to the ligature with tissue scissors.

    f. Break off the disposable cone handle.

E. Post-circumcision Care

1. Circumcisions performed with Mogen or Gomco clamps

Observe carefully for 1–2 hours for any signs of excessive bleeding. Petroleum jelly is used to protect the healing glans and should be reapplied with each diaper change. The baby will usually urinate normally within 6–8 hours following the procedure; it is not necessary to delay hospital discharge to document voiding. Parents should expect the tip of the penis to appear red and have slight yellowish coating intitially, but should report frank bleeding or signs of infection. The healing process will take 7–10 days.

2. Circumcisions performed with the Plastibell

The cone and ligature should not be disturbed and will fall off spontaneously within 5–8 days. The cone should be removed if it remains in place beyond that time. Parents should report any persistent bleeding or signs of infection.

References

1. American Academy of Pediatrics, Task Force on Circumcision: Circumcision Policy Statement. Pediatrics 103:686–693, 1999.
2. Arnett RM, Jones S, Horger EO: Effectiveness of 1% lidocaine dorsal penile nerve block in infant circumcision. Am J Obstet Gynecol 163:1074–1080, 1990.
3. Benini F, Johnston C, Faucher D, et al: Topical anesthesia during circumcision in newborn infants. JAMA 270:850–853, 1993.
4. Blass EM, Hoffmeyer LB: Sucrose as an analgesic for newborn infants. Pediatrics 87:215–218, 1991.
5. Cook LS, Koutsky LA, Holmes KK: Circumcision and sexually transmitted diseases. Am J Public Health 84:197–201, 1994.
6. Fergusson DM, Lawton JW, Shannon FT: Neonatal circumcision and penile problems: An eight-year longitudinal study. Pediatrics 81:537–541, 1988.
7. Fontaine P, Dittberner D, Scheltema K: The safety of dorsal penile nerve block for anesthesia in circumcision. J Fam Pract 39:243–248, 1994.
8. Fontaine P, Toffler W: Dorsal penile nerve block for neonatal circumcision. Am Fam Physician 43:1327–1333, 1991.
9. Holman JR, Lewis EL, Ringler RL: Neonatal circumcision techniques. Am Fam Physician 52:511–518, 1995.
10. Holve RL, Bromberger PJ, Groveman HD, et al: Regional anesthesia during newborn circumcision: Effect on infant pain response. Clin Pediatr 22:813–819, 1983.
11. Howard CR, Howard FM, Weitzman ML: Acetaminophen analgesia in neonatal circumcision: The effect on pain. Pediatrics 93:641–649, 1994.

12. Hughes WT, Buescher ES: Pediatric Procedures, 2nd ed. Philadelphia, W.B. Saunders, 1980, pp 292–296.
13. Kaplan GW: Complications of circumcision. Urol Clin North Am 10:543–549, 1983.
14. Lander J, Brady-Fryer B, Metcalfe JB: Comparison of ring block, dorsal penile nerve block, and topical anesthesia for neonatal circumcision: A randomized clinical trial. JAMA 278:2157–2162, 1997.
15. Laumann EO, Masi CM, Zuckerman EW: Circumcision in the United States: Prevalence, prophylactic effects, and sexual practice. JAMA 277:1052–1057, 1997.
16. Lenhart JG, Lenhart NM, Reid MA, et al: Local anesthesia for circumcision: Which technique is most effective? J Am Board Fam Pract 10:13–19, 1997.
17. Maxwell LG, Yaster M, Wetzel RC, et al: Penile nerve block for newborn circumcision. Obstet Gynecol 70:415–419, 1987.
18. Masciello AL: Anesthesia for neonatal circumcision: Local anesthesia is better than dorsal penile nerve block. Obstet Gynecol 75:834–838, 1990.
19. Schoen EJ, Fischell AA: Pain in neonatal circumcision. Clin Pediatr 30:429–432, 1991.
20. Stang HJ, Gunnar MR, Snellman L, et al: Local anesthesia for neonatal circumcision: Effects on distress and cortisol response. JAMA 259:1507–1511, 1988.
21. Taddio A, Stevens B, Craig K, et al: Efficacy and safety of lidocaine-prilocaine cream for pain during circumcision. N Engl J Med 336:1197–1201. 1997.
22. To T, Agha M, Dick PT, Feldman W: Cohort study on circumcision of newborn boys and subsequent risk of urinary tract infection. Lancet 352:1813-1816, 1998.
23. Williamson PS, Williamson ML: Physiologic stress reduction by a local anesthetic during circumcision. Pediatrics 71:36–40, 1983.

SECTION D.
NEONATAL JAUNDICE

I. Overview

Neonatal jaundice is a common phenomenon—approximately 60% of newborns in the United States appear clinically jaundiced during the first days of life.[1] The family physician can use the infant's history, physical examination, and a few laboratory tests to distinguish benign physiologic jaundice from significant jaundice that may be due to pathologic causes.

Physiologic jaundice is best treated with a conservative approach, including simple monitoring and parental reassurance. Pathologic jaundice, on the other hand, requires more thorough investigation and more aggressive management, especially in preterm or compromised infants. The goal in these cases is to prevent kernicterus, central nervous system damage caused by bilirubin deposition.

Jaundice associated with breastfeeding is the result of physiologic processes, yet it occasionally culminates in significant jaundice. Early hospital discharges appear to be associated with increased hospitalization rates for jaundice in breastfed newborns,[9] and rare cases of kernicterus have occurred in healthy term infants where breastfeeding appeared to be the only etiology.[11,12]

II. Physiologic Jaundice
A. Etiology

Three factors contribute to neonatal jaundice: a high level of bilirubin production, a transient deficiency of bilirubin conjugation, and an increase in enterohepatic circulation. Infants are born with relatively high red cell counts (mean cord blood hemoglobin = 16.5 ± 1.5 g/dl). The subsequent breakdown of heme into iron, carbon monoxide, and biliverdin (which is converted to bilirubin by bilirubin reductase) leads to the formation of 34 mg of bilirubin for each 1 g of hemoglobin reduced. Serum albumin binds bilirubin and carries it to the liver, where the newborn's transient deficiency of the enzyme bilirubin glucuronosyltransferase (BGT or UDPGT) leads to suboptimal hepatic bilirubin uptake and conjugation. Conjugated bilirubin is excreted through the bile into the intestine, where it may be deconjugated by a mucosal enzyme (β-glucuronidase) and reabsorbed into the enterohepatic circulation before it can be excreted with the stool. Newborns have slow intestinal motility due to a paucity of gut flora and relative caloric deprivation in the first days of life, both of which promote physiologic hyperbilirubinemia through increased enterohepatic circulation.[17,31]

Virtually all infants develop some degree of physiologic hyperbilirubinemia. Because bilirubin is a potent antioxidant and peroxyl scavenger, the speculation is that physiologic increases may help the newborn to avoid oxygen toxicity in the days after birth.[22]

B. Diagnosis

1. Clinical assessment

Physiologic jaundice is a clinical diagnosis, based on the appearance of yellow coloration in the infant's skin. The yellow color first appears on the face, indicating a total serum bilirubin level (TSB) of 4–8 mg/dl (68–137 µmol/L). As jaundice deepens and progresses down the trunk and abdomen, the serum bilirubin also increases. By the time the distal extremities are involved, the TSB is likely to be ≥ 15 mg/dl (258 µmol/L).[8]

The clinical assessment may be aided by standardized color guides (Ingram icterometer) or by measurements from a transcutaneous bilirubin meter (Minolta Airshields Jaundice Meter).[3] Serum bilirubin should be measured for confirmation.

2. Characteristics of physiologic jaundice

By definition, physiologic jaundice occurs in healthy infants in whom no pathologic processes such as hemolysis or sepsis are occurring. It has the following characteristics:[22]

   a. Time of onset. Clinical jaundice appears *after* 24 hours of age. A TSB of 8 mg/dl is at the 95th percentile for 24 hours of age. Values ≥ 8 mg/dl at 24 hours are likely to be associated with hemolysis.
   b. Rate of bilirubin increase. The total serum bilirubin level (TSB) rises by less than 5 mg/dl (86 µmol/L) per day.
   c. Peak bilirubin levels. TSB peaks between 3 and 5 days of age, and never exceeds15 mg/dl (258 µmol/L). TSB is composed almost exclusively of unconjugated bilirubin.
   d. Resolution of jaundice. Clinical jaundice resolves within 7–10 days in term newborns and within 2 weeks in preterm newborns.

3. Pathologic jaundice

It is important not to attribute jaundice to physiologic mechanisms when the infant's clinical condition or TSB level warrants additional investigation. Diagnostic testing for pathologic jaundice should be considered for term newborns with a TSB ≥ 12mg/dl and should definitely be performed when the level reaches 15 mg/dl. A transient, reversible depression of brainstem auditory evoked responses occurs at 14.9 mg/dl.[21]

C. Management

1. Physiologic jaundice

No treatment is necessary for strictly physiologic jaundice. Parents generally appreciate reassurance and explanations of how the condition develops.

2. Early infant discharge

With recent trends toward shorter newborn hospital stays (some as brief as 24 hours following delivery), the responsibility for detecting significant jaundice lies with the parents. When early discharge is planned, parents should be instructed to observe for jaundice once the baby is home and to report a rapidly developing color change that extends from the face into the sclera or onto the chest and abdomen. Written parent education materials, neonatal jaundice protocols, and tracking systems can be helpful, but a national survey of head nurses and pediatricians found that only 50–60% of nurseries had such systems in place.[23]

The American Academy of Pediatrics recommends that newborns discharged before 48 hours of age be seen by a health care provider within 2–3 days.[1]

III. Jaundice Associated with Breastfeeding

Breastfeeding is clearly associated with neonatal jaundice. Compared to bottlefed infants, breastfed infants have higher mean serum bilirubin levels during the first week of life, and are more likely to develop hyperbilirubinemia of moderate or significant degree.[19] There are two clinical syndromes: breastfeeding-associated jaundice, also known as "lack of breast milk jaundice" and true breast milk jaundice (Fig. 4). In addition, there may be considerable overlap between the two.

A. Breastfeeding-associated Jaundice

1. Definition

Breastfeeding-associated jaundice is considered an exaggerated form of physiologic jaundice, characterized by levels of unconjugated bilirubin higher than

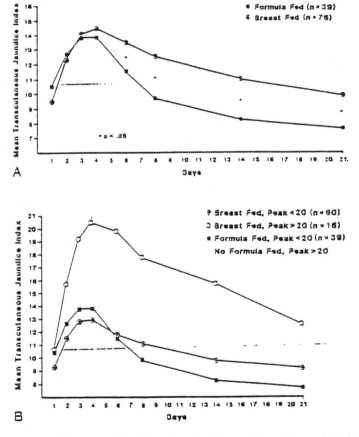

FIGURE 4.   Natural history of jaundice in white breast-fed and formula-fed infants. The transcutaneous jaundice index was measured with the Minolta Jaundice Meter. *A*, The natural history of jaundice in the formula-fed and breast-fed infants. Significant differences in the TcB index were found from days 6 to 21. *B*, Bimodal distribution of jaundice in the breast-fed infants. Twenty-one percent of breast-fed infants had TcB indexes greater than 20 (> 12.9 mg/dl), but in the remaining breast-fed infants the bilirubin pattern was similar to that of the formula-fed infants. (From Kiylahan C, James EJP: Pediatrics 74:364, 1984, with permission.)

expected from physiologic mechanisms alone. It is primarily due to decreased caloric intake and increased enterohepatic circulation of bilirubin.[22] The syndrome has been termed lack of breast milk jaundice because it is a sign of failure to establish an adequate milk supply, and more frequent nursing can actually decrease the likelihood of hyperbilirubinemia.

2. Clinical course

The initial time course for breastfeeding-associated jaundice is similar to that of physiologic jaundice, with TSB levels peaking during the first week of life. The clear majority of breastfed infants experience only mild hyperbilirubinemia; however, 2–7.4% have peak levels exceeding 15–17 mg/dl. Resolution may extend beyond the typical 7–10 days, with prolonged mild jaundice occurring in 25–30% of infants.[13,19]

B. True Breast Milk Jaundice Syndrome

True breast milk jaundice syndrome is less common, occurring in an estimated 0.5–2.5% of breastfed infants. It is distinguished by significant and prolonged unconjugated hyperbilirubinemia. Classically, the syndrome shows a progressive rise in TSB starting from 4 days of age, peaking as high as 20–30 mg/dl by the end of the second week. Elevated levels gradually decline, but may not return to normal for 3–4 months.[19]

C. Pathophysiology

The mechanisms by which breastfeeding causes jaundice are the subject of ongoing investigation. They include the following:

1. Decreased caloric intake

Breastfed infants generally take in fewer calories than bottlefed infants in the first few days of life, due to less frequent feedings, smaller amounts of milk per feeding, or to other factors. Hyperbilirubinemia may result from a direct effect of calorie deprivation or from increased enterohepatic circulation in the presence of slow gut motility.

2. Inhibition of bilirubin conjugation

Components in breast milk may either inhibit bilirubin conjugation or enhance enterohepatic circulation. Lipoprotein lipase, free fatty acids, and β-glucuronidase have been proposed to have such effects. Breast milk may vary in composition from woman to woman, and higher concentrations of these factors (or others yet to be identified) could place infants at greater risk for true breast milk jaundice.[3]

D. Diagnosis

Breastfeeding may be a sole cause for jaundice or may combine with other factors. Before making the diagnosis of breastfeeding-associated jaundice, physicians should use the history, physical examination, and appropriate laboratory studies to evaluate for other contributing conditions.

E. Treatment

Management of breastfeeding-associated jaundice is based upon assumptions that breast milk is optimal infant nutrition and that a mother's decision to nurse her baby should be supported during treatment for hyperbilirubinemia.[16] The overall treatment goal is to prevent TSB from rising above 20–25 mg/dl.[1]

1. Breastfeeding counseling

Encourage mothers to begin breastfeeding as soon as possible and to nurse frequently. Feedings should be on demand, or at least every 3 hours. Request a certified lactation consultant if the mother has difficulty in establishing nursing or there are signs of excessive infant weight loss.

2. Supplementation

Discourage supplementation with dextrose water, which has been associated with decreased breast milk intake and increased bilirubin levels in the first week of life.

TABLE 10. Treatment Options and Outcomes for Jaundiced Breast-fed Newborns

		Treatment*				
		Breast	Formula	B + Photo tx	F + Photo tx	P[†]
% Failing treatment (TSB > 20 mg/dl, 342 mmol/L)		24	19	13	3	0.0685
% Achieving reduction of TSB to < 13.5 mg/dl (< 231 μmol/L) after 48 hours of treatment		0	19	42	45	0.0003
Change in TSB (mean + SD) after 48 hours of treatment	mmol/L	−17 + 32	−34 ± 51	−65 ± 34	−77 ± 41	< 0.0001
	mg/dl	−1.0 ± 1.9	−2.0 + 3.0	−3.8 ± 2.0	−4.5 ± 2.4	

* From Martinez JC, Maisels MJ, Otheguy L, et al: Hyperbilirubinemia in the breast-fed newborn: A controlled trial of four interventions. Pediatrics 91:470–473, 1993, with permission.
[†] Treatments were randomly assigned to 125 term breastfed infants with total serum bilirubin (TSB) ≥ 17 mg/dl (291 μmol/L).
Breast, continue breastfeeding; formula = discontinue breastfeeding, substitute formula; B+ Photo tx, continue breastfeeding and begin phototherapy; F+ Photo tx, substitute formula and begin phototherapy.

3. High bilirubin levels
If it appears that serum bilirubin will rise above 20–25 mg/dl (TSB of 15 mg/dl on the third day of life or 17 mg/dl or greater thereafter), careful management is warranted. Options are to continue breastfeeding and follow TSB levels, to interrupt nursing and substitute formula feedings, or to add phototherapy to either feeding plan. An RCT comparing these treatment options found that the majority of healthy, term, breastfed infants do well with conservative monitoring.[13] However, adding phototherapy achieves a greater and more rapid decline in TSB than can be anticipated with either feeding method alone.[13,21] Table 10 summarizes results from the trial, and can be used to help parents choose an appropriate management plan.

4. Interruption of breastfeeding
When a woman chooses to interrupt breastfeeding, give assurance that nothing is wrong with her milk and that she can resume nursing once the hyperbilirubinemia has resolved. An electric breast pump can be used to maintain her milk supply during the temporary interruption.

5. Checking bilirubin levels
How often to check the bilirubin level depends on the age of the infant and how quickly the TSB is increasing. However, checking once every 24 hours is usually sufficient when breastfeeding is the sole etiology for jaundice. TSB should be documented until a definite decline is noted. Although TSB may rise with the resumption of breastfeeding, it rarely returns to previous maximum levels.

6. Home phototherapy
Home phototherapy units can be used for infants whose jaundice does not become significant until after they are discharged home.[2,3] Clinical assessments and TSB measurements can be facilitated by a visiting nurse. Where home health services are not available or adequate follow-up is in question, re-hospitalization may be necessary for phototherapy. Hospitalization is mandatory for any infant who appears dehydrated, lethargic or otherwise ill.

IV. Pathologic Jaundice
A. Definition and Etiologies
Neonatal jaundice is termed "pathologic" when there is an identifiable etiology beyond the expected physiologic mechanisms. In a population where many women chose to breastfeed, fewer than half of term infants with TSB > 12 mg/dl have a pathologic cause for jaundice.[10]

TABLE 11. Causes of Pathologic Jaundice

Overproduction of bilirubin
  1. Immune-mediated hemolysis (Coombs' test positive)
     ABO incompatibility (the type A or type B infant of a type O mother)
     Rh incompatibility (the Rh positive infant of an Rh negative mother)
     Other blood group incompatibilities (Kell, Duffy, etc.)
  2. Coombs'-negative hemolysis
     Red blood cell membrane defects (spherocytosis and other abnormally shaped RBCs)
     Red blood cell enzyme abnormalities (G6PD, pyruvate kinase, and hexokinase deficiencies)
  3. Non-hemolytic causes of increased bilirubin load
     Extravascular hemorrhage (skin, scalp, central nervous system, adrenal glands)
     Polycythemia

Decreased Rate of Bilirubin Conjugation
  1. Gilbert's syndrome (an autosomal dominant deficiency of bilirubin glucuronosyltransferase; affects 3–6% of the population)
  2. Crigler-Najjar syndrome, types I and II (rare genetic deficiencies of BGT)

Decreased Excretion of Bilirubin
  1. Cholestatic syndromes
  2. Obstruction of the biliary tree
  3. Congenital cirrhosis, hepatitis
  4. Exaggerated enterohepatic circulation (gastrointestinal obstruction, ileus)

Table 11 lists the causes of pathologic jaundice, grouped into three main categories: overproduction of bilirubin, decreased conjugation of bilirubin, and decreased bilirubin excretion.[1,3,22]

B. Diagnosis
  1. Overview
As seen in Table 12,[1,14,22] pathologic jaundice is suspected on clinical grounds and verified by the presence of early high or rapidly rising TSB levels. A prolonged TSB elevation or an elevation of the direct bilirubin fraction also implies a pathologic cause.
  2. Prenatal history
The work-up of pathologic jaundice should begin with a review of the mother's prenatal course and delivery summary. Oxytocin use in labor and maternal diabetes are each associated with increased bilirubin levels in the newborn. Prolonged rupture of membranes or maternal fever may be associated with newborn sepsis and hyperbilirubinemia. Intrauterine growth restriction may be accompanied by polycythemia, which increases the risk of jaundice. Maternal smoking, by contrast, is associated with decreased newborn bilirubin levels.[1]
  3. Ethnicity and family history
Asian infants are more likely than whites or blacks to have TSB > 12 mg/dl: 23% compared to 10–13% and 4%, respectively.[22] Certain causes of jaundice may be seen with increased prevalence in particular ethnic groups. For example, G6PD deficiency is seen in males (it is X-linked) with African, Mediterranean, or Asian backgrounds. It is present in 10–14% of black American males.[1] Gilbert's syndrome is not common in the general U.S. population (prevalence 3–6%), but is seen in 10–19% of the Eastern Scottish population.[14]
  4. Physical findings
    a. Severity of jaundice. Estimate the severity of jaundice based on the extent of yellow coloration in the skin, as described for physiologic jaundice above.
    b. Check for weight loss. A loss of greater than 10% of birth weight during the first week of life is a sign of feeding problems and inadequate caloric intake.
    c. Verify the gestational age. Preterm infants are at increased risk for jaundice, and although infants born at 37 weeks gestation are considered

TABLE 12. Characteristics of Pathologic Jaundice

Characteristics	Suggested Etiologies
Jaundice is clinically apparent in the first 24 hours of life or TSB is increasing by more than 5 mg/dl/day.	Hemolytic disease: 1. ABO incompatibility is the most common etiology 2. Rh incompatibility is less common due to Rh immunoglobulin prophylaxis 3. G6PD deficiency is seen in males of African, Mediterranean, and Asian descent; TSB typically increases later than expected (after 24–48 hours). 4. Hereditary spherocytosis—a family history of anemia, jaundice and gallstones may be present.
The jaundiced infant is also clinically ill: lethargy, poor feeding, apnea, tachypnea, excessive weight loss, vomiting, hepatosplenomegaly, or temperature instability.	Sepsis, congenital infections (e.g., syphilis, TORCH), galactosemia
Direct (conjugated) serum bilirubin exceeds 1.5–2.0 mg/dl.	Cholestasis, biliary atresia, sepsis
Clinical jaundice persists for more than 3 weeks.*	Cholestasis, biliary atresia, Gilbert's syndrome, Crigler-Najjar syndrome 1. Suspect cholestasis when the infant has light-colored stools or dark urine that tests positive for bilirubin.

* True breast-milk jaundice syndrome is also in the differential diagnosis

"term," they are much more likely to develop TSB of > 13 mg/dl than infants born at 40 weeks.[1]
  d. Check for excessive bruising or cephalhematoma. This can lead to an elevation of TSB due to increased red blood cell breakdown.
  e. Assess for lethargy, irritability, hepatosplenomegaly, or other signs of sepsis. These signs are serious indicators of underlying disease and deserve aggressive work-up.
5. Laboratory investigation (Table 13)
  a. Initial work-up. The initial test is a total serum bilirubin level, usually obtained from the infant by heel stick. When the TSB is > 12–15 mg/dl (i.e., in the range where phototherapy would be considered based on the infant's age), additional investigation is necessary.
  b. Coombs' testing. Hospitals are encouraged to save cord blood from infants of mothers with blood types O-positive or Rh-negative. In the event

TABLE 13. Laboratory Investigation for Pathologic Jaundice

Initial evaluation (capillary blood sample obtained from the infant by heelstick)
  Total serum bilirubin

Additional Studies
  When mother's blood type is O-positive or Rh-negative (cord blood sample obtained at delivery)
    Infant blood type
    Direct Coombs' test
  When Hemolysis Is Suspected
    Hemoglobin or hematocrit
    Peripheral smear for red blood cell morphology
    Reticulocyte count
    Glucose-6-phosphatase dehydrogenase (G6PD) screening test
  When Cholestasis or Biliary Atresia Is Suspected
    Direct fraction serum bilirubin
    Imaging studies of hepatobiliary tree

of significant jaundice, the cord blood is used to determine the infant's blood type and a Coombs' test. A positive Coombs' test indicates the presence of maternally produced antibodies to infant red blood cells, typical for immune-mediated hemolysis.

c. Additional testing. When hemolysis is severe, or if there is no blood group incompatibility to explain the jaundice, then further studies should be obtained. A peripheral smear may reveal fragmented red blood cells compatible with hemolysis or abnormally shaped cells as in hereditary spherocytosis. An elevated reticulocyte count and dropping hemoglobin or hematocrit may indicate active hemolysis with the potential for severe jaundice.

V. Treatment of Significant Hyperbilirubinemia
According to the American Academy of Pediatrics, "Few issues in neonatal medicine have generated such long-standing controversy as the possible adverse consequences of neonatal jaundice and when to begin treatment." There is agreement that extreme elevations in TSB are toxic to newborn's central nervous system; however, it is not known at what TSB level or under what clinical circumstances significant risk of brain damage occurs. Factors such as prematurity and active hemolysis significantly increase an infant's risk, and require more aggressive treatment than does the healthy term infant, where a less aggressive approach may suffice.[15]

A. Treatment Guidelines for Healthy Term Newborns
The American Academy of Pediatrics has developed a set of treatment guidelines based on available evidence and derived from consensus where data were lacking (Table 14). The treatment goal is to keep TSB below 25 mg/dl, primarily by using phototherapy. Exchange transfusion is needed for rare cases where intensive phototherapy fails or the TSB is already $\geq$ 30 mg/dl at the time of diagnosis.[1]

B. Treatment Guidelines for Term Infants when Hemolysis Is Present
When hemolysis is present, phototherapy should be considered earlier and at lower levels of TSB: TSB > 10 mg/dl at < 12 hours, TSB $\geq$ 12–14 mg/dl at < 18 hours, and TSB $\geq$15 mg/dl at 24 hours.[22]

TABLE 14. Management of Hyperbilirubinemia in the Healthy Term Newborn
[TSB* Level, mg/dl (mmol/L)]

Age (hrs)	Consider Phototherapy[†]	Phototherapy	Exchange Transfusion if Intensive Phototherapy Fails[‡]	Exchange Transfusion and Intensive Phototherapy
<24[§]	—	—	—	—
25–48	> 12 (170)	> 15 (260)	> 20 (340)	> 25 (430)
49–72	> 15 (260)	> 18 (310)	> 25 (430)	> 30 (510)
>72	> 17 (290)	> 20 (340)	> 25 (430)	> 30 (510)

Adapted from American Academy of Pediatrics, Provisional Committee for Quality Improvement and Subcommittee on Hyperbilirubinemia: Practice parameter: Management of hyperbilirubinemia in the healthy term newborn. Pediatrics 94:560, 1994.
* TSB indicates total serum bilirubin.
[†] Phototherapy at these TSB levels is a clinical option, meaning that the intervention is available and may be used on the basis of individual clinical judgment.
[‡] Intensive phototherapy should produce a decline of TSB of 1–2 mg/dl within 4–6 hours and the TSB level should continue to fall and remain below the threshold level for exchange transfusion. If this does not occur, it is considered a failure of phototherapy.
[§] Term infants who are clinically jaundiced at < 24 hours old are not considered healthy and require further evaluation (see text).

C. Phototherapy

1. Phototherapy

Phototherapy is the standard treatment for significant hyperbilirubinemia because it is effective, safe, and relatively noninvasive.[18] The principle behind phototherapy is that light converts bilirubin into isomeric forms that are less toxic and more easily excreted than native bilirubin itself. The effectiveness of phototherapy is determined by the spectrum of light delivered, the energy output of the light in the blue spectrum (measured in $\mu W/cm^2$), and the surface area of the infant exposed to treatment.[1]

2. Types of phototherapy

No single choice of light for phototherapy is favored by evidence, and commonly used phototherapy units may contain daylight, cool white, blue, or special blue (narrow spectrum) fluorescent tubes.[1] Fiberoptic blankets are as effective as conventional phototherapy units, and they eliminate the need for eye patches and permit more time for mother–infant bonding.[3] Standard phototherapy may be interrupted for feedings or brief parental visits.

3. Intensive phototherapy

Intensive phototherapy differs from standard phototherapy in that more than one light source is typically used, the lights are brought to within 15–20 cm of the infant, and skin exposure is maximized. Special blue tubes in standard fluorescent phototherapy units may be placed above the infant, while additional blue or daylight tubes are used on either side. Similarly, a standard phototherapy unit above the infant with a fiberoptic blanket below is a form of intensive phototherapy that is significantly more effective than single phototherapy.[1,3] For TBS $\geq$ 20–25mg/dl, continuous intensive phototherapy should be employed until a satisfactory decline occurs.

4. Monitoring for side effects

Infants undergoing phototherapy should be carefully monitored for side effects, such as overheating and increased insensible water loss. Retinal damage is a hypothetical concern with overhead lights, for which the infant's eyes are shielded with a soft mask. Less frequently observed side effects include diarrhea, hypocalcemia, riboflavin deficiency, hyperpigmentation, and bronzing.

D. Exchange Transfusion

1. Indications

Exchange transfusion is needed for the rare infant with extreme hyperbilirubinemia unresponsive to intensive phototherapy. In addition to providing a rapid and dramatic decline in TSB levels, an exchange transfusion will remove the majority of sensitized or abnormal red blood cells in cases of hemolysis.[22]

2. Complications of exchange transfusion

These include electrolyte disturbances, hypoglycemia, thrombocytopenia, necrotizing enterocolitis, and cardiac arrest. The mortality rate for exchange transfusion is estimated at 3 per 1000 procedures.[4,7] It is best performed in a referral center by experienced clinicians who have carefully assessed the risks and benefits for the infant involved.

E. Metalloporphyrins

Metalloporphyrins are heme analogs that interrupt bilirubin formation by inhibiting the enzyme heme oxygenase.[17,20] Tin-mesoporphyrin (SnMP) and tin-protoporphyrin (SnPP) have been investigated in clinical trials outside the United States.[6] The intramuscular injection of SnMP (6 μmol/kg) in healthy term or near-term infants, although still considered investigational, is a promising approach to preventing neonatal jaundice.

VI. Adverse Effects of Extreme Hyperbilirubinemia
A. Kernicterus
The term kernicterus was first used in the early 1900s to describe a yellow staining seen on autopsy analysis in the basal ganglia of infants dying with severe jaundice. Kernicterus also refers to the acute and chronic clinical syndromes associated with bilirubin encephalopathy.[3]

1. Acute bilirubin encephalopathy

This occurs in the immediate newborn period. An acute rise in TSB is accompanied by lethargy, poor feeding, high-pitched cry, sensorineural hearing loss, abnormal tone, and an evolving series of neurologic abnormalities. Seizures and death may occur.[3]

2. Chronic bilirubin encephalopathy

This entity develops over months to years following the acute insult. It is characterized by severe neurologic abnormalities, including motor delay, athetoid cerebral palsy, paralysis of upward gaze, sensorineural hearing loss, and dental dysplasia. Cognitive dysfunction and mental retardation can occur.[3]

3. Less severe bilirubin toxicity.

There is ongoing controversy about the existence of a less severe form of bilirubin encephalopathy that is asymptomatic in the newborn period but associated with subtle deficits in hearing, neurodevelopment or intellectual capacity later in life.[1,15]

B. Mechanism of Bilirubin Deposition in the Central Nervous System
Bilirubin is a polar compound that diffuses across the blood–brain barrier in its unbound form. Low serum albumin levels and drugs that displace bilirubin from albumin (such as sulfa drugs, salicylates, and indomethacin) increase the risk for bilirubin toxicity. Other conditions that favor bilirubin passage through the blood–brain barrier include infection, acidosis, anoxia, and hypertonic intravenous infusions. Sick or preterm infants are particularly likely to experience these conditions and are therefore at increased risk for kernicterus as compared to healthy term newborns.[1]

C. Relationship between Kernicterus and Peak Bilirubin Level
In early case reports, kernicterus occurred in infants with significant hemolysis due to Rh or ABO isoimmunization and was avoided when exchange transfusions were used to keep TSB below 20 mg/dl.[5] Currently, there is no evidence to suggest that bilirubin is more toxic to the newborn with hemolysis than to the newborn with a similar TSB level but without hemolysis. Although factors influencing bilirubin toxicity are complex and TSB may not be the most important factor related to risk for a given infant, kernicterus is likely with TSB levels exceeding 30 mg/dl and unlikely with levels less than 20mg/dl.[3]

References
1. American Academy of Pediatrics, Provisional Committee for Quality Improvement and Subcommittee on Hyperbilirubinemia: Practice parameter: Management of hyperbilirubinemia in the healthy term newborn. Pediatrics 94:558–565, 1994.
2. Eggert LD, Pollary RA, Folland DS, et al: Home phototherapy treatment of neonatal jaundice. Pediatrics 76:579–584, 1985.
3. Gourley GR: Bilirubin metabolism and kernicterus. Adv Pediatr 44:173–229, 1997.
4. Hovi L, Siimes MA: Exchange transfusion with fresh heparinized blood is a safe procedure: Experience from 1069 newborns. Acta Pediatr Scand 774:360–365, 1985.
5. Hsia DY, Allen FH, Gellis SS, Drummond LK: Erythroblastosis fetalis, VIII: Studies of serum bilirubin in relation to kernicterus. N Engl J Med 247:668–671, 1952.
6. Kappas A, Drummond GS, Henschke C, et al: Direct comparison of Sn-mesoporphyrin, and inhibitor of bilirubin production, and phototherapy in controlling hyperbilirubinemia in term and near-term newborns. Pediatrics 95:468–474, 1995.

7. Keenan WJ, Novak KK, Sutherland JM et al: Morbidity and mortality associated with exchange transfusion. Pediatrics 75(Suppl):417–421, 1985.
8. Kramer LI: Advancement of dermal icterus in the jaundiced newborn. Am J Dis Child 118:454–458, 1969.
9. Liu LL, Clemens CJ, Shay DK, et al: The safety of newborn early discharge: The Washington state experience. JAMA 278:293–298, 1997.
10. Maisels MJ, Gifford K: Neonatal jaundice in full-term infants: role of breast-feeding and other causes. Am J Dis Child 137:561–562, 1983.
11. Maisels MJ, Newman TB: Jaundice in full-term and near-term babies who leave the hospital within 36 hours: The pediatrician's nemesis. Clin Perinatol 25:295–302, 1998.
12. Maisels MJ, Newman TB: Kernicterus in otherwise healthy, breast-fed term newborns. Pediatrics 96:730–733, 1995.
13. Martinez JC, Maisels MJ, Otheguy L, et al: Hyperbilirubinemia in the breast-fed newborn: A controlled trial of four interventions. Pediatrics 91:470–473, 1993.
14. Monaghan G, Mclellan A, McGeehan A, et al: Gilbert's syndrome is a contributory factor in prolonged unconjugated hyperbilirubinemia of the newborn. J Pediatr 134:441–446, 1999.
15. Newman TB, Maisels MJ: Evaluation and treatment of jaundice in the term newborn: A kinder, gentler approach. Pediatrics 89:809–818, 1992.
16. Osborn LM, Bolus R: Breast-feeding and jaundice in the first week of life. J Fam Pract 20:475–480, 1985.
17. Rubaltelli FF: Current drug treatment options in neonatal hyperbilirubinaemia and the prevention of kernicterus. Drugs 56:23–30, 1998.
18. Scheidt PC, Bryla DA, Nelson KB, et al: Phototherapy for neonatal hyperbilirubinema: Six-year follow-up of the National Institute of Child Health and Human Development Clinical Trail. Pediatrics 85:455–463, 1990.
19. Schneider AP: Breast milk jaundice in the newborn: A real entity. JAMA 255:3270–3274, 1986.
20. Steffensrud S: Tin-metalloporphyrins: An answer to neonatal jaundice? Neonatal Network 17:11–17, 1998.
21. Tan KL: Decreased response to phototherapy for neonatal jaundice in breast-fed infants. Arch Pediatr Adolesc Med 152:1187–1190, 1998.
22. Thilo EH, Rosenberg AA: The newborn infant. In Hay WW, Hayward AR, Levin MJ, Sondheimer JM (eds): Current Pediatric Diagnosis and Treatment, 14th ed. New York, Appleton & Lange, 1999, pp 29–33.
23. Wiley CC, Lai N, Hill C, et al: Nursery practices and detection of jaundice after newborn discharge. Arch Pediatr Adolesc Med 152:972–975, 1998.

SECTION E.
EVALUATION AND MANAGEMENT OF INFECTION IN THE NEWBORN

I. Introduction

Infants in the first month of life can become infected with a variety of bacterial and viral pathogens. There are three main routes of infection—transplacental (blood-borne), ascending (following disruption of the amniotic membranes), and direct contact (passage through an infected birth canal or exposure to infected blood at delivery).[13] Diagnosing a septic infant can be challenging since the symptoms are nonspecific and may initially be subtle. Management strategies may include preventive actions taken at the time of delivery (e.g., cesarean section for active maternal genital herpes, antibiotic prophylaxis for group B streptococcus) and careful monitoring in the newborn nursery for infants at high risk of developing infection. It may involve transfer to an intensive care unit for evaluation and treatment in cases when clinical signs of infection develop.

II. Bacterial Sepsis in Newborns
A. Definitions, Incidence, and Pathogenesis

Bacterial sepsis in newborns is characterized as either early- or late-onset.

1. Early-onset sepsis

Early-onset infections occur during the first week of life, with an incidence of 4–5 cases per 1000 live births.[13] Group B streptococcus (GBS) has been the most common cause of early-onset infection. Gram-negative enteric organisms such as *Escherichia coli* and *Klebsiella pneumoniae* are other common pathogens, and *Haemophilus influenzae* is occasionally responsible.[4,13] Many infants with early-onset disease are infected from birth and manifest symptoms within the first 24 hours of life.[13]

2. Late-onset sepsis

Late-onset infections begin after the first week of life. They may be caused by coagulase-negative staphylococci (especially in infants with central venous lines), *Staphylococcus aureus*, GBS, enterococcus, pseudomonas, and other gram-negative organisms.[13]

B. Risk Factors and Protective Factors

1. Prolonged rupture of membranes and chorioamnionitis (see Chapter 15, section C)

Rupture of the amniotic membranes for over 24 hours increases the rate of neonatal infection to 1 in 100 live births. If chorioamnionitis is present, the rate increases to 1 in 10 live births.[13]

2. Prematurity

Preterm infants are five times more susceptible to infection than term infants. This is due to the immaturity of their cellular and humoral immune systems. In addition, infants born preterm lack a portion of the maternal IgG normally transferred across the placenta during the third trimester.[13]

3. Epidural analgesia

Epidural analgesia has not been shown to be a risk factor for neonatal sepsis. However, the rise in maternal temperature that occurs in association with epidural analgesia can suggest the possibility of chorioamnionitis. In one study of 1657 nulliparous women at term, 14.5% of those who received epidurals developed temperatures > 100.4°F, compared to 1.0% of controls who did not. As a result, infants of the women who received epidurals were four times as likely to be evaluated for sepsis (OR = 4.3, 95% CI = 3.2–5.9) and treated with antibiotics (OR = 3.9, 95% CI = 2.1–6.1).[8]

4. Protective factors

Exclusive breastfeeding has been shown to reduce the incidence of early-onset sepsis in a case-control study (odds ratio 0.33, 95% CI 0.1–0.8).[4]

C. Signs of Sepsis

1. Clinical signs

There are many clinical signs of sepsis in newborns. Unanticipated low Apgar scores,[4] poor perfusion, and hypotension can be signs of sepsis at birth. Respiratory distress is the most common sign during the first 24–48 hours of life. Persistent tachypnea (respiratory rate over 60 breaths/minute), retracting, and failure to maintain adequate oxygenation are the typical clinical picture. Other warning signs include temperature instability (temperatures < 36.5°C or > 37.5°C), sustained tachycardia (heart rate > 160 beats/minute), lethargy, hypotonia, poor feeding, vomiting, abdominal distension and unexplained jaundice.[1,7]

2. Laboratory tests

    a. Presumptive tests. No single laboratory test or panel of tests has achieved success in accurately predicting the presence of infection in at-risk or symptomatic newborns. Many markers have been evaluated for predictive value, including the white blood cell count, absolute neutrophil count, immature/total neutrophil ratio (I:T ratio), C-reactive protein (CRP), and erythrocyte sedimentation rate (ESR).[7] The range of values used to predict infection, as well as positive and negative predictive values of the tests, are shown in Table 15. In general, negative tests are better at excluding infection than positive tests are in predicting infections subsequently confirmed with blood cultures. Other laboratory abnormalities associated with neonatal infection include thrombocytopenia, hypoglycemia, and hyperbilirubinemia.

TABLE 15. Presumptive Tests for Predicting Neonatal Infection[7]

Test	Cut-off Values for Predicting Infection	Positive Predictive Value %	Negative Predictive Value %
WBC	< 5000/mm^3	27	92
ANC	< 1500–1750 mm^3	na	na
I:T ratio	> 20%	11	100
C-reactive protein	Positive (at 0.8 mg/dl)	28	99
ESR	> 10 mm/hr days 0–3; > 15 mm/hr thereafter	24	95

WBC, white blood cell count; ANC, absolute neutrophil count; I:T, immature/total neutrophil ratio; ESR= erythrocyte sedimentation rate; na, data not available from the referenced study. In this study, the tests were performed twice—on admission and 12–24 hours later.

    b. Cultures. Cultures from blood, cerebral spinal fluid, or another normally sterile source are considered standard for documenting neonatal infection.[1] Surface cultures and cultures of gastric aspirates are not sufficiently accurate to be clinically helpful.[5]

    c. Urine GBS antigen test. The result of a single urine latex agglutination test is not helpful for predicting GBS sepsis. The false-positive rates of the test are as high as 30%,[14] while the false-negative rates have been found to be 43%.[3]

    d. Chest x-ray. A chest x-ray is useful for ruling out other causes of respiratory distress, such as a pnuemothorax or congenital anomalies of the heart or lungs. The presence of infiltrates on the chest x-ray is a nonspecific finding, seen with pnuemonia, atelectasis, or excessive interstitial fluid.

    e. Lumbar puncture. The role of lumbar puncture in evaluating asymptomatic newborns at risk for sepsis remains uncertain.[1] Some authors find that lumbar puncture is unnecessary for the term infant with risk factors but no clinical signs of sepsis, since meningitis occurs in at most 4 per 1,000 infants in that situation.[6] Another retrospective study, however, observed that 37% (16 of 43 infants) with culture-proven meningitis would have escaped diagnosis if lumbar puncture had not routinely been performed.[15] The American Academy of Pediatrics states that a lumbar puncture may be performed at the discretion of the physician as part of a full diagnostic evaluation for sepsis.[2]

D. Group B Streptococcal Infections
  1. Rationale for GBS prevention
Because group B streptococcal infections are a leading cause of neonatal morbidity and mortality in the United States, they have been targeted for aggressive preventive measures. In 1996, the CDC issued guidelines for intrapartum antibiotic prophylaxis (IAP) to reduce the vertical transmission of GBS and the subsequent occurrence of early-onset GBS sepsis. Maternal indications for IAP for GBS as well as recommended drugs and doses are described in Chapter 8, section A.

  2. Management of infants whose mothers received IAP or who are GBS-positive
The American Academy of Pediatrics has developed guidelines for managing newborns whose mothers were colonized or at risk for colonization with GBS at the time of delivery. These guidelines are based on expert opinion, as other evidence is not yet available. An algorithm for empirical management of infants born to mothers receiving intrapartum antibiotics for GBS is given in Figure 5. It is important to remember that the majority will be term infants, without symptoms,

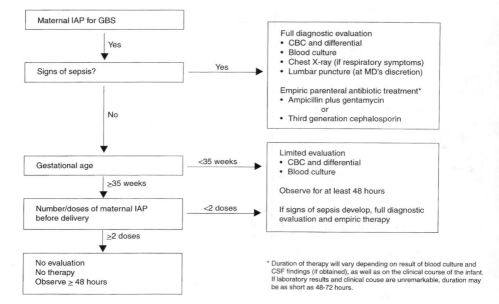

FIGURE 5. Empiric management of newborns whose mothers receive intrapartum antibiotic prophylaxis (IAP) against early-onset group B streptococcal infection. (Adapted from American Academy of Pediatrics Committee on Infectious Diseases and Committee on Fetus and Newborn: Revised guidelines for prevention of early-onset group B streptococcal (GBS) infection. Pediatrics 99:493, 1997.)

whose mothers received two or more doses of penicillin or ampicillin. These infants can be regarded as healthy, low-risk newborns requiring nothing more than 48 hours of hospital observation.[2]

  a. Monitoring vital signs and clinical activity. A minimum stay of 48 hours in the newborn nursery is recommended for any infant whose mother had a positive culture for GBS prenatally or who received antibiotics for GBS prophylaxis during labor.[2] GBS risk factors should be documented on the infant's record and regular vital signs obtained. Clinical signs of sepsis are those described above.

  b. Risk factors that require further infant evaluation for sepsis. In addition to monitoring the infant's vital signs and activity, further evaluation may be required depending on:
    i. adequacy of maternal antibiotic doses
    ii. infant's gestational age
    iii. clinical signs of GBS infection

  c. Adequacy of maternal antibiotic doses. Intrapartum antibiotics are effective in preventing early onset GBS disease, defined as onset within the first 7 days of life, when the mother has received at least two doses. In one study, infants of GBS-colonized mothers who had received intravenous ampicillin more than 4 hours prior to delivery (i.e., two or more doses) showed no laboratory or clinical evidence of GBS infection; by comparison, one dose alone was not fully protective.[9]

  d. Gestational age. Premature infants are at a 10–15-fold increased risk for developing GBS sepsis compared to term infants.[11] In addition, signs of sepsis may be subtle in premature infants. Infants less than 35 weeks' gestation who are high risk for GBS by virtue of maternal history require at least a limited laboratory evaluation with blood culture and a complete blood count with differential.

e. Signs of GBS infection. Early-onset GBS disease presents as bacteremia (80% of cases), pneumonia (7%), or meningitis (6%).[10] More than 95% of infants with early-onset GBS show symptoms within 48 hours of birth,[11] with the majority of cases at less than 12 hours.

3. Effectiveness of IAP for GBS

According to a meta-analysis of five clinical trials, comprehensive strategies for intrapartum antibiotic prophylaxis against GBS have been successful in reducing the rates of infant colonization and early-onset neonatal infection.[12] A multicenter epidemiologic surveillance study has also documented a decline in incidence of early-onset GBS disease coincident with wider use of intrapartum antibiotics.[10] Age- and race-adjusted annual incidence of GBS sepsis was 1.8 cases of per 1000 live births in 1990, resulting in 310 deaths.[2] By 1998, the incidence had declined to 0.6 per 1000, with an estimated 200 neonatal deaths prevented.[10]

E. Treatment

1. Transfer

Any infant with a clinical picture suggesting sepsis, pneumonia, or meningitis should be transferred from the normal newborn nursery to a level 2 or 3 nursery for a full diagnostic evaluation and empiric antibiotic treatment.

2. Recommended antibiotics

The initial choice of antibiotic is aimed at broad-spectrum coverage appropriate for GBS and other common pathogens. Recommended options include the combination of ampicillin 100 mg/kg/d divided every 12 hours, plus gentamicin 2.5 mg/kg/dose every 12–24 hours depending on gestational age, or cefotaxime 100 mg/kg/d divided every 12 hours.[2] The antibiotic choice can be adjusted based on results of cultures and sensitivities. Sepsis is treated for 10–14 days. Meningitis requires 21 days of treatment.[13]

III. Viral Infections in Newborns

Viral infections in newborns may be acquired either in utero (congenital infection) or at the time of delivery. Congenital infections include cytomegalovirus, rubella, varicella, and syphilis. Examples of perinatally acquired infections include herpes simplex, hepatitis, and HIV. Perinatal aspects of these infections are discussed in Chapter 8, section A.

References

1. Allen SR: Management of asymptomatic term neonates whose mothers received intrapartum antibiotics—Part 2: Diagnostic tests and management strategies. Clin Pediatr 36:617–624, 1997.
2. American Academy of Pediatrics Committee on Infectious Diseases and Committee on Fetus and Newborn: Revised guidelines for prevention of early-onset group B streptococcal (GBS) infection. Pediatrics 99:489–495, 1997.
3. Becker JA, Ascher DP, Mendiola J, et al: False-negative urine latex particle agglutination testing in neonates with group B streptococcal bacteremia. Clin Pediatr 32:467–471, 1993.
4. Bhutta ZA, Yusuf K: Early-onset neonatal sepsis in Pakistan: A case-control study of risk factors in a birth cohort. Am J Perinatol 14:577–581, 1997.
5. Dobson SRM, Isaacs D, Wilkinson AR, et al: Reduced use of surface cultures for suspected neonatal sepsis and surveillance. Arch Dis Child 67:44–47, 1992.
6. Fielkow S, Reuter S, Gotoff SP: Cerebrospinal fluid examination in symptom-free infants with risk factors for infection. J Pediatr 119:971–973, 1991.
7. Gerdes JS, Polin RA: Sepsis screen in neonates with evaluation of plasma fibronectin. Pediatr Infect Dis J 6:443–446, 1987.

8. Lieberman E, Lang JM, Frigoletto F, et al: Epidural analgesia, intrapartum fever, and neonatal sepsis evaluation. Pediatrics 99:415–419, 1997.
9. Pylipow M, Gaddis M, Kinney JS: Selective intrapartum prophylaxis for group B streptococcus colonization: Management and outcome of newborns. Pediatrics 93:631–635, 1994.
10. Schraig SJ, Zywicki S, Farley M, et al: Group B streptococcal disease in the era of intrapartum antibiotic prophylaxis. N Engl J Med 342:15–20, 2000.
11. Schuchat A, Deaver-Robinson K, Plikaytis BD, et al: Multi-state case-control study of maternal risk factors for neonatal group B streptococcal disease. Pediatr Infect Dis J 13:623–629, 1994.
12. Smaill F: Intrapartum antibiotics for group B streptococcal colonisation (Cochrane Review). In The Cochrane Library, Issue 3. Oxford, Update Software, 2000.
13. Thilo EH, Rosenberg AA: The newborn infant. In Hay WW, Hayward AR, Levin MJ, Sondheimer JM (eds): Current Pediatric Diagnosis and Treatment, 14th ed. New York, Appleton & Lange, 1999, pp 61–64.
14. Williamson M, Fraser SH, Tilse M: Failure of the urinary group B streptococcal antigen test as a screen for neonatal sepsis. Arch Dis Child Fetal Neonatal Ed 73:F109–F111, 1995.
15. Wiswell TE, Baumgart S, Gannon CM et al: No lumbar puncture in the evaluation for early neonatal sepsis: Will meningitis be missed? Pediatrics 95:803–806, 1995.

SECTION F.
INFANT FEEDING AND NUTRITION

Family physicians play important roles in providing parents with information about infant nutritional requirements and optimal feeding practices. The physician may also help by supporting the mother's decision to bottle- or breastfeed. Qualified nursing personnel and trained lactation consultants can enhance the physician's efforts by working closely with mothers and infants in the immediate postpartum period.

I. Breastfeeding
A. Advantages for Infants
Human breast milk is widely recognized as the ideal source of infant nutrition. It provides adequate calories for optimal growth and development, appropriately distributed among protein, fats, and carbohydrates. In addition, colostrum and breast milk together contain many immunologic factors that are not present in commercial formulas—including secretory IgA, lysozyme, lactoferrin, bifidus factor, and macrophages.[5] Infants fed human milk have been shown in epidemiologic studies to have a decreased incidence of diarrhea, lower respiratory infection, otitis media, bacterial meningitis, urinary tract infection, and necrotizing enterocolitis. In addition, an infant diet of human milk appears to confer a measure of protection against certain chronic illnesses, including insulin-dependent diabetes mellitus, Crohn's disease, ulcerative colitis, lymphoma, and allergic conditions.[3] A detailed discussion of the advantages of breastfeeding appears in Chapter 3, section D.
B. Prevalence
In the late 1990s, 64% of mothers breastfed their infants in the early postpartum period and 29% continued for 6 months. National goals as outlined in Healthy People 2010 are to increase the percent of women who breastfeed to 75% in the early postpartum period, 50% at 6 months, and 25% at one year.[10] Factors influencing breastfeeding rates are discussed in Chapter 19, section C.
C. Breastfeeding Routines[3] (see also Chapter 3, section D)
1. Initiating breastfeeding
Breastfeeding should be initiated as soon as possible post-partum. Many mother–infant pairs are able to begin nursing within the first hour of life.
2. Rooming-in
Rooming-in is desirable because it enhances the full-time, exclusive nature of the early breastfeeding experience.

3. On-demand feeding

An on-demand feeding schedule is optimal. Infant signs of hunger include increased alertness and activity, mouthing, and rooting. Crying is a late sign of hunger.

Breastfed infants require frequent feedings. (The gastric emptying time for breast milk is 1.5 hours, compared to nearly 4 hours for formula.) Mothers should be prepared initially to nurse their infants every 2 to 2.5 hours, or approximately 8–12 times in 24 hours.

4. Supplementation

No supplements such as formula, water, or dextrose solutions should be given to breastfeeding newborns unless there is a specific medical indication.

5. Early discharge

The American Academy of Pediatrics recommends that when a breastfeeding infant is discharged less than 48 hours after birth, there should be follow-up at 2 to 4 days of age for evaluation of successful breastfeeding behavior.[3]

D. Pumping and Storing Breast Milk

1. Role of pumps

Women may experience difficulty in pumping a significant volume of breast milk before letdown is well established. Hospital-style electronic pumps can be helpful, particularly in the early postpartum period.

2. Storage

Pumped breast milk can be safely stored at room temperature for 8 hours, or kept in the refrigerator at 0°–4°C for 72 hours with no degradation of its many beneficial constituents.[7] Freezing allows the milk to be stored for up to 6 months, although cellular activity and concentrations of vitamins B_6 and C are decreased.[7] A clean plastic or glass container may be used, although glass has the potential to break with freezing. Milk may be thawed in the refrigerator or under running water. Once thawed, any milk not used within 24 hours should be discarded.[6]

E. Contraindications to Breastfeeding

1. Maternal conditions

Mothers who are unable to discontinue illicit drug use, those taking certain medications (radioactive isotopes, antimetabolites, cancer chemotherapy agents, and a few others),[1] and those with active infectious tuberculosis should not breastfeed. Women who are positive for the human immunodeficiency virus (HIV) have a small chance of transmitting infection to their infants through breast milk and in the U.S. are generally counseled not to breastfeed.[3] Mothers positive for hepatitis B surface antigen (HBsAg) who have a strong desire to breastfeed may do so, provided the infant received appropriate vaccination within 12 hours of birth (see section A).[5]

2. Infant conditions

Galactosemia in the infant is one widely recognized contraindication to breastfeeding; otherwise, infant contraindications are rare. Human milk is the preferred feeding for preterm infants and infants with most medical conditions. When direct breastfeeding is not possible, pumped breast milk should be considered the first alternative.[3]

F. Vitamin and Mineral Supplements for the Breastfed Infant

1. Vitamin K

Low levels of vitamin K in breast milk make it advisable for the infant to receive the standard dose of parenteral vitamin K in the newborn nursery.[4]

2. Vitamin D

Vitamin D may be given as a supplement to infants at high risk of deficiency, such as those not exposed to adequate sunlight or those with mothers who are vitamin D-deficient.[3]

3. Thiamine (B_1), cobalamin (B_{12}), and folate

Deficiencies of B_1, B_{12} and folate develop uncommonly in breastfed infants; they are usually associated with problems in the mother's dietary intake or absorption of these vitamins.[5]

  a. Thiamine deficiency. This condition may develop if the mother is alcoholic or has a poor diet.

  b. B_{12} deficiency. This may occur in infants of mothers with untreated pernicious anemia or an unsupplemented vegetarian diet.

  c. Maternal folate deficiency. This deficiency can result in a similar deficiency in the infant, particularly in preterm infants.

4. Iron

Iron is well absorbed by breastfed infants, who acquire 0.06 mg/kg per day of iron from breast milk. This daily intake, combined with iron stores accumulated in utero, gives the healthy breastfed infant enough iron to meet ongoing requirements without supplementation for the first 6 months of life.[2] Certain high-risk infants, or those with documented anemia, are candidates for iron supplementation. For example, infants of poorly controlled diabetics and small-for-gestational-age and preterm infants are born with reduced iron stores and may be at risk.[2]

5. Fluoride

Although the addition of fluoride to municipal water supplies has been an important public health measure for reducing dental caries among U.S. children, excessive supplementation can lead to dental fluorosis (cosmetic dental changes ranging from white striations to brownish-gray strains). Fluoride supplements are not recommended for infants less than 6 months of age. This applies to both bottle- and breastfed infants, regardless of the amount of fluoride in the municipal water supply.[3]

II. Bottlefeeding

Bottlefeeding with commercial infant formula fails to confer the nutritive, immunologic, and developmental advantages of breastfeeding. It is an alternative to consider when breastfeeding is unacceptable to the mother, when breastfeeding has failed despite best attempts at education and management of common minor difficulties, or when maternal circumstances such as illness or employment dictate. Commercial infant formulas are manufactured either from cow's milk or soy-based protein. Formulas are patterned as closely as possible after human breast milk and are fortified with selected vitamins and minerals.

A. Preparation and Storage of Infant Formula[6]

1. Types of infant formula

Infant formula comes in three types: ready to feed, liquid concentrate, and powder. Ready-to-feed formula is conveniently pre-diluted, and is the most expensive. Concentrated formula must be mixed 1:1 with water. Powdered formula is the most economical choice, prepared as one scoop to 2 ounces of water.

2. Formula preparation

Boiling the water is not necessary when sanitized city water is used. To alleviate concerns of lead contamination from water pipes, parents may let tap water run for 2 minutes before mixing it with formula.

3. Warming formula

Once prepared, formulas may be heated by warm running water, in a bottle warmer, or on the stove. Microwave heating is sometimes discouraged because it may cause "hot spots" in formula; at a minimum, thorough mixing is required after heating.

4. Shelf life of opened formula

Once opened, cans of liquid formula or concentrate should be refrigerated and used within 48 hours. Diluted formula should be used within 24 hours.

5. Bottlefeeding routines

During the first days of life, formula-fed newborns will take ½ to 1 ounce every 3–5 hours. By the end of the first week, amounts have increased to 1–3 ounces per feeding. By the end of the first month, a typical feeding schedule will be 2–4 ounces, 7–8 times a day.

B. Vitamin and Mineral Fortification

1. Iron

Infant formulas are classified as low-iron or iron-fortified. Iron-fortified formulas range in concentration from 10–12 mg/L, which are adequate amounts to meet requirements for the first 12 months of life (assuming the addition of appropriate solid foods in the second 6 months). Low-iron formulas contain 1.1–4.5 mg/L, a range that fails to meet minimum iron requirements for infants and results in unacceptably high rates of iron deficiency by age 9 months.[2] Controlled studies have found no difference between low-iron and iron-fortified formulas in the occurrence of infant gastrointestinal disturbances such as fussiness, cramping, colic, reflux or gas.[8,9] Iron-fortified formulas are therefore the preferred option.

2. Fluoride

Ready-to-feed formulas have fluoride concentrations less than 0.3 ppm, the minimum standard beyond which supplementation is recommended. Infants older than 6 months who are maintained exclusively on ready-to-feed formulas with no additional fluoride intake from fluoridated municipal water or other sources therefore require fluoride supplementation. The concentration of fluoride in bottled waters is variable. Parents should be discouraged from using bottled water for preparing powdered or concentrated formula.[6]

References

1. American Academy of Pediatrics Committee on Drugs: The transfer of drugs and other chemicals into human milk. Pediatrics 93:137–150, 1994.
2. American Academy of Pediatrics Committee on Nutrition: Iron fortification of infant formulas. Pediatrics 104:119–123, 1999.
3. American Academy of Pediatrics Work Group on Breastfeeding: Breastfeeding and the use of human milk (RE9727). Pediatrics 100:1035–1039, 1997.
4. Greer FR: Vitamin K status of lactating mothers and their infants. Acta Paediatr Suppl 430:95–103, 1999.
5. Howard CR, Weitzman M: Breast or bottle: Practical aspects of infant nutrition in the first 6 months. Pediatr Ann 21:619–621, 1992.
6. Krebs NF, Hambidge KM: Normal childhood nutrition and its disorders. In Hay WW, Hayward AR, Levin MJ, Sondheimer JM (eds): Current Pediatric Diagnosis and Treatment, 14h ed. New York, Appleton & Lange, 1999, pp 246–271.
7. Lawrence RA: Storage of human milk and the influence of procedures on immunological components of human milk. Acta Paediatr 88:14-18, 1999.
8. Nelson SE, Ziegler EE, Copeland AM, et al: Lack of adverse reactions to iron-fortified formula. Pediatrics 81:360–364, 1988.
9. Oski FA: Iron-fortified formulas and gastrointestinal symptoms in infants: A controlled study. Pediatrics 66:168–170, 1980.
10. U.S. Department of Health and Human Services. Healthy People 2010: Understanding and improving health. January 2000. http://www.health.gov/healthypeople/default.htm

SECTION G.
BONDING AND FAMILY ADAPTATION

I. Background

Bonding is defined as a positive, emotionally based relationship between infant and parent that is long-term, reciprocal, and includes the concept of attachment. Secure infant attachment develops over time as a mother or other primary caretaker who is sensitive to infant behavioral cues consistently and appropriately meets the infant's needs.[4] By age 12–18 months, the infant develops a characteristic attachment style that can be objectively judged to be either secure or insecure. The importance of attachment cannot be overstated. Investigations have repeatedly shown that infants whose relationship with their parents can be characterized as secure look more competent as toddlers and preschoolers. In fact, some authorities consider security of attachment to be of paramount importance to mental health across the life span.[14,15]

Early studies of bonding indicated that maternal-infant contact within the first 3 hours of birth, combined with extended contact in a rooming-in arrangement, could lead to significant positive effects on subsequent maternal behavior.[8] Additional research over the past 20 years, however, has been unable to substantiate whether there is a "sensitive period" after birth during which bonding must take place, how long the sensitive period may last, and how much and what type of maternal-infant contact is optimal for bonding.[11] Nevertheless, it is highly consistent with the philosophy of family-centered perinatal care to provide opportunities for appropriate physical contact and to educate parents regarding the physiologic and emotional responses of infants and parents throughout pregnancy, birth, and postpartum period. Family physicians may find themselves in a position to review and modify existing hospital routines that arbitrarily interrupt the bonding process.

II. Prenatal Bonding
A. Origins of Maternal Attachment
Maternal attachment to the infant may begin to develop during the prenatal period.[11,13] The family physician can assess the level of emotional attachment by talking to the mother about her emotional acceptance of the pregnancy, the amount of social support she has for child-rearing, what fantasies she has for her baby's future, and what physical preparations she has made for the infant's arrival. Failure to exhibit expected responses may be a clue to a high-risk situation in which additional social services or supports may be needed.

B. Paternal Attachment before Birth
It has become common to invite the father to prenatal visits. Both parents appear to be emotionally affected by experiences such as hearing the fetal heartbeat or viewing the infant via ultrasound. However, the outcomes of such experiences on paternal attachment have not been well studied.

III. Bonding after Birth
A. Sensory Components
1. Tactile sensation

Tactile sensation plays a key role in the bonding process. Parents tend to touch their newborns in a specific pattern, fondling the hands and feet before touching the body, implying an innate process. Tactile stimulation enhances the parent–child relationship from the beginning, providing relaxation and comfort. Direct skin-to-skin contact has been recommended.[8,11] In a trial designed to test the hypothesis that increased physical contact promotes secure infant attachment, mothers of newborns were randomized to receive either a soft infant carrier or a plastic car seat when discharged from the hospital. Infants whose mothers kept them in close body contact with the soft carrier were significantly more likely to be securely attached at 1 year of age.[3]

2. Mother's voice

The mother's voice is familiar to the infant from many months of in utero perception. Tone, pitch, cadence, and accent all contribute to familiarity and comfort. Newborns show a significant preference for voices speaking the language they heard in utero.[5] Parents may be encouraged to talk, hum, or sing to the newborn.

3. Eye contact

This plays an important role in initial parent–infant bonding. Mothers and their infants exhibit a preference for viewing one another at close range with eyes aligned, the en face position. Drops or ointments used to prevent newborn conjunctivitis can cause irritation and tearing. Instillation may be postponed for 1 hour, until after the initial bonding experiences with mother and father.[11] Parents should be informed that the baby focuses best at a distance of several inches, roughly from the crook of the parent's arm to the face.

4. Nursing and bonding

Mother's milk is surely among the strongest stimuli for attachment, having psychobiologic effects beyond its nutritive value. Although breastfeeding is a powerful bonding influence, it is not strictly essential. Mothers who choose to bottlefeed should be particularly encouraged to engage in other bonding behaviors.[12]

B. Emotional Components

Most mothers, though certainly not all, develop maternal feelings for their infants the first time they hold the baby. The typical experience is a surge of affection followed by a feeling that the baby belongs to her. The emotional bonding response may be delayed due to medical emergencies or under conditions of maternal addiction or depression. Parents should be assured that a satisfying bonding experience can still occur after such conditions have stabilized.[12,13] In cases of cesarean section delivery under regional anesthesia, the mother should be given the opportunity to view and touch her infant while still in the operating room.

C. Rooming In

Rooming in should be encouraged because of the extended opportunities it allows for parent–infant contact.

IV. Bonding and Attachment Issues for the Father and Other Family Members

A. Paternal Bonding

No conclusive statements can be made about the effects of paternal birth attendance, early contact, and extended contact on the father's subsequent involvement with the infant.[9] Many of the factors involved in maternal bonding may also experienced by the father. Voice, eye, and body contact, with its accompanying warmth, motion, and breathing rhythm, can be encouraged for the father as he interacts with his baby in the delivery room and thereafter.

B. Sibling Bonding

Sibling visits can be encouraged in the immediate postpartum period, although the effects of visits on sibling attachment to the new baby are largely unstudied.[1] It is prudent for child with a fever or symptoms of an acute illness, such as upper respiratory infection or gastroenteritis, to be excluded from early visits.[1] Healthy siblings may be taught how to touch, stroke, and speak to the baby within the first days of birth. Allowing a brother or sister of appropriate age to participate in infant care such as feeding or dressing may facilitate positive attachment. Possible sibling jealousy should be anticipated, and clear limits should be set against hitting or rough handling. Sibling classes, analogous to birth preparation classes for parents, are available in some communities. They have not definitively been shown to decrease sibling rivalry or alter reactions to the newborn.[2]

C. Extended Family

The grandmother may be a key support person, particularly for adolescent mothers. One observational study found that infants who were insecurely attached to adolescent mothers were securely attached to the maternal grandmothers who had a significant care-taking role.[10]

V. Marital Adaptation (see Chapter 20, section D)

The first month of the infant's life is a redefining period in the parents' relationship, characterized by vulnerability as well as the potential for growth. Lack of sleep, continuing constraints on the sexual relationship, and new physical, emotional, and financial responsibilities may affect both father and mother. Family physicians may explore issues of marital adjustment during both postpartum and well-infant visits. Satisfactions inherent in the bonding process and adequate support from an extended social network may serve to counteract the frustrations inherent in new parenting roles.[6,7]

References

1. American Academy of Pediatrics and American College of Obstetricians and Gynecologists. Postpartum and follow-up care. In Guidelines for Perinatal Care, 4th ed. 1997, pp 162–164.
2. Anderberg GJ: Initial acquaintance and attachment behavior of siblings with the newborn. J Obstet Gynecol Neonatal Nurs 17:49–54, 1988.
3. Anisfeld E, Casper V, Nozyce M, et al: Does infant carrying promote attachment? An experimental study of the effects of increased physical contact on the development of attachment. Child Dev 61:1617–1627, 1990.
4. Bowlby J: Attachment and Loss, Vol. 1, Attachment. New York, Basic Books, 1982.
5. Fifer WP, Moon CM: The role of mother's voice in the organization of brain function in the newborn. Acta Paediatr Suppl 397:86–93, 1994.
6. Gjerdingen DK, Froberg DG, Fontaine P: The effects of social support on women's health during pregnancy, labor and delivery, and the postpartum period. Fam Med 23:370–375, 1991.
7. Gjerdingen DK, Chaloner KM: The relationship of women's postpartum mental health to employment, childbirth, and social support. J Fam Pract 38:465–472, 1994.
8. Klaus MH, Jerauld R, Kreger NC, et al: Maternal attachment: Importance of the first post-partum days. N Engl J Med 286:460–463, 1972.
9. Palkovitz R: Changes in father-infant bonding beliefs across couples' first transition to parenthood. Matern Child Nurs J 20:141–154, 1992.
10. Patterson DL: Adolescent mothering: Child–grandmother attachment. J Pediatr Nurs 12:228–237, 1997.
11. Symanski ME: Maternal–infant bonding: Practice issues for the 1990s. J Nurse Midwifery 37:67S–73S, 1992.
12. Troy NW: Early contact and maternal attachment among women using public health care facilities. Appl Nurs Res 6:161–166, 1993.
13. United States Department of Health and Human Services: Children and mental health. In Mental Health: A Report of the Surgeon General, 1999. http://www.nimh.nih.gov/mhsgrpt/chapter3/sec1.html.
14. Vanzendoorn MH, Juffer F, Duyvesteyn MGC: Breaking the intergenerational cycle of insecure attachment: A review of the effects of attachment-based interventions on maternal sensitivity and infant security. J Child Psychol Psychiatry 36:225–247, 1994.
15. Wright JC, Binney V, Smith PK: Security of attachment in 8–12-year-olds: A revised version of the separation anxiety test, its psychometric properties and clinical interpretation. J Child Psychol Psychiatry 36:757–774, 1995.

SECTION H.
GENERAL CARE OF THE NEONATE

Parents of healthy babies should leave the hospital with basic written information on home care and feeding. The pre-discharge interview should include reviewing the instructions with the mother or both parents.

I. Cord Care

Parents should clean baby's cord once or twice a day, using rubbing alcohol on a cotton swab. The cord will fall off in 1–3 weeks. A slight bloody discharge is normal, both before and after the cord falls off. Pyogenic granuloma, a firm pink nodule developing in the umbilicus after the cord falls off, may be treated with silver nitrate cautery.

II. Penis/Circumcision Care

A. Circumcision Healing

A circumcised penis should heal within a week to 10 days. During healing the glans oozes small amounts of blood or yellowish serum. Petroleum jelly should be applied to the tip of the penis at each diaper change until it heals, to prevent sticking to the diaper.

B. Care of the Uncircumcised Penis

No special care is necessary for the uncircumcised penis during the first month of life. Parents should be instructed not to retract the foreskin forcibly.[1]

C. Bathing

1. Bathing in the first weeks of life

The newborn requires only sponge bathing two to three times a week until the cord falls off. After that, the baby may be bathed in a small tub, using mild soap if necessary. Overzealous washing with soap can lead to drying of the skin.

2. Use of powder, oil, and lotions

Powder, oil, and lotion are generally unnecessary and are not recommended because they can clog pores and theoretically increase the risk of contact dermatitis from perfumes, dyes, and other chemicals.

3. Treatment of "cradle cap"

Baby shampoo and a soft scalp brush are helpful for dislodging the scales of seborrhea or "cradle cap."

III. Sleeping

A. Newborn Sleeping Patterns

Newborns sleep 10–12 hours out of 24, waking every 2–4 hours for feeding. They will gradually sleep less often for longer periods, and be awake longer. At 12–13 pounds, they may sleep 8–9 hours at a time, or through the night.

B. Sleeping Position

Healthy term newborns should be placed on their backs to sleep in order to decrease the risk of sudden infant death syndrome (SIDS).[5,7,8] Soft thick bedding, pillows, and compressible toys should be avoided. No airtight materials should be within reach. Side sleeping is less desirable, as infants may roll onto their stomachs from their sides. The "Back to Sleep" campaign initiated in 1994 by the National Institute of Child Health and Human Development and the American Academy of Pediatrics has improved public awareness of the link between SIDS and prone (stomach) sleeping.[5,9] These recommendations do not apply to preterm newborns, however, who may be more vulnerable to respiratory problems when put to sleep on their backs.[6]

IV. Crying

A crying baby may be hungry, overfed, hot, cold, wet, tired, or just want to be held. When the problem is corrected, the baby usually stops crying and goes to sleep. However, many babies have a fussy period, usually late in the day. At such times, special handling may include walking, rocking, background noise, low lighting, or a trip in the stroller or car.

V. Car Seats

Laws in all 50 states require children to be restrained in car seats when traveling. Infants less than 20 pounds should be in rear-facing infant seats. Proper use of infant safety seats can reduce hospitalizations and fatalities by approximately 70%.[2]

VI. Pacifiers

During the early months, pacifiers can provide the baby sucking comfort after a full stomach or for short periods of fussiness at sleep time. They are handy, harmless, and often effective. Pacifiers are preferable to thumb sucking because they can be eliminated after 6–12 months, and the habit broken.

VII. Burping and Vomiting
A. Burping
Burping expels air swallowed during feeding. Parents typically "burp the baby" after feeding about 5 minutes, holding the baby upright against the shoulder, or prone across the knees, and gently patting or rubbing its back. If the baby has not burped in 3–5 minutes, continue feeding and try again.
B. "Spitting Up"
Spitting up is normal and can be reduced by gentle handling, feeding smaller amounts, and by placing the baby in an upright position after feeding. Projectile vomiting should be reported to the doctor if it occurs repeatedly.
C. Hiccups
Hiccups are caused by a full stomach pressing on the diaphragm, causing it to contract rhythmically and involuntarily. Hiccups may continue for an hour, but are harmless. Burping the baby or offering additional sips of warm water, milk, or formula may interrupt the hiccups.

VIII. Bowel and Bladder Function
A. Normal Infant Bowel Movements
Bowel movements may occur after every feeding or as infrequently as every few days. The typical breastfed infant's stools will be yellow, soft, and "seedy" in appearance. Stools of formula-fed infants are more formed and brown in color. Parents should understand that variation in color is common and rarely signifies pathology.
B. Constipation
If the stools appear as small, hard pellets, the baby is constipated and corrective action, such as giving the baby a little warm water, should be taken. Parents should not use enemas or bowel stimulants without physician supervision.
C. Frequency of Urination
The baby should urinate every 2–4 hours.

IX. Fever
A. Significance of Fever in Infancy
Fever may be a sign of serious illness during the first month of life. The rate of bacterial infection has been found to be roughly 4% when the temperature is 38.1–39°C, 8% for 39.1–39.9°C and 18% for 40°C or more.[3] Parents should report to the physician a rectal temperature over 38.8°C.
B. Thermometers
Every household with an infant should be equipped with a thermometer. Glass thermometers with mercury, digital thermometers, and tympanic thermometers all give accurate measurements. Glass thermometers can be used by the oral, rectal, or axillary routes; however, they are slow to register (2 minutes to obtain a rectal temperature, 3 minutes for oral, and 5–6 minutes for axillary). The axillary route is less accurate, and the rectal measurement becomes uncomfortable and embarrassing for older children. Liquid crystal strips applied to the forehead and temperature-sensitive pacifiers have been studied and found to be inaccurate.[4]
C. Antipyretics
Liquid formulations of acetaminophen or ibuprofen can be used for managing fever in infants older than 2 months.[4]

References

1. American Academy of Pediatrics: Newborns: Care of the Uncircumcised Penis. AAP Professional Publication, Elk Grove IL.
2. American Academy of Pediatrics. Policy Statement: Safe transportation of newborns at hospital discharge. Pediatrics 104:986–987, 1999.
3. Bonadio WA, Romine K, Gyuro J: Relationship of fever magnitude to rate of serious bacterial infection. J Pediatr 116:733–735, 1990.
4. Brayden RM, Headley RM: Ambulatory pediatrics. In Hay WW, Hayward AR, Levin MJ, Sondheim JM (eds): Current Pediatric Diagnosis and Treatment, 14th ed. New York, Appleton & Lange, 1999, pp 215–217.
5. Hirschfield JA: The "Back to Sleep" campaign against SIDS. Am Fam Physician 51:611–612, 1995.
6. Martin RJ, DiFiore JM, Korenke CB, et al: Vulnerability of respiratory control in healthy preterm infants placed supine. J Pediatr 127:609–614, 1995.
7. Oyen N, Markestad T, Skjaerven R, et al: Combined effects of sleeping position and prenatal risk factors in sudden infant death syndrome: The nordic epidemiologic SIDS study. Pediatrics 100:613–621, 1997.
8. Willinger M, Hoffman HJ, Hartford RB: Infant sleep position and risk for sudden infant death syndrome: Report of a meeting held January 13 and 14, 1994, National Institutes of Health, Bethesda, MD. Pediatrics 95:814–819, 1994.
9. Willinger M, Hoffman HJ, Wu KT, et al: Factors associated with the transition to non-prone sleep positions of infants in the United States. JAMA 280:329–335, 1998.

CHAPTER 19

Postpartum Biomedical Concerns

SECTION A.
DELAYED POSTPARTUM HEMORRHAGE

Elizabeth G. Baxley, M.D.

Late postpartum bleeding is defined as excessive vaginal bleeding that occurs more than 24 hours after delivery. This postpartum complication occurs most commonly as a result of sub-involution of the former placental site, but less frequently also may be the result of partial retention of placental tissue or blood clots. Retained placental fragments that do not cause immediate postpartum hemorrhage undergo necrosis and fibrin deposition, leading to formation of a placental polyp. As the eschar of the polyp detaches from the myometrium, a brisk late postpartum hemorrhage may occur. Other less common causes of delayed postpartum hemorrhage include ruptured varix, submucosal leiomyomata, or genital tract hematomas.[1]

I. Diagnosis
The diagnosis of late postpartum hemorrhage is made when heavier bleeding, in excess of normal lochia rubra, develops after the first postpartum day. Once hemorrhage is noted, a bleeding source must be identified. The episiotomy site and vagina should be explored for hematomas, and the uterine size should be assessed by bimanual examination.

If a bleeding source is not found on examination or if the patient does not respond adequately to therapeutic measures to control bleeding, laboratory tests to measure clotting function should be ordered, including platelet count, prothrombin time, partial thromboplastin time, fibrinogen, and fibrin split products.

Ultrasound can be used to exclude retained placental fragments as the cause of hemorrhage in the majority of cases. Good correlation has been demonstrated between ultrasound findings, clinical examination, and patient response to treatment.[5] Ultrasound can be used to look for placental tissue, leading to quick evacuation of the uterus when found while helping to avert unnecessary curettage when retained placental fragments are not discovered. When postpartum bleeding is moderate but not severe enough to require immediate surgical intervention, ultrasound may be a helpful diagnostic tool.[5]

II. Treatment
Initial therapy is directed at controlling the bleeding. Oxytocin, in concentrations of 20–24 units per liter of fluid, given intravenously at a rate of 250 ml/hour, or methylergonovine, at a dose of 0.2 mg given intramuscularly, are commonly used drug regimens for postpartum hemorrhage. Prostaglandin E_2 vaginal suppositories, or intramuscular or intramyometrial injection of 0.25 mg of prostaglandin F_2, have been shown to work in refractory cases of bleeding.[1,3] Misoprostol is another prostaglandin that may be effective in treating postpartum hemorrhage. It can be given either orally or rectally, and has additional advantages of being inexpensive and stable in harsh environments. It has been studied only in reduction of postpartum hemorrhage during the third stage of

labor, where results of its effectiveness have been contradictory when compared to traditional uterotonics.[2,4,6,7,8,9] It has not been studied in delayed postpartum hemorrhage.

Adequate blood replacement, appropriate anesthesia, and surgical assistance should be obtained as needed. Curettage is usually effective in stopping immediate hemorrhage and may be helpful in identifying the cause of bleeding if placental fragments or large blot clots are retrieved. In some cases, angiographic embolization of the involved vessel is effective when curettage has failed. In severe cases of hemorrhage, uterine packing and/or surgical intervention are necessary, often with ligation of the uterine and/or hypogastric artery. Occasionally, subtotal or total hysterectomy must be performed.

References

1. Andrinopoulos GC, Mendenhall HW: Prostaglandin F_{2a} in the management of delayed postpartum hemorrhage. Am J Obstet Gynecol 146:217–219, 1983.
2. Cook CM, Spurrett B, Murray H: A randomized clinical trial comparing oral misoprostol with synthetic oxytocin or syntometrine in the third stage of labour. Aust N Z J Obstet Gynaecol 39:414–419, 1999.
3. Goldstein AI, Kent DR, David A: Prostaglandin E_2 vaginal suppositories in the treatment of intractable late-onset postpartum hemorrhage: A case report. J Reprod Med 28:425–426, 1983.
4. Gülmezoglu AM: Prostaglandins for prevention of postpartum haemorrhage (Cochrane Review). In The Cochrane Library, Issue 2, 2000. Oxford, Update Software.
5. Lee CY, Madrazo B, Drukker BH: Ultrasonic evaluation of the postpartum uterus in the management of postpartum bleeding. Obstet Gynecol 58:227–232, 1981.
6. O'Brien P, El-Refaey H, Gordon A, et al: Rectally administered misoprostol for the treatment of postpartum hemorrhage unresponsive to oxytocin and ergometrine: A descriptive study. Obstet Gynecol 92:212–214, 1998.
7. Surbek DV, Fehr PM, Hosli I, et al: Oral misoprostol for third stage of labor: A randomized placebo-controlled trial. Obstet Gynecol 94:255–258, 1999.
8. Walder J: Misoprostol: Preventing postpartum haemorrhage. Modern Midwife 7:23–27, 1997.
9. Young DC: Misoprostol use in pregnancy: An update. JSOGC 239–245, 1999.

SECTION B.
POSTPARTUM ENDOMETRITIS

Elizabeth G. Baxley, M.D.

Postpartum endometritis is the most common puerperal infection. It occurs in 1.2–2.5% of patients following vaginal delivery, and in 20–38.5% of women who undergo cesarean section, depending on the risk factors that led to operative delivery.[14] Postpartum fever less than 101.1°F in the first 24 hours after delivery often resolves spontaneously.[9] However, a diagnosis of endometritis should be suspected when a woman develops persistent fever in the postpartum period and another site of infection is not found.

I. Etiology
A. Causative Agents
Endometritis occurs as an ascending infection of normal vaginal organisms. The majority of cases are polymicrobial in origin, with a mixture of aerobic and anaerobic organisms isolated (Table 1). Gram-positive aerobic cocci, predominantly streptococci, are most common. Other less common aerobic organisms include *Escherichia coli* and *Enterococcus*. *Enterococcus* has been isolated in up to one-fourth of women who receive cephalosporin prophylaxis before delivery.[4] Group A beta-hemolytic streptococci rarely have been found to present as a syndrome of toxic shock syndrome in the postpartum period.[10,17]

TABLE 1. Commonly Isolated Organisms in Women with Endometritis

Aerobes	Anaerobes
Gram-positive cocci	Gram-positive cocci
Group B streptococcus	*Peptococcus* sp.
Group A streptococcus	*Peptostreptococcus* sp.
Enterococcus	Gram-positive bacilli
Streptococcus sp. (other)	*Clostridium* sp.
Staphylococcus sp.	Gram-negative bacilli
Gram-negative cocci	*Bacteroides bivius*
Escherichia coli	*Bacteroides fragilis*
Klebsiella pneumoniae	*Bacteroides* sp. (other)
Proteus mirabilis	

From Cox S, Gilstrap L: Postpartum endometritis. Obstet Gynecol Clin North Am 16(2):1989, with permission.

Anaerobic gram-negative bacilli make up approximately one-third of isolates, with *Bacteroides* being most common. *Gardnerella vaginalis* and other anaerobes that are typically associated with bacterial vaginosis also should be considered likely pathogens. These women are more likely to have severe endometritis or develop a wound infection.[25] *Chlamydia*, *Mycoplasma*, and herpes simplex virus have infrequently been implicated in postpartum endometritis, but the clinical significance of these organisms remains unclear.[9]

B. Pathogenesis

The pathogenesis of postpartum endometritis is unknown, but appears to result from an interaction between maternal host defense mechanisms, the size of the inoculum, and the virulence of the organisms involved.[4] The flora of vaginal organisms during pregnancy is the same as that during the non-gravid state. However, the pH of the vagina is low during pregnancy, and the acidic environment prevents overgrowth of many of these organisms. After delivery, the vagina changes from being acidic to alkaline, which favors the growth of aerobic organisms.

Progressive necrosis of endometrial and placental remnants creates a favorable environment for multiplication of organisms. After abdominal delivery, the combination of an ischemic wound and serosanguineous fluid collection provides an optimal culture medium. This contributes to the 20-fold increase in rates of endometritis seen after cesarean section, even when controlled for other risk factors.[4]

II. Risk Factors

A. Route of Delivery

The dominant predictor of postpartum endometritis is cesarean delivery.[15,16] Labor duration, rupture of membranes, and internal fetal monitoring also function as facilitators of puerperal infection.[15,16] There is wide variation in reported rates of endometritis following abdominal delivery. In patients considered to be at low risk, as in elective repeat cesarean sections, the incidence may be as low as 10%. However, when operative delivery follows prolonged labor and rupture of membranes, and in women in whom a large number of vaginal examinations have been done, endometritis rates approach 90–95%.[4] Duration of surgery in patients undergoing abdominal delivery is associated with endometritis rates in a directly proportional fashion. Amnioinfusion during labor appears to significantly decrease the incidence of postpartum endometritis in patients subsequently undergoing cesarean delivery.[13]

In contrast, women who are readmitted for postpartum endometritis after initial hospital discharge (late-onset endometritis) have more often delivered vaginally.

These women were more likely to also have had spontaneous rupture of membranes, a shorter latent period, and have fewer bilateral tubal ligations, although route of delivery was the only significant maternal variable associated with late-onset endometritis.[2]

B. Length of Labor

The length of a woman's labor correlates positively with risk for endometritis, presumably due to increased contamination and colonization of the lower uterine segment as a result of frequent cervical checks.

C. Rupture of Membranes

Positive amniotic fluid cultures have been reported in 36–100% of women with membrane rupture longer than 24 hours, although this appears to relate more to corresponding long labor length. When the effect of length of labor has been removed, rupture of membranes alone has not been confirmed as an independent risk factor for endometritis.[4]

D. Vaginal Examinations and Internal Fetal Monitoring

There is little evidence to support higher endometritis rates as a result of internal fetal monitoring. Studies that have reported an association between these practices and endometritis have selected women who have had longer labors, more vaginal examinations, and a protracted period of ruptured membranes.[4]

E. Additional Risk Factors

Postpartum anemia, maternal age less than 17 years, obesity, and manual removal of the placenta or uterine exploration after placental delivery have been implicated as contributing risk factors in the development of postpartum endometritis.[7]

III. Diagnosis

A. History and Clinical Examination

Postpartum endometritis is a clinical diagnosis, suggested primarily by fever and the exclusion of extrapelvic sources of infection. Its onset is usually heralded by fever exceeding 100.4°F (38°C), and is often accompanied by lower abdominal pain and uterine tenderness, typically on the second or third postpartum day. The patient may have associated foul-smelling lochia, although this is not a consistent finding. It is rare to find a palpable mass distinct from the tender uterus on initial examination.

B. Differential Diagnosis

Other causes of postpartum fever that need to be considered in the evaluation of endometritis are breast engorgement, mastitis, urinary tract infection, pneumonia or atelectasis, wound infection, intravenous site phlebitis, and viral syndrome. As such, the clinical examination should be comprehensive in nature, including auscultation of the lungs and palpation of the breasts, back, and extremities. Examination of abdominal or perineal wounds also should include looking for abscess or cellulitis. Septic pelvic thrombophlebitis also may cause postpartum fever, and should be considered when a woman fails to respond to conventional therapy for endometritis.

C. Laboratory Studies

Leukocytosis in the range of 15,000 to 30,000 is typical for women with postpartum endometritis. However, this leukocytosis is difficult to interpret in view of the physiologic leukocytosis of the early puerperium. Genital cultures are frequently contaminated and rarely provide clinically useful information in treating patients with endometritis. Likewise, blood cultures are positive in only 5–10% of patients and rarely implicate a single causative agent.[4] Culture findings are not available at the time treatment is initiated, which further limits their usefulness. However, urine cultures should be collected routinely in postpartum patients with fever to rule out a urinary tract source.

D. Imaging Studies

In women with puerperal fever refractory to antimicrobial therapy, CT and MR imaging have proved superior to sonography in evaluation for septic pelvic thrombosis.[24]

IV. Prevention of Endometritis

Prophylactic antibiotics often are used at the time of cord clamping to prevent postpartum endometritis in women undergoing cesarean section. Their use has *not* been associated with any reduction in perioperative morbidity in women undergoing elective cesarean delivery.[22]

However, in women *at risk* for postpartum endometritis (e.g., prolonged membrane rupture), prophylatic antibiotics may be of some benefit. Single-dose antibiotic prophylaxis with ampicillin/sulbactam, cefazolin, or cefotetan is as effective as standard triple-dose therapy for uninfected, at-risk women undergoing cesarean section.[18] Single-dose ampicillin + sulbactam provides better prophylaxis than single-dose ampicillin in women undergoing cesarean section with rupture of membranes.[21] Cefazolin prophylaxis, followed by an extended-spectrum cephalosporin in women with infectious morbidity, has been shown to be associated with a higher incidence of wound infection, thus necessitating caution in the use of this combination.[15,16]

Prophylactic use of antibiotics (cefazolin, ampicillin or penicillin + gentamicin) by way of amnioinfusion also has been studied in labors complicated by meconium-stained amniotic fluid or clinical evidence of chorioamnionitis. The use of antibiotics in amnioinfusions did *not* significantly reduce rates of maternal or neonatal infection.[6,19]

Overall, the growing body of literature on prophylactic antibiotic use in pregnancy has yielded conflicting results. Because the answer to this frequently encountered clinical question is uncertain, a review of the results of randomized double-blind placebo-controlled trials of prophylactic antibiotic administration in pregnancy is underway by the Cochrane Collaboration.[1]

V. Treatment

A. Antibiotic Choices

Once endometritis is diagnosed, treatment should be initiated with parenteral antibiotics. Broad-spectrum coverage is necessary because of the polymicrobial nature of the disease, but there is no consensus on the safest and most efficacious regimen.[4] The gold standard to which all newer antibiotic regimens are compared is that of clindamycin in combination with an aminoglycoside. The combination of gentamicin and clindamycin is appropriate for the treatment of endometritis.[3,8] When used, once-daily dosing of gentamicin (4.5 mg/kg) has been shown to achieve therapeutic peak levels without drug accumulation and with substantial cost savings.[12,23] Regimens with activity against penicillin-resistant anaerobic bacteria are better than those without. There is no evidence that any one regimen is associated with fewer side effects.[8]

Because of the broad-spectrum coverage achieved with second- and third-generation cephalosporins, there is a trend toward single-agent therapy for endometritis, which offers the advantages of lower toxicity and less pharmacy and nursing time, thereby reducing cost of therapy (Table 2). Additionally, ampicillin-sulbactam as a single agent has been demonstrated to be as effective and well-tolerated as combination clindamycin plus gentamicin for the treatment of endometritis.[11,20] Because of the frequency of anaerobic involvement, metronidazole or tetracycline are often added if there is no initial response from single-drug therapy.

B. Length of Treatment

Parenteral antibiotics should be continued until the patient has been afebrile for 24–36 hours. A rapid response to broad-spectrum intravenous therapy is achieved in more than 90% of patients.[5] RCTs have shown no benefit from oral antibiotic therapy following successful parenteral treatment for endometritis, which has led to the conclusion that this common practice is unnecessary and not indicated.[5,8,14]

TABLE 2.   Summary of Studies of Single-agent and Combination Therapy
for Endometritis

Study	Cure Rate Single Agent	Clindamycin (Percent)	Gentamicin	Cure Rate (Percent)
Cunningham et al. (1979)	Cefamandole	87	—	—
Gall and Hill (1980)	Cefamandole	85	—	—
Sweet et al. (1979,83)	Cefoxitin	92	—	—
	Piperacillin	91	—	—
Herman et al. (1986)	Cefoxitin	75	Yes	76
Hemsell et al. (1983)	Cefotaxime	97.5	Yes	95
Gilstrap et al. (1986)	Cefoperazone	92	Yes	94
Gibbs et al. (1983)	Moxalactam	93	Yes	96
Gilstrap et al. (1984)	Piperacillin	85	Yes	100
Faro et al. (1987)	Mezlocillin	87	Yes	92
	Cefoxitin	82	Yes	92

From Cox S, Gilstrap L: Postpartum endometritis. Obstet Gynecol Clin North Am 16(2):1989, with permission.

C. Treatment Failure

Bacterial pathogen resistance is a rare cause of failed response to antibiotic therapy. When a patient fails to respond to appropriate parenteral antibiotic therapy for postpartum endometritis, additional diagnoses should be considered. Other pelvic pathologies that can present similarly to endometritis include cellulitis or true pelvic abscess, wound infection following cesarean section, infection or abscess involving the episiotomy and deeper vaginal tissue, and septic pelvic thrombophlebitis. The latter usually occurs 7–10 days after delivery and is characterized by persistent spiking temperatures that respond to heparin therapy.

VI. Summary

Postpartum endometritis is the most common cause of puerperal infection. It occurs more frequently in women undergoing operative delivery. The infection is usually polymicrobial, with a predominance of anaerobes. The diagnosis is based predominantly on the clinical examination and the exclusion of other causes of postpartum fever. The majority of patients respond to conventional therapy, irrespective of culture results. Antibiotic therapy should be parenteral and broad-spectrum, and single-agent therapy has been shown to be safe and effective.

References

1. Adetoro O, Hofmeyr GJ: Prophylactic antibiotic administration in pregnancy to prevent infectious morbidity and mortality [Protocol]. Issue 3, 2000, The Cochrane Library, Oxford, Update Software.
2. Atterbury JL, Groome LJ, Baker SL, et al: Hospital readmission rates for postpartum endometritis. J Matern Fetal Med 7:250–254, 1998.
3. Brumfield CG,. Hauth JC, Andrews WW: Puerperal infection after cesarean delivery: evaluation of a standardized protocol. Am J Obstet Gynecol 182:1147–1151, 2000.
4. Cox SM, Gilstrap LC: Postpartum endometritis. Obstet Gynecol 16:363–371, 1989.
5. Dinsmoor MJ, Newton ER, Gibbs RS: A randomized, double-blind, placebo-controlled trial of oral antibiotic therapy following intravenous antibiotic therapy for postpartum endometritis. Obstet Gynecol 77:60–62, 1991.
6. Edwards RK, Duff P: Prophylactic cefazolin in amnioinfusions administered for meconium-stained amniotic fluid. Infect Dis Obstet Gynecol 7:153–157, 1999.
7. Ely JW, Rijhsinghani A, Bowdler NC, et al: The association between manual removal of the placenta and postpartum endometritis following vaginal delivery. Obstet Gynecol 86:1002–1006, 1995.
8. French LM, Smaill FM: Antibiotic regimens for endometritis after delivery (Cochrane Review). The Cochrane Library, Issue 4, 2000, Oxford, Update Software.

9. Hollier LM, Scott LL, Murphree SS, et al: Postpartum endometritis caused by herpes simplex virus. Obstet Gynecol 89:836–838, 1997.
10. Jorup-Ronstrom C, Hofling M, Lundberg C, et al: Streptococcal toxic shock syndrome in a postpartum woman: Case report and review of the literature. Infection 24:164–167, 1996.
11. McGregor JA, Crombleholme WR, Newton E, et al: Randomized comparison of ampicillin-sulbactam to cefoxitin and doxycycline or clindamycin and gentamicin in the treatment of pelvic inflammatory disease or endometritis. Obstet Gynecol 83:998–1004, 1994.
12. Mitra AG, Whitten MK, Laurent SL, et al: A randomized, prospective study comparing once-daily gentamicin versus thrice-daily gentamicin in the treatment of puerperal infection. Am J Obstet Gynecol 177:786–792, 1997.
13. Moen MD, Besinger RE, Tomich PG, et al: Effect of amnioinfusion on the incidence of postpartum endometritis in patients undergoing cesarean delivery. J Reprod Med 40:383–386, 1995.
14. Morales WJ, Collins EM, Angel JL, et al: Short course of antibiotic therapy in treatment of postpartum endomyometritis. Am J Obstet Gynecol 161:568–572, 1989.
15. Newton ER, Prihoda TJ, Gibbs RS: A clinical and microbiologic analysis of risk factors for puerperal endometritis. Obstet Gynecol 75:402–406, 1990.
16. Newton ER, Wallace PA: Effects of prophylactic antibiotics on endometrial flora in women with postcesarean endometritis. Obstet Gynecol 92:262–268, 1998.
17. Noronha S, Yue CT, Sekosan M: Puerperal group A beta-hemolytic streptococcal toxic shock-like syndrome. Obstet Gynecol 88:728–733, 1996.
18. Noyes N, Berkeley AS, Freedman K, et al: Incidence of postpartum endomyometritis following single-dose antibiotic prophylaxis with either ampicillin/sulbactam, cefazolin, or cefotetan in high-risk cesarean section patients. Infect Dis Obstet Gynecol 6:220–223, 1998.
19. Parilla BV, McDermott TM: Prophylactic amnioinfusion in pregnancies complicated by chorioamnionitis: A prospective randomized trial. Am J Perinatol 15:649–652, 1998.
20. Resnick E, Harger JH, Kuller JA: Early postpartum endometritis: Randomized comparison of ampicillin/sulbactam vs. ampicillin, gentamicin and clindamycin. J Reprod Med 39:467–472, 1994.
21. Rijhsinghani A, Savopoulos SE, Walters JK, et al: Ampicillin/sulbactam versus ampicillin alone for cesarean section prophylaxis: A randomized double-blind trial. Am J Perinatol 12:322–324, 1995.
22. Rizk DE. Nsanze H. Mabrouk MH, et al: Systemic antibiotic prophylaxis in elective cesarean delivery. Internat J Gynaecol Obstet 61:245–251, 1998.
23. Sunyecz JA, Wiesenfeld HC, Heine RP: The pharmacokinetics of once-daily dosing with gentamicin in women with postpartum endometritis. Infect Dis Obstet Gynecol 6:160–162, 1998.
24. Twickler DM, Setiawan AT, Evans RS, et al: Imaging of puerperal septic thrombophlebitis: Prospective comparison of MR imaging, CT and sonography. Am J Roentgenol 169:1039–1043, 1997.
25. Watts DH, Eschenbach DA, Kenny GE: Early postpartum endometritis: The role of bacteria, genital mycoplasmas, and *Chlamydia trachomatis*. Obstet Gynecol 73:52–60, 1989.

SECTION C.
BREASTFEEDING

Patricia A. Payne, CNM, MPH

The number of women who breastfeed has not increased enough to meet public health goals. The Healthy People 2000 goal was breastfeeding in 75% of women.[1] The percentage of women who breastfed at hospital discharge in 1995 was 59.4%. Breastfeeding has not been adopted as frequently as desired despite its increased social acceptance, easy availability and cost-effectiveness, capacity to promote bonding, and superior nutritional and immunologic value to the nursing baby. Physician support is important to the mother who decides to nurse her infant. However, breastfeeding is not always a natural, trouble-free process, and the physician must be familiar with common breast disorders that may occur during lactation, with a goal of preventing premature discontinuation of breastfeeding (Table 3).

I. Successful Breastfeeding
Successful breastfeeding is largely dependent on a mother's confidence in her ability to breastfeed. She must be capable of providing the proper environment to nurse and be prepared physically and emotionally for the experience. In addition to determination and

TABLE 3. Summary of Prevention and Treatment of Breast Disorders in Nursing Mothers

Disorder	Prevention	Treatment
Nipple irritation, chafing, fissures	Regular feedings, manual breast emptying; avoiding soaps and chemicals; using lanolin or cocoa butter	Frequent nursing pad changes; leaving nipples open to air; using sunlamp one minute twice daily
Superficial bacterial skin infection	Routine breast care	Topical or systemic antibiotics; culture and determine micro-organism sensitivity if condition is unresolved after therapy
Superficial monilial skin infection	Routine breast care; frequent nursing pad changes, avoiding moisture accumulation	Topical antifungal cream; check infant for thrush or diaper dermatitis and treat
Herpes simplex infection	Avoiding contact with herpes labialis lesions	Nonsteroidal anti-inflammatory drugs; topical acyclovir (Zovirax); manual breast emptying; avoiding direct contact between lesion and infant
Macromastia		Corticosteroids; nonsteroidal anti-inflammatory drugs; bromocriptine (Parlodel); surgical intervention
Milk stasis; noninfectious inflammation	Regular feedings, manual breast emptying	Massage, warm compresses, breast emptying
Mastitis (infectious, sporadic, epidemic puerperal)	Preventing and treating noninfectious inflammation and milk stasis	Regular feedings, breast emptying, massage, warm compresses; culture milk and determine micro-organism sensitivity; antibiotics (penicillinase-resistant penicillins, cephalosporins)
Abscess	Preventing and treating mastitis	Incision and drainage; antibiotics
Fibrocystic breast disease		Nonsteroidal anti-inflammatory drugs; may continue breast feeding
Breast masses; neoplasia	Regular physician breast examination; monthly self-breast examination for detection	Diagnostic needle aspiration of newly discovered masses; breast biopsy of solid masses; standard treatment of neoplasia (mastectomy, radiation, etc.)

From Olsen C, Gordon R: Breast disorders in nursing mothers. Am Fam Physician, 41:1509–1516, 1990, with permission.

commitment, a nursing mother needs adequate knowledge about how to breastfeed and support from her family during the process. Breastfeeding is, in part, considered successful if the mother is relaxed, pain-free, and enjoys nursing. Other measures of successful breastfeeding are an infant who is gaining weight (averaging ½ ounce per day), resting adequately between feedings, and enjoying periods of quiet wakefulness without crying. Up to 50% of mothers discontinue breastfeeding within the first 14 days. When this happens, the woman's family and physician should be prepared to deal with the potential disappointment, feelings of failure, and guilt that may occur as a result.[8]

II. Breastfeeding Preparation
Breastfeeding preparation begins when women or children enter a "breastfeeding-friendly" office that includes posters, books, and information about breastfeeding. Discussions with pregnant women should be initiated early in their prenatal care. In addition to the psychological preparation, education and preparation promote prevention and help to avoid most of the common problems encountered in breastfeeding. A thor-

ough breast examination and assessment of nipples for suitability for breastfeeding should be a standard part of an initial prenatal examination as well as a follow-up exam in the third trimester after breast changes have occurred.[11] The physician should check for lumps or cysts and look for flat or inverted nipples. Although there are relatively few contraindications to breastfeeding, one must rule out the coexistence of breast cancer, potentially harmful maternal medications, and infections such as hepatitis C, cytomegalovirus, and HIV, which may preclude safe nursing.[10] Limited research has been devoted to assessing the outcome of nipple preparation, and there are conflicting data in support of its effectiveness in the published literature.[7,14] One theory is that desensitization of the nipple may result in less overall pain when the mother begins to breastfeed, and can be accomplished by nipple rolling, prenatal expression of colostrum, allowing air exposure to the nipple, and friction against a terry cloth towel or the inside of clothing while not wearing a bra.[6] Use of hydrous lanolin or A and D ointment may help keep the nipples soft and pliable; soaps, alcohol, and other drying agents should be avoided. Women with a known tendency toward premature delivery should avoid breast stimulation, because this practice may result in uterine contractions. Although there is controversy about the effectiveness of breast and nipple preparation, it does allow the woman to become familiar and comfortable with handling her own breasts.

III. Common Breastfeeding Problems

When breastfeeding problems occur, the physician must take a good history, paying particular attention to any coexistent physical or emotional problems in the mother, as well as determine the feeding schedule and activity of the baby. The physician also must examine the breasts for the presence of superficial skin infections, nipple cracking, and indurated or infected lobes. Frequently, the diagnosis of breastfeeding problems is made from observing the mother as she nurses. Two common problems associated with discontinuation of breastfeeding are nipple pain and a perception of inadequate milk supply.

A. Nipple Soreness/Pain

The majority of breastfeeding mothers have sore nipples, especially when nursing their first child. This problem, which is unrelated to the frequency or duration of feedings, unnecessarily halts breastfeeding in many cases. Although it is not medically serious, it is very distressing to mothers. Nipple irritation is a transient phenomenon that is usually worst on the third postpartum day and gradually decreases thereafter. Mothers may be reassured that it often diminishes or resolves as nipples become accustomed to suckling. Nipple pain, however, is not part of the normal process and usually indicates a problem. It is one of the most common reasons women stop breastfeeding. For indepth review of proper positioning, readers are encouraged to use breastfeeding textbooks with multiple diagrams, such as *Breastfeeding: A Guide for the Medical Profession* by Lawrence (Mosby, 1994) or *Breastfeeding and Human Lactation* by Riordan and Auerbach (Jones and Bartlett, 1993).

The most common causes of nipple pain are improper positioning and faulty sucking. When talking with mothers and observing the nursing infant, physicians should look for the following:

1. Position of the infant's tongue. The tongue should be positioned under the nipple (Fig. 1). A short frenulum, tight lips instead of flanged lips around the nipple, absence of a noisy drawing of milk while feeding, and excessive drawing of the infant's cheeks due to inadequate suction are signs of improper positioning. The baby's whole body should be facing the mother, rather than just his head, and the baby's shoulders should be rounded forward to maximize head and tongue control.

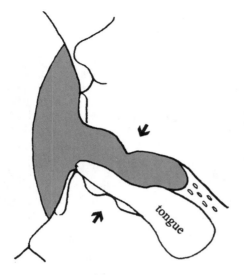

FIGURE 1. Correct latch-on. Notice how far the nipple goes into the mouth. (From Wiggins PK: Breastfeeding: A Mother's Gift, 2nd ed. Franklin, VA, L.A. Publishing Company, 1998, with permission.)

2. Frequent changes in the infant's positioning for nursing. This facilitates healing and proper emptying of all milk ducts. Three positions are typically used in this regard: side-lying (mother's abdomen to infant's abdomen), sitting (cradling the infant, preferably with pillow support to alleviate maternal bending), and cross nursing or the "football hold," with the baby's body and legs underneath the mother's arm, as if she were carrying a football.

3. "Gumming" the nipple. Likewise, proper breaking of suction, by inserting a maternal finger in the baby's mouth before discontinuing a feeding, must occur to prevent nipple damage.

4. Signs of infection. The physician should look for signs of monilial, bacterial, or HSV infection, and examine the infant for oral thrush or diaper candidiasis.[12] Maternal exposure to antibiotics in labor may increase the risk of monilial infections that may be associated with nipple pain or burning.[3]

B. Treatment of Nipple Soreness

Patient support and education are the cornerstones of treatment for nipple soreness. The physician should *not* recommend less frequent nursing, as this causes the infant to suck more vigorously, which causes further pain and trauma. Soap, alcohol, benzoin, and other drying agents should be avoided. Topical therapy with hydrous lanolin or A and D ointment may be helpful. Leaving the nipples exposed to air after feeding and frequent changing of nursing pads prevent excessive moisture that can irritate the nipple. Some lactation consultants also recommend exposure to heat or sun lamps for brief (1–2-minute) periods each day.

C. Breast Engorgement and Milk Stasis

Breast engorgement is a common problem in breastfeeding mothers, particularly primiparas.

1. Within the first 48 hours after delivery. This is initially a result of vascular congestion rather than milk production, and it is not alleviated by additional nursing or breast pump use. Ice packs may help improve breast pain associated with this early engorgement.

2. Engorgement after milk production begins. This is more common and is associated with incomplete emptying of the milk glands. Symptoms include tender, swollen breasts (engorgement) or presence of a more localized tender, firm area of the breast (milk stasis). In cases of milk stasis, there are fewer than

10 leukocytes per milliliter of milk, and cultures are sterile. In either case, symptoms persist only a few days and the outcome is good. Lactation can and should continue without interruption.

D. Treatment of Engorgement

1. Early and frequent feedings. These feedings, as well as breast massage, decrease the incidence and degree of engorgement. By stretching already tender skin, engorgement can exacerbate nipple soreness.

2. Manual expression of a small amount of milk prior to nursing. This will help to relieve the engorgement and will make it easier for the baby to grasp the nipple.[2]

3. Warm compresses, frequent nursing, and massage of the affected area(s). These are usually sufficient treatment recommendations.

4. Raw washed cabbage leaves. These can be used for 20 minutes on a limited basis to decrease inflammation.[13]

5. Use of nipple shields. This is controversial. In fact, by reducing stimulation to the nipple and areola, they risk decreasing the milk supply, changing the infant's suckling patterns, and causing more nipple pain and damage.[16] Although nipple shields may have a place in nursing for mothers with flat or inverted nipples, they should not be prescribed for a woman with normal breast anatomy.

E. Inadequate Milk Supply

Mothers frequently stop nursing when they fear that they have an inadequate milk-supply. It is important to provide all mothers with normal signs so they are reassured their baby is getting enough milk (Table 4). True inadequacy of milk is rare.[2] Milk production is directly related to nipple stimulation. Therefore, the supply will increase by increasing the frequency of nursing and completely emptying the breast at each feeding.

F. Maternal Fatigue

The most common cause of decreased milk supply is maternal fatigue. As long as the infant is gaining weight appropriately, avoid recommending formula supplementation, as this will decrease the infant's suckling strength and the length and frequency of sucking, which in turn will lower breast milk production further. Consider the feeding schedule of the newborn, and ensure that the baby is nursing at least every 3 hours, or eight times in 24 hours. The mother should be relaxed and have adequate intake of calories and fluids. Rest and relaxation are important components

TABLE 4. How to Tell Whether Your Breastfeeding Baby Is Getting Enough Milk

Your milk should "come in" at 2–4 days after delivery.

Your baby should latch on correctly to your breast and suck rhythmically for at least 10 minutes on each breast.

Your baby should appear satisfied after nursings and probably will fall asleep at the second breast.

Your newborn baby should nurse at least eight times in each 24 hours.

Your breasts should feel full before each feeding and softer after your baby has nursed.

Your baby should urinate six or more times a day.

Your baby's bowel movements should look yellow—somewhat like a mixture of cottage cheese and mustard—by the fourth or fifth day of life.

Your baby should have four or more bowel movements each day.

Your nipples may be slightly tender for the first several days of nursing.

After 2 or 3 weeks, you may be aware of the sensations associated with the milk ejection or milk let-down reflex.

Once your milk has come in, your breastfed baby should gain about 1 oz each day for the first few months of life.

From Neifert M: Early assessment of the breastfeeding infant. Contemp Pediatrics, October 1996, with permission.

of adequacy of milk supplies, and the physician should support periods of mandated rest for the nursing mother. Parents need to know about growth spurts that can be misinterpreted as lack of milk instead of a need to increase the supply further.

G. Medications to Avoid

Mothers should avoid medications that may effect their milk supply. However, most drugs are acceptable for use while nursing. It is important that physicians do not find themselves ill-prepared to counsel a breastfeeding mother who needs to make a decision about using a medication while breastfeeding. Without sufficient knowledge, a more conservative approach may be used and cause a mother to stop nursing when, in actuality, the risks associated with use of a medication are minimal. Consideration must be given to the actual level of exposure based on the milk-to-plasma ratio and rate of clearance of the drug.[9] Well known resources include Hale[6] and Briggs,[5] which are available in hard copy or through PerinatalNetwork.com, a website sponsored by international obstetric associations including ACOG. Drugs are categorized according to their level of risk to infants.

H. Determining if Milk Supply Is Adequate

Infant test weights can be an effective way to determine if the milk supply is adequate.[11] If supplemental feeding is necessary, supplementary systems or finger feeds should be used to avoid nipple confusion (Fig. 2).[8] A supplemental feeder system can be used indefinitely for mothers with a low milk supply or infants with conditions that inhibit sucking, such as Down syndrome or premature infants.

I. Painful Let-Down Sensations

Milk let-down is controlled by a nerve reflex from the breast to the hypothalamus that causes the release of oxytocin by the posterior pituitary gland.[4] Within minutes of suckling, oxytocin levels peak and cause myoepithelial cells surrounding the alveoli to contract and expel breast milk. Breast filling also is known to happen

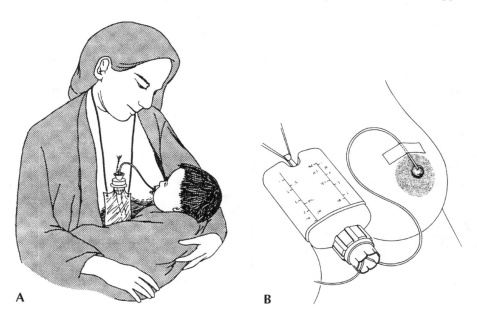

A   **B**

FIGURE 2.   A, Lact-Aid Nursing Trainer System (Lact-Aid International, Inc.). **B**, Lactation Supplementer by Medela, which provides additional nourishment to the infant while suckling at the underproducing breast. (From Lawrence RA: Breastfeeding: A Guide for the Medical Profession, 4th ed. St. Louis, Mosby, 1994, with permission.)

when the sights and sounds that induce the neural-hormonal reflex response occur (i.e., mother thinking about her infant, or hearing an infant cry). Similarly, fatigue, stress, smoking, and excessive caffeine intake inhibit the reflex, and milk production is reduced. Most mothers do not find the sensation of let-down to be particularly painful, although it may be described as deep, shooting pains that occur during feedings. This problem is not serious or pathologic, and mothers can be reassured that it will usually disappear quickly when breastfeeding is established. If let-down is incomplete or inadequate, this may also cause a similar breast pain because the infant is having to suck more vigorously. Milk let-down may be facilitated by having the mother go to a quiet room away from distractions where she can relax and apply warm compresses to the breast. In more severe cases of inadequate let-down, Syntocinon, an oxytocin nasal spray, may be applied 1 minute before breastfeeding begins. This medication has a rebound effect, so it should be used sparingly and tapered until discontinued.

J. Noninfectious Inflammation

Noninfectious inflammation is characterized by persistent tenderness, swelling, erythema, and heat of the breast.[12] This is frequently a precursor to bacterial mastitis and is sometimes referred to as milk stasis. Diminished milk secretion is common in noninfectious inflammation. Breast milk samples have greater than 10 leukocytes but less than 10 bacteria per milliliter of fluid. The bacteria that are found in these samples are most often thought to be skin contaminants. Regular emptying of the breast usually shortens the duration of symptoms and results in a lower rate of progression to mastitis.[15] Mothers can massage a tender area while nursing or hand expressing to empty a clogged duct and avoid bacterial growth and subsequent mastitis. Hand expression in a warm shower or warm compresses combined with massage while nursing may alleviate the problem (see section D).

K. Afterbirth Pains

For some women, especially multiparas, afterbirth pains are stimulated by breastfeeding. These may equal labor contractions in quality and intensity. Breathing and relaxation techniques such as those taught for use in labor and delivery help to promote a calm, relaxed frame of mind and may reduce pain associated with this postpartum uterine activity.[16] Mild analgesics (acetaminophen, nonsteroidal anti-inflammatory agents) also are helpful to block this pain response and thereby permit a more relaxed feeding session. Multiparous women often experience severe after-pains and may benefit from analgesics as soon after birth as possible.

L. Coexistent Breast Disease

1. Fibrocystic breast disease. This is a common, benign breast disorder characterized by multiple, nodular cystic lesions that are usually bilateral and tender to palpation.[12] The presence of fibrocystic disease is not a contraindication to breastfeeding. Treatment is symptomatic, primarily by use of analgesics (acetaminophen, nonsteroidal anti-inflammatory agents).

2. Breast carcinoma. This is discovered during pregnancy and lactation in 2–3 per 1000 women and is a contraindication to breastfeeding.[12] Neoplastic breast nodules are usually recognized at a more advanced stage in pregnant or lactating women than in nonpregnant women. This is thought to occur because pregnant and breastfeeding women delay seeking medical attention for breast problems and because physicians often fail to perform adequate breast examinations in pregnant women. Alteration of immune function may occur during pregnancy, and the high estrogen levels present during pregnancy may stimulate tumor growth in estrogen receptor–positive tumors. For these reasons, women with breast cancer diagnosed during pregnancy or lactation generally have a poorer prognosis than women diagnosed outside of the peripartum period.[12]

IV. Breastfeeding and Return to Work
The success of breastfeeding after the mother returns to work is directly related to the length of maternity leave, as it generally requires 6 to 8 weeks to establish lactation. The infant should suck three times a day, and the mother should express milk in between, completely emptying the breast, to ensure adequate milk supply if no supplementation is planned. Breast pumps may provide breast stimulation and allow for collection for milk for the infant during the hours that the mother is at work. Alternatively, the mother may choose to continue nursing for three to four feedings each day and supplement with formula while away from her baby. Preparation for this option consists of dropping one feeding at a time for a period of several days. In this manner, the woman's body can adjust to a partial schedule of nursing and will not have breast engorgement or leaking during the work day. Physicians can play a significant role in helping women prepare to return to work and to communicate with employers in their community about the importance of breastfeeding support for working mothers. Mothers require adequate break time, pumping equipment and facilities, and support from their coworkers.

References
1. American Academy of Pediatrics Work Group on Breastfeeding: Breastfeeding and the use of human milk. Pediatrics 100:1035–1039, 1997.
2. Andolsek KM: Obstetric Care: Standards of Prenatal, Intrapartum, and Postpartum Management. Philadelphia, Lea & Febiger, 1990, p 293.
3. Bodley V, Power D: Long-term treatment of a breastfeeding mother with fluconazole-resolved nipple pain caused by yeast: a case study. J Human Lactation 12:307–311, 1997.
4. Borovies DL: Assessing and managing pain in breast-feeding mothers. Am J Matern Child Nurs 9:272–276, 1984.
5. Briggs GG, Freeman RK, Yaffe S, et al: Drugs in Pregnancy and Lactation: A Reference Guide to Fetal and Neonatal Risk, 5th ed. Baltimore, Williams & Wilkins, 1998.
6. Hale T: Medications and Mother's Milk. Pharmasoft Medical Publishers, 2000.
7. Hewat RJ, Ellis DJ: A comparison of the effectiveness of two methods of nipple care. Birth 14:41–43, 1987.
8. International Lactation Consultant Association: Evidence-Based Guidelines for Breastfeeding Management during the First Fourteen Days. April 1999, International Lactation Consultant Association.
9. Ito S: Drug therapy for breast-feeding women. N Engl J Med 343:118–125, 2000.
10. Lawrence RA: Given the benefits of breastfeeding, are there any contraindications? Clin Perinatol 26:479–490, 1990.
11. Neifert MR: Clinical aspects of lactation: Promoting breastfeeding success. Clin Perinatol 265:281–306, 1999.
12. Olsen CG, Gordon R: Breast disorders in nursing mothers. Am Fam Physician 41:1509–1516, 1990.
13. Renfrew MJ, Lang S: Cabbage leaves for breast engorgement (Cochrane Review). The Cochrane Library, Issue 4, 2000, Oxford, Update Software.
14. Storr GB: Prevention of nipple tenderness and breast engorgement in the postpartum period. J Obstet Gynecol Neonatal Nurs 17:203–209, 1988.
15. Thomsen AC, Espersen T, Maigaard S: Course and treatment of milk stasis, noninfectious inflammation of the breast, and infectious mastitis in nursing women. Am J Obstet Gynecol 149:492–495, 1984.
16. Walker M: Functional assessment of infant breast-feeding patterns. Birth 16:140–147, 1989.

SECTION D.
MASTITIS

Elizabeth G. Baxley, M.D.

I. Definition and Incidence
Lactation mastitis is an acute mammary cellulitis involving the periglandular connective tissue of the breast.[9] It is an uncommon complication of breastfeeding that occurs in approximately 2–3% of nursing mothers.[7] Risk factors for lactation mastitis include

improper nursing techniques, nipple cracking and pain during feeding, breast trauma, blocked ducts, engorgement/stasis, maternal fatigue or high levels of stress, poor diet, and professional, technical, or managerial occupations in both parents.[3,4,7,11] Women with a history of mastitis following an earlier pregnancy have a higher rate of recurrence in subsequent periods of nursing.[4]

A. Pathophysiology

The most frequently isolated etiologic agent in lactation mastitis is *Staphylococcus aureus*, which gains access through an irritated or cracked nipple. Milk stasis often precedes infection by offering a favorable substrate for bacterial multiplication. Prevention, therefore, is aimed at preventing and treating milk stasis and noninfectious inflammation by frequent feedings, nipple care, and a gradual increase in the duration of nursing at each breast.

B. Clinical Presentation

Mastitis commonly presents 2–4 weeks after breastfeeding begins with an abrupt onset of fever, chills, and flu-like muscle aches. Usually there is an associated segmental erythema of the breast, induration, and pain. On clinical examination, a demarcated, V-shaped division of inflammation between the lobes of the breasts may be found. The segmental anatomy of the breast accounts for the typical wedge of inflammation with its apex at the nipple and its base toward the periphery of the duct.[1] Although it is unlikely to encounter purulent drainage from affected ducts, milk samples can be submitted for culture and sensitivity if available or needed to direct treatment. Bacteria that are commonly isolated from breast milk samples are listed in Table 5.

II. Treatment

Women with a clinical presentation suggestive of mastitis should be treated with antibiotics within the first 48 hours of the onset of symptoms.[6] A good clinical response can be achieved in most cases even if cultures are not obtained or results are not available. The aim of treatment for mastitis is to prevent complications and allow lactation to continue.[12]

Antibiotic therapy with either a penicillinase-resistant penicillin or a first- or second-generation cephalosporin should be continued for 10 days. Shorter courses have been associated with relapse.[10] Although *Staphylococcus aureus* is the most frequently isolated organism, patients have generally good clinical response to penicillin even when resistant bacteria are isolated by culture. Mothers of infants less than 1 month of age should avoid use of sulfonamides.

In addition to antibiotic therapy, treatment should include regular breast emptying, massage, and warm compresses for symptomatic relief of pain. Analgesics, including codeine-containing preparations, can be used when discomfort is severe. Mastitis need not halt breastfeeding or lactation, as breast engorgement may contribute to abscess

TABLE 5. Bacteria in Milk of Nursing Mothers with Infectious Mastitis

Frequently Isolated	Infrequently Isolated
Staphylococcus aureus	Enterobacter cloacae
Coagulase-negative staphylococci	Serratia marcescens
Beta-hemolytic streptococci	Pseudomonas aeruginosa
Streptococcus faecalis	Haemophilus influenzae
Escherichia coli	Klebsiella pneumoniae
Diphtheroids	Bacteroides fragilis

From Olsen C, Gordon J: Breast disorders in nursing mothers. Am Fam Physician 41:1509–1516, 1990, with permission.

formation.[9] Illness in the newborn does not appear to result from sporadic mastitis in the mother.[2,10] Maintaining lactation during mastitis may enhance the resolution of inflammation by reducing congestion, thereby shortening the duration of symptoms and improving outcomes.[8]

III. Breast Abscess

Breast abscess develops in approximately 5–11% of women with lactation mastitis.[2] An increased incidence is noted after abrupt weaning and subsequent milk stasis, or if antibiotic treatment is delayed more than 24 hours after onset of mastitis. Breast abscesses are typically situated peripherally in the breast. The prime insult is blockage of a lactiferous duct or sinus with inspissated secretions, resulting in retention of milk in the sector of breast parenchyma served by the blocked duct.[1]

Clinically, breast abscess presents similarly to mastitis, but exquisite tenderness is present in the region of the abscess. Ipsilateral axillary lymphadenitis is usually not a prominent feature.[1] Fluctuation may be present but should not be expected. Ultrasound examination of the breast when persistent induration, swelling, or tenderness is present aids in the diagnosis of breast abscess.[5,6]

Treatment includes antibiotic therapy as for mastitis, incision and drainage, and wound packing. Breast abscess is usually considered a relative contraindication to breastfeeding and lactation often ceases spontaneously in women who develop acute puerperal breast abscess.[1]

References

1. Benson EA: Management of breast abscesses. World J Surg 13:753–756, 1989.
2. Devereux WP: Acute puerperal mastitis: Evaluation of its management. Am J Obstet Gynecol 108:78–81, 1970.
3. Fetherston C: Risk factors for lactation mastitis. J Hum Lact 14:101–109, 1998.
4. Foxman B, Schwartz K, Looman SJ: Breastfeeding practices and lactation mastitis. Soc Sci Med 38:755–761, 1994.
5. Hayes R, Michell M, Nunnerley HB: Acute inflammation of the breast—the role of breast ultrasound in diagnosis and management. Clin Radiol 44:253–256, 1991.
6. Johnson PE, Hanson KD: Acute puerperal mastitis in the augmented breast. Plast Reconstr Surg 98:723–725, 1996.
7. Kaufmann R, Foxman B: Mastitis among lactating women: Occurrence and risk factors. Soc Sci Med 33:701–705, 1991.
8. Marshall BR, Hepper JK, Zirbel CC: Sporadic puerperal mastitis: An infection that need not interrupt lactation. JAMA 233:1377–1379, 1975.
9. Niebyl JR, Spence MR, Parmley TH: Sporadic (nonepidemic) puerperal mastitis. J Reprod Med 20:97–100, 1978.
10. Olsen CG, Gordon R: Breast disorders in nursing mothers. Am Fam Physician 41:1509–1516, 1990.
11. Riordan JM, Nichols FH: A descriptive study of lactation mastitis in long-term breastfeeding women. J Hum Lact 6:53–58, 1990.
12. Thomsen AC, Espersen T, Maigaard S: Course and treatment of milk stasis, noninfectious inflammation of the breast, and infectious mastitis in nursing women. Am J Obstet Gynecol 149:492–495, 1984.

SECTION E.
THYROIDITIS

Elizabeth G. Baxley, M.D.

Thyroid dysfunction is a frequently encountered postpartum disorder, with a prevalence of 4–6% in the first year after delivery.[4,8,9,11,12,13,14] The most common syndrome seen at this time is postpartum thyroiditis (PPT), although women who have been previously treated for Graves' disease may experience reactivation of the illness in the postpartum period.[8,9]

PPT is an autoimmune disorder characterized by a destructive lymphocytic infiltration of the thyroid gland, and often manifests as transient hyperthyroidism between 1 and 3 months postpartum and hypothyroidism between 3 and 6 months postpartum.[15] The incidence of PPT is highest in Hispanics, less common in Caucasian women, and uncommon among African-Americans.[5] Rates of thyroid dysfunction are not dependent upon age, parity, or breastfeeding, but a family history of thyroid disorders is common.

I. Diagnosis

The majority of women with PPT have a brief, often asymptomatic, thyrotoxic phase, followed by a more long-lasting symptomatic hypothyroid phase.[20] The onset of thyroiditis typically begins around the fourth postpartum week, with symptoms peaking at 8–12 weeks. Symptoms are typically subtle and insidious in onset, making it difficult to distinguish between PPT and other presenting complaints frequently encountered during the postpartum period, such as fatigue, weight gain, dry skin, constipation, loss of initiative, memory impairment, depression, anxiety, and emotional lability. Because of this, PPT is often underdiagnosed and can be associated with significant morbidity.

Women whose lethargy persists beyond several weeks must be evaluated with respect to thyroid function. Thyroid enlargement may be found on physical examination, although a persistent goiter is uncommon. Patients who have a symptomatic thyrotoxic phase in the early stages of PPT experience an abrupt onset of neck pain and tenderness, fatigue, and palpitations. Occasionally, this presents as panic attacks or postpartum psychosis.[2]

The syndrome of PPT is strongly associated with the presence of thyroid microsomal antibodies (MCAb) or thyroid peroxidase antibodies (TPO-Ab) in maternal serum.[20] The diagnosis is based on the observation of abnormal thyroid function tests in a postpartum women who has elevated thyroid peroxidase antibodies.[17] During the hypothyroid phase of PPT, TSH levels are elevated, peaking at 4–6 months. The severity of symptoms usually follows the trend of TSH variation. Patients who do have elevated TSH levels should be followed expectantly by repeating TSH and thyroid antibody levels every 8–12 weeks until these values return to normal.[5,21]

Diffuse or multifocal hypoechogenicity of the thyroid is also seen on ultrasound, correlating with lymphocytic infiltration of the thyroid gland.[11–14,17] When needed, the thyrotoxic phase may be distinguished from Graves' disease by the finding of low, rather than high, uptake of radioactive iodine or technetium in the thyroid.[20] For women in whom an I[131] scan is necessary for diagnosis, breastfeeding should be interrupted for 36 hours to reduce the infant's exposure to I[123] radioactivity.[16]

II. Screening

Since PPT is characterized as a postpartum exacerbation of subclinical autoimmune thyroid disease, some immunologic abnormalities can be observed before the onset of thyroid dysfunction. Studies have shown that 50% of thyroid peroxidase antibody (TPOAb)-positive pregnant women will develop postpartum thyroid dysfunction (PPTD), leading some to suggest that screening should play a role in predicting which women will develop PPTD.[1,7,11–14,17] Yet the benefit of screening presently remains controversial because of a lack of knowledge about how to screen, when to screen, and whether or not treatment makes a difference for women with unrecognized mild or moderate thyroid dysfunction.[1] No prospective diagnostic and therapeutic trials have been published that indicate whether or not a screening program would be beneficial.[1]

Thyroid peroxidase antibody screening, although readily available, easily reproducible, and relatively cheap, has a low positive predictive value (30–52%).[1] Nearly half of all TPO-Ab-positive women do not develop PPT, and up to 39% of women who develop PPT may have been antibody-negative.[1,11–14] The Canadian Task Force on the Periodic Health Examination (1994) and the United States Preventive Services Task Force (1996) both recommend against general screening.[3,18] They do recommend that clinicians remain alert for signs and symptoms that suggest thyroid dysfunction and have a low threshold for evaluating thyroid status in high-risk patients. The American Thyroid Association leans more toward universal screening, recommending TSH screening in certain high-risk groups, including "postpartum women at 4–8 weeks."[19]

Screening with TSH determinations at 3 and 6 months postpartum may be valuable in women with other autoimmune disorders such as women with a prior history of PPT (69% prevalence of recurrence) and type 1 diabetes mellitus (25–25% prevalence of PPT).[1,20] All postpartum women with depression are potential candidates for testing for thyroid dysfunction.[1]

III. Treatment

Women with mild to moderate thyroid dysfunction may have minimal symptoms and may not even present to a provider. Of women who do seek medical attention, not all require treatment, which should be tailored to the symptoms. Treatment should be reserved for symptomatic women with laboratory evidence of thyroid dysfunction, and is not indicated for patients with elevated thyroid antibody titers alone.[8]

Treatment of PPT is relatively simple, consisting of beta-blockers for moderate to severe symptoms in the hyperthyroid phase, and levothyroxine for the hypothyroid phase.[1,20] Levothyroxine is continued for 12–18 months after diagnosis. Thyroid replacement improves symptoms but does not alter the course of the illness.[10]

Permanent hypothyroidism is uncommon, occurring in only 1–2% of patients with PPT. High thyroid antibody titers and low radioactive iodine uptake herald a more severe hypothyroid phase and greater likelihood of persistent hypothyroidism. In most cases, normal thyroid function returns within one year. Relapse of PPT with subsequent pregnancies occurs in up to 70% of women. Peak antibody levels and duration of illness are similar in each relapse for individual patients. In addition, 25–30% of women develop permanent hypothyroidism.[1,11–14] Recent data indicate that 50% of women who have developed PPT will be hypothyroid 7–9 years later.[11] Factors predictive of long-term thyroid dysfunction include a hypothyroid form of PPTD, TSH > 20 mU/L, and higher TPOAb levels during the postpartum period (relative risk = 32).[17]

References

1. Amino N, Tada H, Hidaka Y, et al: Therapeutic controversy: Screening for postpartum thyroiditis. J Clin Endocrinol Metab 84:1813–1821, 1999.
2. Bokhari R, Bhatara VS, Bandettini F, et al: Postpartum psychosis and postpartum thyroiditis. Psychoneuroendocrinology 23:643–650, 1998.
3. Canadian Task Force on the Periodic Health Examination: The Canadian guide to clinical preventive health care. Ottawa, Canada Communication Group, 1994, pp 611–618.
4. Gerstein HC: How common is postpartum thyroiditis: A methodologic overview of the literature. Arch Intern Med 150:1397–1400, 1990.
5. Hayslip GC, Fein HG, O'Donnell VM, et al: The value of serum antimicrosomal antibody testing in screening for symptomatic postpartum thyroid dysfunction. Am J Obstet Gynecol 159:203–209, 1988.
6. Heath GC: Postpartum thyroiditis. J Natl Med Assoc 80:1231–1235, 1988.
7. Hidaka Y, Tada H, Amino N: [Postpartum autoimmune thyroid syndrome]. Jpn J Clin Med 57:1775–1778, 1999.
8. Jansson R, Dahlberg PA, Karlsson FA: Postpartum thyroiditis. Baillieres Clin Endocrinol Metab 2:619–635, 1988.
9. Jansson R, Dahlberg PA, Winsa B, et al: The postpartum period constitutes an important risk for the development of clinical Graves' disease in young women. Acta Endocrinol 116:321–325, 1987.
10. Kampe O, Jansson R, Karlsson FA: Effects of L-thyroxine and iodide on the development of autoimmune postpartum thyroiditis. J Clin Endocrinol Metab 70:1014–1018, 1990.
11. Lazarus JH: Clinical manifestations of postpartum thyroid disease. Thyroid 9:685–689, 1999.

12. Lazarus JH, Ammari F, Oretti R, et al: Clinical aspects of recurrent postpartum thyroiditis. Br J Gen Pract 418:305–308, 1997.
13. Lazarus JH, Hall R, Othman S, et al: The clinical spectrum of postpartum thyroid disease. Q J Med 89:429–435, 1996.
14. Lazarus JH, Parkes AB, Premawardhana LD, et al: Screening for postpartum thyroiditis. J Clin Endocrinol Metabol 84:495–496, 1999.
15. Lucas A, Pizarro E, Granada ML, et al: Postpartum thyroiditis: Epidemiology and clinical evolution in a non-selected population. Thyroid 10:71–77, 2000.
16. Morita S, Umezaki N, Ishibashi M, et al: Determining the breast-feeding interruption schedule after administration of ^{123}I-iodide. Ann Nucl Med 12:303–306, 1998.
17. Premawardhana LD, Parkes AB, Ammari F, et al: Postpartum thyroiditis and long-term thyroid status: Prognostic influence of thyroid peroxidase antibodies and ultrasound echogenicity. J Clin Endocrinol Metab 85:71–75, 2000.
18. Report of the U.S. Preventive Services Task Force, 2nd ed: Screening for thyroid disease. In Guide to Clinical Preventive Services: An Assessment of the Effectiveness of 169 Interventions. Washington, DC, U.S. Government Printing Office, 1996, pp 209–218.
19. Surks MI, Chopra IJ, Mariash CN, et al: 1990 American Thyroid Association guidelines for the use of laboratory tests in thyroid disorders. JAMA 263:1529–1532, 1990.
20. Terry AJ, Hague WM: Postpartum thyroiditis. Semin Perinatol 22:497–502, 1998.
21. Vargas MT, Briones-Urbina R, Gladman D, et al: Antithyroid microsomal autoantibodies and HLADRS are associated with postpartum thyroid dysfunction: Evidence supporting an autoimmune pathogenesis. J Clin Endocrinol Metab 67:327–333, 1988.

SECTION F.
CONTRACEPTION

Elizabeth G. Baxley, M.D.

I. Introduction

Discussion of postpartum contraception should ideally begin during prenatal visits. However, this discussion often does not occur until after childbirth. In one study, only 4% of women reported that they had discussions of postpartum contraception antenatally.[5] Eighty-four percent had discussed contraception in the immediate postpartum period in the hospital, but felt that this discussion was brief, limited, and frequently held as the mother was leaving the hospital. Only 50% of women left the hospital with contraceptive supplies.[5]

Women are particularly motivated to prevent conception just after the birth of a new baby.[2] Decisions about family planning methods will largely depend on the woman's number of children, overall state of health, and whether or not she is breastfeeding. Experience with previous birth control methods as well as religious background of the couple may influence this decision. Thus, recommendations should be individualized for each woman and take into account how issues of lactation and child spacing affect contraceptive choices.[13]

A. Reproductive Stages and Contraceptive Method

The time from first childbirth to completion of the desired family typically represents approximately 10% of a woman's reproductive life.[3] Contraceptive goals during this period are to space the pregnancies while preserving the ability to conceive and bear more children. The frequency of intercourse between pregnancies is less than during other reproductive stages but the predictability is high, making it somewhat less important that the contraceptive method be coitus-independent.[3]

B. Resumption of Sexual Activity Following Delivery

Women have historically been advised not to resume sexual intercourse until 6 weeks after delivery. In actuality, sexual activity may be resumed when the perineum is comfortable and when bright red bleeding has subsided, which generally occurs before the traditional 6-week postpartum visit. In most cases it is probably safe to resume intercourse 3 weeks following an uncomplicated delivery, although few women are ready to do so at that time.

The desire and willingness to resume sexual activity vary greatly, depending on the state of healing of perineal lacerations, lactation-related vaginal atrophy, and return of libido, which is often delayed secondary to fatigue. Most couples begin having regular intercourse by 3 months following delivery, though some begin earlier. Thus, it is important to attempt to reach a decision prior to leaving the hospital. The period of anovulatory infertility lasts only 5 weeks in nonlactating women, and up to 8 weeks or more in women who breastfeed without supplementation.

C. Choice of Contraception

1. Natural family planning

The natural, or rhythm, method of family planning depends on the couple anticipating the fertile period of the menstrual cycle and abstaining from intercourse during this time. Couples using natural family planning require intensive training to recognize periods of fertility or infertility based upon specified qualities of the cervical mucus. Along with an increase in basal body temperature at the time of ovulation, cervical mucus thickens and loses its elasticity after the rise in progesterone at the onset of the postovulatory, or infertile, phase.[19] This method requires daily attention and a high degree of motivation by both partners and has a reported failure rate of 4–5 per 100 women-years when properly used. Its use by nonlactating women is difficult until regular menses have resumed. In breastfeeding women, hormonal suppression often alters cyclic symptoms, making interpretation difficult.[3]

2. Lactational amenorrhea (LAM)

In the first 6 months after birth, provided there is little or no supplemental feeding for the infant, breastfeeding will provide ≥ 98% contraceptive effectiveness.[4,7,12,18] Suckling induces a reduction in gonadotropin-releasing hormone, luteinizing hormone, and follicle-stimulating hormone release, resulting in amenorrhea. When breastfeeding is used exclusively and amenorrhea exists, ovulation does not usually occur before 6 months postpartum, and fertility remains low.[7,18] This contraceptive effect is quite effective, but not universal, as 5–10% of women using LAM become pregnant. A higher percentage of nursing mothers who have reinitiated menses become pregnant. Those women should be advised to use additional supplemental contraception for complete protection.

LAM is particularly well suited for couples interested in natural family planning or who have religious preferences to avoid other methods. It also gives women and their partners time to decide upon a longer-term method of contraception to use at the end of the puerperium.[18] Overall patient satisfaction with lactational amenorrhea (LAM) is high, up to 83.6% in a large multicenter study.[9]

3. Barrier methods

Barrier methods of contraception, which include the diaphragm, condom, and vaginal sponge, all have in common a requirement of substantial motivation on the part of the couple. However, because the timing of intercourse is more predictable after the birth of a child, any one of these methods may serve as a suitable form of birth control for parents of infants and small children.

  a. Diaphragm. The diaphragm is often a preferred form of reversible contraception for older women, especially those not yet ready to consider sterilization for themselves or their partners. The reported failure rate for diaphragm users is quite variable, from 2.4 to 19.6 per 100 women-years.

  Patients must be fitted with an appropriately sized diaphragm, which should not be any sooner than the 6-week postpartum visit, or longer to ensure proper fitting. This is necessary even in women who previously used this form of contraception prior to pregnancy. A diaphragm that fits too tightly may place pressure against the urethra, resulting in an inability to empty the bladder completely and higher rates of urinary tract infection. In breastfeeding mothers, anovulation leads to vaginal dryness and tightness, which may make the proper insertion of the diaphragm more difficult than in women who are not lactating. The diaphragm should be used with a spermicidal lubricant, which can aid in problems of vaginal dryness while providing greater contraceptive effectiveness.

b. Condoms. The use of condoms, alone or in combination with spermicide, is often advised for women who want to postpone a decision about sterilization or oral contraceptive therapy until the postpartum visit. Reported failure rates are similarly variable, from 1.6 to 21 per 100 women-years. Latex condoms should be recommended, as HIV and some hepatitis B subparticles may pass through natural skin condoms. Use of condoms containing nonoxynol-9 provide better protection against sexually transmitted diseases and have been shown to kill infectious agents, including HIV, in vitro.

c. Vaginal sponge. This is an over-the-counter, single-use product that acts primarily as a release for spermicide, and only secondarily as a barrier contraceptive. It provides protection against pregnancy for 24 hours, and its effectiveness rate is similar to that of other vaginal contraceptives. Vaginal sponges need no fitting, but there is a tendency for them to tear during removal. Women should be advised to examine them after each use, as a retained portion may predispose to infection.

4. Combination oral contraceptives

In women who choose not to breastfeed, oral contraceptives may be started as early as 2 weeks following delivery. Beginning pills sooner than this time increases the risk of puerperal thromboembolism, as oral contraceptive use is associated with a decrease in antithrombin III levels, which can be clinically significant when coupled with the hypercoaguable state of pregnancy and the early puerperium.

The effect of combination oral contraceptives on lactation is controversial. Lactation is known to be suppressed with oral estrogen doses of 50 mg or greater. However, the more commonly used low-dose combination oral contraceptives when begun 1 month after lactation is fully established, have been associated with only a small decrease in lactation performance and infant weight gain when compared to controls. The amount of estrogen the infant receives in breast milk from women on low-dose oral contraceptive pills is not harmful to the newborn if a breastfeeding mother desires to use this method of contraception.[10] If, however, breastfeeding motivation is marginal, the slight reduction in breast milk induced by oral contraceptives may be sufficient to discourage continued nursing, and another method should be sought.[10]

5. Progesterone-only contraceptives

Progesterone-only methods of contraception constitute a viable and popular choice for breastfeeding mothers, since they do not interfere with lactation. Since progesterone withdrawal is the likely stimulus that initiates lactogenesis, it is best for natural progesterone levels to drop before a progestin-only contraceptive is initiated.[11] Medroxyprogesterone has been shown to have no detrimental effect on the duration of lactation or timing of introduction of formula within the first four months postpartum.[6]

a. Progesterone-only pills. Progesterone-only contraceptive pills consist of a microdose of progestin given daily in a continuous fashion and are indicated for women who are breastfeeding and for those who need to avoid estrogen. Under the influence of chronic progesterone exposure, cervical mucus becomes scant, thick, and relatively impermeable to sperm. Ovulation is prevented in 15–40% of cycles, and normal endometrial development is inhibited. The reported failure rate for this type of oral contraception is 2.5 per 100 women-years. The low progesterone dose means that a high degree of compliance is essential, as the likelihood of accidental pregnancy with a missed dose is much higher than seen with combination oral contraceptives. The most common side effect of progesterone pills is the absence of regular menses and most women experience irregular, breakthrough bleeding.

b. Injectable or implantable contraception. Long-acting injectable forms of medroxyprogesterone acetate have been used for contraception for over 40 years.[14] Current injectable or implantable forms of birth control, Depo-Provera and Norplant, are designed to prevent pregnancy by releasing a constant small dose of progesterone. Use of long-acting forms of medroxyprogesterone acetate in adolescents has been associated with higher rates of continued use and lower rates of rapid repeat pregnancy than those seen with oral contraceptives.[1,8,17] They do not appear to affect the use of health care services, sexual activity, condom use, or the rate of sexually transmitted diseases.[8,17]

i. Depo-Provera

Depo-Provera is medroxyprogesterone at a dose of 150 mg injected deep intramuscularly every 3 months. This method has a failure rate of less than 1.0%, and has been shown to have good continuation rates. It may be used within 5 days postpartum if a woman is not breastfeeding, and at 6 weeks postpartum if a woman is breastfeeding. Menstrual irregularities are very common, the most predominant of which is amenorrhea, which occurs in up to 60% of users at the end of 1 year and 70% at 2 years. Weight gain is also common, and contraceptive continuation may be enhanced by counseling concerning management of body weight concerns.[8] The drug may remain in the bloodstream for weeks to months, often resulting in a delay in fertility (median time 10 months) after use has been discontinued.

ii. Norplant

Norplant is a set of six small capsules of an elastomer containing levonorgestrel that are inserted subcutaneously through a trocar.[14] Insertion requires a small incision in the upper arm using local anesthesia and is easily accomplished in an ambulatory office or clinic setting. The implants release progesterone into the circulation at a relatively constant rate, with a total monthly progesterone dose that is less than that provided by oral contraceptives. Postpartum, serum levonorgestrel peak during the first week after insertion at 2,000 pg/ml, and decline to approximately 250 pg/ml by the 8th week.[15] It provides effective contraception for 5 years, with an annual pregnancy rate of less than 1% and a continuation rate of 50% after 5 years, and is safe for use in breastfeeding mothers.[14]

The main side effect associated with Norplant is irregular menstrual bleeding. As with Depo-Provera, weight gain is commonly encountered. Other side effects that may be reported include headaches, alopecia, and abdominal discomfort.[15] Fertility returns to normal promptly after removal, which is done in an office surgical procedure that is of variable difficulty and length.

6. Intrauterine device (IUD)

In early 1986, IUDs were withdrawn from the U.S. market due to rising liability costs that stemmed from infectious complications. Since that time, it has been demonstrated that there is no apparent increase in infectious risk with IUD usage compared with other contraceptive methods *among monogamous women at low risk for sexually transmitted diseases.*[16] As a result, the use of the IUD has regained some popularity in recent years. Two are now available for use: Progestasert, with a reservoir that releases progesterone; and Paragard, a copper IUD. The addition of bioactive materials, such as copper or progesterone, has not significantly reduced the pregnancy rates but has reduced the risk of expulsion or abnormal bleeding.[4]

The IUD may be an ideal choice of postpartum contraception for women who are not sexually promiscuous and who are not yet ready to consider sterilization. It carries a failure rate of 1 to 6 per 100 women years. The risk of uterine perforation, a potential complication of IUD use that occurs in up to 8 in 1000 insertions, is highest when the insertion is performed within the first 8 weeks after delivery. The first postpartum week is associated with fewer perforations but an unacceptably high rate of expulsion, up to 21%. Most authorities recommend delaying IUD insertion until the 6th to 8th postpartum week. If there is any doubt about the adequacy of involution of the uterus, it is best to postpone placement for 2 to 3 additional weeks and reassess the condition.[4] The IUD is safe for use in breastfeeding mothers, and nursing has not been shown to increase the risk of expulsion or other complications.

7. Sterilization

Worldwide, sterilization is the most frequently used method of birth control in postpartum women. The failure rate associated with tubal sterilization is 0.5–1.0%. The puerperium is a convenient time for tubal ligation procedures to be performed, at the time of cesarean section or within the first 24–48 hours after vaginal delivery, without prolonging postpartum hospitalization.

Puerperal sterilization has been associated with an increased incidence of grief and guilt as compared to interval sterilization.[4] Postponing the procedure until 6–8 weeks after delivery provides time to ensure that the infant is healthy and gives parents a chance to review the implications of their decision. Laparoscopic tubal ligation can be done on an outpatient basis at this point with minimum morbidity or disruption of family routines or breastfeeding.

Vasectomy is the alternative sterilization procedure that should be discussed with couples. With a failure rate of 3 to 4 per 1000 procedures, this can be done as an outpatient with local anesthesia.[4] The success of the procedure is confirmed by postoperative semen analysis.

References

1. Berenson AB, Wiemann CM: Contraceptive use among adolescent mothers at 6 months postpartum. Obstet Gynecol 89:999–1005,1997.
2. Debrovner CH, Winikoff B: Trends in postpartum contraceptive choice. Obstet Gynecol 63:65–70, 1984.
3. Forrest JD: Contraceptive needs through stages of women's reproductive lives. Contemp Obstet Gynecol 31:12–22, 1988.
4. Gabbe SG, Niebyl JR, Simpson JL (eds): Postpartum care. In Obstetrics: Normal and Problem Pregnancies, 2nd ed. New York, Churchill Livingstone, 1991, pp 766–769.
5. Glasier AF, Logan J, McGlew TJ: Who gives advice about postpartum contraception? Contraception 53:217–220, 1996.
6. Hannon PR, Duggan AK, Serwint JR, et al: The influence of medroxyprogesterone on the duration of breast-feeding in mothers in an urban community. Arch Pediatr Adolesc Med 151:490–496, 1997.
7. Hardy E, Santos LC, Osis MJ, et al: Contraceptive use and pregnancy before and after introducing lactational amenorrhea (LAM) in a postpartum program. Adv Contracept 14:59–68, 1998.

8. Hellerstedt WL, Story M: Adolescent satisfaction with postpartum contraception and body weight concerns. J Adolesc Health 22:446–452, 1998.
9. Hight-Laukaran V, Labbok MH, Peterson AE, et al: Multicenter study of the lactational amenorrhea method: II. Acceptability, utility, and policy implications. Contraception 55:337–346, 1997.
10. Kelsey JJ: Hormonal contraception and lactation. J Hum Lact 12:315–318, 1996.
11. Kennedy KI, Short RV, Tully MR: Premature introduction of progestin-only contraceptive methods during lactation. Contraception 55:347–350, 1997.
12. Labbok MH, Hight-Laukaran V, Peterson AE, et al: Multicenter study of the lactational amenorrhea method: I. Efficacy, duration, and implications for clinical application. Contraception 55:327–336, 1997.
13. Mintzer M: Contraception. In Sloan PD (ed): Essentials of Family Medicine. Baltimore, Williams & Wilkins, 1988, pp 175–190.
14. Mishell DR: Contraception. N Engl J Med 320:777–787, 1989.
15. Molland JR, Morehead DB, Baldwin DM, et al: Immediate postpartum insertion of the Norplant contraceptive device. Fertil Steril 66:43–48, 1996.
16. Pitkin RM: The return of the IUD. Obstet Gynecol 72:119–124, 1988.
17. Polaneczky M, Slap G, Forke C, et al: The use of levonorgestrel implants (Norplant) for contraception in adolescent mothers. N Engl J Med 331:1201–1206, 1994.
18. Vekemans M: Postpartum contraception: The lactational amenorrhea method. Eur J Contracept Reprod Health Care 2:105–111, 1997.
19. Zinaman MJ: Why you should know about natural family planning. Contemp Obstet Gynecol 31:69–86, 1988.

CHAPTER 20

Postpartum Psychosocial Concerns

Dwenda Gjerdingen, M.D.
Janis E. Byrd, M.D.

SECTION A.
MATERNAL ADJUSTMENT

Women may experience a variety of psychological disorders after childbirth, from the milder and more common transient *blues*, to severe depression and psychosis. The relatively high prevalence of mood disorders during the months after childbirth is reflected in the finding that the rate of admission to a psychiatric hospital is greater during the 12 months after childbirth than at any other time in a woman's life.[8] Mood disorders after pregnancy are significantly underdiagnosed and undertreated. A heightened surveillance for mental disorders is called for during this period.

The fact that women are at increased risk for mood disorders in the postpartum period suggests that gonadal steroids may play a role in the pathogenesis of depression in women. Neurotransmitter and neuroendocrine studies have been generally unfruitful, although changes in the sensitivities of serotonin receptors have been documented. Further evidence for a biologic component comes from family history studies. In women with postpartum mood disturbances, at least one family member met criteria for a past or present psychiatric disorder in 71% of cases, and positive family histories for major depressive disorder and alcoholism were found in 48% and 30%.[46] This association is much higher than in the population at large and may indicate a potential genetic or familial component. Other potential etiologic theories include lack of social supports, unsatisfactory marital relationship (or being unmarried), negative life events, occupational instability, lack of prior experience with children, unplanned pregnancy and antenatal pessimism, and a poor relationship with the woman's mother.[46]

I. Postpartum Blues

Postpartum blues are commonly experienced by new mothers, with prevalence rates of 26% to 85%, depending on the diagnostic criteria used.[46] Symptoms, which are usually short-lived, begin within the first week after birth, peak around day 5, and usually resolve by 12 days postpartum. These symptoms include dysphoria, mood lability, crying, anxiety, insomnia, poor appetite, and irritability.[46] Although the blues are considered a simple adjustment disorder of childbirth, they also are known to be a risk factor for subsequent postpartum depression.[48] Although symptoms usually resolve spontaneously, women often are helped by reassurance and support.

II. Postpartum Depression

Of all women who give birth, approximately 10% to 20% suffer with postpartum depression.[46] The prevalence rate varies with the length of the period observed and the diagnostic instruments employed. Physicians often fail to recognize this disorder, delaying diagnosis and treatment.

625

A. Risk Factors

Risk factors for postpartum depression appear to be multiple and include the following.

1. Psychological
   - Positive family history for depression[48]
   - Personal psychiatric history[48]
   - Postpartum blues[48]
   - History of premenstrual mood changes prior to conception.[49]
2. Social
   - Less emotional support from the partner and others[22]
   - High levels of marital concerns
   - Less satisfaction with partner participation in household chores[22]
   - Marital conflict[48]
   - Stressful life events during pregnancy
   - Little personal involvement in recreational activities[22,48]
3. Physical
   - Poor general health[22]
   - Fatigue[22]
   - Sleep disturbances[22]
   - Use of intramuscular progesterone contraceptive[36]
   - Thyroid dysfunction[24,36,46]
4. Infant
   - Infant health problems[22]
   - Child care stressors, such as feeding or sleep problems[48]
   - Perceptions of a temperamentally difficult infant[48]
5. Employment characteristics
   - Short leave (≤ 6 weeks)
   - Long work hours
   - Fewer work rewards[30]

B. Signs and Symptoms

Because postpartum depression is a type of major depressive disorder, with symptoms beginning sometime during the first 4 weeks after delivery, the clinical characteristics are those of major depression (Table 1). The *postpartum onset* modifier also can be applied to manic or mixed episodes of major depressive disorder, bipolar I disorder, bipolar II disorder, or to brief psychotic disorder.[2] Although this definition specifies an onset within the first postpartum month, women remain at increased risk for depression for several months after delivery.[22] The duration of depressive symptoms in childbearing women is similar to that of nonchildbearing women: 44% and 47% continue to show symptoms at 6 months follow-up.[55]

C. Screening and Diagnostic Measures

Visits should be scheduled sooner than the traditional 6 weeks for patients considered at high risk for developing postpartum depression. The moderately depressed mother often experiences guilt and embarrassment secondary to her sense of failure, and this may limit her ability to call her physician or admit the symptoms of her depression. In this regard, the importance of talking with family members cannot be overstated. Home visits may be appropriate to assess the new mother's parenting skills and to determine how she is coping.

1. Role of history and physical examination
   A careful history and physical examination should be done on all women presenting with postpartum mood symptoms. Important components of the history are the psychiatric history, including previous postpartum episodes, a family history of Axis I disorders, and stressful life events. Recording the woman's current symptoms enables the provider to rate these prospectively over the course of follow-up.

TABLE 1. Criteria for Major Depressive Episode

Five or more of the symptoms listed below, together with these qualifications:
  Must include symptom no. 1 or 2
  Symptoms are present nearly every day for the same 2-week period
  Symptoms represent a change from baseline
  Symptoms produce clinically significant distress or change in functioning
  Symptoms are not due to drugs, another medical condition, or bereavement (unless prolonged, i.e. > 2 months)
  Symptoms do not meet criteria for a mixed episode

Symptoms
1. Depressed mood most of the day
2. Markedly diminished interest or pleasure in all, or almost all, activities most of the day
3. Marked decrease or increase in appetite, resulting in significant unintentional weight loss or weight gain (i.e., > 5% body weight in 1 month)
4. Insomnia or hypersomnia
5. Psychomotor agitation or retardation
6. Fatigue or loss of energy
7. Feelings of worthlessness or inappropriate guilt
8. Decreased ability to think or concentrate
9. Recurrent thoughts of death or recurrent suicidal thoughts (with or without a plan)

Adapted from American Psychiatric Association: Diagnostic and Statistical Manual of Mental Disorders, 4th ed. Washington, D.C., American Psychiatric Association, 1994.

2. Edinburgh Postpartum Depression Scale

Although DSM IV criteria constitute the gold standard for the clinical diagnosis of postpartum depression in the United States, the most widely used screening tool for postpartum depression in large populations is the Edinburgh Postnatal Depression Scale. This scale, consisting of 10 statements (Table 2) relating to mood, has been validated, computerized, and used as a telephone screen. Mothers who score above a threshold of 12/13 (out of 30) are likely to be suffering from a major depressive illness (sensitivity, 86%; specificity, 78%).[16]

3. Exclude other common medical conditions

Women who are thought to be depressed should be evaluated for thyroid dysfunction because depression frequently is associated with the hypothyroid phase of postpartum thyroiditis, seen in 5% to 10% of postpartum women.[1] This condition is marked by an elevated level of thyroid-stimulating hormone and often thyroid microsomal autoantibodies. Treatment of postpartum thyroid dysfunction is crucial to the effective management of postpartum depression in these patients. Postpartum depression also may be associated with anemia; a hemoglobin or hematocrit should be ordered, particularly when depressed patients specify fatigue as a primary complaint.

D. **Management Recommendations**

1. Antidepressant drugs versus psychotherapy

Postpartum depression generally has been treated with antidepressant medications, psychotherapy, or both. A randomized controlled trial tested the efficacy of medications versus psychotherapy and found both to be effective.

When comparisons were made among four treatment groups (fluoxetine or placebo, plus one or six sessions of counseling), the greatest improvement was seen in patients treated with fluoxetine or six psychotherapy sessions, as opposed to placebo and one psychotherapy session. There appeared to be no additional benefit from combining fluoxetine and psychotherapy.[3]

In addition to fluoxetine, a variety of other antidepressants may be used to treat postpartum depression (Table 3). Of the three classes of antidepressants shown in this table, the tricyclic antidepressants produce the most side effects

TABLE 2.   Edinburgh Postnatal Depression Scale

In the past 7 days:

1. I have been able to laugh and see
   the funny side of things
     As much as I always could
     Not quite so much now
     Definitely not so much now
     Not at all

2. I have looked forward with enjoyment
   to things
     As much as I ever did
     Rather less than I used to
     Definitely less than I used to
     Hardly at all

*3. I have blamed myself unnecessarily
   when things went wrong
     Yes, most of the time
     Yes, some of the time
     Not very often
     No, never

4. I have been anxious or worried for
   no good reason
     No, not at all
     Hardly ever
     Yes, sometimes
     Yes, very often

*5. I have felt scared or panicky for
   no very good reason
     Yes, quite a lot
     Yes, sometimes
     No, not much
     No, not at all

*6. Things have been getting on top of me
     Yes, most of the time I haven't been able
       to cope at all
     Yes, sometimes I haven't been coping
       as well as usual
     No, I have been coping quite well
     No, I have been coping as well as ever

*7. I have been so unhappy that I have
   had difficulty sleeping
     Yes, most of the time
     Yes, sometimes
     Not very often
     No, not at all

*8. I have felt sad or miserable
     Yes, most of the time
     Yes, quite often
     Not very often
     No, not at all

*9. I have been so unhappy that I have
   been crying
     Yes, most of the time
     Yes, quite often
     Only occasionally
     No, never

*10. The thought of harming myself has
   occurred to me
     Yes, quite often
     Sometimes
     Hardly ever
     Never

Note. Response categories are scored 0, 1, 2, and 3 according to increased severity of the symptom. Items marked with an asterisk are reverse scored (3, 2, 1, and 0). The total score is calculated by adding together the scores for each of the 10 items.

From Cox JL, Holden JM, Sagovsky R: Detection of postnatal depression: Development of the 10-item Edinburgh Postnatal Depression Scale. Br J Psychiatry 150:782–786, 1987.

Note. Users may reproduce the scale without further permission, provided they respect copyright by quoting the names of the authors, the title, and the source of the paper in all reproduced copies.

and carry the greatest risk of toxicity when taken in overdose quantities. Although selective serotonin reuptake inhibitors (SSRIs) are tolerated better than tricyclic antidepressants, there are fewer data available about their effects on nursing infants.

2. Antidepressant therapy for breastfeeding women

For women who are breastfeeding and taking antidepressant medications, there is insufficient evidence regarding the potential long-term effects on the child. There are more limited data on short-term effects of antidepressants, particularly tricyclics, on nursing infants. A review of the literature using 15 published reports on antidepressant therapy in breastfeeding mothers concluded that amitriptyline, nortriptyline, desipramine, clomipramine, and sertraline were not found in quantifiable amounts in nurslings, and no adverse events had been reported for nursing infants.[57,58] A study found controversial results with the use of fluoxetine with breastfeeding.[42] When potential risks and benefits have been weighed and the decision has been made to use antidepressant therapy, these are the drugs of choice for breastfeeding women, based on currently available information.

TABLE 3. Use of Antidepressants in Postpartum Depression[1]

Antidepressant[2]	Starting Dose (mg)	Usual Dosage Range (mg/day)	Anticholinergic Effects	Sedation	Effects on Breastfed Infant[3]
Selective Serotonin Reuptake Inhibitors					
Fluoxetine (Prozac)	20 qd	20–80	–	–	Adverse[4]
Paroxetine (Paxil)	20 qd	20–50	1+	2+	–
Sertraline (Zoloft)	50 qd	50–200	–	–	Adverse not seen[5]
Citalopram (Celexa)	20 qd	20–40	–	–	–
Tricyclic Antidepressants					
Tertiary Amines					
Amitriptyline (Elavil)	25 qd	75–300	4+	4+	Adverse not seen[5]
Doxepin (Sinequan)	25 qd	75–300	3+	4+	Adverse[6]
Imipramine (Tofranil)	25 qd	75–300	3+	3+	–
Secondary Amines					
Desipramine (Norpramin)	25 qd	75–300	2+	2+	Adverse not seen[5]
Nortriptyline (Pamelor)	25 qd	50–200	3+	3+	Adverse not seen[5]
Other Antidepressants					
Bupropion (Wellbutrin; Wellbutrin SR)	100 bid/ 150 qd	300–450 ($\div$3)/ 300 ($\div$2)	1+	–	–
Trazodone (Desyrel)	50 tid	50–600	–	3+	–
Venlafaxine (Effexor; Effexor XR)	37.5 bid/ 37.5–75 qd	75–375/75–225	+/–	2+	–
Nefazodone (Serzone)	100 bid	300–600	+/–	2+	–
Mirtazapine (Remeron)	15 qd	15–30	2+	2+	–

[1] Table adapted from Jermain (ref)
[2] The antidepressants in this table do not constitute an inclusive list.
[3] If no comment, insufficient data are available.
[4] Substantial levels found in 6-week-old infant; long half-life (Wisner 1996).
[5] "Adverse not seen" means that non-quantifiable drug levels were seen in infant's serum, and no adverse effects were seen in nurslings. Most studies have not looked at potential delayed effects on older infants and children.
[6] Metabolites were found in nursing infants; infants appeared sedated (Wisner 1996).

Doxepin should be used with caution in breastfeeding women based on reports of neonatal sedation and high serum levels of this drug or its metabolites in nursing infants (see Table 3). In general, many antidepressants are excreted into breast milk, and the American Academy of Pediatrics classifies most antidepressants as drugs "whose effects on the nursing infant are unknown, but may be of concern."[9] For non–breastfeeding women, SSRIs generally are considered as first-line therapy.[31]

3. Estrogen therapy

Clinicians and researchers have used high-dose estrogen as prophylaxis for postpartum depression in high-risk women and as primary therapy for postpartum depression with some success.[25,45] In a double-blind RCT, women diagnosed with depression within 3 months after giving birth were treated with transdermal 17 β-estradiol, 200 μg daily (equivalent to two 0.1-mg dose Estraderm patches) for 3 months, followed by 3 months of transdermal estrogen (same dose) plus cyclic progesterone, 10 mg daily for 12 days each month. The women showed a more rapid and prolonged improvement in depression scores than a blinded, placebo-treated comparison group.[25] Although estrogen therapy is not considered standard of care for postpartum depression in the United States, it might be considered for women with recurrent or resistant postpartum depression. Estrogen therapy is not recommended for breastfeeding women because it is associated with decreased milk production.

4. Other recommendations
   a. At postpartum and well-child visits: All women should be screened for depression by asking about their mood. Patients and their family members should be advised to notify their provider if they note significant, persistent mood changes between visits.
   b. After depression is diagnosed: The physician should advise regular physician visits; evaluate for suicide potential at each visit; and counsel the patient to curtail stress (e.g., heavy workloads), to obtain support, and to maintain a regular exercise program. Women who do not show improvement with these initial measures may require antidepressant therapy or psychological or psychiatric referral.
   c. Women with postpartum depression who desire contraception: The physician must be aware of the potential negative impact of progesterone-containing contraceptives on mood. Although such contraceptives are not contraindicated for depressed patients, their impact on mental well-being should be monitored.

III. Postpartum Psychosis

Postpartum psychosis occurs in 0.1% to 0.2% of women who have given birth, a frequency approximately 40% higher than that of women in the general population.[46,51] Its onset is usually rapid and dramatic and occurs within the first 4 weeks after delivery.[48] In most cases, postpartum psychosis is believed to be an episodic presentation of a manic-depressive illness.[46] Initial symptoms may be manic in nature, with inability to sleep for several nights, agitation, restlessness, expansive or irritable mood, and avoidance of the infant. Symptoms may progress to include incoherence or loosening of association, delusions, hallucination, and grossly disorganized or catatonic behavior. Often the delusional content reflects themes of childbirth.[29] Postpartum psychosis constitutes a medical emergency because patients with severe psychosis are at risk for suicide or infanticide.[46] With appropriate treatment, 95% of patients improve within 3 months.[51] For patients who do not receive antimanic therapy, however, there is a greater risk of recurrent affective instability in subsequent months.[13] For women who have had a previous episode of postpartum psychosis, the risk of recurrence is 13% to 20%.[28]

IV. Management Recommendations

A. Hospitalization
In most cases, women should be hospitalized with suicide precautions.

B. Pharmacologic Treatment
Pharmacologic treatment may consist of one or a combination of the following agents: lithium, carbamazepine, antipsychotics, or antidepressants.

C. Breastfeeding
For breastfeeding women, the American Academy of Pediatrics considers lithium to be contraindicated because of neonatal complications, including cyanosis, electrocardiogram abnormalities, and hypotonia. Carbamazepine levels in the nursing infant usually remain low, and the American Academy of Pediatrics considers the drug to be compatible with breastfeeding.[34]

SECTION B.
PATERNAL ADJUSTMENT

I. Epidemiology and Natural History

Fathers may experience emotional disturbances after the birth of an infant, although the prevalence of such disorders in fathers is thought to be less than in mothers. In a review of studies focusing on fathers in the first 2 months postpartum, a psychiatric morbidity rate of at least 10% was reported.[4] Specific psychiatric conditions seen in new fathers include depression, psychosis, impulsive behavior disorders, anxiety disorders, neurotic disorders, sexual deviancy, and problem drinking.[4,35] Apart from these discrete diagnoses, fathers may experience a variety of nonspecific emotional symptoms, as evidenced by a longitudinal study comparing new fathers with male controls. In the early postpartum period, the fathers, compared with controls, reported significantly more problems with fatigue, irritability, headaches, difficulty concentrating, insomnia, nervousness, and restlessness.[12]

II. Risk Factors

Risk factors contributing to psychiatric problems in fathers include having a depressed partner; work-related stress; economic pressures; and receiving little support from in-laws, other relatives, and friends.[4,60] Depression in new fathers generally follows a course similar to that seen in depressed mothers or other individuals.

III. Management Recommendations

A. Paternal Assessment

The physician should ask about paternal well-being during routine postpartum or well-child visits.

B. Risk Assessment

Routinely screening fathers whose partners are known to be depressed should be considered because there is a 50% prevalence rate of psychiatric morbidity among fathers who have partners with psychiatric problems.[4]

C. Treatment

Fathers with moderate to severe depression usually benefit from measures similar to those used in treating maternal depression, including antidepressant therapy, psychotherapy, social support, and exercise.

SECTION C.
MARITAL ADJUSTMENT

Not only is the arrival of a child frequently stressful for the mother and father as individuals, but also it tends to be stressful on the marriage, as documented by multiple studies revealing general marital decline across the transition to parenthood.[6,18,37,52,56] For some couples, this decline is minimal, whereas for others it constitutes a major crisis and may extend into the second year after childbirth.[15] For couples with adequate support systems, the period of distress may be shorter.

I. Changes in Marital Structure and Roles

When investigators have attempted to identify specific changes in marital structure and interaction that occur during the transition to parenthood, they have found that the presence of children is associated with several variables that potentially compromise marital satisfaction: lower marital interaction, greater dissatisfaction with finances and the division of labor, and a more traditional division of labor.[56]

There is good evidence that these marriage-influencing factors are themselves importantly linked. For example, research has documented the importance of husbands' participation in household chores and child care to their wives' satisfaction with the marriage.[27,43,50,54,59] As important as this support is, however, it appears to decline progressively after childbirth, as evidenced by longitudinal data showing couples' gravitation toward more traditional division of household labor over the first postpartum year.[24]

There is less information about how dual-earner couples' relationships are affected by childbirth. Given the volume of their total workload, however, it is possible that sharing the work of the household and family is even more crucial to the stability of the marriage than for single-earner couples.

II. Changes in Sexual Relationship

The sexual relationship of a couple often changes after the birth of a child. Most women report decreased sexual desire and less frequent sexual activity in the second trimester of pregnancy and at 1 month postpartum, with gradual recovery by 1 year postpartum.[11] On average, non–breastfeeding women resumed intercourse at 6.9 weeks after the birth compared with 7.8 weeks for breastfeeding mothers. There was wide variation: 19% had resumed intercourse within the first month, and 19% did not resume intercourse until 4 months postpartum or later. More women with cesarean deliveries than with vaginal deliveries (27% versus 18%) had resumed intercourse by 1 month postpartum. Although there was a slight decrease in satisfaction with the sexual relationship at 1 month postpartum, men and women were moderately satisfied with their sexual relationship at all intervals, on average. The reduced activity and lack of desire for sexual intimacy is likely related to multiple demands of caring for a newborn, resulting in distraction, irregular schedules, and fatigue, as well as vaginal discomfort from episiotomies, lacerations, and dry vaginal mucosa from hormonal alterations, especially in breastfeeding mothers.

In contrast, fathers generally do not appear to lose interest in sexual activity during this time, but their sexual activity declines in response to their partners' disinterest.[21] This male/female discordance in sexual desire may contribute to marital distress.

III. Management Recommendations

The physician should offer the following advice to partners:
- Regularly affirm their care and support of one another.
- Plan ways in which they will show tangible support, particularly through the sharing of family and household responsibilities. It is important that these issues be addressed early, perhaps before childbirth, because early postpartum marital dissatisfaction is a portent of subsequent family maladjustment.[53]
- Give accurate information about changes in the sexual relationship during prenatal visits. Anticipatory guidance may prevent the development of long-term problems.
- Because of the value of breastfeeding for the infant, it is especially important that couples understand the hormonal effects of breastfeeding so as not to terminate it prematurely or assume a problem in their relationship.

SECTION D.
SIBLING ADJUSTMENT

Sibling reactions to the birth of a sibling vary by the gender of the infant and sibling, the length of time since the birth, and the age of the sibling. Same-sex sibling dyads have been reported to show more problematic behaviors. Problems tend to diminish as time progresses; siblings older than 6 years of age show fewer negative behaviors than do younger siblings.[47]

I. Birth Impact on Mother's Relationship to the Older Sibling

Direct observations of families before and after the birth of a second child reveal changes in mothers' interactions with the older siblings after the arrival of the infant. After childbirth, mothers tend to decrease the attention they give to older siblings and to increase their negative interactions with this child.[17] These changes may explain, at least partially, the negative behaviors of older children after the arrival of a new infant.

II. Reactions of a Sibling to the Birth
Children may react to the birth of a sibling in various ways:
- Attention-seeking behavior
- Imitating behaviors
- Direct aggression or confrontation (with the mother or infant)
- Regression
- Anxiety behaviors
- Maturity and independence.[26,47]

III. Management Recommendations
Both parents should give focused, positive attention to the older child regularly. Parents can be encouraged to find ways to include an older child in providing care to the infant.

SECTION E.
SINGLE-PARENT FAMILIES

The stresses felt by single-parent families are likely even greater than for those of two-parent families because the burdens of financial support, child care, household chores, and other work responsibilities generally rest on a single individual.

I. Management Recommendations
The physician should be sensitive to the pressures felt by single parents, which may be manifested in late arrival for appointments or difficulty administering multiple-dose drug regimens to children.

The physician should encourage participation in or development of support networks for assistance with child care, household chores, and other responsibilities and for recreational activities.

The physician should screen for mental disorders that may stem from the stress caused by trying to manage multiple competing responsibilities.

SECTION F.
SPECIAL FAMILY SITUATIONS

I. Adolescent Mothers
A. Epidemiology
Adolescent motherhood is becoming increasingly common: The number of infants born to single adolescent women doubled during the period from 1984 through 1996.[5] Nearly 1 in 10 births in the United States is to a single adolescent mother, many of whom confront multiple stressors as they assume their parenting roles.[39] With minimal life experience and preparation, they face the adult challenges of providing financial support, protection, love, nutrition, and other needs for a completely dependent child.
B. Psychological Consequences
The added stress of parenting a newborn may have adverse psychological consequences for both the mother and the infant. The infant or child may be at risk for child abuse. In a nationally representative sample of 1997 mothers, the younger the mother, the greater the rate of child abuse.[14]
C. Adolescent Outcomes
Decades ago, it was common for a new adolescent mother to place her child for adoption. This has been a much less common decision in recent years. Namerow et al.[41] looked at 406 single teenage girls who had just given birth and examined the consequences of placing their newborns for adoption versus parenting them. Girls

who relinquished their infants for adoption showed more favorable outcomes after 4 years on a broad variety of sociodemographic and social psychological parameters. They attained higher educational levels, were more likely to be employed and consequently less likely to be on welfare, were more often married, had had fewer abortions, and had lower depression and higher life satisfaction scores. The girls who gave up their infants for adoption were slightly less confident about their decision, compared with those who kept their infants. Although 4 years of follow-up may not be sufficient to measure all of the consequences of a teenage mother's relinquishing or caring for an infant, this study suggests that benefits may be realized from a teenage mother's decision to consider adoption as an alternative to parenting.[41]

II. Violence

In some communities, violence is the leading cause of injuries and death among women of childbearing age.[21] Women who are pregnant or who have recently given birth are commonly the subjects of violence, which is often administered by a male partner, family member, or friend. In a study of 276 women from an urban setting (89% married and 92% African-American) interviewed three times during pregnancy and at 6 months postpartum, the proportion of women who documented moderate-to-severe violence was 19% before delivery and 25% in the postpartum period. Factors that have been associated with battering include stress, low self-esteem, anxiety, depression, isolation, and alcohol and drug use; protective factors include being older, having a confidant, and having social support from friends.[21] The prevalence of violence in expectant and new mothers underscores the importance of screening for violence in women during the prenatal and postpartum periods and for providing information to women about ways to avoid and respond to violence.

III. Adoption

It is estimated that 2% to 4% of American families have an adopted child.[44] The process of adoption affects several individuals: relinquishing parents and their families, adopting parents and their families, and the adopted child.

A. Relinquishing Parents

Most of the available information on relinquishing parents relates to the mother, and these data indicate that relinquishing mothers, although usually of normal mental health, often manifest symptoms of anxiety and depression before and after the adoption.[40] They undergo a grief process that may be stronger than that felt by bereaved parents, and this grief has a tendency to resurface in the future, especially during certain events, such as the child's birthday or Mother's Day.[44]

It is not known whether ongoing contact with the relinquished child serves to relieve or aggravate the process of grieving. The decision to place a child for adoption is one that produces feelings of loss for biologic parents and often for extended family members as well. Support and counseling are beneficial.

B. Adopting Parents

There is little information available about the well-being of adoptive parents after the arrival of the child, and the few data that exist apply primarily to new adoptive mothers. Although adoptive mothers do not undergo a process of physical recovery similar to that of biologic mothers, they encounter similar parental demands, resulting in fatigue, less readiness to work at a job, and less activity with household chores and recreational or social functions.[24] Parents who adopt children with special needs face additional challenges, including those related to their children's health, development, behavior, and education.[33]

C. Adopted Children

Although adoptive children often are advantaged in terms of their childhood experiences, standards of health care, family material conditions, and family stability, they also may be emotionally vulnerable. This vulnerability may be expressed in early years or later, in adolescence, through conduct disorders, juvenile offending, and substance abuse.[19]

D. Management Recommendations
1. Relinquishing parents

Relinquishing parents should be encouraged to discuss feelings that result from giving up a child.

2. Adoptive parents

The following advice should be offered to adoptive parents.

    a. When to begin talking to the child about the adoption: It is recommended that these discussions begin during the child's preschool years, if possible, realizing that children do not understand completely the meaning of adoption until adolescence.[10]

    b. Ethnic background: The child should be educated about his or her ethnic background, especially if it is different from that of the adoptive parents.

    c. Potential later request: It is common that the child will want to pursue the identity of his or her biologic parents at a later date.

    d. Adolescent emotional turmoil: Parents should anticipate that the adolescent years will be turbulent.

3. Use of language

In communicating with relinquishing and adoptive parents, the physician should use language that is nonjudgmental. Phrases such as "placing or arranging for adoption," "choosing to raise," "deciding to parent," "biologic parent," "birthparent," and "adoptive parent" are preferred over "putting up, giving up, or surrendering for adoption," "keeping the baby," and "real or natural parent."[32]

4. Obtain support

The physician should be familiar with local resources, support groups, state laws, and literature regarding adoption. Adoptive Families of America is a national support group for adoptive families.

SECTION G.
RETURN-TO-WORK ISSUES

Employment has become the norm for new mothers in the United States: 1.9 million working women become pregnant each year, and most women with preschool and older children are in the workforce.

I. Family and Medical Leave Act
In 1993, the federal Family and Medical Leave Act (FMLA) became law, guaranteeing 12 weeks of job-protected parental leave for mothers and fathers. The employee has a right to return to the same job or a job comparable in pay and responsibility. The employer must also continue employer-provided group health insurance, an important consideration for families with a new infant. Small businesses (those with < 50 employees) are excluded, leaving many parents uncovered.

A serious limitation of the FMLA is that it made no provision to require that this leave be paid. Often, employees substitute accumulated paid vacation and personal leave time first, before personally enacting the FMLA. Economic issues appear to be the strongest influence in determining when a woman returns to work.

II. Length of Leave
In the Wisconsin Maternity Leave and Health (WMLH), a longitudinal study of more than 500 mothers and fathers observed from the second trimester of pregnancy through

the first postpartum year, mothers took an average of 10.69 weeks of leave.[30] Of these women, 66% said their leave periods were too short. The most common reason women gave for not taking more leave was that they could not afford to do so. Fathers in the WMLH study took an average of 4.21 days, usually taken as sick, vacation, or discretionary days, as opposed to parental leave. In Sweden, after 15 years of strong government encouragement and more generous benefits, the percent of eligible fathers taking leave rose from 3% to 44%. It is unlikely that either parent in the United States would be able to take full advantage of the FMLA unless national policy guarantees *paid* leave.

III. Infant Feeding Practices

Infant feeding practices are an important issue for women planning to return to work. In the WMLH study, 23.9% of women said the decision to stop breastfeeding was related to their return to work. Accommodation of breastfeeding by the employer is currently required in only one state. Whether breastfeeding is a right versus a choice is currently being litigated and is complicated by antidiscrimination law requiring equal treatment for men and women. In contrast, mothers in China are allowed to nurse twice a day during the infant's first year with nurseries provided at the work site. Advice that may be provided to women who want to continue breastfeeding after returning to work includes the following: The mother should:

- Discuss breastfeeding plans with her manager, including possible flexible hours, part-time work, use of break or lunch times, and places where they may pump.
- Consider finding a daycare provider near work or one who will cooperate with breastfeeding plans.
- Make sure that breastfeeding is well established before return to work.
- Practice pumping and expressing milk by hand before returning to work.
- Join a breastfeeding support group, take a lactation class, or consult with a lactation consultant.
- Breast-feed more frequently when at home to maintain milk supply.

IV. Infant Development

Optimal leave for infant development has been controversial and conflicting in the psychological literature.[30] In the WMLH study, shorter leaves were associated with more negative affect and behavior. There were significant associations with other risk factors, such as depression, more physical health symptoms, and difficult infant temperament.

V. Summary

Employment of mothers is a reality for most families in the United States, and unpaid leave is driving a rapid return to work for many, often contributing to early discontinuation of breastfeeding. Cultural biases as well as economic issues hinder most fathers from taking advantage of their guaranteed parental leave. Job-guaranteed parental leave is a significant advance, however, especially benefiting poor and working-class women of color who were most vulnerable to job loss before FMLA.

Acknowledgment

The authors wish to acknowledge Ita Killeen, M.D., for her contributions to the section on adoption.

References

1. American College of Obstetricians and Gynecologists: Thyroid disease in pregnancy. Int J Gynecol Obstet 43:82–88, 1993. (ACOG Technical Bulletin, No. 181, June 1993.)
2. American Psychiatric Association: Diagnostic and Statistical Manual of Mental Disorders, 4th ed (DSM-IV). Washington, D.C., American Psychiatric Association, 1994.

3. Appleby L, Warner R, Whitton A, et al: A controlled study of fluoxetine and cognitive-behavioural coun-selling in the treatment of postnatal depression. BMJ 314:932–936, 1997.
4. Ballard C, Davies R: Postnatal depression in fathers. Int Rev Psychiatry 8:65–71, 1996.
5. Barratt MS, Roach MA, Morgan KM, et al: Adjustment to motherhood by single adolescents. Fam Relations 45:209–215, 1996.
6. Belsky J, Spanier GB, Rovine M: Stability and change in marriage across the transition to parenthood. J Marriage Fam 45:567–577, 1983.
7. Blanton TL, Deschner J: Biological mothers' grief: The postadoptive experience in open versus confi-dential adoption. Child Welfare 69:525–535, 1990.
8. Brandon S: Depression after childbirth. BMJ (Clin Res) 284:613–614, 1982.
9. Briggs GG, Freeman RK, Yafee SJ: Drugs in Pregnancy and Lactation, 5th ed. Baltimore, Williams & Wilkins, 1998.
10. Brodzinsky DM, Singer LM, Braff AM: Children's understanding of adoption. Child Dev 55:869–878, 1984.
11. Byrd JE, Hyde JS, DeLamater JD, et al: Sexuality during pregnancy and the year postpartum. J Fam Pract 47:305–308, 1998.
12. Clinton JF: Physical and emotional responses of expectant fathers throughout pregnancy and the early postpartum period. Int J Nurs Stud 24:59–68, 1987.
13. Cohen LS, Sichel DA, Robertson LM, et al: Postpartum prophylaxis for women with bipolar disorder. Am J Psychiatry 152:1641–1645, 1995.
14. Connelly CD, Straus MA: Mother's age and risk for physical abuse. Child Abuse Negl 16:709–718, 1992.
15. Cowan CP, Cowan PA, Heming G, et al: Transitions to parenthood: His, hers, and theirs. J Fam Issues 6:451–481, 1985.
16. Cox JL, Holden JM, Sagovsky R: Detection of postnatal depression: Development of the 10-item Edinburgh Postnatal Depression Scale. Br J Psychiatry 150:782–786, 1987.
17. Dunn J, Kendrick C: The arrival of a sibling: Changes in patterns of interaction between mother and first-born child. J Child Psychol Psychiatry 21:119–132, 1980.
18. Dyer ED: Parenthood as crisis: A re-study. Marriage Fam Living 25:196–201, 1963.
19. Fergusson DM, Lynskey M, Horwood LJ: The adolescent outcomes of adoption: A 16-year longitudinal study. J Child Psychol Psychiatry 36:597–615, 1995.
20. Fischman SH, Rankin EA, Soeken KL, et al: Changes in sexual relationships in postpartum couples. J Obstet Gynecol Neonatal Nurs 15:58–63, 1984.
21. Gielen AC, O'Campo PJ, Faden RR: Interpersonal conflict and physical violence during the childbearing year. Soc Sci Med 39:781–787, 1994.
22. Gjerdingen DK, Chaloner KM: The relationship of women's postpartum mental health to employment, childbirth, and social support. J Fam Pract 38:465–472, 1994.
23. Gjerdingen DK, Chaloner K: Mothers' experience with household roles and social support during the first postpartum year. Women Health 21:57–74, 1994.
24. Gjerdingen DK, Froberg DG: The fourth stage of labor: The health of birth mothers and adoptive moth-ers at six-weeks postpartum. Fam Med 23:29–35, 1991.
25. Gregoire AJP, Kumar R, Everitt B, et al: Transdermal oestrogen for treatment of severe postnatal depres-sion. Lancet 347:930–933, 1996.
26. Griffin EW, de la Torre C: Sibling jealousy: the family with a new baby. Am Fam Physician 28:143–146, 1983.
27. Hawkins AJ, Roberts TA, Christiansen SL, et al: An evaluation of a program to help dual-earner couples share the second shift. Fam Relations 43:213–220, 1994.
28. Herzog A, Detre T: Psychotic reactions associated with childbirth. Dis Nerv Syst 37:229–235, 1976.
29. Hopkins J, Marcus M, Campbell SB: Postpartum depression: A critical review. Psychol Bull 95:498–515, 1984.
30. Hyde JS, Essex MJ, Clark R, et al: Parental leave: Policy and research. J Soc Issues 52:91–109, 1996.
31. Jermain DM: Treatment of postpartum depression. Am Pharmacy NS 35:33–38, 45, 1995.
32. Kaunitz AM, Grimes DA, Kaunitz KK: A physician's guide to adoption. JAMA 258:3537–3541, 1987.
33. Kramer L, Houston D: Supporting families as they adopt children with special needs. Fam Relations 47:423–432, 1998.
34. Kuller JA, Katz VL, McMahon MJ, et al: Pharmacologic treatment of psychiatric disease in pregnancy and lactation: Fetal and neonatal effects. Obstet Gynecol 87:789–794, 1996.
35. Lacoursiere RB: Fatherhood and mental illness: A review and new material. Psychiatr Q 46:109–124, 1972.
36. Lawrie TA, Hofmeyr GJ, De Jager M, et al: A double-blind randomised placebo controlled trial of post-natal norethisterone enanthate: The effect on postnatal depression and serum hormones. Br J Obstet Gynaecol 105:1082–1090, 1998.
37. LeMasters EE: Parenthood as crisis. Marriage Fam Living 19:352–355, 1957.

38. Melina LR: Making Sense of Adoption: A Parent's Guide. New York, Harper & Row, 1989.
39. Mylod DE, Whitman TL, Borkowski JG: Predicting adolescent mothers' transition to adulthood. J Res Adolesc 7:457–478, 1997.
40. Najman JM, Morrison J, Keeping D, et al: Social factors associated with the decision to relinquish a baby for adoption. Community Health Studies 14:180–189, 1990.
41. Namerow PB, Kalmuss D, Cushman LF: The consequences of placing versus parenting among young unmarried women. Marriage Fam Rev 25:175–197, 1997.
42. Nulman I, Koren G: The safety of fluoxetine during pregnancy and lactation. Teratology 53:304–308, 1996.
43. Perry-Jenkins M, Folk K: Class, couples, and conflict: Effects of the division of labor on assessments of marriage in dual-earner families. J Marriage Fam 56:165–180, 1994.
44. Rosenberg KF, Groze V: The impact of secrecy and denial in adoption: Practice and treatment issues. Families in Society 78:522–530, 1997.
45. Sichel DA, Cohen LS, Robertson LM, et al: Prophylactic estrogen in recurrent postpartum affective disorder. Biol Psychiatry 38:814–818, 1995.
46. Steiner M: Perinatal mood disorders: Position paper. Psychopharmacol Bull 34:301–306, 1998.
47. Stewart RB, Mobley LA, Van Tuyl SS, et al: The firstborn's adjustment to the birth of a sibling: A longitudinal assessment. Child Dev 58:341–355, 1987.
48. Stowe Z, Nemeroff CB: Women at risk for postpartum-onset major depression. Am J Obstet Gynecol 173:639–645, 1995.
49. Sugawara M, Toda MA, Shima S, et al: Premenstrual mood changes and maternal mental health in pregnancy and the postpartum period. J Clin Psychol 53:225–232, 1997.
50. Suitor JJ: Marital quality and satisfaction with the division of household labor across the family life cycle. J Marriage Fam 53:221–230, 1991.
51. Susman JL: Postpartum depressive disorders. J Fam Pract 43 (suppl):S17–S24, 1996.
52. Tomlinson PS: Spousal differences in marital satisfaction during transition to parenthood. Nurs Res 36:239–243, 1987.
53. Tomlinson PS, Irvin B: Qualitative study of women's reports of family adaptation pattern four years following transition to parenthood. Issues Mental Health Nurs 14:119–138, 1993.
54. Watson WJ, Watson L, Wetzel W, et al: Transition to parenthood: What about fathers? Can Fam Phys 41:807–812, 1995.
55. Whiffen VE, Gotlib IH: Comparison of postpartum and nonpostpartum depression: Clinical presentation, psychiatric history and psychosocial functioning. J Consult Clin Psychol 61:485–494, 1993.
56. White LK, Booth A, Edwards JN: Children and marital happiness. J Fam Issues 7:131–147, 1986.
57. Wisner KL, Perel J, Blumer J: Serum sertraline and N-desmethylsertraline levels in breast-feeding mother-infant pairs. Am J Psychiatry 155:690–692, 1998.
58. Wisner KL, Perel JM, Findling RL: Antidepressant treatment during breast-feeding. Am J Psychiatry 153:1132–1137, 1996.
59. Zammichieli ME, Gilroy FD, Sherman MF: Relation between sex-role orientation and marital satisfaction. Personality and Social Psychology Bulletin 14:747–754, 1988.
60. Zelkowitz P, Milet TH: Stress and support as related to postpartum paternal mental health and perceptions of the infant. Infant Mental Health J 18:424–435, 1997.

Appendix A

Interpretation of Summary Tables

Readers of this book will find repeated references to randomized controlled trials (RCTs). They will also frequently encounter summary tables that graphically depict the results of combined randomized studies that have undergone meta-analyses.

We have chosen this approach for one simple reason. Randomized controlled studies clearly provide the strongest scientific evidence as to the effectiveness of a given treatment or intervention by minimizing the potential for bias or confounding.

Our colleagues who have created the Oxford Perinatal Database over the past 15 years deserve much credit for having organized, by subject area, systematic meta-analyses of all published and unpublished RCTs in the world. These results are now quite accessible via the Cochrane Pregnancy and Childbirth Database published twice yearly on software diskettes by the British Medical Journal and managed in the United States by the American College of Physicians. This source of evidence has been used extensively throughout the book.

A summary table examines a given intervention and its effect on measurable clinical outcomes by combining all of the available data from randomized trials of acceptable quality and performing a meta-analysis. Combining data across clinical trials greatly enhances the ability to detect an effect, either positive or negative, of an intervention by increasing the "statistical power" of the analysis. This is particularly important when the outcome being studied is uncommon or rare, such as perinatal mortality. An example of a meta-analysis detecting an important effect on an infrequent outcome (perinatal mortality) is demonstrated in the following summary table which examines the impact of induction at 41+ weeks' gestation compared with control treatment of ongoing antenatal surveillance.

Individual RCTs of this intervention demonstrated a "nonsignificant" trend of routine induction at 41+ weeks' gestation to improve perinatal survival rates. When these studies are combined, the trend of improved fetal survival becomes statistically significant.

To interpret this summary table the reader must note a few key factors. First, the vertical line in the middle of the table represents an **odds ratio** of one, which indicates the intervention neither improves nor worsens study outcomes. In any given study, there are a range of responses or odds ratios to a given intervention represented by a **confidence interval**. The horizontal bars that are adjacent to a given outcome represent the confidence interval created by the meta-analysis. A confidence interval that lies completely to the left of the vertical line (identifying an odds ratio of one) indicates that the intervention is effective in improving the clinical outcome at a 95% confidence interval or a P value of less than .05. Conversely, a confidence interval that lies cleanly to the right of the vertical line indicates that the intervention leads to a "significant" worsening of the clinical outcome.

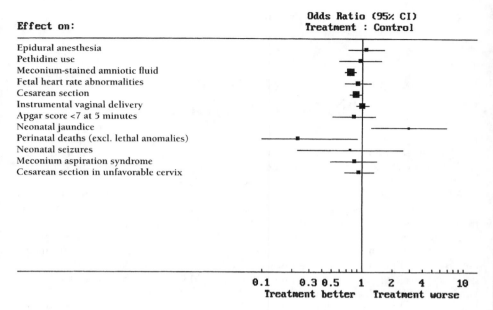

FIGURE. Postterm pregnancy. Elective induction of labor at 41+ weeks' gestation (13 trials reviewed). (From Crowley P: Elective induction of labour at 41+ weeks gestation. In Enkin MW, Keirse MJNC, Renfrew MJ, Neilson JP (eds): Pregnancy and Childbirth Module. Cochrane Database of Systematic Reviews: Review No. 04144. Cochrane Updates on Disk. Oxford, Update Software, 1994, with permission.)

APPENDIX B

Analysis of Risking Instruments

As with any screening test, risk scoring systems should be evaluated by their sensitivity, specificity, positive predictive value (PPV), negative predictive value (NPV), and reliability.

1. **Sensitivity and specificity.** The sensitivity of a test can be seen as the proportion of those individuals with a condition, in which the test is *positive*. Typically, screening tests such as newborn metabolic screens seek high sensitivity, possibly at the expense of specificity. Specificity is the proportion of those *without* the condition, in which the test is *negative*. Tests which determine definitive diagnosis (such as follow-up newborn metabolic testing) seek high specificity, also possibly at the expense of sensitivity.

2. **Positive and negative predictive value.** Positive and negative predictive value represent the likelihood a patient might or might not, respectively, develop a condition with a positive test. Predictive values are typically dependent on the incidence of a condition within a population, with higher incidence resulting in higher predictive values. Maternal serum alpha-fetoprotein testing for fetal neural tube defects, for example, yields higher predictive values in Wales (where the test was developed), where there is a high incidence of fetal neural tube defects, than in the U.S., where the incidence is lower. Pregnancy risk assessment can be expected to have higher predictive values, therefore, in a population which has a high incidence of poor pregnancy outcome, than in a population which has a low incidence.

3. **Reliability.** Reliability is the consistency of the scoring instrument when applied more than once to the same individual. Reliability directly affects the quality of data used in risk calculation. Important determinants of reliability include not only the design of the instrument but also the clinical situation in which it is applied and the staff who apply it.

Calculation of Sensitivity, Specificity, Positive Predictive Value, and Negative Predictive Value

Risk Assessment:	Poor Pregnancy Outcome:	
	Yes	No
High Risk	True Positive	False Positive
Low Risk	False Negative	False Negative

Sensitivity = TP/(TP 1 FN)
Specificity = TN/(TN 1 FP)
PPV = TP/(TP 1 FP)
NPV = TN/(TN 1 FN)

APPENDIX C

Summary of Recommendations for Immunization during Pregnancy

Immunobiologic Agent	Risk from Disease to Pregnant Women	Risk from Disease to Fetus or Neonate	Type of Immunizing Agent	Risk from Immunizing Agent to Fetus	Indications for Immunization during Pregnancy	Dose Schedule*	Comments
LIVE VIRUS VACCINES							
Measles	Significant morbidity, low mortality; not altered by pregnancy	Significant increase in abortion rate; may cause malformations	Live attenuated virus vaccine	None confirmed	Contraindicated (see immune globulins)	Single dose SC, preferably as measles-mumps-rubella[†]	Vaccination of susceptible women should be part of post-partum care
Mumps	Low morbidity and mortality; not altered by pregnancy	Probable increased rate of abortion in first trimester	Live attenuated virus vaccine	None confirmed	Contraindicated	Single dose SC, preferably as measles-mumps-rubella	Vaccination of susceptible women should be part of post-partum care
Poliomyelitis	No increased incidence in pregnancy, but may be more severe if it does occur	Anoxic fetal damage reported; 50% mortality in neonatal disease	Live attenuated virus (oral polio vaccine [OPV]) and enhanced-potency inactivated virus (e-IPV)[‡] vaccine	None confirmed	Not routinely recommended for women in U.S., except persons at increased risk of exposure	*Primary:* 2 doses of e-IPV SC at 4–8 week intervals and a 3rd dose 6–12 months after the 2nd dose *Immediate protection:* 1 dose OPV orally (in outbreaks setting)	Vaccine indicated for susceptible pregnant women traveling in endemic areas or in other high-risk situations

Rubella	Low morbidity and mortality; not altered by pregnancy	High rate of abortion and congenital rubella syndrome	Live attenuated virus vaccine	None confirmed	Contraindicated	Single dose SC, preferably as measles-mumps-rubella	Teratogenicity of vaccine is theoretic, not confirmed to date; vaccination of susceptible women should be part of post-partum care
Mumps	Significant morbidity and mortality; not altered by pregnancy	Unknown	Live attenuated virus vaccine	Unknown	Contraindicated except if exposure is unavoidable	Single dose SC	Postponement of travel preferable to vaccination, if possible
Influenza	Possible increase in morbidity and mortality during epidemic of new antigenic strain	Possible increased abortion rate; no malformations confirmed	Inactivated virus vaccine	None confirmed	Women with serious underlying diseases; public health authorities to be consulted for current recommendations	One dose IM every year	
Rabies	Near 100% fatality; not altered by pregnancy	Determined by maternal disease	Killed virus vaccine	Unknown	Indications for prophylaxis not altered by pregnancy; each case considered individually	Public health authorities to be consulted for indications, dosage, and route of administration	
Hepatitis B	Possible increased severity during third trimester	Possible increase in abortion rate and prematurity; neonatal hepatitis can occur; high risk of newborn carrier state	Recombinant vaccine	None reported	Pre- and post-exposure for women at risk of infection	Three- or four-dose series IM	Used with hepatitis B immune globulin for some exposures; exposed newborn needs vaccination as soon as possible

(Table continued on following page.)

Immunobiologic Agent	Risk from Disease to Pregnant Women	Risk from Disease to Fetus or Neonate	Type of Immunizing Agent	Risk from Immunizing Agent to Fetus	Indications for Immunization during Pregnancy	Dose Schedule*	Comments
			INACTIVATED BACTERIAL VACCINES				
Cholera	Significant morbidity and mortality; more severe during third trimester	Increased risk of fetal death during third-trimester maternal illness	Killed bacterial vaccine	None confirmed	Indications not altered by pregnancy; vaccination recommended only in unusual outbreak situations	Single dose SC or IM, depending on manufacturer's recommendations when indicated	
Plague	Significant morbidity and mortality; not altered by pregnancy	Determined by maternal disease	Killed bacterial vaccine	None reported	Selective vaccination of exposed persons	Public health authorities to be consulted for indications, dosage, and route of administration	
Pneumococcus	No increased risk during pregnancy; no increase in severity of disease	Unknown	Polyvalent polysaccharide vaccine	No data available on use during pregnancy	Indications not altered by pregnancy; vaccine used only for high-risk individuals	In adults, 1 SC or IM dose only; consider repeat dose in 6 years for high-risk individuals	
Typhoid	Significant morbidity and mortality; not altered by pregnancy	Unknown	Killed or live attenuated oral bacterial vaccine	None confirmed	Not recommended routinely except for close, continued exposure or travel to endemic areas	*Killed:* *Primary:* 2 injections SC at least 4 weeks apart. *Booster:* Single dose SC or ID (depending on type of product used) every 3 years. *Oral:* *Primary:* 4 doses on alternate days *Booster:* Schedule not yet determined	

TOXOIDS

	Effect on Mother	Effect on Fetus/Neonate	Vaccine/Globulin	Adverse Effects	Indications	Dose	Comments
Tetanus-diphtheria	Severe morbidity; tetanus mortality 30%, diphtheria mortality 10%; unaltered by pregnancy	Neonatal tetanus mortality 60%	Combined tetanus-diphtheria toxoids preferred; adult tetanus-diphtheria formulation	None confirmed	Lack of primary series, or no booster within past 10 years	*Primary:* 2 doses IM at 1–2 month interval with a 3rd dose 6–12 months after the 2nd. *Booster:* Single dose IM every 10 years after completion of primary series	Updating of immune status should be part of antepartum care

SPECIFIC IMMUNE GLOBULINS

	Effect on Mother	Effect on Fetus/Neonate	Vaccine/Globulin	Adverse Effects	Indications	Dose	Comments
Hepatitis B	Possible increased severity during third trimester	Possible increase in abortion rate and prematurity; neonatal hepatitis can occur; high risk of newborn carrier state	Hepatitis B immune globulin	None reported	Postexposure prophylaxis	Depends on exposure; consult Immunization Practices Advisory Committee recommendations (IM)	Usually given with HBV vaccine; exposed newborn needs immediate post-exposure prophylaxis
Rabies	Near 100% fatality; not altered by pregnancy	Determined by maternal disease	Rabies immune globulin	None reported	Postexposure prophylaxis	Half dose at injury site, half dose in deltoid	Used in conjunction with rabies killed virus vaccine
Tetanus	Severe morbidity; mortality 21%	Neonatal tetanus mortality 60%	Tetanus immune globulin	None reported	Postexposure porphylaxis	One dose IM	Used in conjunction with tetanus toxoid
Varicella	Possible increase in severe varicella pneumonia	Can cause congenital varicella with increased mortality in neonatal period; very rarely causes congenital defects	Varicella-zoster immune globulin (obtained from the American Red Cross)	None reported	Can be considered for healthy pregnant women exposed to varicella to protect against maternal, not congenital, infection	One dose IM within 96 hours of exposure	Indicated also for newborns of mothers who developed varicella within 4 days prior to delivery or 2 days following delivery;

(Table continued on next page.)

Immunobiologic Agent	Risk from Disease to Pregnant Women	Risk from Disease to Fetus or Neonate	Type of Immunizing Agent	Risk from Immunizing Agent to Fetus	Indications for Immunization during Pregnancy	Dose Schedule*	Comments
Tetanus-diphtheria (cont.)							approximately 90–95% of adults are immune to varicella; not indicated for prevention of congenital varicella
STANDARD IMMUNE GLOBULINS							
Hepatitis A	Possible increased severity during third trimester	Probable increase in abortion rate and prematurity; possible transmission to neonate at delivery if mother is incubating the virus or is acutely ill at that time	Standard immune globulin	None reported	Postexposure prophylaxis	0.02 ml/kg IM in one dose of immune globulin	Immune globulin should be given as soon as possible and within 2 weeks of exposure; infants born to mothers who are incubating the virus or are acutely ill at delivery should receive one dose of 0.5 ml as soon as possible after birth
Measles	Significant morbidity, low mortality; not altered by pregnancy	Significant increase in abortion rate; may cause malformations	Standard immune globulin	None reported	Postexposure prophylaxis	0.25 ml/kg IM in one dose of immune globulin, up to 15 ml	Unclear if it prevents abortion; must be given within 6 days of exposure

* Abbreviations: SC = subcutaneously; PO = orally; IM = intramuscularly; ID = intradermally.
† Two doses necessary for adequate vaccination of students entering institutions of higher education, newly hired medical personnel, and international travelers.
‡ Inactivated polio vaccine recommended for nonimmunized adults at increased risk.

From Cunningham F, MacDonald P, Gant N (eds): Williams Obstetrics, 19th ed. Norwalk, CT, Appleton & Lange, 1994; ACOG Technical Bulletin 160, October 1991, with permission.

APPENDIX D

Measuring Clinical Effectiveness

Appendix A provides an overview of how to interpret a Cochrane Library Summary Table. Any clinical outcome that has a confidence interval that excludes unity (an odds ratio of one) is statistically significant at the level indicated (90%, 95%, etc.) If the confidence level (horizontal bar) is located to the left of unity (odds ratio = 1), it means that the intervention results in improved clinical outcomes. Conversely, if the confidence interval is situated to the right of unity, the intervention results in a statistically significant worsening of the designated clinical outcome.

There is, however, a difference between an intervention that is statistically significant and one that is clinically significant. There is an epidemiologic tool that can be used to demonstrate clinical utility or effectiveness. This tool is the *number needed to treat* (NNT) or in some cases the *number needed to harm* (NNH).

What we use to demonstrate statistical significance is the odds ratio (OR) and its surrounding confidence interval. For example, an odds ratio of 0.5 with a confidence interval of 0.30 to 0.70 indicates that the intervention results in a *relative* decrease in the odds of experiencing the clinical outcome of 50%. The formula for calculating an odds ratio is experimental event rate (EER)/control event rate (CER) = EER/CER. If the 95% confidence interval is that listed above, then the clinician would know with 95% certainty that, at best, there would be a *relative* decrease in the odds of an adverse outcome of 70% and at worst a 30% *relative* decrease in the odds of an adverse outcome. This type of statistical improvement may, at times, lead the clinician to overestimate its clinical effectiveness. The following example illustrates this point.

Intervention A compared to control B results in a decrease in the adverse outcome from an incidence of 5 per 10,000 to 2.5 per 10,000.

Example 1   Experimental Event Rate   Control Event Rate
                     2.5/10,000 = 0.00025   5.0/10,000 = 0.00050

                     Odds Ratio = EER/CER = 0.5

Take an intervention with the same odds ratio but with a clinical condition whose incidence is much higher.

Example 2   Experimental Event Rate   Control Event Rate
                     25/100 = 0.25   50/100 = 0.50

                     Odds Ratio = EER/CER = 0.5

Both of these interventions result in the same odds ratio. To determine which intervention will result in increased clinical significance, the clinician needs to calculate the absolute risk reduction (ARR) that occurs with a given treatment intervention. The formula for this is CER − EER = ARR. Using the above examples:

Example 1   CER (0.00050) − EER (0.00025) = 0.00025 or a 0.025% absolute risk reduction

Example 2   CER (0.50) − EER (0.25) = 0.25 or a 25% absolute risk reduction

Although both of these interventions result in the same odds ratio, there is a thousand-fold improvement in the clinical effectiveness in example 2. The utility of calculating the ARR lies in its direct translation to the number needed to treat (NNT). The NNT refers to the number of patients who will require a given intervention to prevent a given adverse clinical outcome. The formula for NNT is simply the inverse of the ARR or 1/ARR. Using the above examples:

Example 1   NNT = 1/ARR = 1/0.00025 = 4000

Four thousand patients would require the intervention to prevent *one* adverse outcome.

Example 2   NNT = 1/ARR = 1/0.25 = 4

Four patients would require the intervention to prevent *one* adverse outcome.

Similarly, when a given intervention results in a statistical increase in an adverse outcome, the absolute risk increase (ARI) can be calculated using the formula CER – EER = ARI. The number needed to harm (NNH) refers to the number of patients receiving the intervention that results in one adverse outcome; thus, it is the inverse of ARI or 1/ARI.

Throughout this text, we have attempted to identify the ARR/ARI and NNT/NNH of interventions so that the clinician can decide if the clinical benefit of a given intervention justifies the costs and potential risks to patients.

References

1. McQuay HJ, Moore RA: Using numerical results from systematic reviews in clinical practice. Ann Intern Med 126:712–720, 1997.
2. Zapletal E, Lemaitre D, Menard J, et al: The number needed to treat: A clinically useful nomogram in its proper context. BMJ 312:426–429, 1996.

Index

Entries in **boldface** type indicate complete chapters.

Warfarin, avoidance in pregnancy, 40, 206
Water delivery, 394–395
Weight gain, pregnancy
  body mass index changes in pregnancy, 57–58
  components of, 59
  management of excessive or inadequate gains, 60
  recommendations, 59–60
WIC program, 96
Work return
  breastfeeding, 614, 636
  Family and Medical Leave Act, 635–636
  infant development impact, 636

Work return (cont.)
  leave length, 636

X-linked disorders, 108
X-ray
malpresentations and malpositions, 480
  radiation exposure in pregnancy, 6

Zavanelli maneuver, dystocia delivery, 446
Zidovudine, human immunodeficiency virus
  management, 267–268
Zinc, preconception supplementation, 4